Two week loan
Benthyciad pythefnos

Please return on or before the due date to avoid overdue charges
*A wnewch chi ddychwelyd ar neu cyn y dyddiad a nodir ar eich llyfr os
gwelwch yn dda, er mwyn osgoi taliadau*

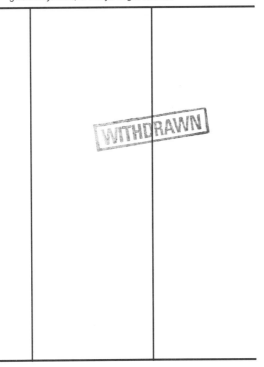

http://library.cardiff.ac.uk
http://llyfrgell.caerdydd.ac.uk

Reviews in Food and Nutrition Toxicity

Volume 1

Reviews in Food and Nutrition Toxicity

Edited by Victor R. Preedy,
Department of Nutrition and Dietetics,
King's College London, UK
and
Ronald R. Watson, Arizona Prevention
Center, USA

Taylor & Francis
Taylor & Francis Group

LONDON AND NEW YORK

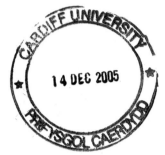
First published 2003 by Taylor & Francis
11 New Fetter Lane, London EC4P 4EE

Simultaneously published in the USA and Canada
by Taylor & Francis Inc,
29 West 35th Street, New York, NY 10001

Taylor & Francis is an imprint of the Taylor & Francis Group

© 2003 Taylor & Francis

Typeset in 10/12pt Goudy by Graphicraft Limited, Hong Kong
Printed and bound in Great Britain by MPG Books Ltd, Bodmin

British Library Cataloguing in Publication Data
A catalogue record for this book is available from the British Library

Library of Congress Cataloging in Publication Data
Reviews in food and nutrition toxicity / edited by Victor R.
Preedy and Ronald Watson.
    p. cm.
  Includes bibliographical references and index.
  Contents: Vol. 1. Toxic and pathological aspects.
  1. Nutrition policy. I. Preedy, Victor R. II. Watson, Ronald R.
(Ronald Ross)

  TX359.R484 2003
  363.8′561—dc21

                                        2002044375

ISBN 0-415-28025-7

Contents

Contributors

Maurizio Aceto, University of Eastern Piedmont, Alessandria, Italy

Yumi Akiyama, Hyogo Prefectural Institute of Public Health and Environmental Sciences, Kobe, Japan

S.H. Arshad, St Mary's Hospital, Isle of Wight, UK

Elisa V. Bandera, The Cancer Institute of New Jersey, New Brunswick, NJ, USA

B.J. Bray, University of Otago, Dunedin, New Zealand

Roland N. Dickerson, University of Tennessee, Health Sciences Center, Memphis, TN, USA

Jefferson Fowles, Institute of Environmental Science and Research, Porirua, New Zealand

Charles R. Geist, University of the Virgin Islands, St Thomas, VI, USA

Anita M. Hartmann, University of Alaska, Fairbanks, AK, USA

Patricia M. Heavey, University of Ulster, Coleraine, UK

Erika Isolauri, University of Turku, Finland

Iris Koch, Royal Military College of Canada, Kingston, Ontario, Canada

Lawrence H. Kushi, Kaiser Permanente, Oakland, CA, USA

Judy S. Lakind, LaKind Associates LLC, Catonsville, MD; Penn State College of Medicine, Hershey, PA, USA

Danièle Lucas, University of Bretagne Occidentale, Brest, France

David Mantle, University of Newcastle upon Tyne, UK

Christopher A. Ollson, Royal Military College of Canada, Kingston, Ontario, Canada

O.S.A. Oluwole, University of Ibadan, Nigeria

A.O. Onabolu, International Institute of Tropical Agriculture, Ibadan, Nigeria

Jennifer Potten, Royal Military College of Canada, Kingston, Ontario, Canada

Victor R. Preedy, King's College, University of London, UK

Dani' K. Rapp, University of Alaska, Fairbanks, AK, USA

Kenneth J. Reimer, Royal Military College of Canada, Kingston, Ontario, Canada

Patrizia Restani, University of Milan, Italy

R.J. Rosengren, University of Otago, Dunedin, New Zealand

Ian R. Rowland, University of Ulster, Coleraine, UK

Seppo Salminen, University of Turku, Finland

Leonard Sax, Montgomery Centre for Research in Child and Adolescent Development, Maryland, USA

Daren A. Scroggie, Uniformed Services University of the Health Sciences, Bethseda, MD, USA

Joanne K. Tobacman, University of Iowa, Iowa City, IA, USA

C. Venter, David Hide Asthma and Allergy Research Centre, St. Mary's Hospital, Isle of Wight, UK

Richard M. Wilkins, University of Newcastle upon Tyne, UK

Atte von Wright, Institute of Applied Biotechnology, University of Kuopio, Finland

Naoki Yoshioka, Hyogo Prefectural Institute of Public Health and Environmental Sciences, Kobe, Japan

1 Toxicity of herbal beverages

Anita M. Hartmann, Dani' K. Raap, and Charles R. Geist

Scope of application

Taking herbs is an old, enduring means of treating human illnesses. By one World Health Organization estimate, nearly 80% of the world's population use herbal medicine for some aspect of their primary healthcare (EHP, 1998). In 1994, the US Congress reduced FDA control over herbs and other dietary supplements, making them more accessible to a thriving American market. The executive director of the American Botanical Council estimates that 30% of US adults use some type of herbal product, and by year 2000, annual sales exceeded $5-billion (EHP, 1998). Worldwide, herbal remedies are rapidly gaining popularity as a result of dissatisfaction with conventional medicines (Bateman et al., 1998). Although it is a widely held belief that herbal preparations are "natural" and therefore intrinsically harmless, their effects can be very powerful, potentially toxic, or fatal.

One reason why safety claims cannot always be based on traditional empiricism is that not all herbal preparations are firmly rooted in traditional medicine (De Smet, 1995). Virtually all our knowledge is derived from human exposures leading to acute toxicities, and little information is available from prior animal experimentation (Kozyrskyi, 1997; Sheehan, 1998). While longstanding traditional experience may tell much about striking and predictable symptoms of acute toxicity, it is a less reliable tool for the detection of reactions which are inconspicuous or develop gradually, have a prolonged latency period, or occur uncommonly (De Smet, 1995). Well-organized monitoring of human populations, such as occurs for drugs, is virtually non-existent for herbal preparations, and thus important toxicities having long latencies are particularly difficult to associate to herb-related factors (e.g. tobacco-smoking, lung cancer; diethylstilbestrol, reproductive tract cancers).

The toxicity of any herbal beverage depends on numerous factors: main content constituents, difficulties identifying plants or plant mixtures, variability in plant quality, adulteration or contamination, preparation methods, and consumer characteristics such as gender, age, genetics, concomitant health problems, and current use of other drugs (Bateman et al., 1998; De Smet, 1995; Huxtable, 1990; Knudsen et al., 2002; Vilon, 1997; Zasshi, 2002), and so forth.

The majority of Chinese herbal preparations are safe, and important Western medicines have been derived from them. Nearly all serious poisonings are due to the few preparations containing aconitine, podophyllin, or anitcholinergics, or other drugs and contaminants (Chan and Critchley, 1996). Decoctions prepared from aconitine sources (e.g. *Aconitum carmichaeli, Aconitum kusnezoffii, Tripterygium wolfordii*) damage the liver through effects on liver lactate dehydrogenase activity (Chan *et al.*, 1995).

The most commonly reported sequela associated with all herbal preparations is hepatotoxicity. Predisposing factors include female gender, and use of agents that induce cytochrome P450 enzymes (Stedman, 2002). Thus far, over 300 plant species, many used for making herbal teas, have been found to contain pyrrolizidine alkaloids whose toxicity was recognized over 40 years ago. These compounds have an inhibitory effect on the Krebs cycle, and can cause a range of liver effects including minor transaminase elevations, acute or chronic hepatitis, steatosis, cholestasis, hepatocellular lysis, zonal or diffuse hepatic necrosis, hepatic fibrosis and cirrhosis, veno-occlusive disease, or acute liver failure requiring transplantation (Larrey, 1994; Stedman, 2002).

Contents of herbal beverages

A herb, in the botanical sense, is any seed plant whose stem withers away to the ground after each season's growth (Agnes and Guralnik, 2001). But in ordinary conversation, most people use the term "herbal" as referring to any plant used as a medicine, seasoning, or flavoring. In this sense then, herbs include flowering plants, shrubs, trees, moss, fern, algae, seaweed, and fungus. In most cultures, herbs are used not only as a part of the treatment of disease, but also in the enhancement of life, physically, emotionally, and spiritually (ASA, 2000). Caution is needed because Chinese herbal preparations include numerous non-plant substances, for example insects such as cicadae, centipedes, and scorpions (Reid, 1993); animals such as antelope, pangolin, earthworm, and turtle (Reid, 1993); and mineral sources such as Glauber salt, gypsum, rhinoceros horn, and gall stones from water buffalo (Reid, 1993). The Chinese character *dan*, associated with Taoist alchemy, is often attached to preparations employing very potent, often toxic, ingredients.

Any product can contain dangerous or harmful adulterants and contaminants, and herbal preparations are no exception. Health Canada has found that certain Chinese herbal preparations contain undeclared prescription drugs such as diethylstilbestrol (DES), indomethacin, and alprazolam, which could cause serious health problems if not taken under medical supervision (Canadian Press, 2002). In particular, DES is a nonsteroidal estrogen and known carcinogen that has been declared unsafe for humans at any dose. Moreover, research chemists in the Division of Natural Products at the Center for Food Safety and Applied Nutrition have found that some herbal preparations contain potentially toxic substances such as diazepam, camphor, and mercury or other toxic heavy metals;

and that botanicals may also be contaminated with pesticides, excreta, molds, and other adulterants (EHP, 1998; Ernst, 2002).

We limit this review to beverages, those liquid preparations for drinking (Agnes and Guralnik, 2001), which are derived from plant sources, concentrating on the ability of the plant derivative to act as a poison or toxin, or to produce disease or ill-health. In this review, we attempt to follow the recommendations put forth at the International Workshop to Evaluate Research Needs on the Use and Safety of Medicinal Herbs (NIEHS, Raleigh, NC, 1998) which is to refer to herbs by their correct, accepted Latin binomials. Since some unusual herbal teas have potentially serious toxic effects, an important challenge is to identify correctly which particular plant is being prepared, as there are many thousands of botanicals in use today. Although some species are highly nutritious (Denning-Barnes, 2002), other similar species are poisonous (Ridker, 1989).

One common cause of toxicity from herbal beverages is mistaken plant identity. For example, the gummy barks of *Acacia senegal* and *Acacia nilotica* have been used by British, American, French, Moors, Bushmen, and Hottentots as syrup bases, sometimes diluted with orange-flower water as demulcents in cough remedies. However, the gummy bark of *Robinia pseudoacacia* has been found to be poisonous, having strong emetic and purgative actions, among foraging animals and also in young boys who chewed the bark and swallowed the juice (Grieve, 1971). A more serious example occurred in the early 1990s, in which a European weight-loss clinic incorrectly used *Aristolochia westlandi* (guang fang ji) instead of the correct herb *Stephania tetrandra* (han fang ji) and several illnesses resulted that were attributed to aristolochic acid, which produces renal hypocellular interstitial fibrosis, renal failure, and urothelial carcinoma (Cosyns *et al.*, 2001).

The source of the plant material may also contribute to toxicity. Even when the same extraction methods are used, there can be wide variation in the final product (Hartmann *et al.*, 2000; Miller, 2000). In ginseng, for example, ginsenoside extraction methods have found *Panax quinquefolius* in American ginseng, *Panax ginseng* in Oriental ginseng, and *Panax pseudoginseng* (var. *notoginseng*) in Sanchi ginseng, but Panax-species ginsenosides were not detected in Siberian ginseng (Lui, 1989 as reviewed by Miller, 2000); Siberian ginseng contains *Eleutherococcus senticosus*. This distinction is particularly important when considering herb–drug interactions, since the eleutherosides have been associated with falsely elevated digoxin levels in the absence of digoxin-toxicity symptoms, presumably because of eleutheroside interaction with the digoxin assay (McRae, 1996 as reviewed by Miller, 2000).

Knowing one name for a toxic plant offers little safety, since the identical plant may be known by several names. One example is comfrey (*Symphytum officinale*), whose tea preparation is used in Western Europe as a treatment for diarrhea; comfrey's common names include knitbone, boneset, blackwort, or bruisewort (Grieve, 1971). Although distribution is banned in Germany and Canada, comfrey remains freely available in the United States. Comfrey is one of the hundreds of plants associated with hepatotoxicity due to pyrrolizidine alkaloids (e.g. lasiocarpine, symphytine, and their related N-oxides); these highly reactive pyrroles act as powerful alkylating agents and produce a non-thrombotic obliteration of small hepatic veins which leads to cirrhosis and eventual liver failure (Stickel and Seitz, 2000).

Moreover, the identical name may refer to different plants having different toxic capacities. For example, a 31-year old man believed he was taking the hallucinogenic plant, mandrake (*Mandragora officinarum*), but was soon hospitalized for severe vomiting; a chromatographic identification of podophyllotoxin in a sample of the plant determined that it was probably *Podophyllum peltatum*, which is also called mandrake (Frasca, Brett and Yoo, 1997).

Toxicities from herbal beverages with correctly identified plants include hepatitis from *Teucrium chamaedrys* (germander) infusions (Perez Alvarez et al., 2001) and from Jin Bu Huan (lycopodium) (Woolf et al., 1994), and diffuse gastrointestinal symptoms from kombucha (Hartmann et al., 2000; Srinivasan et al., 1997). Although the gastrointestinal system is most commonly affected, other body systems also exhibit symptoms of toxicity. For example, ma huang is a herbal source of ephedrine, which has been linked with myocardial infarction, sudden death, and stroke (Samenuk et al., 2002). A woman died as a result of drinking tea prepared from oleander leaves (*Nerium oleander*), which inactivate the Na–K–ATPase pump producing hyperkalemia and cardiac arrhythmias (Haines et al., 1985). Dickstein and Kunkel (1980) reports similar cardiac glycoside toxicity from brewing tea made from foxglove (*Digitalis purpurea*). Yet other plants, for example *Passiflora incarnata L*, produce combinations of symptoms involving several body systems, such as gastrointestinal (nausea, vomiting, diarrhea), cardiovascular (prolonged QTc, nonsustained ventricular tachycardia), and neurological (drowsiness). And while not toxic *per se*, extracts from some plants can exacerbate preexisting conditions; for example, stringbush (*Wikstroemia chamaedaphne*) is shown to be a tumor promoting agent on uterine cervical carcinoma in mice (Lin et al., 1991).

Preparation methods

The modes of preparation, administering plants or extracts to ensure maximum efficacy, and maintaining consistency from one batch to another have always been central to the practice of pharmacy. Extraction procedures, i.e. water-based, alcohol-based, oil-based, or acid-based, how much heat and for how long, have long been known to produce variations in quality as well as toxicity (Crellin and Philpott, 1990; Lee et al., 2000). The useful parts of some plants (e.g. roots of *Triptergygium wilfordii hook*, leaves of *Garcinia hanburyii*) have toxins that require careful processing to minimize toxicity; improper processing can be an important cause of poisoning (Kong et al., 1996; Pyatt et al., 2000; Zhang et al., 1983).

Moreover, toxic constituents of plants can survive the extraction procedure. For example, four Chinese women died from portal hypertension and hepatic veno-occlusive disease that developed after drinking an unidentified "Indian" tea; pyrrolizidine alkaloids were identified in the raw leaves as well as the brewed tea (Kumana *et al.*, 1985). Additionally, the length of the extraction procedure can increase or decrease the amounts of harmful toxins. In one example (Lee *et al.*, 2000), boiling the ma huang herb for two hours reduced the toxic content and produced an extract with a high ephedrine-to-toxins ratio. Botanical stimulants such as ma huang have disposition characteristics similar to their pharmacological counterparts (e.g. ephedrine) and can produce significant cardiovascular responses even after a single dose (Haller *et al.*, 2002). In another example, directions for preparing chuan wu tou (*Aconitum carmechaeli*) are to "brew a long time" (Reid, 1993). Aconitine poisoning often follows ingestion, and is marked by nausea, vomiting, paresthesias of the mouth or extremities, and ventricular extrasystoles (Chan *et al.*, 1993). Aconitine is one of several pharmacologically active deterpenoid alkaloids and is highly toxic. Aconitine suppresses the inactivation of voltage-dependent Na^+ channels by binding to neurotoxin binding site 2 of the alpha-subunit of the channel protein (Ameri, 1998).

Once extracted, the liquid can be added to other vehicles, such as honey, to make herbal syrups (Weiss and Weiss, 1985). In Chinese herbal medicine, there are eight traditional methods of mixing herbal medications of which two are beverages: broth and medicine-wine (Reid, 1993).

Broth techniques are the most common, and oldest, method of preparing herbs. Herbal medicine teas (tisanes, infusions, and decoctions) are strong, requiring about one ounce of dried herb per pint of water. By comparison, commercially-prepared tea bags are only about one-seventh of that ratio (Weiss and Weiss, 1985). Infusions and tisanes are made by steeping the herbs in hot water until the useful properties are extracted (Viereck, 1987). The popular "sun tea" infusion method of soaking herbs in water placed in the summer sun produces beverages nearly as strong. Toxins, contaminants, and adulterants are also extracted as part of the process. Decoctions involve simmering herbs in water, and are primarily used with coarse plant parts, e.g. bark, stems, heavy leaves (Weiss and Weiss, 1985). Herbs, singly or in mixtures, are placed into a clean vessel along with three to four cups of water, covered, and boiled until half the liquid has evaporated. The liquid is strained, cooled, and consumed in divided portions over a day. Whatever therapeutic or toxic ingredients are in the broth are absorbed quickly after digestion and take effect quite rapidly. A technique that produces stronger beverages is to place the herbs in a small covered bowl with only a little water and then steam the bowl in a steamer. The resultant "medicine dew" is a concentrated liquid that is strong and fast-acting. But the broth technique which produces the strongest beverage is to mash fresh herbs with scant water. The resultant "medicine-juice" is strong and active (Reid, 1993).

The alcohol-based extraction methods include tinctures and medicine-wine. To make a tincture, about four ounces of powdered herbs are added to one pint of spirits (e.g. brandy, vodka, or gin), and shaken daily over the two-week extraction period. Several drops to one tablespoon is the recommended dose.

Even herbalists recommend caution with tinctures because they are so potent (Weiss and Weiss, 1985). "Fluid extracts" which are available commercially are up to ten times more potent than the tinctures with which they are often confused (Weiss and Weiss, 1985).

The medicine-wine preparation method involves steeping herbs in strong alcohol for up to six months. One to two ounces are drunk at bedtime (Reid, 1993). Alcohol is a powerful solvent which can leach out toxic as well as therapeutic constituents of the herbs. Moreover, alcohol alone causes health problems for some people, as well as having potentially toxic interactive effects with prescription pharmaceuticals such as anxiolytics or analgesics.

Lipid-soluble components, both therapeutic and toxic, result from oil-based extraction which can be performed either cold or with added heat. The usual strength is two ounces of dried herb per pint of oil (e.g. almond, olive, sunflower, sesame). Cold extraction involves soaking for three days. Heat extraction requires bringing the herbs-in-oil to 200°F for one hour, then cooling (Weiss and Weiss, 1985). Oil extraction preparations can be consumed as well as applied topically.

Acid-extraction involves soaking large handfuls of herbs in strong cider vinegar, approximately six handfuls of herb per gallon; soaking times vary from four days to four weeks. After straining, depending on intended use, other ingredients may be added such as camphor or salts (Meyer, 1993). These, too, may be applied either topically as an astringent, or consumed as a beverage.

Developmental concerns

Research on potential toxic developmental effects of early exposure to herbal beverages is severely lacking. The concern lies with the developing physiological systems. Any toxic substance that targets a specific biological system has the potential for interfering with the development of that system. Hence, the developing organism is not only susceptible to immediate effects, but is also at risk of permanent physiological damage. Furthermore, organisms at any stage of development (fetus, neonate, infant, child, adolescent) have a heightened sensitivity to toxicity. Ingestion of any beverage containing toxicants will likely result in a higher dose of the preparations per unit body weight, putting the developing organism at greater risk than an adult consuming the same volume. Additionally, a developing system lacks the necessary hepatic enzymes responsible for the metabolism of many toxic substances.

Prior to having the skills necessary to obtain beverages voluntarily, a developing child or animal is at the mercy of what is provided. *In utero*, the developing fetus is exposed to most substances consumed by the mother. Immediately after birth, the neonatal mammal will typically receive its nourishment through milk provided by the mammary glands of the mother, or through a surrogate source (such as infant formula). Once consumption of beverages becomes voluntary, herbal sources may increase.

In humans, preparations can be knowingly provided by the mother, as when herbal substances are used with the intention of easing various ailments during pregnancy or in the infant after birth. Alternatively, certain elements may enter the developing system unknowingly, for example based on lack of knowledge of the presence of the substance, or due to lack of education regarding transfer of substances through the placenta. More importantly, it is likely that there is no research on the effects of the substance on the fetus or baby. Hence, the safety of most ingested herbal preparations on development is not known. Whatever the route or timing of exposure in humans, it is typically without the knowledge of potential toxicity to the developing system.

For example, over 50% of pregnant Chinese women have reported ingesting herbal beverages during pregnancy, mainly in the form of teas (e.g. five-flower tea), in order to alleviate common pregnancy ailments such as urinary frequency, indigestion, and constipation, as well as to facilitate delivery and provide energy for labor (Fok, 1985, as reported in Chan, 1994). In addition, 89% of Chinese mothers have reported giving herbal preparations to their infants, typically in the form of milk preparations in place of formula, flower teas, and cool teas (Sung, 1988, as reported in Chan, 1994). While potential toxicity has not been investigated in most of these herbal beverages, it has been reported that Yin-chen (*Artemisia scoparia*), a herbal extract used in pediatric units to treat neonatal jaundice, displaces bilirubin from its serum protein binding (Yueng, 1993, as reported in Chan, 1994). Hence, perinatal exposure has been discouraged. Comfrey root, which is used for tea and is readily available in healthfood stores, have been shown to increase the incidence of liver damage and cancer in laboratory animals, and to be associated with hepatic veno-occlusive disease in Chinese youth (see review by Panter and James, 1990). Specific developmental effects have been found in laboratory animals after exposure to colchicine (autumn crocus). Effective in the treatment of gout, colchicine prevents mitosis, specifically inhibiting spindle formation (Panter and James, 1990). Hence, effects on development would be especially critical.

In animals, there has been much more research on the toxicity of substances contained in the milk of lactating females. Most of the research has focused on domesticated animals grazing on plants known to contain herbal toxins (Panter and James, 1990). Toxicity has been found in cattle, sheep, goats, and even dogs and cats. Many of the substances become concentrated in the milk due to pH differences between the plasma and the mammary milk. The milk is typically more acidic, hence basic compounds (e.g. plant alkaloids) accumulate in the milk. The level of toxicity to the female consuming the substance is not at as high a risk as the nursing offspring. Exposure through the milk will likely be at higher concentrations and processed by a system not yet able to handle fully the metabolism of toxic substances. Hence, signs of toxicity after milk consumption typically appear before symptoms in the lactating female. The concern for humans arises when ingestion of that same milk occurs (e.g. from goats or cattle). While handling practices of bulk-produced milk (which dilute the plant toxicants) and controlled grazing procedures have eliminated most of the health risk for herbal toxins, there is still great risk from milk produced at home for farming families.

Table 1.1 Examples of plant toxins contained in milk, their source, and reported effects in humans (as reported in Panter and James, 1990)

Toxin	Sources	Usual effects
Pyrrolizidine alkaloids	Tansy (*Tanacetum vulgare L.*) Ragwort (*Ambrosia artemisiifolia L.*)	Cancer, neural degeneration Liver toxicosis
Piperidine alkaloids	Poison-hemlock (*Conium maculatum*)	Teratogen: skeletal defects in offspring
Glucosinolates	Crucifers (*Brassica oleracae*)	Thyroid enlargement, liver necrosis, kidney lesions, reduced growth rate
Indolizine alkaloids	Locoweed (*Astragalus pachypus*)	Neural lesions, lack of coordination, head shaking

For example, in the southern and midwestern United States, cattle typically ingest white snakeroot (*Eupatorium rugosum*) while grazing. The toxin, tremetol, is the source of "trembles" in cattle (a condition characterized by sluggishness, decreased appetite, and trembling in the hindquarters) and "milk sickness" in humans (a debilitating condition of weakness, decreased appetite, abdominal pain, and severe vomiting). About 10–20% of exposures are in high enough concentrations to result in death (Panter and James, 1990). Other toxicants from plant sources that can be passed through milk, and their effects, are noted in Table 1.1.

Herb–drug interactions

Plants contain many active ingredients, not all of which are toxic *per se*, but which may contribute to adverse drug–plant interactions (Saxe, 1987). There are thousands of herbal products currently on the market, and countless others locally gathered and used. We present common herbs with known or suspected drug–plant interactions (ASA, 2000; MFMER, 1998–2000; Miller, 2000). We also present in Table 1.2 certain common drugs along with known and suspected herb–drug interactions.

Cayenne (*Capsicum frutescens*) preparations should not be used in conjunction with asthma preparations containing theophylline, or with angiotensin-converting enzyme (ACE) inhibitors, nor in combination with drugs used in diabetic kidney disease, heart failure, or hypertension, because cayenne increases the absorption and effect of these drugs. Cayenne also increases the likelihood of developing a cough when taken with ACE inhibitors.

Chamomile (*Matricaria chamomilla*) contains coumarin and should not be used in conjunction with anticoagulation therapeutics such as warfarin. Additionally, those with a known allergy to ragweed often manifest cross-allergenicity

Table 1.2 List of common pharmacological agents and potentially interactive plants used in herbal beverages (as reviewed by Miller, 2000)

Drug	Interactive herbs	Effects
Alpazolam	*Piper methysticum*	Prolonged sedation, coma
Corcosteroids Cyclosporine	*Astralagus* species *Echinacea* species *Glycyrrhiza glaba*	Offset or minimize immunosuppressive effects
Digoxin	*Adonis vernalis* *Apocynum androsaemifolium* *Apocynum cannabinum* *Asclepias tuberosa* *Convallaria majalis* *Cystisus scoparius* *Digitalis lanata* *Eleutherococcus senticosus* *Leonurus cardiaca* *Scilla maritime* *Scrophularia nodosa* *Strophantus komba* *Uzarae radix*	Various: all the listed plants contain cardiac glycosides which can have additive effects leading to cardiac dysrhythmias
Iron	*Hypericum perforatum* *Serenoa serrulata* and *repens* *Tanacetum parthenium*	Plants contain tannin which inhibits iron absorption
Levothyroxine	*Cochlearia armoracia*	Depresses thyroid function; reduces effectiveness of thyroid replacement drugs
Nonsteroidal anti-inflammatory drugs	*Arctostaphylos uva-ursi* *Cetraria islandica* *Chamaelirium luteum* *Coffea arabica* *Cola arcuminata* and *nitida* *Ruta graveolens* *Schinus terebinthifolia* and *molle* *Symplocarpus foetidus* *Trillium erectum* *Quilla saponaria*	Additive effects of the plants exacerbate the gastric irritant effects of NSAIDs
Phenobarbital	*Artemisia* species *Salvia officianalis* *Primrose vulgaris*	Plants contain thujone or gamolenic acid, both of which lower seizure threshold
Phenytoin	*Centella asiatica* *Convulvulus pluricaulis* *Nardostachys jatamansi* *Nepeta hinostana* and *elliptica* *Onosma bracteatum*	Diminishes effectiveness of seizure control; action involves reducing plasma drug levels
Warfarin	*Allium sativa* *Gingko biloba* *Panax* species *Tanacetum parthenium* *Zingiber officinale roscoe*	Some have additive effects that may increase bleeding; others (panax) inhibit drug's anti-clotting effectiveness

to chamomille, manifesting in abdominal cramps, tongue thickness, tight sensation in the throat, angioedema of lips and eyes, diffuse pruritus, generalized urticaria, and upper airway obstruction due to pharyngeal edema.

Echinacea (*Echinacea purpurea, angustifolia* and *pallida*) has been associated with tachyphylaxis and hepatotoxicity when used for longer than eight weeks, although the mechanism is not well understood, since echinacea lacks the 1,2-unsaturated necrine ring system associated with hepatotoxicity of pyrrolizidine alkaloids. Hepatotoxicity may also occur when it is used in combination with other drugs known to affect the liver (e.g. anabolic steroids, amiodarone, methotrexate, or ketoconazole).

Feverfew (*Tanacetum parthenium Schulz-Bip.*) has been shown to inhibit platelet activity which increases bleeding, and should not be used in combination with other anticoagulants such as warfarin. In those taking feverfew for migraine headache control, its effectiveness can be reduced when taken with NSAIDs (nonsteroidal anti-inflammatory drugs), presumably mediated through prostaglandin inhibition effects.

Garlic (*Allium sativa*) can induce hypotension, and thus may compound the effect of prescription antihypertensive agents. While garlic is commonly taken to reduce serum cholesterol and triglyceride levels, concomitant effects include inhibition of spermatogenesis and decreased platelet aggregation which has been associated with spontaneous spinal epidural hematoma in the elderly. Garlic has also been associated with elevated prothrombin times, and thus caution is needed by those taking warfarin.

Ginger (*Zinbiber officinale Roscoe*) has powerful effects on reducing nausea, vomiting, and vertigo, but ginger is also associated with mutagenesis of *Escherichia coli* which can result in abdominal cramping and diarrhea. Furthermore, ginger has been found to be a potent inhibitor of thromboxane synthetase, and thus prolongs bleeding time. This results in adverse implications for pregnant women and persons taking anticoagulation agents such as warfarin, aspirin, ticlopidine, dipyridamole, or clopidogrel.

Gingko (*Gingko biloba*) has been linked with spontaneous hyphema, and bilateral subdural hematomas, attributed to ginkgolide-B which is a potent platelet-inhibiting factor that is needed to induce arachidonate-independent platelet aggregation. Thus, gingko should not be used in conjunction with aspirin, nonsteroidal anti-inflammatory drugs, or anticoagulants such as heparin or warfarin. Epileptics taking anticonvulsants (e.g. carbamazepine, phenytoin, or Phenobarbital) are advised to avoid gingko because of gingko toxin, a neurotoxin, present in the leaf which can diminish the effectiveness of neuroleptics and reduce seizure control.

Ginseng (*Panax ginseng*) toxicity is difficult to evaluate, in part because of the different chemical constituents in the various species. Adverse effects associated with ginseng include insomnia, headache, hypertension, epistaxis, and vomiting. Ginseng has a moderate estrogen effect which may interact with oral contraceptives or hormonal replacement therapy; ginseng has been associated with onset of vaginal bleeding in post-menopausal elderly women, disordered endometrial proliferation, and mastalgia with diffuse breast nodularity. Ginseng may cause decreased effectiveness of warfarin, heparin, aspirin, and nonsteroidal anti-inflammatory drugs due to the antiplatelet components of *Panax* species. Other effects such as CNS stimulant activity, sleeplessness, and nervousness suggest a steroidal-like mechanism of action for ginseng which should be avoided in patients being treated for manic-depressive disorders and psychosis, or those receiving the antidepressant phenelzine sulfate.

Goldenseal (*Hydrastis canadensis*) is an aquaretic, but most herbalists refer to it as a diuretic. This is an important distinction because with diuretics (e.g. hydrochlorothiazide), sodium is excreted along with water, whereas with aquaretics such as goldenseal, sodium is not excreted. Consequently, goldenseal may actually worsen edema and hypertension, and may diminish the effectiveness of antihypertensives.

Kava (*Piper methysticum*) should not be taken in conjunction with alcohol, sedatives, sleeping pills, antipsychotics, anti-anxiety agents or drugs used in Parkinson's disease. Kava itself can be addictive, and its toxicity is increased when taken in combination with alcohol. The active ingredient, a pyrone, has been found to have synergistic effects with alprazolam inducing disorientation, lethargy, and coma.

Licorice (*Glycyrrhiza glaba*) compounds such ascarbenoxoline, the hemi-succinate derivative of glycyrrhizic acid which inhibits 11-beta-hydroxysteroid dehydrogenase, and has been associated with pseudoaldosteronism, sodium retention, and hypertension. Thus, licorice can reduce the effectiveness of antihypertensives such as spirinolactone. Chronic ingestion of licorice has also been associated with potassium loss leading to hypokalemia and tetraparesis; this can interact with electrolyte therapies such as are used in conjunction with furosemide therapy in congestive heart failure.

Saw palmetto (*Serenoa serrulata* and *repens*) is prudently avoided in conjunction with hormonal therapies (e.g. oral contraceptives, hormone replacement therapy) since additive effects may occur. The hexane extract of saw palmetto has been identified as the active ingredient which has predominantly antiandrogenic activity and *in vivo* estrogen activity.

St John's wort (*Hypericum perforatum*) contains at least 10 constituents or groups of compounds that may contribute to its pharmacologic effects, including naphthodianthroms, flavonoids, xanthose, and bioflavonoids. The mechanism of action is uncertain, but has been characterized as a monoamine oxidase inhibitory or a selective-serotonin reuptake inhibitor.

The US National Institutes of Health's Office of Alternative Medicine has a study in progress to define better its characteristics and effectiveness. Until those or similar results are available, it is prudent to avoid concomitant use of St John's wort with MAOIs (e.g. phenelzine) or with betasympathomimetic amines (e.g. ma huang, pseudephedrine HCl), and similarly with SSRIs (e.g. fluoxetine and paroxetine).

Valerian (*Valerian officinalis*) is a potent soporific and mild hyponotic, which can have additive effects when mixed with alcohol. Valerian has been shown to prolong thiopental- and pentobarbital-induced sleep, and should be avoided in anticipation of surgical anesthesia and by those taking barbiturates.

Conclusion

Several excellent additional resources for further information are presented in Table 1.3.

While herbal beverages remain popular, pleasantly satisfying, and for the most part safe, certain gaps in our knowledge remain to be filled, some urgently so (van Ornum and Weber, 2002). Standardization in nomenclature, and monitoring for adulteration, are needed to address the wide inter-product and intra-product variation and composition of active constituents. Also needed are

Table 1.3 Internet databases change much faster than print resources. The following websites were current, active, and accurate at the time this manuscript was prepared. Each is an informative, authoritative resource with much more information than could be included here. Numerous others exist.

- US Dept of Health and Human Services, National Institutes of Health (NIH)
  http://www.nih.gov/health/
  Links to consumer information, clinical databases, health literature references, and other Federal agencies such as Food and Drug Administration
- NIH Office of Dietary Supplements – IBIDS database
  http://dietary-supplements.info.nih.gov/databases/ibids.html
  International Bibliographic Information on Dietary Supplements (IBIDS) is a database of published, international, scientific literature on dietary supplements including vitamins, minerals, botanicals
- HerbMed, project of the Alternative Medicine Foundation, Inc.
  http://www.herbmed.org
  An interactive, electronic herbal database that provides hyperlinked access to the evidence-based, scientific information underlying the use of herbs for health. A recent search for "toxicity" retrieved 169 documents
- Ethnobotanical Resource Directory
  http://cieer.org/directory.html
  CIEER (Center for International Ethnomedicinal Education and Research) attempts to unify global information regarding ethobotanical research and documentation. The directory has over 150 active links in 12 areas, including databases
- Medline Plus for Herbal Medicine, NIH/NCCAM (also available in Spanish)
  http://www.nlm.nih.gov/medlineplus/herbalmedicine.html
  The primary US National Institutes of Health (NIH) organization for research on herbal medicine is NCCAM, National Center for Complementary and Alternative Medicine. Links include: latest news, clinical trials, alternative therapies, research, specific conditions and aspects, and other US federal agencies such as Alternative Medicine Foundation, and the National Toxicology Program
- USDA Food and Nutrition Information Center
  http://www.nal.usda.gov/fnic/etext/ds_herbinfo.html
  USDA, United States Department of Agriculture. Active links to herbal information from American Botanical Council, Mayo Clinic, Center for Science in the Public Interest, US Pharmacopeia, and many others

more scientifically based studies evaluating safety issues in general as well as during development. Importantly, studies targeting herb–drug interactions would serve public safety.

Acknowledgment

Thanks are due to Nancy McGrath-Hanna for her research assistance.

References

Agnes, M. (editor in chief) and Guralnik, D.B. (editor in chief, emeritus) (2001) *Webster's New World College Dictionary*, 4th edn, Foster City, CA: IDG Books Worldwide.

Ameri, A. (1998) The effects of *Aconitum* alkaloids on the central nervous system. *Progress in Neurobiology*, **56**: 211–235.

ASA (American Society of Anesthesiologists) (2000) What you should know about herbal use and anesthesia. *Medem Medical Library*. San Francisco, CA: Medem.

Bateman, J., Chapman, R.D., and Simpson, D. (1998) Possible toxicity of herbal remedies. *Scottish Medical Journal*, **43**: 7–15.

Canadian Press (2002) Health Canada warns some Chinese herbs contain undeclared prescription drugs. http://www.nlm.gov/medlineplus/news/fullstory_8175.html, 19 June.

Chan, T.Y. (1994) The prevalence use and harmful potential of some Chinese herbal medicines in babies and children. *Veterinary and Human Toxicology*, **36**: 238–240.

Chan, T.Y. and Critchley, J.A. (1996) Usage and adverse effects of Chinese herbal medicines. *Human & Experimental Toxicology*, **15**: 5–12.

Chan, W.Y., Ng, T.B., Lu, J.L., Cao, Y.X., Wang, M.Z., and Liu, W.K. (1995) Effects of decoctions prepared from *Aconitum carmichaeli*, *Aconitum kusnezoffii* and *Tripterygium wilfordii* on serum lactate dehydrogenase activity and histology of liver, kidney, heart and gonad in mice. *Human & Experimental Toxicology*, **14**: 489–493.

Chan, T.Y., Tomlinson, B., and Critchley, J.A. (1993) Aconitine poisoning following ingestion of Chinese herbal medicines: a report of eight cases. *Australia and New Zealand Journal of Medicine*, **23**: 268–271.

Cosyns, J.P., Dehoux, J.P., Guiot, Y., Goebbels, R.M., Robert, A., Bernard, A.M., and van Ypersele de Strihou, C. (2001) Chronic aristolochic acid toxicity in rabbits: a model of Chinese herbs nephropathy? *Kidney International*, **59**: 2164–2173.

Crellin, J.K. and Philpott, J. (1990) *Herbal Medicine Past and Present, Vol. II – a Reference Guide to Medicinal Plants*. London: Duke University Press.

Denning-Barnes, A. (2002) Sharing the tundra's bounty: Native nutritionist instructs on use of local herbs. *Fairbanks Daily News-Miner*, 11 June, D-1.

De Smet, P.A. (1995) Health risks of herbal remedies. *Drug Safety: an International Journal of Medical Toxicology and Drug Experience*, **13**: 81–93.

Dickstein, E.S. and Kunkel, F.W. (1980) Foxglove tea poisoning. *American Journal of Medicine*, **69**: 167–169.

EHP (1999) Medicinal herbs: NTP extracts the facts. *Environmental Health Perspectives*, **107**, 12. http://ehpnet1.niehs.nih.gov/docs/1099/107-12/niehsnews.html, December.

EHP (1998) Supplemental information; Herbal health. *Environmental Health Perspectives*, **106**. http:ehpnet1.niehs.nih.gov/docs/1998/106-12/forum.html#net/ and /106-12/niehsnews.ntml, 12 December.

Ernst, E. (2002) Toxic heavy metals and undeclared drugs in Asian herbal medicines. *Trends in Pharmacological Sciences*, **23**: 136–139.

Fisher, A.A., Purcell, P., and LeCouteur, D.G. (2000) Toxicity of *Passiflora inarnata* L. *Journal of Toxicology and Clinical Toxicology*, **38**: 63–66.

Frasca, T., Brett, A.S., and Yoo, S.D. (1997) Mandrake toxicity: a case of mistaken identity. *Archives of Internal Medicine*, **157**: 2007–2009.

Grieve, M. (1971) *A Modern Herbal: the Medicinal, Culinary, Cosmetic, and Economic Properties, Cultivation, and Folk-lore of Herbs, Grasses, Fungi, Trees & Shrubs with All Their Modern Scientific Uses*, 2 vols. New York: Dover Publications.

Haines, B.E., Bessen, H.A., and Wightman, W.D. (1985) Oleander tea: draught of death. *Annals of Emergency Medicine*, **14**: 350–353.

Haller, C.A., Jacob, P., and Benowitz, N.L. (2002) Pharmacology of ephedra alkaloids and caffeine after single-dose dietary supplement use. *Clinical Pharmacology and Therapeutics*, **71**: 421–432.

Hartmann, A.M., Burleson, L.E., Holmes, A.K., and Geist, C.R. (2000) Effects of chronic kombucha ingestion on open-field behaviors, longevity, appetitive behaviors and organs in C57-BL/6 mice: a pilot study. *Nutrition*, **16**: 755–761.

Huxtable, R.J. (1990) The harmful potential of herbal and other plant products. *Drug Safety 1990 Supplement*, **5**: 126–136.

Knudsen, V.K., Rasmussen, L.B., Haraldsdottir, J., Ovesen, L., Bulow, I., Knudsen, N., Jorgensen, T., Laurberg, P., and Perrild, H. (2002). Use of dietary supplements in Denmark is associated with health and former smoking. *Public Health Nutrition*, **5**: 463–468.

Kong, L., Ye, D., Wang, S., Xu, Y., and Bian, J. (1996) Acute toxicity and anti-inflammatory effect of processed products of gamboges. *China Journal of Chinese Materia Medica*, **21**: 214–216.

Kozyrskyi, A. (1997) Herbal products in Canada: how safe are they? *Canadian Family Physician*, Apr., **43**: 697–702.

Kumana, C.F., Ng, M., Lin, J.H., Ko, W., Wu, P.C., and Todd, D. (1985) Herbal tea induced hepatic veno-occlusive disease: quantification of toxic alkaloid exposure in adults. *Gut*, **26**: 101–104.

Larrey, D. (1994) Liver involvement in the course of phytotherapy. *Medical Press, Paris, France*, **23**: 691–693.

Lee, M.K., Cheng, B.W., Che, C.T., and Hsieh, D.P. (2000) Cytotoxicity assessment of Mahuang (ephedra) under different conditions of preparation. *Toxicology Science*, **56**: 424–430.

Lin, Z.X., Lu, G.Z., Jiang, S.W., Zhou, L.X., and Han, Y.L. (1991) Effects of tumor promoting herb *Wikstroemia chamaedaphe* extract on V79 cells and WB liver cells: I. Correlation between cellular growth and gap junctional intercellular communication. *Journal of Experimental Biology*, **24**: 307–315.

MFMER (Mayo Foundation for Medical Education and Research) (1998–2000) Herb and drug interactions. www.MayoClinic.com

Meyer, J.E. (reprinted 1993 by D.C. Meyer) *The Herbalist*. Glenwood, IL: Meyerbooks.

Miller, L.G. (2000) Herbal medicinals – selected clinical considerations focusing on known or potential drug–herb interactions. *Alternative Medicine: an Objective Assessment*. Chicago, IL: American Medical Association.

Minter, S. (1993) *The Healing Garden: a Natural Haven for Body, Senses and Spirit*. Boston, MA: Charles E. Tuttle.

Panter, K.E. and James, L.F. (1990) Natural plant toxicants in milk: a review. *Journal of Animal Science*, **68**: 892–904.

Perez Alvarez, J., Saez-Royuela, F., Gento Pena, E., Lopez Morante, A., Velasco Oses, A., and Martin Lorente, J. (2001) Acute hepatitis due to ingestion of *Teucrium chamadedrys* infusions. *Gastroenterology and Hepatology*, **24**: 240–243.

Pyatt, D.W., Yang, Y., Mehos, B., Le, A., Stillman, W., and Irons, R.D. (2000) Hematotoxicity in the Chinese herbal medicine *Tripterydium wilfordii* hook f in CD34-positive human bone marrow cells. *Molecular Pharmacology*, **57**: 512–518.

Reid, D.P. (1993) *Chinese Herbal Medicine*. Boston, MA: Shambala Publications.

Ridker, P.M. (1989) Health hazards of unusual herbal teas. *American Family Physician*, **39**: 153–156.

Samenuk, D., Link, M.S., Homoud, M.K., Contreras, R., Theohardes, T.C., Wange, P.J., and Estes, N.A. (2002) Adverse cardiovascular events temporally associated with ma huang, an herbal source of ephedrine. *Mayo Clinic Proceedings*, **77**: 12–16.

Saxe, T.G. (1987) Toxicity of medicinal herbal preparations. *American Family Physician*, **35**: 135–142.

Sheehan, D.M. (1998) Herbal medicines, phytoestrogens and toxicity: risk:benefit considerations. *Proceedings of the Society for Experimental and Biological Medicine*, **217**: 379–385.

Shlosberg, A. and Egyed, M.N. (1983) Examples of poisonous plants in Israel of importance to animals and man. *Archives of Toxicology*, Supplement 6: 194–196.

Srinivasan, R., Smolinske, S., and Greenbaum, D. (1997) Probably gastrointestinal toxicity of kombucha tea: is this beverage healthy or harmful? *Journal of General Internal Medicine*, **12**: 643–644.

Stedman, C. (2002) Herbal hepatotoxicity. *Seminars on Liver Disease*, **22**, 2: 195–206.

Stickel, F. and Seitz, H.K. (2000) The efficacy and safety of comfrey. *Public Health & Nutrition*, **3**: 501–508.

Van Ornum, M. and Weber, C. (2002) Pharmacology Update – Dietary supplements: applying the knowledge. *Journal of Neuroscience Nursing*, **34**: 160–164.

Viereck, E.G. (1987) *Alaska's Wilderness Medicines: Healthful Plants of the Far North*. Edmonds, WA: Alaska Northwest.

Vilon, C. (1997) Belgian (Chinese herb) neuropathy: why? *Journal of Belgian Pharmacology*, **52**: 7–27.

Weiss, G. and Weiss, S. (1985) *Growing & Using Healing Herbs*. Emmaus, PA: Rodale Press.

Woolf, G.M., Petrovic, L.M., Roiter, S.E., Wainwright, S., Vilamil, F.G., Katkov, W.N., Michieletti, P., Wanless, I.R., Stermitz, F.R., and Beck, J.J. (1994) Acute hepatitis associated with the Chinese herbal product jin bu huan. *Annals of Internal Medicine*, **121**: 729–735.

Zasshi, Y. (2002) The plant origins of herbal medicines and their quality evaluation. *Journal of the Pharmaceutical Society of Japan*, **122**: 363–379.

Zhang, Y.G., Chieh, C.H.I., and Chih, H.T. (1983) An experimental pathologic study on acute *Triptergium wilfordii* poisoning in rats. *Poisonous Plant Toxicity*, **3**: 360–362.

2 Arsenic in vegetables

An evaluation of risk from the consumption of produce from residential and mine gardens in Yellowknife, Northwest Territories, Canada

Iris Koch, Christopher A. Ollson, Jennifer Potten, and Kenneth J. Reimer

Summary

The soil arsenic concentrations in Yellowknife, Northwest Territories, Canada, are above national averages as a result of both the natural geology of the region and the release of arsenic-containing waste during local gold mining processes. The presence of elevated soil arsenic concentrations raised concerns about the safety of arsenic levels in residentially grown vegetables. Accordingly, the arsenic levels in voluntarily donated residential vegetables and fruits were studied. The possibility that residential soil had been historically augmented with arsenic contaminated waste from the mines prompted the study of worst-case scenario gardens. For the latter study, two gardens were constructed: one on mine property, and one using soil from a nearby lakeshore that was contaminated with arsenic.

Following washing procedures similar to those used in typical food preparation, vegetables and fruits were dried, ground, and acid-digested. Total arsenic concentrations were determined in the acid digests by hydride generation–atomic absorption spectrometry (HG-AAS) and arsenic levels in dried and ground soils from each garden were determined by neutron activation analysis (NAA).

The concentration of arsenic in soils from the residential gardens was 33 ± 14 mg/kg, which is within the range of the natural or background concentration in the soil of the Yellowknife area. A higher average arsenic concentration of 200 ± 140 mg/kg was determined in garden soils collected from a mine townsite property, which is no longer used residentially. The soils from the lake garden and mine garden contained elevated arsenic levels of 720 ± 220 mg/kg and 1560 ± 660 mg/kg respectively, which are concentrations typical of the sampled areas.

A significant finding is that arsenic concentrations in produce from Yellowknife residential gardens are almost always an order of magnitude greater than those found in like foods in a Canadian diet survey (Dabeka *et al.*, 1993). The highest arsenic concentrations were found in leafy vegetables such as lettuce (maximum 0.27 mg/kg fresh weight) and berries (maximum 0.44 mg/kg fresh weight). Arsenic levels in vegetables grown in the lake and mine gardens were two orders of magnitude higher than in Yellowknife residential produce, with maxima of 46 mg/kg fresh weight in beets from the lake garden and 330 mg/kg fresh weight in onions from the mine garden.

The study of bioaccumulation and translocation factors (BAFs and TFs) revealed a general trend towards greater BAFs for below-ground plant parts with increasing soil arsenic concentrations. The TF data supported this by exhibiting lower values with increasing soil concentrations. These trends suggest that for these vegetables root sequestration of arsenic may be a tolerance mechanism for exposure to high arsenic levels.

The potential risk of adverse effects from the consumption of this arsenic-containing produce was evaluated by using a risk assessment approach recommended by Health Canada (1995). The goal was to determine if the estimated daily intake of arsenic exceeds the provisional maximum daily intake (PMDI) of 2.1 µg/kg per day recommended by the Food and Agriculture Organization/World Health Organization (FAO/WHO).

The risk calculation, which incorporated the consumption of other arsenic-containing foods as well as the garden produce, revealed that the PMDI is not exceeded when Yellowknife residential produce is consumed. On the other hand, the PMDI would be exceeded in most cases should the lake or mine produce be ingested, assuming that all of the arsenic in the produce is absorbed into the body. The risk was lowered by the incorporation of a bioaccessibility factor that was obtained from an extraction process that modeled gastric dissolution of arsenic. The reduction in risk (i.e. the lowering of EDIs to levels below the PMDI) was significant only for produce from the lake garden.

Therefore no increase in risk is posed to the residents consuming garden vegetables from their gardens in Yellowknife. However, produce grown in soils similar to those used in the lake and mine gardens would not be safe to eat.

Introduction

Arsenic in Yellowknife

Arsenic is a ubiquitous, naturally occurring element in the environment, ranking in abundance twentieth in the earth's crust, fourteenth in seawater, and twelfth in the human body. In spite of its ubiquity, arsenic is still nearly synonymous with poison, as some arsenic compounds were used for that purpose for centuries. While arsenic is often associated with adverse effects, its toxicity is actually dependent on its chemical form, or species (i.e. the specific combination of arsenic with other elements) (Shiomi, 1994). For example, arsenobetaine, an organoarsenic compound that is found in marine animals (Francesconi and Edmonds, 1997) and mushrooms (Koch *et al.*, 2000b; Kuehnelt *et al.*, 1997;

Table 2.1 Names, abbreviations, and chemical structures of some common arsenicals

Name	Abbreviation	Chemical formula
Arsenate, arsenic acid	As(V)	$AsO(OH)_3, [AsO_2(OH)_2]^-,$ $[AsO(OH)_3]^{2-}, [AsO_4]^{3-}$
Arsenite, arsenous acid	As(III)	$As(OH)_3, [AsO(OH)_2]^-,$ $[AsO_2(OH)]^{2-}, [AsO_3]^{3-}$
Monomethylarsonic acid	MMA	$CH_3 AsO(OH)_2$
Dimethylarsinic acid	DMA	$(CH_3)_2AsO(OH)$
Arsenobetaine	AB	$(CH_3)_3As^+CH_2COO^-$

Slejkovec *et al.*, 1997), is much less toxic than arsenic trioxide, an inorganic form of arsenic (and the main historical poison). Some common forms of arsenic are summarized in Table 2.1.

Arsenic can be introduced to the environment naturally as a result of the weathering of rocks that contain arsenic-rich minerals, and geothermal activities (Matschullat, 2000). It can also enter the environment anthropogenically as a consequence of its industrial use, through the application of arsenic-containing pesticides, and through mining and smelting activities (Matschullat, 2000). A very important example of the latter is gold mining.

Yellowknife, located in the Northwest Territories, Canada (see Figure 2.1) has been an active gold mining community since 1938. The gold in Yellowknife ore is found with arsenopyrite (FeAsS), an arsenic-containing iron sulfide. Consequently, the milling of the arsenic-rich ore generates a considerable amount of arsenic waste. This waste can enter the environment in the form of solid waste (waste rock and tailings), liquid effluent, and aerial emissions from the roaster stack.

As a result of both the anthropogenic inputs of arsenic from gold mining and the natural inputs from the weathering of arsenic-containing minerals, the arsenic levels in the Yellowknife area are elevated compared with the typical Canadian background concentration range of 5 to 14 mg/kg in soils. In previous studies, the background levels have been estimated to range from 3 to 150 mg/kg in Yellowknife (Ollson, 2000; Reimer, 2002).

Arsenic in food

Epidemiological studies of populations consuming drinking water with high natural arsenic concentrations (up to 1000 µg/L or more) suggest a relationship between elevated levels of arsenic exposure and the prevalence of skin, bladder and lung cancers (Chiou *et al.*, 1995; Tsuda *et al.*, 1995). In most regions of Canada, the concentration of arsenic in drinking water (usually of the order of 1 µg/L) is much lower than the provisional maximum allowable concentration of 25 µg/L (CCME, 1999). Even in Yellowknife, where elevated levels of

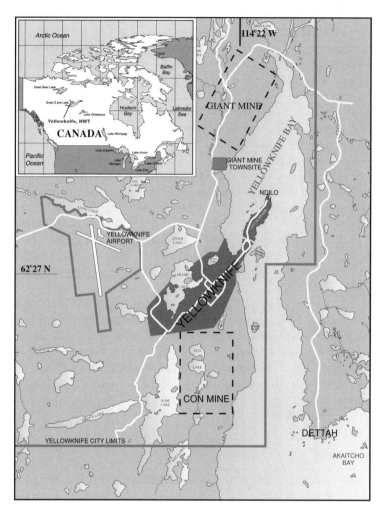

Figure 2.1 Location of Yellowknife city and mines.

arsenic occur in lakes in and surrounding the city, the arsenic concentration in the municipal supply of drinking water (obtained from a different watershed area) is less than 1 µg/L and is therefore safe to drink. Under these circumstances, the main contribution of arsenic to the human diet comes from food, and cumulative exposure is the primary concern. Indeed, total diet studies conducted by the US Food and Drug Administration (FDA) determined that food contributes 93% of the total arsenic intake in the US human diet. Of that 93%, seafood contributes 90% (Adams *et al.*, 1994, Subcommittee on Arsenic in Drinking Water, 1999) and such foods generally contain non-toxic organoarsenic compounds (e.g. arsenobetaine and arsenosugars). Other foods, such as vegetables, rice, poultry, and mushrooms, contain much lower levels of arsenic, and due to limitations in analysis methods, the arsenic in these foods has been very difficult to characterize (Subcommittee on Arsenic in Drinking Water, 1999). In cases where the growing environment contained elevated levels of arsenic, vegetables contained predominantly inorganic arsenic (Helgesen and Larsen, 1998; Pyles and Woolson, 1982).

A comprehensive survey of the arsenic content in Canadian foods was published in 1993 and is used throughout this report for comparison to our findings (Dabeka *et al.*, 1993). This survey found that the arsenic concentrations ranged from low µg/kg levels in milk and dairy products, soups, vegetables, fruit, fruit juices, and other beverages; to double digit µg/kg levels in meat and poultry, bakery goods and cereals, fats and oils, sugar and candy, and miscellaneous foods; to low mg/kg levels in fish and shellfish. In summary, all foods other than fish and shellfish contained arsenic at levels less than 50 µg/kg. From these values, the average daily intake of arsenic by a Canadian adult was calculated to be 40% of the provisional maximum daily intake (PMDI) recommended by the Food and Agriculture Organization/World Health Organization (FAO/WHO), of 2.1 (µg of arsenic)/(kg of body weight) per day, or 15 µg/kg per week (FAO/WHO, 1999; WHO, 2002).

In 1979 a survey of arsenic in Yellowknife vegetables was published, summarizing total arsenic levels in a variety of vegetables and fruits sampled from five general areas in Yellowknife (Soniassy, 1979). Arsenic levels ranged from 0.05 mg/kg fresh weight in pea pods to 2.05 mg/kg fresh weight in green onions, with an average overall concentration of 0.32 mg/kg fresh weight ($n = 42$). It was noted that the levels of the arsenic were similar to those found in previous years, but no attempt was made to predict human health risk from the consumption of the produce in this report.

Risk assessment

If a contaminant level exceeds those that constitute national criteria, such as the soil and water guidelines established by Canadian Council of Ministers of the Environment (CCME, 1999), then further investigation of the contamination is recommended, including sampling of garden vegetables. In the case of Yellowknife the majority of soil samples collected from the city exceed the recommended soil quality guideline of 12 mg/kg (CCME, 1999).

There are several ways that an assessment of risk to human health posed by a route of exposure can be conducted. In this study, the guidelines specified by Health Canada (1995) were used. The approach of this method is to determine the estimated daily intake (EDI) by all possible pathways, and then to compare this EDI with a tolerable daily intake (TDI) for non-carcinogenic substances, or with a risk-specific dose (RsD) for carcinogenic substances.

The TDI used in this study is derived from the provisional tolerable weekly intake (PTWI) of 15 µg/kg per week (corresponding to a provisional maximum daily intake, PMDI, of 2.1 µg/kg per day) of inorganic arsenic (FAO/WHO, 1999), specifically recommended for the intake of arsenic from food. This PTWI/PMDI was recommended by the Joint FAO/WHO Expert Committee on Food Additives (JECFA) in their last toxicological evaluation of food contaminants in 1988, in spite of the limited knowledge of adverse health effects (if any) from intake of arsenic through food, and it provides an initial basis for risk characterization.

Regulatory authorities have frequently assumed that 100% of the arsenic ingested is absorbed. However, experimental work using arsenic-contaminated soils has revealed that arsenic oral accessibility from most solid-phase compounds was substantially lower than from air or water because the arsenic was incompletely dissolved in the gastrointestinal tract (Ruby *et al.*, 1996). Therefore, it is necessary to account for incomplete absorption and accessibility of arsenic when attempting to assess accurately potential health effects associated with arsenic exposure.

An extraction process that mimics human gastrointestinal digestion has been developed to estimate the amount of a contaminant that is accessible to an individual as a result of digestive dissolution (Hamal *et al.*, 1998; Rodriguez *et al.*, 1999; Ruby *et al.*, 1996). For simplicity, this process will be referred to as gastric fluid extraction (GFE). We propose that the amount of arsenic available by using GFE can be utilized to calculate more accurately human health risk.

Although arsenic is a carcinogen, we will not consider the cancer risks associated with the consumption of vegetables grown in Yellowknife gardens. Such an evaluation should include estimated doses of arsenic from air, drinking water, soil ingestion, food, and skin absorption (water and soil) (Health Canada, 1995) and is a topic for future study.

Study objectives

Following the reporting of elevated levels of arsenic in soils in the Yellowknife area, concerns arose regarding the safety of garden produce grown in that area. In response, a study of the arsenic content of residential garden produce was initiated. Moreover, the possibility existed that some residents unknowingly augmented their gardens with soil that had been contaminated with mine waste. In order to model a worst-case exposure scenario (e.g. residential use of mine soil that has not been remediated), a vegetable garden was planted in Yellowknife in arsenic-contaminated soil from the Con Mine and adjoining Rat Lake areas.

The main objective of this study was to assess the potential human health risk associated with the consumption of vegetables grown in Yellowknife residential soils, and on arsenic contaminated mine soil. To do this, the following specific objectives were met:

1   levels of total arsenic in soil and produce from residential Yellowknife gardens and mine soils were quantified;
2   uptake of arsenic from soil by plants was determined, to study any biological responses to high soil arsenic concentrations;
3   estimated daily intakes were calculated and compared to the international standard described above.

Methods

Locations of gardens in the Yellowknife area

Vegetables and soil samples were collected from 10 gardens in the Yellowknife area. In order to protect the privacy of the garden owners who donated their vegetables, each location was assigned a number between 1 and 10. Locations 2 through 10 were taken from residential gardens from different areas in Yellowknife. Location 1 is a group of samples taken from two locations from residences no longer in use on a mine townsite (Giant Mine Townsite, Figure 2.1). Even though sample locations were based largely on the voluntary participation of residents, most areas from around the city were successfully represented.

The location of the mine garden was on mine property (Con Mine, Figure 2.1) in a sheltered low-lying area known to contain elevated levels of arsenic in the soil. Soil from the shore of a small lake adjacent to the mine property was used as well (referred to as the lake garden), as the soil from this area was believed to have been used to augment gardens in the area.

The soil composition of the gardens was noted at each location, and consisted of black organic soils. Residential soils had been amended with mulching agents.

Mine and lake garden preparation

The mine and lake vegetable gardens were prepared at the end of June 2001 without any amendments with mulching agents or lime. The mine plot, which consisted of two adjoining rectangles (5 × 6 m and 2 × 3 m), was tilled with shovels from 0 to 40 cm to homogenize and aerate the soil.

The lake garden, consisting of soil in planter boxes, was constructed by first homogenizing a 4 m^2 patch of soil from 0 to 60 cm. Equal amounts of gravel were placed in the bottom of five 1 × 0.3 × 0.3 m planter boxes to enhance drainage, and the boxes were filled with approximately equal amounts of the homogenized lake soil. The planters were kept adjacent to the mine garden plot for the entire growth period.

The most common vegetables found in Yellowknife residential gardens were selected as the varieties to be grown in the mine and lake gardens, and the vegetable seeds and bulbs were obtained from a garden store in June 2001. Fourteen rows of vegetables were planted in the mine plot (mustard, Swiss chard, beets, radish, peas × 2, Grand Rapids lettuce, Prize Head lettuce, carrots, beans, white onions × 2, white potatoes × 2), while each lake soil planter contained a single vegetable type (beets, radish, Grand Rapids lettuce, carrots, beans). In total, 11 types of vegetables were planted. The seeds and bulbs were planted according to the spacing and depth instructions on each package. The plants were fertilized twice in June (following planting) using 10–20–10 (NPK) outdoor garden formula (Miracle Grow®). Constant rainfall during the summer precluded further application of fertilizer or watering.

Sampling and analysis of soil samples

The soil sampling program was designed to obtain samples that, when composited, would be representative of each garden as a whole. Each sample was collected with a plastic scoop, stored in a plastic bag and kept frozen during transport and until analysis. Residential garden soils were sampled when vegetable samples were collected, and mine and lake gardens were sampled prior to planting in June.

For each residential garden three to five samples were collected, one from each corner (or end, depending on the size and shape of the garden) and one from the center of the garden. In areas where only one plant was collected, only one soil sample was collected. Samples were obtained at the depths between 0 and 20 cm or between 0 cm and bedrock, if bedrock occurred at a shallower depth. The mine garden plot was divided into a 1 × 1 m grid system and samples were collected from 0 to 20 cm at each intersection of grid lines. A soil sample was collected from the center of each lake soil planter box from 0 to 20 cm.

A random number generator (Urbaniak and Lestick, 1997) was used to select 30% of the soil samples collected from the mine plot, which were then analyzed. All lake and composite (residential, mine and lake garden) soil samples were analyzed.

Soils were air-dried at room temperature for two to three days and then ground into a homogeneous powder using a coffee grinder or a mortar and pestle. The grinding tool was rinsed three times with 2–3 g of each new sample, which was then discarded, before homogenizing the bulk of the sample.

Composite samples were prepared from soil samples that were collected from the same garden, by adding an equal portion of each dried and ground soil sample to total 20 g (e.g. 4 g soil × five samples = 20 g). Field duplicates were included by using half the normal amount for each duplicate (e.g. as for the example above, for 4 g soil samples, 2 g of each duplicate). The composite sample was then homogenized as described above.

Neutron activation analysis (NAA) in the SLOWPOKE-2 reactor located at RMC was used to determine the total concentration of arsenic in all soil samples. Each dried and ground sample was weighed (1–2 g) into a 1.5 mL polyethylene vial and heat-sealed. The samples were irradiated at a flux of $5 × 10^{11}/cm^2$ per s for two hours, cooled for 80–120 h, and then counted for 2 h using a GMC HpGe detector coupled with a Nuclear Data μ-multichannel analyzer (MCA).

Sampling and analysis of plant samples

Residential gardens were sampled in September 2000. Mine and lake gardens were sampled in August 2001, by uprooting the entire plant. After they were collected, residential garden samples were washed with tap water as if they were being prepared for consumption. Root vegetables were gently scrubbed with a brush to remove all dirt and each sample was carefully inspected visually to ensure that cleaning was thorough. Mine and lake garden plants, because of their small size, were subjected to a more rigorous cleaning regime that included careful separation of all plants, washings in at least three changes each of tap water and deionized distilled water (DDW) and meticulous visual inspection. Samples were then dried with Kim™ towels and stored frozen in plastic bags until further processing.

Samples were chopped while frozen, then frozen completely with liquid nitrogen, and then ground and homogenized in a blender. A portion of the frozen ground sample was weighed and then dried in a 70°C oven overnight. When dry, the sample was reweighed, and homogenized briefly in the blender or by using a mortar and pestle.

A quantity of 0.5 g of each dried sample was accurately measured (±0.0001 g) into a glass 50 mL test tube. A Teflon™ boiling stone and 10 mL of ultrapure nitric acid (Seastar Baseline) were added, and the samples were heated in a heating block from room temperature to 100°C for 1 h and then heated at 140°C for 6 h. The samples were then cooled, and 2 mL of hydrogen peroxide was added. The samples were heated at 140°C for another 1.5 h, then cooled and diluted to approximately 25 g (±0.01 g).

Analysis was carried out by diluting the samples 10-fold with 1 mol/L HCl (Fluka, puriss p.a.) and introducing them to a SOLAAR 969 atomic absorption spectrometer (AAS), outfitted with an EC90 furnace via a VP90 hydride generation (HG) system (all from Thermo Instruments Canada), in which AsH$_3$ was generated with a reducing solution of 1% w/v NaBH$_4$ (Aldrich) and 0.1% NaOH (Aldrich). The arsenic in the samples was quantified by using calibration curves constructed from matrix matched standards (Aldrich ICP/DCP arsenic standard).

Gastric fluid extraction (GFE) of mine and lake garden plants

The dried, homogenized mine and lake garden plant samples were extracted with 20 g of a synthetic gastric fluid containing 1.25 g/L pepsin (Sigma) and 8.77 g/L NaCl (Fluka, puriss p.a.) that had been titrated to pH 1.8 with HCl (Fluka, puriss p.a.) by shaking for one hour at 272 rpm and 37°C. Samples were then centrifuged for 30 min at 3000 rpm, and the supernatant was filtered (no. 4 filters, Whatman). A 2 g aliquot of the resulting extract was digested on a hot plate with 1 mL of ultrapure nitric acid (Seastar Baseline) and then diluted to 5 g with DDW. The digested extracts were analyzed by using hydride generation–atomic absorption spectroscopy (HG-AAS) in the same manner as the plant digests.

Statistical analysis

For statistical analyses Systat® 10 and Microsoft Excel® were used. Prior to conducting analysis of variance (ANOVA) tests, data were normalized by log transformation.

Quality assurance/quality control (QA/QC)

Quality assurance/quality control (QA/QC) measures were undertaken to ensure that the data were of high quality. Field duplicate soil samples were collected every 10 samples and these duplicates were treated as separate samples. During analysis, every batch of soil and plant samples (18–19 in a batch) included two duplicate analyses, one or two standard reference materials (SRMs) (GSS5, GSR6, NIST Montana 2710 or NRC MESS-3 for soils; Pine Needles NIST 1575 and Bush Branches GBW07603), and one blank. The blank consisted of an empty vial for soils, and 10 mL nitric acid + 2 mL H_2O_2 for plants, and they were treated in the same manner as the rest of the samples. Grinding blanks were also prepared from Ottawa sand (soils) and DDW (plants). During HG-AAS analysis, calibration was conducted after every tenth sample, and an external QC check prepared from a separate arsenic (V) source ($K_2HAsO_4·7H_2O$, Aldrich) was included after every fifth sample. The external QC checks were within ±10% of the correct value.

For soils, the measured and certified values of SRMs agreed within 5%, except for one trial that was within 20%; all of these results were considered to be excellent or acceptable. For plants, agreement was within 15% or better, which was considered to be acceptable.

Relative standard deviations (RSDs) for field duplicates of soils ranged from 1.9% to 9%, which indicates good homogeneity during the sampling procedure. Analytical precision (obtained from the analytical duplicates) for soils ranged from 5% to 6% RSD, which is considered to be excellent.

Analytical precision for plants ranged from 2% to 49% RSD, with a mean RSD of 16%. This mean RSD is within the acceptable limit for analytical precision (20%), indicating that the analysis was conducted with good precision. For samples containing arsenic levels greater than approximately 0.5 mg/kg, the RSD ranged from 2% to 22%, indicating that the lower precision (i.e. higher RSD) was exhibited only at lower arsenic concentrations.

The precision of the GFE procedure ranged from 0.6% to 55% RSD, with a mean of 21%. Again, higher RSDs were observed for samples containing lower amounts of arsenic.

Soil blanks (empty vials) and a grinding blank of Ottawa sand contained no detectable arsenic (<3 mg/kg). Plant digestion and grinding blanks contained no detectable arsenic (<0.11 mg/kg dry weight).

Based on the accuracy and precision results reported above, a 20% error was estimated. All values were thus reported with significant figures such that this uncertainty is in the last significant figure; calculated values (e.g. means) were reported with an extra significant figure.

Results and discussion

Arsenic concentrations in soils

Arsenic concentrations in residential, mine and lake garden soils are summarized in Table 2.2. The average arsenic concentration in the residential gardens

Table 2.2 Arsenic concentrations ([As]) in soils from Yellowknife gardens

Garden location	[As] (mg/kg dry weight)
Residential 1	200
Residential 2	28
Residential 3	24
Residential 4	55
Residential 5	30
Residential 6	35
Residential 7	29
Residential 8	27
Residential 9	12
Residential 10	56
Mine	1600
Lake planters	700

Table 2.3 Results from analysis of single samples within gardens compared with composite samples, to show spatial homogeneity of garden soils (concentrations are dry weight)

Garden	n	Mean (mg/kg)	Standard deviation (mg/kg)	% RSD	Composite (mg/kg)
Residential 2	3	28	14	52	nd
Mine	8	1560	660	42	1600
Lake	5	720	220	31	700

nd = not determined; RSD = relative standard deviation.

was 33 ± 14 mg/kg, ranging from 12 to 56 mg/kg. Samples that were not included in this average were collected from garden location 1, which was an abandoned garden on the Giant Mine Townsite. The average arsenic concentrations were much higher in this area with an average of 200 ± 140 mg/kg, ranging from 81 to 350 mg/kg. These samples are considered separately because they are from a currently non-residential area.

Soil from the mine garden contained more arsenic (1600 mg/kg) than that from the lake garden (700 mg/kg), which is statistically confirmed by a *t*-test even when the spatial variability in the gardens is taken into account (Table 2.3) ($n = 13$, $t = 4.36$, $p < 0.05$).

Analysis of individual samples from residential garden 2, the mine garden and the lake garden was carried out to ascertain the degree of variability that might be expected in a garden as a result of the sampling method used. The results are summarized in Table 2.3 and indicated that the spatial precision (i.e. percent relative standard deviation, RSD) ranged up to 50%. The composite samples for the mine and lake gardens are within 2.5 percentage points of the mean values. These results indicate that the sampling method was adequately spatially representative, and that the composite analyses of the soils collected from the remaining gardens are a good estimate of the arsenic concentrations in each garden.

All soils contained arsenic at levels that are above the CCME soil guideline of 12 mg/kg (CCME, 1999). Arsenic concentrations found in residential garden soil samples from the city were consistent with previously reported background concentrations (3 to 150 mg/kg) in the Yellowknife area (Ollson, 2000; Reimer *et al.*, 2002); those from residential garden 1 were slightly higher. The levels in the mine and lake gardens are elevated above the local background, and are consistent with those previously reported in humic soils collected on the mine property (1140 ± 1190 mg/kg) (Hough, 2001) and from the shores of the lake (580 to 1000 mg/kg) (Ollson, 2000).

Arsenic concentrations in vegetables

Concentrations of total arsenic were determined in 23 different edible vegetable and fruit types and the results are summarized in Table 2.4. All arsenic concentrations in vegetables in this study are reported as fresh weight, since produce is most commonly consumed in the fresh (not dried) form.

In the residential gardens, leafy vegetables and greens, in general, contained the highest concentrations of arsenic, although the highest arsenic concentration in all the residential produce was found in Saskatoon berries (0.44 mg/kg fresh weight). The lowest concentrations of arsenic were below the analytical limit of detection in several residential samples, including potatoes, cabbage, peas, rhubarb, garlic, broccoli and zucchini. While below-ground vegetables, above-ground vegetables and fruits did not differ statistically in arsenic content for residential produce, in the lake and mine gardens, root (below-ground) vegetables contained the highest amounts of arsenic. Onions from the mine garden contained the highest concentration of arsenic of all the samples analyzed (330 mg/kg fresh weight), and beets, another root vegetable, contained the most arsenic in the lake garden (90 mg/kg). These findings are consistent with the general arsenic distribution in plants of the highest concentrations in roots, intermediate values in the above-ground shoots and leaves, and lowest levels in the edible seeds and fruits (Yan-Chu, 1994).

The arsenic concentrations in Yellowknife residential garden vegetables were almost always an order of magnitude greater than those found in a survey of foods from supermarkets across Canada (Dabeka *et al.*, 1993). Conversely, arsenic levels in residential vegetables collected for this study were approximately four to five times lower than those determined previously in Yellowknife (Soniassy, 1979). Lettuce and berries are the exceptions, as they appear to contain comparable concentrations of arsenic in both studies.

The arsenic concentrations in edible parts of the vegetables grown in the mine and lake gardens are much higher than those found in the residential gardens, and those reported in other studies conducted with elevated soil arsenic. Vegetables grown in loam soil treated with 100 mg/kg arsenic acid contained only trace quantities of arsenic (<0.01 mg/kg dw) (Pyles and Woolson, 1982). Carrots

Table 2.4 Arsenic concentrations ([As], mg/kg fresh weight) in edible vegetables; n = 1 for lake and mine gardens, except where indicated

| Plant | n | Residential gardens | | | Lake garden | Mine garden |
		Minimum	Maximum	Average		
Carrot	6	0.020	0.07	0.045	1.3	
White and red potatoes	8	<0.02	0.07	0.031		15
Radish	1			0.17	1.8	31
Garlic	1			<0.03		
Garlic greens	1			0.11		
Onion	2	0.017	0.041	0.029		330
Onion greens	2	0.15	0.18	0.17		19
Beets	3	0.02	0.19	0.081	46	90
Beet greens	4	0.1	0.29	0.18	1.3	10
Lettuce	5	0.06	0.27	0.13	8	7.2*
Swiss chard	2	0.06	0.09	0.075		8
Kale	1			0.16		
Dill	1			0.07		
Italian parsley	1			0.10		
Oregano	1			0.23		
Cabbage	3	<0.01	0.09	0.043		
Kohlrabi	1			0.044		
Broccoli	1			<0.02		
Rhubarb	5	<0.01	0.05	0.020		
Celery	1			0.05		
Celery leaves	1			0.29		
Beans	3	0.016	0.026	0.02		
Peas	3	<0.02	0.036	0.019		1.5
Tomatoes	1			0.009		
Zucchini	1			<0.005		
Saskatoon berries	2	0.15	0.44	0.30		
Pin cherries	1			0.09		
Below ground	21	<0.02	0.19	0.048	17	120
Above-ground shoots	30	<0.01	0.29	0.104	4.7	12
Above-ground fruits	11	<0.02	0.44	0.073		1.5
Average of all (SD)				0.080 (0.086)	12 (20)	57 (105)

SD = standard deviation.
*Mean of two lettuce varieties (9.0 and 5.4 ppm).

grown in soil amended with different quantities of arsenic exhibited stunted growth with increasing soil arsenic content, with a maximum accumulation of arsenic in the carrots of 1.85 mg/kg dry weight (soil concentration of 338 mg/kg), while no carrots grew in soils containing more than 400 mg/kg arsenic (Helgesen and Larsen, 1998). Not surprisingly, carrots did not grow in the mine garden, where the soil concentration was 1600 mg/kg, but they did grow in the lake soil in the carrot planter, which contained 540 mg/kg of arsenic.

The results summarized in Table 2.4 suggest that the concentration of arsenic in garden produce increases with increasing concentration in the associated soil. Examination of this relationship[1] reveals that a linear correlation appears

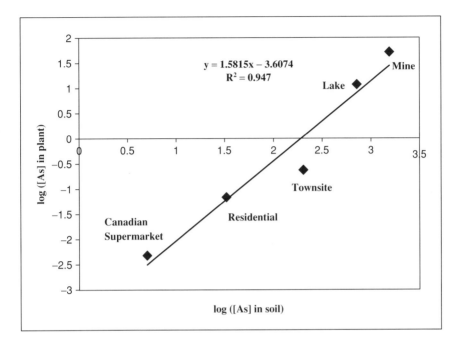

Figure 2.2 Relationship of log soil arsenic concentrations and log plant arsenic concentrations. [As] = arsenic concentration (mg/kg). Canadian supermarket values were estimated by using a typical Canadian soil concentration of 5 mg/kg and an average concentration in vegetables (Dabeka *et al.*, 1993) of 0.0048 mg/kg.

to exist between the log values of the average plant and soil concentrations (Figure 2.2). However, analysis of variance (ANOVA) of the concentrations revealed that while significant differences were present between mine, lake and residential soils, only mine plants were statistically different from residential plants in arsenic concentration ($p < 0.05$). These results are a reflection of the variability in the data, which is consistent with previous findings in Yellowknife that did not establish clear relationships between soil and plant arsenic (Hough, 2001). Considering that the soil types were all the same in the present study, the variability is likely a result of the different uptake behaviors of the plants studied.

It is important to note that during the summer of 2001, when the mine and lake gardens experiments were underway, an unusually large amount of rain fell in Yellowknife. Moreover, the mine garden was situated in a depression and did not drain well; hence some of the mine plants were partially (potatoes and carrots) or fully (onions) submerged in a pool of water. On the other hand, the lake planters appeared to drain well and consequently the plants accumulated more biomass and appeared healthier than the mine garden plants. The effect of the saturated conditions on the plant uptake of arsenic is unknown at this time.

Plant arsenic uptake

To understand how plants behave in contaminated soils in a predictive fashion, a study of how plants take up arsenic at different concentrations was conducted. Bioaccumulation factors (BAFs) were calculated as defined by equation (1).

$$\text{BAF} = \frac{([\text{As}]_{\text{plant}} \text{ in mg/kg fresh weight})}{([\text{As}]_{\text{soil}} \text{ in mg/kg dry weight})} \tag{1}$$

This calculation of BAF uses the fresh weight arsenic concentrations in plants to include the potential dilution effect of water content and to represent accurately the natural state of the plants. Dry weight soil concentrations are used because the wet and dry weights of soils were not found to differ by more than 20%, which is within the analytical error of the methods used.

When possible, translocation factors (TFs) from roots to shoots within the same plant were also calculated, as defined by equation (2) and with both concentrations in mg/kg fresh weight.

$$\text{TF} = \frac{[\text{As}]_{\text{shoot}}}{[\text{As}]_{\text{root}}} \tag{2}$$

The BAF data were examined with respect to above-ground (shoot) and below-ground (root) types of plants, as well as location (residential, lake, and mine). These data are summarized in Figure 2.3a, where an increasing trend in BAFs is observed for below-ground plants with increasing soil arsenic content. The highest mean BAF, observed in the below-ground plants from the mine garden, was significantly different from all other means, as determined by ANOVA and the below-ground mean BAFs were all different from each other. The results of ANOVA for this data set are summarized in Table 2.5; probabilities lower than 0.05 (italicized) indicate statistically significant differences between groups of data. Statistically significant differences were not observed between above- and below-ground BAFs for any other gardens, or between above-ground BAFs between neighboring gardens. However, mine BAFs were significantly different from residential BAFs. These trends imply that the ratios of plant arsenic to soil arsenic increase slightly in above-ground plants, and increase significantly with increasing soil arsenic in roots. The higher BAFs in roots, while subject to great variability, suggest that at extremely high soil arsenic concentrations, arsenic may be sequestered in the roots. Others have suggested that plants may compartmentalize arsenic in their root cells as a method to increase plant tolerance (Carbonell-Barrachina et al., 1999). However, it is not known how root tissues tolerate extremely high concentrations of arsenic without exhibiting symptoms of toxicity (Creger and Peryea, 1994).

This trend is supported by the translocation (TF) data. TFs are greatest for residential vegetables, and lowest for mine vegetables (Figure 2.3b). This observation is statistically significant for the residential TFs compared with the mine but not the lake TF data set, and the other two data sets are not significantly

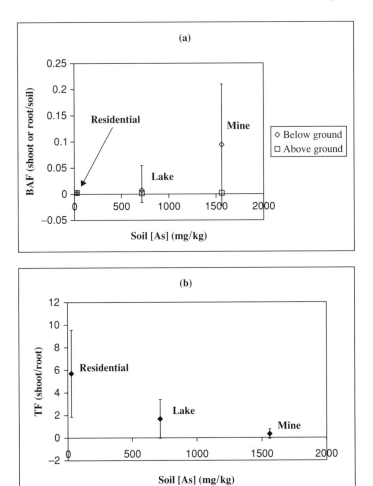

Figure 2.3 (a) Mean bioaccumulation factor (BAF) vs soil arsenic concentration (mg/kg dry weight) of below-ground and above-ground parts of plants. Error bars (± standard deviation) are for below-ground plants only; those for above-ground plants are <0.0036. (b) Mean translocation factor (TF) vs soil arsenic concentration (mg/kg dry weight) for the three gardens.

different from each other (ANOVA results, Table 2.6). The decrease in translocation from roots to shoots with increasing soil arsenic concentrations is likely a protective exclusion mechanism for these plants (Marin *et al.*, 1993).

Gastric fluid extraction (GFE)

Gastric fluid extraction (GFE) was conducted on the plants that contained high levels of arsenic to estimate the portion of arsenic that might be bioaccessible to

Table 2.5 ANOVA results for bioaccumulation factors (BAFs) of above-ground (shoots) and below-ground (roots) plants from soil, from the three gardens: matrix of pairwise comparison probabilities following Bonferroni adjustment. Italicized numbers ($p < 0.05$) indicate that a statistical difference exists

	n	Lake above	Lake below	Mine above	Mine below	Residential above	Residential below
Lake above	5	1					
Lake below	5	1	1				
Mine above	8	1	1	1			
Mine below	8	0.006	0.03	0.005	1		
Residential above	41	0.48	0.101	0.025	0	1	
Residential below	21	0.088	0.016	0.003	0	1	1

Table 2.6 ANOVA results for translocation factors (TFs) from residential, lake and mine gardens: matrix of pairwise comparison probabilities following Bonferroni adjustment. Italicized number ($p < 0.05$) indicates that a statistical difference exists

	n	*Lake TF*	*Mine TF*	*Residential TF*
Lake TF	5	1		
Mine TF	8	0.205	1	
Residential TF	6	0.251	*0.002*	1

Table 2.7 Arsenic concentrations ([As], mg/kg fresh weight) and extraction efficiency (EE) from gastric fluid extraction of edible parts of plants from mine and lake gardens

Plant	Mine garden			Lake garden		
	Plant [As]	Gastric fluid extractable [As]	%EE	Plant [As]	Gastric fluid extractable [As]	%EE
Carrots				1.3	0.17	13
Red potatoes	15	6	37			
Radishes	31	6	19	1.8	0.27	15
Onion	330	0.18	0.1			
Onion greens	19					
Beets	90			46	33	68
Beet greens	10			1.3	0.5	12
Prize Head lettuce	9	7	78			
Grand Rapids lettuce	5	1.0	19	8		
Swiss chard	8	10	120			
Peas	1.5	1.0	70			
Average (SD)		4.4 (3.6)	49 (42)		8.4 (16)	27 (27)
Average % EE of all plants from both gardens (SD)						41 (38)

SD = standard deviation.

the human gastrointestinal tract. The results for edible plants are summarized in Table 2.7.

Sample size sufficed for the extraction of only a limited number of samples ($n = 7$ for mine garden, $n = 4$ for lake garden). Most extraction efficiencies were less than 100%, although they ranged from less than 1% to 100% and averaged 41%. This finding is consistent with GFE extraction efficiencies for other plants from Yellowknife (Koch *et al.*, 2002). No statistically significant differences were found in GFE extracted arsenic amounts or extraction efficiencies between the two gardens (*t* test, $p > 0.05$).

Risk posed by the consumption of Yellowknife garden vegetables

Given that the levels of arsenic in Yellowknife vegetables from residential gardens are typically 10 times higher than the national average, the question is:

are they safe for human consumption? Moreover, to what extent does the risk increase for the mine and lake gardens?

The risk assessment approach was to determine whether the increase in the estimated daily intake (EDI), through the consumption of arsenic-containing vegetables grown in Yellowknife, causes the provisional maximum daily intake (PMDI) recommended by FAO/WHO (2.1 µg/kg per day) to be exceeded.

The EDI of arsenic from vegetables was calculated as described by equation (3).

$$EDI = ED_f = \frac{CF \times CR \times EF \times PH \times AF}{BW} \tag{3}$$

where:

EDI = estimated daily intake

ED_f = estimated dose from food: as µg of the contaminant eaten per kg of body weight per day (µg/kg per day)

CF = concentration of arsenic in food: the concentration of the contaminant in the food group is expressed as µg/g (mg/kg)

CR = consumption rate: the amount of each individual food consumed per day expressed as grams per person per day (g/person per day)

EF = exposure factor: indicates how often the individual has eaten the contaminated food in a year (unitless, with a maximum value of 1.0)

PH = percentage of the food that is home-grown. Health Canada suggests that for residential gardens this amount is 7% (i.e. PH = 0.07)

AF = accessibility factor: indicates the fraction that is accessible following ingestion and digestion in the human gastrointestinal tract (unitless, with a maximum value of 1.0)

BW = body weight: the average body weight in kilograms (kg) based on an individual's age group.

To put these data into the perspective of the typical Canadian diet, total EDIs were also calculated. This calculation consisted of adding the garden vegetable EDIs to the amounts of arsenic that are estimated to be ingested by Canadians from the consumption of all foods (Dabeka *et al.*, 1993).

Several assumptions were made in the risk calculation.

1   For the purposes of the worst-case scenario for human health risk assessment, 100% of the arsenic is assumed to be inorganic. Previous studies have shown that inorganic arsenic forms are predominant in terrestrial plants from Yellowknife (Koch *et al.*, 2000a).

2   The concentration of arsenic in the food is the average for each garden (Table 2.4) (expressed as fresh weight), since only a limited number of plants were successfully grown in the mine and lake gardens.

3   The consumption averages for daily intake of all vegetables were taken from the Human Health Risk Assessment for Priority Substances (Health Canada, 1994) and are based on a nutritional survey conducted from 1970 to 1972 and published in 1977 (National Health and Welfare, 1977).

4   Eleven categories based on age, sex, weight, and differing daily consumption rates are published (Health Canada, 1995); these were summarized into four categories for the EDI calculation for the garden produce, because body weights and food intakes are the same for males and females at 12–19 years of age, and for all males and females older than 20 years. However, the 11 categories were used in the calculation of total EDIs, because the Canadian EDIs differ for each category (Dabeka *et al.*, 1993). These categories are generalized, since an obvious range of weights and daily consumption rates exists that cannot be taken into consideration in this model.

5   Residential, mine and lake garden produce were considered to be home-grown food and therefore the recommended value of 7% (i.e. 0.07) was used for PH.

Two scenarios were generated by calculating EDIs with two accessibility factors for each of the three garden types. For Scenario 1, all the arsenic was assumed to be accessible (AF = 1) and for Scenario 2, the arsenic was assumed to be only as accessible as the GFE method predicts. In the latter case, the mean GFE extraction efficiencies were used for the mine garden (49%, AF = 0.49) and the lake garden (27%, AF = 0.27), and the overall mean was used for the residential gardens (41%, AF = 0.41) from Table 2.7.

The EDIs from the consumption of garden vegetables are summarized in Table 2.8, and total EDIs, which incorporate arsenic from all food sources, are found in Table 2.9. The general trends that emerge from these data are that in all cases the EDIs for children in the age groups 1–4 years and 5–11 years are higher than those of all the other age and gender groups. This is the result of a smaller body weight (20–25% of other age groups) for these groups combined with a consumption rate that is not proportionally smaller (≥50% of other age groups). In addition, the EDI of arsenic tends to be slightly higher on average for males in all categories. This can be attributed to higher consumption rates of foods. These findings are not surprising, as these trends are also true for the Canadian averages (Dabeka *et al.*, 1993).

In all cases, the consumption of vegetables from Yellowknife residential gardens does not significantly increase the EDI, and does not increase the total EDIs above the PMDI specified by FAO/WHO. At the other extreme, the consumption of mine-grown garden vegetables causes the EDIs to exceed the PMDI in all age and weight groups and for both scenarios.

When Scenario 1 is assumed for the lake garden, the PMDI is exceeded for all age groups. However, the use of the GFE extractable amounts for the accessibility factor causes the total EDIs to decrease so that the PMDI is exceeded only for toddlers and children. This is an interesting result as it highlights the mitigating effect of using a less conservative AF. However, considering that the extraction efficiency from GFE ranged up to 100%, it may be prudent to continue to use the more conservative estimates.

Thus, although residents of Yellowknife may be consuming vegetables that contain arsenic concentrations that are approximately 10 times greater than

Table 2.8 Estimated daily intakes (EDIs) of arsenic (μg/kg) from consumption of vegetables grown in Yellowknife gardens. Italicized numbers exceed the PMDI of 2.1 μg/kg per day

Consumption rates and body weights

Category	Toddler	Child	Teen male/female	Adult male/female
Age (years)	1 to 4	5 to 11	12 to 19	20+
Weight (kg)	13	27	57	70
Canadian average consumption of vegetables (g/person per day)*	125	198	250	250

Most conservative – all arsenic bioaccessible (Scenario 1)

	Average [As] in produce (mg/kg fresh weight)	AF	Estimated daily intake of arsenic (μg/kg)			
Residential	0.080	1	0.054	0.041	0.025	0.020
Lake	12	1	*7.9*	*6.0*	*3.6*	*2.9*
Mine	57	1	*38*	*29*	*18*	*14*

Less conservative – limited arsenic bioaccessibility (Scenario 2)

	Average [As] in produce (mg/kg fresh weight)	AF	Estimated daily intake of arsenic (μg/kg)			
Residential	0.080	0.41	0.022	0.017	0.010	0.008
Lake	12	0.27	*2.1*	*1.6*	0.97	0.79
Mine	57	0.49	*19*	*15*	8.6	7.0

*Health Canada (1995).

those found in vegetables from Canadian supermarkets, there is no indication that this consumption incurs an increased health risk.

On the other hand, the consumption of vegetables grown in the lake and mine gardens is considered to be unsafe.

Conclusions

Arsenic concentrations in residential garden soils from Yellowknife are within the previously reported background concentrations for the area, with Giant Mine Townsite soils being six to seven times higher than other residential soils. The mine and lake garden soils, while elevated in arsenic concentration, are typical of their locations.

The concentrations of arsenic in produce from Yellowknife residential gardens are approximately 10 times higher than those found in produce from supermarkets

Table 2.9 Total estimated daily intakes (EDIs) of arsenic (µg/kg) from consumption of vegetables grown in Yellowknife gardens, adding Canadian EDIs (Dabeka et al., 1993: 14). Italicized numbers are above the PMDI of 2.1 µg/kg per day; (1) = Scenario 1; (2) = Scenario 2

Category	Child M/F		Male				Female				M/F
Age	1–4	5–11	12–19	20–39	40–64	65+	12–19	20–39	40–64	65+	All ages
Weight (kg)	13	27	57	70	70	70	57	70	70	70	70
Canadian estimated daily arsenic intakes (µg/kg)*	1.15	1.11	0.72	0.83	0.61	0.51	0.56	0.49	0.75	0.37	0.54
Residential (1)	1.20	1.15	0.74	0.85	0.63	0.53	0.58	0.51	0.77	0.39	0.56
Lake (1)	9.02	7.11	4.31	3.76	3.54	3.44	4.15	3.41	3.68	3.29	3.47
Mine (1)	39.5	30.4	18.2	15.1	14.9	14.8	18.1	14.7	15.0	14.6	14.8
Residential (2)	1.17	1.12	0.73	0.84	0.62	0.52	0.57	0.50	0.76	0.38	0.55
Lake (2)	3.27	2.73	1.69	1.62	1.40	1.30	1.53	1.28	1.54	1.16	1.33
Mine (2)	19.9	15.4	9.29	7.81	7.60	7.49	9.13	7.47	7.74	7.35	7.53

*Dabeka et al., 1993.

across Canada. The produce grown in the more elevated soils contain arsenic concentrations two orders of magnitude greater than those in residential produce.

While the mine garden produce contained higher levels, on average, than the lake garden produce, the great variability in arsenic content precludes the prediction of plant arsenic content based on soil arsenic concentration. The examination of bioaccumulation and translocation factors, while revealing the propensity for arsenic to be accumulated in the roots rather than the shoots, also did not allow for any generalized predictions.

The risk assessment, consisting of a comparison of estimated daily intakes (including intakes from sources other than local produce) to a safe level recommended by FAO/WHO, reveals that locally grown Yellowknife produce from residential gardens is safe to eat. However, vegetables from the lake and mine gardens should not be consumed.

Acknowledgments

We would like to thank the families who donated vegetables from their gardens and thus made this work possible, as well as Mike Borden from Miramar Con Mine for his assistance with the mine gardens. We would also like to thank Christopher Hough and Niki Sharma for their field and laboratory assistance. Financial support through the Summer Work Experience Program (SWEP, Queen's University), Natural Sciences and Engineering Research Council of Canada (NSERC), the Department of National Defence Academic Research Program (DND-ARP), and Health Canada and Environment Canada's Toxic Substances Research Initiative (TSRI Grant #295) is gratefully acknowledged.

Note

1 Canadian supermarket values were estimated by using a typical Canadian soil concentration of 5 mg/kg (CCME, 1999) and the average concentration of vegetables in Dabeka et al. (1993) of 0.0048 mg/kg.

References

Adams, M.A., Bolger, P.M., and Gunderson, E.L. (1994) Dietary intake and hazards of arsenic. In W.R. Chapell, C.O. Abernathy, and C.R. Cothern (eds), Arsenic exposure and Health. Northwood, UK: Science and Technology Letters.
Canadian Council of Ministers of the Environment (CCME) (1999) Canadian Environmental Quality Guidelines. Winnipeg: Canadian Council of Ministers of the Environment.
Carbonell-Barrachina, A., Burlo, F., Valero, D., Lopez, E., Martinez-Romero, D., and Martinez-Sanchez, F. (1999) Arsenic toxicity and accumulation in turnip as affected by arsenic chemical speciation, Journal of Agriculture and Food Chemistry, 47: 2288–2294.
Chiou, H.Y., Hsueh, Y.M., Liaw, K.F., Horng, S.F., Chiang, M.S., Pu, Y.S., Lin, J.S., Huang, C.H., and Chen, C.J. (1995) Incidence of internal cancers and ingested inorganic arsenic: a seven year follow-up study in Taiwan, Cancer Research, 55: 1296–1300.

Creger, T. and Peryea, F. (1994) Phosphate fertilizer enhances arsenic uptake by apricot liners grown in lead-arsenate-enriched soil, *Horticultural Science*, **29**: 88–92.

Dabeka, R.W., McKenzie, A.D., Lacroix, G.M.A., Cleroux, C., Bowe, S., Graham, R.A., Conacher, H.B.S., and Verdier, P. (1993) Survey of arsenic in total diet food composites and estimation of the dietary intake of arsenic by Canadian adults and children, *Journal of AOAC International*, **76**: 14–25.

Food and Agricultural Organization of the United Nations and the World Health Organization (FAO/WHO) (1999) *Summary of Evaluations performed by the Joint FAO/WHO Expert Committee on Food Additives (JECFA): Arsenic*. Washington, DC: ILSI Press International Life Sciences Institute. http://jecfa.ilsi.org/evaluation.cfm?chemical= ARSENIC&keyword=ARSENIC (accessed 15 July 2002).

Francesconi, K.A. and Edmonds, J.S. (1997) Arsenic and marine organisms, *Advances in Inorganic Chemistry*, **44**: 147–189.

Hamal, S., Buckley, B., and Lioy, P. (1998) Bioaccessibility of metals in soils from different liquid to solid ratios in synthetic gastric fluid, *Environmental Science and Technology*, **32**: 358–362.

Health Canada (1994) *Human Health Risk Assessment for Priority Substances: Canadian Environmental Protection Act*, En40-215/41E, Ottawa: Health Canada.

Health Canada (1995) *Investigating Human Exposure to Contaminants in the Environment: a Handbook for Exposure Calculations*, H49-96/1-1995E. Ottawa: Health Canada.

Helgesen, H. and Larsen, E.H. (1998) Bioavailability and speciation of arsenic in carrots grown in contaminated soil, *Analyst*, **123**: 791–796.

Hough, C. (2001) *Characterization of arsenic in a short terrestrial food chain: Yellowknife Northwest Territories*. MSc thesis, Royal Military College of Canada.

Koch, I., Hough, C., Mousseau, S., Mir, K., Rutter, A., Ollson, C., Lee, E., Andrewes, P., Granhchino, S., Cullen, W.R., and Reimer, K.J. (2002) Sample extraction for arsenic speciation, *Canadian Journal of Analytical Sciences and Spectroscopy*, **47**: 109–118.

Koch, I., Wang, L., Ollson, C.A., Cullen, W.R., and Reimer, K.J. (2000a) The predominance of inorganic arsenic species in plants from Yellowknife, Northwest Territories, Canada, *Environmental Science and Technology*, **34**: 22–26.

Koch, I., Wang, L., Reimer, K.J., and Cullen, W.R. (2000b) Arsenic species in terrestrial fungi and lichens from Yellowknife, NWT, Canada, *Applied Organometallic Chemistry*, **14**: 245–252.

Kuehnelt, D., Goessler, W., and Irgolic, K.J. (1997) Arsenic compounds in terrestrial organisms. I. Collybia maculata, Collybia butyracea, and Amanita muscaria from arsenic smelter sites in Austria, *Applied Organometallic Chemistry*, **11**: 289–296.

Marin, A., Pezeshki, S., Masschelen, P., and Choi, H. (1993) Effect of dimethylarsenic acid on growth, tissue arsenic, and photosynthesis of rice plants, *Journal of Plant Nutrition*, **16**: 865–880.

Matschullat, J. (2000) Arsenic in the geosphere – a review, *Science and the Total Environment*, **249**: 297–312.

National Health and Welfare (1977) *Food Consumption Patterns Report*. Ottawa: Nutrition Canada, Department of National Health and Welfare.

Ollson, C.A. (2000) *Arsenic contamination of the terrestrial and freshwater environment impacted by mining operations, Yellowknife, NWT*. MSc thesis, Royal Military College of Canada.

Pyles, R.A. and Woolson, E.A. (1982) Quantitation and characterization of arsenic compounds in vegetables grown in arsenic acid treated soil, *Journal of Agricultural and Food Chemistry*, **30**: 866–870.

Reimer, K.J., Ollson, C.A., and Koch, I. (2002) An approach for characterizing arsenic sources and risk at contaminated sites: application to gold mining sites in Yellowknife, NWT, Canada. In Y. Cai and O.C. Braids (eds), *Symposium Series No. 835, Biogeochemistry of Environmentally Important Trace Elements*. Washington, DC: Oxford University Press.

Rodriguez, R., Basta, N., Casteel, S.W. and Pace, L.W. (1999) An in vitro gastrointestinal method to estimate bioavailable arsenic in contaminated soils and solid media, *Environmental Science and Technology*, **33**: 642–649.

Ruby, M.V., Davis, A., Schoof, R., Eberle, S., and Sellstone, C.M. (1996) Estimation of lead and arsenic bioavailability using a physiologically based extraction test, *Environmental Science and Technology*, **30**: 422–430.

Shiomi, K. (1994) Arsenic in marine organisms: chemical forms and toxicological aspects. In J.O. Nriagu (ed.), *Arsenic in the Environment Part II: Human Health and Ecosystem Effects*. New York: Wiley.

Slejkovec, Z., Byrne, A.R., Stijve, T., Goessler, W., and Irgolic, K.J. (1997) Arsenic compounds in higher fungi, *Applied Organometallic Chemistry*, **11**: 673–682.

Soniassy, R. (1979) *Arsenic in vegetables grown in Yellowknife, NWT*. Unpublished report prepared for Health and Welfare Canada and for the Standing Committee on Arsenic Pollution. Yellowknife: Water Resources Division, Northern Affairs Program, Department of Indian Affairs and Northern Development.

Subcommittee on Arsenic in Drinking Water, Committee on Toxicology, Board on Environmental Studies and Toxicology, Commission on Life Sciences, National Research Council (1999) *Arsenic in Drinking Water*. Washington, DC: National Academy Press.

Tsuda, T., Babzono, A., Yamamoto, E., Kurumetani, N., Ogawa, T., Kishi, Y., Aoyama, H. (1995) Ingested arsenic and internal cancer: a historical cohort study followed for 33 years, *American Journal of Epidemiology*, **141**: 198–209.

Urbaniak, G. and Lestik, M. (1997) *Research Randomizer*, Geoffrey C. Urbaniak and S. Plous. http://www.randomizer.org (accessed 12 July 2001).

World Health Organization (WHO), Water and Sanitation, *Guidelines for Drinking Water Quality: Arsenic*. World Health Organization. www.who.int/water_sanitation_health/GDWQ/Chemicals/arsenicfull.htm (accessed 15 July 2002).

Yan-Chu, H. (1994) Arsenic distribution in soils. In J. Nriagu (ed.), *Arsenic in the Environment, Part 1: Cycling and Characterization*. New York: Wiley.

3 Cyanogenic compounds in cassava and exposure to cyanide

O.S.A. Oluwole and A.O. Onabolu

Cassava plant

Cassava (*Manihot esculenta* subsp. *esculenta*) (Allem, 1994; Olsen and Schaal, 1999) is a major source of calories in many countries in the tropics (Nweke *et al.*, 2002). It is estimated that half a billion people in the tropical regions of Africa, Latin America and Asia depend on cassava roots for their supply of energy (Cock, 1985; FAO/IFAD, 2000). Cassava is valued in farming systems in the tropics because the times of planting and harvesting are flexible (Cock, 1982; Coursey, 1973; Coursey and Haynes, 1970). Cassava grows in relatively poor soils, and can be inter-cropped with many other crops (Cock, 1982, 1985). Its production of calories per unit of land, and per unit of labour time, is higher than maize, rice, wheat, and potatoes (Cock, 1982, 1985).

The production of cassava in the world was 179 million metric tonnes of fresh roots in 2001, 60% of which was produced in Nigeria, Brazil, Thailand, Indonesia, and the Democratic Republic of Congo (FAO, 2002). Currently about 50% of the world production of cassava is from Africa. Nigeria, which produces about 19% of the world's total and 36% of Africa's total, is the largest producer of cassava in the world (FAO, 2002). Although cassava is used largely as food, its use for livestock feed, and for raw materials in the food, textile, and paper industries, is increasing (FAO/IFAD, 2000). Cassava is also becoming a major export commodity (FAO/IFAD, 2000).

Cassava roots and leaves are processed to various foods (Coursey, 1973; Coursey and Haynes, 1970; Lancaster *et al.*, 1982). Although cassava root is an excellent source of dietary energy, it is a poor source of protein, minerals and vitamins (Cock, 1982, 1985). Cassava roots contain about 32% carbohydrate, but only about 1% protein on a wet weight basis (Cock, 1985; Lancaster *et al.*, 1982). However, cassava leaves contain about 7% protein and 14% carbohydrates (Bokanga, 1994c; Lancaster and Brooks, 1983).

Cyanogenesis and classification of cassava

Cassava roots and leaves contain linamarin and lotaustralin, two cyanogenic glucosides that are present in a ratio of 97 to 3 (Nartey, 1968, 1981), but the concentration of cyanogenic glucosides is higher in the leaves than in the roots (Bokanga, 1994a; Nambisan and Sundaresan, 1994). In the roots, concentration of cyanogenic glucosides is higher in the cortex than in the parenchyma (Cock, 1985; Nambisan and Sundaresan, 1994). Cassava also contains two enzymes, linamarase (Conn, 1969) and α-hydroxynitrile lyase (White *et al.*, 1998), which are involved in the release of cyanide from the cyanogenic glucosides (McMahon *et al.*, 1995; White *et al.*, 1998). Linamarase catalyzes the hydrolysis of the glucosides (Conn, 1994; Vetter, 2000), while α-hydroxynitrile lyase catalyzes the decomposition of acetone cyanohydrin to acetone and hydrogen cyanide (Vetter, 2000). Linamarase is located in the cell wall, while glucosides are located inside vacuoles in the cytoplasm (Kakes, 1990; McMahon *et al.*, 1995; Mkpong *et al.*, 1990; Poulton, 1990; Vetter, 2000). Thus, the enzymes and the cyanogenic glucosides are not in contact unless cassava tissue is disrupted (McMahon *et al.*, 1995; Vetter, 2000).

Cassava is often classified into two groups, bitter and sweet, based on the taste of the roots (Allem, 1994; Nweke and Bokanga, 1994; Pereira *et al.*, 1981; Sinha and Nair, 1968; Sundaresan *et al.*, 1987). Several studies have shown that the level of cyanogenic glucosides in bitter cassava is usually higher than in sweet cassava (Nweke and Bokanga, 1994; Sundaresan *et al.*, 1987). However, some bitter cassava varieties have been found to have low levels of cyanogenic glucosides, while some sweet cassava varieties have been found to have high levels of cyanogenic glucosides (Bokanga, 1994b). It appears that the level of cyanogenic glucosides in cassava is a continuum, since the level of cyanogenic glucoside in a cassava variety can change depending on time of planting, climate, fertility of the soil, and geographical location (de Bruijn, 1973; Kayode, 1983; Lancaster *et al.*, 1982). Another classification of cassava, which employs the absolute level of cyanogenic glucosides in roots, classified fresh cassava roots containing less than 50 mg HCN eq./kg wet weight as *innocuous*, fresh roots containing 50–100 mg HCN eq./kg wet weight as *moderately poisonous*, and fresh roots containing more than 100 mg HCN eq./kg wet weight as *dangerously poisonous* (Bolhius, 1954; McKey and Beckerman, 1993).

It has been shown that free cyanide is rarely detectable in fresh roots of cassava (Bokanga, 1995). However, cyanide is released from cyanogenic glucosides in cassava after hydrolysis (McMahon *et al.*, 1995; White *et al.*, 1998). When cassava roots or leaves are crushed, cyanogenic glucosides in the vacuoles and linamarase in the cell wall come into contact, and the glucosides are hydrolyzed to cyanohydrins, usually acetone cyanohydrin (Conn, 1994; McMahon *et al.*, 1995). This reaction is dependent on pH that is above 5 and temperature that is above 35°C (Vetter, 2000). Acetone cyanohydrin can decompose spontaneously to hydrogen cyanide and acetone when the pH is above 5 or the temperature is above 35°C (McMahon *et al.*, 1995). The decomposition of acetone cyanohydrin can also be catalyzed by α-hydroxynitrile lyase (Vetter, 2000). Since α-hydroxynitrile lyase has been shown not to be expressed in cassava roots (White *et al.*, 1998), it appears that only one step in the breakdown of cyanogenic glucosides in the roots is enzymatic.

Processing of cassava and removal of cyanogenic compounds

The usage of cassava roots as food depends on the level of cyanogenic glucosides (Cock, 1985; Lancaster *et al.*, 1982). Although cassava roots of the sweet type can be eaten raw, cassava roots of the sweet and bitter types are usually pro-cessed before consumption (Cock, 1985; Lancaster *et al.*, 1982). Cassava roots of the sweet type can be boiled or roasted. Boiling of whole cassava roots usually does not achieve significant reduction of cyanogenic glucosides (Cooke and Maduagwu, 1978; Nambisan and Sundaresan, 1985; Ravi and Padmaja, 1997), but if small pieces of the roots are boiled, 70–75% of the initial level of cyanogenic glucosides may be lost (Nambisan and Sundaresan, 1985). Boiling and roasting are not effective methods to process cassava roots which contain high levels of cyanogenic compounds, because the enzyme linamarase is inactiv-ated by heat (Ravi and Padmaja, 1997).

Cassava roots of the bitter type are usually processed extensively before they are eaten (Cock, 1985; Hahn, 1989; Lancaster *et al.*, 1982; Nweke *et al.*, 2002). Fermentation, sun drying, and soaking are the major methods of processing cassava of the bitter type (Hahn, 1989; Nweke and Spencer, 1995). The methods of processing cassava roots used in any particular community appear to be dictated by availability of water, technology, and market for the foods (Nweke and Spencer, 1995). In addition to reduction of cyanogenic glucosides in the roots during processing (Dufour, 1989, 1994; Hahn, 1989), foods processed from cassava roots have longer shelf life than fresh roots, which deteriorate rapidly after harvest (Montaldo, 1973; Nweke *et al.*, 2002). The sensory qualities of the foods also improve significantly compared with raw cassava roots (Bokanga, 1995; Nweke, 1994; Sanni *et al.*, 1994).

Whole, grated, or partially dried cassava roots can be fermented (Oke, 1994; Oyewole, 1990; Westby and Choo, 1994). Extensive disruption of cassava root tissues, which occurs during grating of the roots, facilitates contact between cyanogenic glucosides and linamarase and subsequent hydrolysis (Bainbridge *et al.*, 1998; Jones *et al.*, 1994; Vasconcelos *et al.*, 1990). The rate of hydrolysis of the glycosides is determined by the amount of linamarase in the roots and the duration of contact between linamarase and glucosides (Vasconcelos *et al.*, 1990). High pH, which may occur during fermentation, may inhibit the activity of linamarase, and the spontaneous breakdown of cyanohydrin (Fomunyam *et al.*, 1985; Oke, 1994). It has been shown that cyanohydrins are the main cyanogenic compounds that often remain in foods produced from fermented grated cassava mash (Bokanga, 1995; Onabolu, 2001).

In some communities peeled cassava roots that have been partially dried are fermented (Essers *et al.*, 1995a; Onabolu *et al.*, 1999). Partial drying reduces moisture to levels that prevent the growth of bacteria, but encourages the growth of moulds (Essers *et al.*, 1995a). Rupture of cassava root cells by enzymes produced by the moulds facilitates contact between cyanogenic glucosides and linamarase (Essers *et al.*, 1995a, 1995b). The pH achieved during this type of fermentation enhances the action of linamarase and the spontaneous breakdown of cyanohydrins formed from the hydrolysis of glucosides (Essers *et al.*, 1995a; Nok and Ikediobi, 1990).

Peeled or unpeeled whole cassava roots, or cassava roots sliced into chips, may be dried in the sun (Cooke and Maduagwu, 1978; Nambisan and Sundaresan, 1985). The size of roots that are dried has been shown to correlate with the levels of cyanogenic compounds in the dried product (Cooke and Coursey, 1981; Nambisan and Sundaresan, 1985). Large pieces of dried cassava roots have been shown to contain lower levels of cyanogenic compounds than smaller pieces (Cooke and Coursey, 1981; Mahungu *et al.*, 1987). This observation is probably due to slower drying of large pieces of roots compared with the rapid drying of thin slices of roots, which retain high levels of unhydrolyzed cyanogenic glucosides.

Cassava can also be processed by soaking whole roots, peeled or unpeeled, in water (Oke, 1994; Westby, 1994). Swelling and rupture of the cells of cassava roots, which occur when the roots absorb water, facilitate the contact of the glucosides and linamarase, and hydrolysis of the glucosides to cyanohydrins and glucose (Ayernor, 1985; Maduagwu, 1983; Oyewole and Odunfa, 1992). Cyanogenic glucosides leach out when the cells rupture during soaking (El Tinay *et al.*, 1984). Endogenous enzymes as well as enzymes produced by microorganisms have been suggested to contribute to disruption of the tissues of soaked cassava roots (Ampe and Brauman, 1995).

Methods of processing cassava roots that involve soaking of whole roots, peeled or unpeeled, have been shown to be associated with lower levels of cyanogenic compounds in the final foods than fermentation of grated roots (Hahn, 1989; Muzanila *et al.*, 2000). Drying of whole roots, or roots cut into pieces, is associated with higher levels of cyanogenic compounds in cassava foods than soaking or fermentation methods (Ernesto *et al.*, 2000; Muzanila *et al.*, 2000).

After processing of cassava roots, several foods in flour, granular or wet pulp form, which are not ready for consumption, are produced (Nweke and Spencer, 1995). Generally they are stored for days, weeks, or months before meals that are consumed are made from them. Hydrogen cyanide and free cyanide ions are rarely detectable in cassava flours, or meals of cassava foods (Onabolu *et al.*, 2001a, 2002; Tuboku-Metzger, 1969; Ukhun and Iwenor, 1989), but several studies have shown that unhydrolyzed and partially hydrolyzed cyanogenic compounds remain in the finished products (Muzanila *et al.*, 2000; Oduro *et al.*, 2000; Onabolu *et al.*, 2001). However, it has been shown that further reduction of cyanogenic compounds in cassava foods occurs during storage (Onabolu *et al.*, 2002) and when final preparation of meals of cassava food involves boiling or application of heat (Onabolu *et al.*, 2002).

In countries where cassava leaves are consumed, young tender leaves are boiled for 15–30 min in water after pounding to fine particles (Bokanga, 1994c). Various ingredients can be added to improve taste (Bokanga, 1994c). Pounding disrupts the cells of cassava leaves and brings the cyanogenic glucosides into contact with linamarase. Hydrolysis of the glucosides in cassava leaves is more rapid than in cassava roots because cassava leaves contain much higher levels of linamarase than cassava roots, and because the near neutral pH of the pounded leaves is optimal (Bokanga, 1994c). The level of cyanogenic compounds in foods prepared from cassava leaves is usually much lower than in foods prepared from cassava roots.

Exposure to cyanide from cassava roots and cassava foods

The relationship of consumption of cassava foods and the development of neurological syndromes has been investigated for about 100 years (Clark, 1935; Money, 1958; Moore, 1937), but causal association has not been established. The unhydrolyzed and partially hydrolyzed cyanogenic compounds in foods processed from cassava roots are the sources of cyanide, which is implicated in the causation of neurological and other medical syndromes (Oluwole et al., 2002a, 2002b).

Indicators and measures of exposure to cyanide from cassava foods

There is no definition of the amount of cyanogenic compounds in cassava foods, or the amount of cyanide that is released from cassava food, that constitutes exposure or that will induce lesions. There is little information about the amount of cyanide which can be released and absorbed from given amounts of specific cassava foods. A study showed that only about 10% of the total cyanide that can be released from the cyanogenic compounds present in a cassava food was absorbed into systemic circulation of subjects (Oluwole et al., 2002b). Since cassava foods are in different forms, the variation of the amount of cyanide that can be released from specific cassava foods is expected to be wide.

Exposure to cyanide from cassava foods has been measured using the frequency of intake of cassava foods (Onabolu et al., 2001a; Osuntokun, 1971), the levels of cyanogenic compounds in cassava foods (Onabolu et al., 2001a), the levels of metabolites of cyanide in body fluids (Monekosso and Wilson, 1966; Osuntokun, 1971; Tylleskär et al., 1992), and the levels of cyanide in the blood (Osuntokun et al., 1970). The frequency of intake of cassava foods is not a very reliable measure of exposure to cyanide because of the wide variation of the levels of cyanogenic compounds in different cassava foods. Some communities where the levels of cyanogenic compounds in their cassava foods are very high have been shown to have high exposure to cyanide, although the frequency of intake of cassava foods is relatively low (Oluwole et al., 2002a; Onabolu et al., 2001a).

Thiocyanate, the major metabolite of cyanide, has been used in several studies to assess exposure to cyanide quantitatively (Foss and Lund-Larsen, 1986; Galanti, 1997; Monekosso and Wilson, 1966; Tylleskär et al., 1992). Thiocyanate is, however, produced in several tissues and is present in healthy subjects under physiological conditions (Arlandson et al., 2001; van Dalen et al., 1997). Cyanide has also been shown to be produced in healthy subjects, and is present in healthy controls in some studies (Osuntokun et al., 1970; Tylleskär et al., 1992).

Thus, the presence of cyanide or thiocyanate in subjects who do not consume cassava foods does not necessarily indicate the intake of foods that contain cyanogenic compounds.

The physiological levels of the metabolites of cyanide, in subjects who do not take cassava foods, should be taken into consideration when assessment of exposure to cyanide is made. A study of 21 communities within two large ethnic groups in Nigeria showed good correlation between the levels of thiocyanate in the urine and the intake of *gari* (Oluwole, 2002), a popular cassava food in West African countries. The mean (95% CI) urine thiocyanate was 36 µmol/l (29–43) for subjects who did not consume *gari*, 52 µmol/l (45–58) for subjects who consumed *gari* 1–7 times per week, 71 µmol/l (64–78) for subjects who consumed *gari* 8–14 times per week, and 100 µmol/l (83–117) for subjects who consumed *gari* more than 15 times per week.

The assessment and comparison of exposure to cyanide from cassava foods between communities is complicated by the differences in the methods of processing cassava foods in different parts of the tropics, and different types of meals that are produced from cassava foods. In Nigeria, significant differences have been shown between the levels of cyanogenic compounds in a cassava food produced in different parts of the country (Onabolu *et al.*, 2001a). The frequency of consumption of cassava foods also varies widely between ethnic groups (Onabolu *et al.*, 2001a). While studies in East and Central Africa suggest that intensity of cultivation, food shortages, and drought are the major determinants of high intake of cassava foods (Banea *et al.*, 1992, 1997; Rosling and Tylleskar, 1996), studies in Nigeria, the largest producer of cassava roots in the world, did not find intensity of production of cassava roots (Onabolu *et al.*, 2001b), food shortages, or droughts as the determinants of high intake of cassava foods (Onabolu *et al.*, 2001a) in Nigerian communities. Furthermore, insufficient processing of cassava roots is not the major cause of high levels of cyanogenic compounds in cassava foods in Nigeria (Onabolu *et al.*, 2002). Prolonged fermentation of cassava mash, which is carried out in some communities in Nigeria, has been shown to be associated with high levels of cyanogenic compounds in cassava foods because of the high acidity that develops during long fermentation (Oluwole *et al.*, 2002a).

Absorption and metabolism of cyanide released from cassava foods

Although the kinetics of cyanide released from salts of cyanide and compounds such as sodium nitroprusside are well studied (Schulz, 1984), the kinetics of cyanide released from foods processed from cassava roots has not been well studied. The kinetics of cyanide is dependent largely on the chemistry of the cyanide compound, and the mode of entry of the compound into the body. Cyanide peaked in the plasma in 10 to 20 min, and was eliminated in less than 2 h when KCN was given orally (Schulz, 1984), while cyanide from the smoke of cigarettes peaked in about 5 min and returned to baseline value within 30 min (Lundquist *et al.*, 1987).

A study showed that concentrations of cyanide rose in the plasma about four hours after ingestion of a meal of *gari* and returned to baseline after about 12 hours (Oluwole, 2002; Oluwole *et al.*, 2002b). The sites of the hydrolysis and absorption of cyanide released from cyanogenic compounds in cassava foods are not known, but it has been suggested that hydrolysis takes place at the alkaline pH of the small intestine by the action of β-glucosidase enzymes of the microbial flora (Fomunyam *et al.*, 1984). The longer transit time of cyanide which is absorbed from cyanogenic compounds in *gari*, a cassava food, compared with cyanide released from salts of cyanide is probably due to prior digestion of the food before hydrolysis of the cyanogenic compounds.

Cyanide is metabolized by enzymatic and non-enzymatic pathways to several less toxic compounds, which include thiocyanate, 2-iminothiazolidine-4-carboxylic acid, cyanate, formate, and CO_2 by enzymatic and non-enzymatic pathways (Isom and Baskin, 1998). Thiocyanate, which is the major metabolite of cyanide, is produced from transfer of sulfur to cyanide in reactions that are catalyzed by sulfur transferases such as rhodanese, which is a mitochondrial enzyme (Isom and Baskin, 1998), and mercaptopyruvate sulfur transferase (Nagahara *et al.*, 1999), which is a cytosolic enzyme. Although rhodanese is considered the major enzyme for the detoxification of cyanide to thiocyanate, thiosulfate, its main substrate, has been shown to penetrate membranes poorly (Way, 1988). It has also been shown that the efficacies of mercaptopyruvate and thiosulfate to antagonize cyanide are almost identical.

It has been proposed that other enzymes such as thiosulphate reductase, which form persulphides that react non-enzymatically with cyanide ions, may participate in the metabolism of cyanide to thiocyanate (Isom and Baskin, 1998). Cystathionase γ-lyase has been shown to form bis (2-amino-2-carboxyethyl) trisulfide (thiocystine), which acts as a more efficient sulfur donor for rhodanese than thiosulfate (Isom and Baskin, 1998). 2-iminothiazolidine-4-carboxylic acid, a tautomer of 2-aminothiazolidine-4-carboxylic acid, is formed from cysteine and cyanide in a non-enzymatic pathway (Lundquist *et al.*, 1995; Smith, 1996). In addition, HCN is also eliminated in the breath (Isom and Baskin, 1998).

Carbonyl compounds such as sodium pyruvate, glyceraldehydes, and ketoglutarate (Way, 1984, 1988) have been reported to antagonize cyanide. Cyanide reacts with these compounds to form cyanohydrin derivatives (Way, 1988), rather than the indirect actions of nitrites. Pyruvate is also able to distribute to the site of localization of cyanide because it has specific carriers (Way, 1988). Cobalt-containing compounds such as hydroxocobalamin also antagonize cyanide (Klassen, 1996).

Cyanide also binds to plasma proteins such as albumin (Kanthasamy *et al.*, 1994), which has been shown to function as a sulfurtransferase, by forming a carrier complex with sulfane sulfur which reacts with cyanide to generate thiocyanate (Westley, 1988). Free thiols have also been shown to act like rhodanese (Westley, 1988). Cyanide also binds to oxidized glutathione (Brimer, 1988). It appears that there are multiple efficient pathways for the detoxification of cyanide (Isom and Baskin, 1998; Way, 1988). Although the roles of albumin, thiols, and carbonyl compounds at physiological conditions are not well defined, they may play major roles in the sequestration and the metabolism of cyanide.

Following acute exposure to cyanide, methemoglobin is considered the first line of defense against cyanide toxicity (Klassen, 1996) because methemoglobin sequesters cyanide as cyanmethemoglobin (Way, 1988). Nitrites are used clinically to induce the formation of methemoglobin (Klassen, 1996). Since the inhibition of the production of methemoglobin does not diminish the cyanide antagonistic properties of nitrites, the role of methemoglobin in the sequestration of cyanide prior to metabolism has been disputed (Way, 1988). Furthermore, the methemoglobin generating action of nitrites is slower than their antagonism of cyanide (Way, 1988).

Sulfur substrates and metabolism of cyanide released from cassava foods

Neurological diseases that have been attributed to exposure to cyanide from cassava foods have been reported largely from populations where food intake is suboptimal (Osuntokun, 1981; Rosling and Tylleskar, 2000). It has been suggested that inadequate intake of amino acids such as cysteine and methionine, which contain sulfur, may be related to the pathogenesis of these neurological diseases (Cliff et al., 1985; Osuntokun et al., 1968). The finding of high levels of the metabolites of cyanide in these communities (Ministry of Health Mozambique, 1984a; Osuntokun, 1971; Tylleskär et al., 1992), however, suggests that substrates required for the metabolism of cyanide are not lacking in the population. Recently a study which measured low molecular weight thiols in the plasma of subjects with ataxic polyneuropathy did not find any difference in the levels of thiols in cases and controls living in the same community (Oluwole, 2002). Furthermore, experimental studies have shown that the formation of thiocyanate is not impaired in laboratory animals on low sulfur amino acids (Tor-Agbidye et al., 1999) or low protein diet (Swenne et al., 1996).

Toxicity of cyanide

Concentration of cyanide less than 150 µmol/l is reported not to be associated with symptoms, while cyanide concentration of 150 to 250 µmol/l is associated with headaches, palpitations, and hyperventilation. Metabolic acidosis and coma occur when the concentration of cyanide is 250 to 350 µmol/l (Schulz, 1984). Fatal poisoning occurs when the concentration of cyanide is about 300 to 3000 µmol/l (Schulz, 1984). Clinical signs of toxicity of cyanide include hyperventilation, agitation, headache, nausea and vertigo, and convulsions. The capacity of the body to sequester and detoxify large amounts of cyanide without symptoms of toxicity is demonstrated in subjects who receive sodium nitroprusside, which contains 44% w/w cyanide ions (Friederich and Butterworth, 1995; Schulz, 1984). Reports of toxicity of cyanide are few following routine use of sodium nitroprusside (Kazim and Sun, 1996; Przybylo et al., 1995).

Reports of fatalities from acute toxicity of cyanide are rare in communities where cassava foods are consumed. With the exception of a few cases (Akintowa *et al.*, 1994; Ruangkanchanasetr *et al.*, 1999), the levels of cyanide were not measured in the presumed cases of acute cyanide poisoning from cassava foods (Rosling and Tylleskar, 2000). Blood cyanide levels ranged from 43 to 67 μmol/l in one series of cases (Akintowa *et al.*, 1994), much less than the range of toxicity of cyanide (Schulz, 1984). The levels of cyanide found in some cases reported as acute poisoning (Ruangkanchanasetr *et al.*, 1999) were much lower than the levels found in healthy subjects in communities where cassava foods are the staple (Osuntokun *et al.*, 1970; Tylleskär *et al.*, 1992). Low occurrence of acute toxicity of cyanide following meals of cassava foods is probably due to the presence of low levels of cyanogenic compounds in meals of cassava foods compared with the high levels of cyanogenic compounds in fresh cassava roots and the intermediate food products from which the meals of cassava foods are prepared (Bainbridge *et al.*, 1998; Gidamis *et al.*, 1993).

Neurological syndromes such as amblyopia, ataxic polyneuropathy, and konzo, and medical conditions such as diabetes mellitus and mucopolysaccharidosis have been attributed to the effects of cyanide from cassava foods. It has been suggested that the clinical effects of cyanide may be related to exposure to sublethal doses of cyanide chronically (Osuntokun, 1981). In addition to cyanide, metabolites of cyanide such as thiocyanate, cyanate, and iminothiazolidine-4-carboxylic acid have been suggested as possible neurotoxicants for the induction of konzo and ataxic polyneuropathy (Spencer, 1999; Tor-Agbidye *et al.*, 1999).

Thiocyanate, which has been shown to disrupt tubulin (Lakshmy and Srinivasarao, 1997), may possibly be involved in the induction of neuropathy. Cyanate has been associated with peripheral neuropathy (Ohnishi *et al.*, 1975). Although cyanate has been shown to be high when rats on low sulfur amino acid diet were exposed to cyanide (Tor-Agbidye *et al.*, 1999), the role of this minor metabolite in the development of ataxic polyneuropathy is yet to be demonstrated, since the formation of thiocyanate is not impaired in humans even in starvation (Davis *et al.*, 1988).

2-iminothiazolidine-4-carboxylic acid injected into the ventricles of mice induced seizure activity, while loss of CA-1 pyramidal neurons and proliferation of astrocytic glial cells surrounding the CA-1 sublayer (Bitner *et al.*, 1995) were induced in rats following intraventricular injection. Cyanide has also been shown to generate a cyanohydrin adduct, 2-hydroxyl-3-(3,4-dihydroxyphenyl) propionitrile, in rat phaeochromocytoma cells (Kanthasamy *et al.*, 1994). It has been suggested that this compound may be responsible for the neurotoxicity of cyanide in acute intoxication, which is followed by dystonia and parkinsonism (Kanthasamy *et al.*, 1994).

Neuropathology of acute cyanide toxicity

Neuropathological effects of cyanide are attributed to inhibition of cytochrome oxidase, the terminal enzyme of the respiratory chain (Graham, 1992). In addition, the breakdown of glycogen is increased, but glucose is shunted to the pentose phosphate pathway (Way, 1988). Cyanide also affects calcium transport and lipid peroxidation (Way, 1988). Following acute intoxication of cyanide, the brain appears normal, grossly, unless death is delayed for hours, when oedema, hyperaemia, petechial, subarachnoid and subdural hemorrhages, and necrotic foci of white matter and globus pallidus have been reported (Ellison and Love, 1997, Graham, 1992). Microscopic changes that are seen when death is delayed for a few days or weeks include necrosis of white matter, gliosis of the cerebral cortex, and loss of Purkinje cells of the cerebellum (Ellison and Love, 1997), and destructive changes in the globus pallidus and putamen (Uitti et al., 1985).

Several cases of parkinsonism and dystonia have been reported to follow acute cyanide poisoning from attempted suicide (Carella et al., 1988; Rosenberg, Myers et al., 1989; Uitti et al., 1985). CT imaging showed bilateral lucencies in the putamen and external globus pallidus (Grandas et al., 1989). MR imaging has also shown multiple areas of low signal intensities in the globus pallidus and putamen, while PET study with 6-fluorodopa showed functional impairment of dopaminergic neurons in a subject who developed several parkinsonism following acute cyanide intoxication (Rosenberg et al., 1989). Neuropathological and neuroimaging studies of subjects who are exposed to subtoxic doses of cyanide chronically from cassava foods are not available.

Neurological diseases attributed to exposure to cyanide from cassava foods

Endemic ataxic polyneuropathy

The clinical syndrome of ataxic polyneuropathy, which is sometimes referred to as Strachan syndrome, has been contrasted with the clinical description by Strachan (Oluwole et al., 2000). Ataxic polyneuropathy has been described in sporadic (Osuntokun, 1971), endemic (Osuntokun, 1971), and epidemic forms (Roman, 1998a). Sporadic cases have been described from several regions of the world (Cockerell and Ormerod, 1993; Dalakas, 1986), but the endemic form has been reported from some communities in southwestern Nigeria (Osuntokun, 1968, 1971).

The major neurological features of endemic ataxic polyneuropathy are sensory polyneuropathy, sensory gait ataxia, optic atrophy, and neurosensory deafness (Money, 1959; Osuntokun, 1968). Onset is usually gradual and maximum disability is reached in months or years, but a seasonal fluctuation of severity is common (Oluwole et al., 2000; Osuntokun, 1968). Cases were first reported from Nigeria in the mid-1950s (Money, 1958; Money and Smith, 1955). Prevalence ranged from 9% to 27% in the endemic area in Nigeria in the 1950s and 1960s (Monekosso and Annan, 1964; Money, 1958; Osuntokun, 1971), but a recent study of one community in the endemic area in Nigeria, which showed prevalence of 60 per 1000 in 2000 compared with 22 per 1000 in 1968 (Oluwole et al., 2000), and incidence of 63 per 10 000 person-years (Oluwole, 2002), suggest that occurrence of ataxic polyneuropathy may still be high in the endemic area. Age-specific prevalence was highest in the fourth and fifth decades in the 1950s (Money, 1959), but in the seventh and eighth decades in the late 1990s (Oluwole, 2002; Oluwole *et al.*, 2000).

Reduction of visual acuity, bilateral pallor of the optic disc, and concentric constriction of the visual fields were present in a subset of subjects (Osuntokun and Osuntokun, 1971). Audiometry showed loss of hearing in the low and high frequencies with minimal impairment in the middle frequencies in mild cases, but loss in all frequencies in advanced cases (Osuntokun *et al.*, 1970c). Electron microscopic study of teased nerve fibers suggests predominant loss of myelinated fibers. Motor nerve conduction studies showed slowing of conduction velocity in the peroneal nerves (Osuntokun, 1970). There is, however, no information on sensory nerve conduction studies. The latency of the visual evoked potentials was prolonged in cases in a recent study (Oluwole, 2002).

The endemic area in Nigeria is populated by an ethnic group of the Yoruba tribe (Osuntokun, 1971). Comparison of the intake of cassava foods in an endemic community and a non-endemic community showed high intake of cassava foods and higher metabolites of cyanide in plasma and urine in the endemic community (Osuntokun and Monekosso, 1969). High consumption of cassava foods, almost exclusive of other major sources of calories, has been observed in several communities in the endemic area (Money, 1958; Osuntokun, 1971). The level of thiocyanate in subjects with ataxic polyneuropathy seen in the 1960s averaged about 113 μmol/l (SD 38) in the plasma (Monekosso and Wilson, 1966; Osuntokun, 1981). A study which showed that the level of thiocyanate fell when cassava foods were removed from the diet of subjects (Osuntokun, 1968) confirmed exposure to cyanide but not a causal association of ataxic polyneuropathy and exposure to cyanide.

The pattern of consumption of cassava foods in the endemic communities observed in recent studies (Oluwole, 2002) was similar to the pattern that was reported in the 1950s and 1960s (Osuntokun, 1971). However, several communities in the non-endemic area in Nigeria have been shown to have higher exposure to cyanide from cassava foods than communities in the endemic area (Onabolu *et al.*, 2001a). The prevalence of ataxic polyneuropathy in one non-endemic community, where exposure to cyanide from cassava food is high, was found to be very low (Oluwole *et al.*, 2002a). A case–control study nested in an incident study in one community in the endemic areas showed no difference in the intake of cassava foods and of exposure to cyanide in cases and controls who lived in the same community (Oluwole, 2002). These recent studies do not suggest that exposure to cyanide has a causal role in the development of ataxic polyneuropathy.

There is no known treatment for endemic ataxic polyneuropathy. Clinical trials with improved diet and B vitamin supplements (Monekosso *et al.*, 1964), and trials of hydroxocobalamin and riboflavin for 24 weeks (Osuntokun *et al.*, 1970b), and hydroxocobalamin and cysteine for 48 weeks (Osuntokun *et al.*, 1974) did not change the clinical status of the subjects. Although previous studies suggest that endemic ataxic polyneuropathy seen in Nigeria is benign, a recent study showed higher mortality in cases compared with controls in a follow-up study (Oluwole, 2002).

Konzo

Konzo is a neurological syndrome characterized by subacute onset of weakness of the limbs, which usually starts in the lower limbs followed by weakness of the upper limbs within hours to days (Howlett et al., 1990; Tylleskär et al., 1993). Slurring of speech and visual disturbances develop, usually after the limbs have been affected (Howlett et al., 1990; Tylleskär et al., 1993). The tetraparesis, which is worse in the lower limbs, is spastic. The patients usually recover some function, some being able to walk with support, but functional impairment is more common (Howlett, Brubaker et al., 1990; Tylleskär et al., 1993).

Konzo has been reported from Mozambique (Essers et al., 1992; Ministry of Health Mozambique, 1984a, 1984b), Democratic Republic of Congo (Tylleskär et al., 1991), Tanzania (Howlett et al., 1992), and the Central African Republic (Rosling and Tylleskär, 1996; Tylleskär et al., 1994). There are unpublished reports of occurrence of konzo in Cameroon and Uganda. Cassava foods are the staple in all the affected areas (Rosling and Tylleskär, 1996). The level of thiocyanate in the plasma was 329 mol/l (SD 125) in one study (Ministry of Health Mozambique, 1984a). High levels of thiocyanate have, however, been reported in some of these communities without epidemics of konzo.

The neuropathology of konzo is not known. Magnetic resonance imaging did not show gross abnormalities in some subjects, but impairment of central conduction of nerve impulses was detected using a transcranial magnetic stimulator (Tylleskär et al., 1993). Conduction of nerve impulse to the arm muscles was completely absent when the motor cortex was stimulated, but was present when the C7 level was stimulated at the neck (Tylleskär et al., 1993). Peripheral nerve conduction studies showed low amplitude of sensory nerve potentials, and increased threshold of temperature perception (Tylleskär et al., 1993). These studies suggest that both central and peripheral nerves are involved in konzo (Tylleskär et al., 1993). One subject had temporal pallor of the optic disc, and atrophy of the papillomacular nerve fiber layer (Tylleskär et al., 1993).

The role of cyanide in the causation of konzo is also not clear. Konzo has not been reported from several parts of Africa where the intake of cassava foods and exposure to cyanide from cassava foods are high. The occurrence of sporadic cases of konzo is also not associated with drought, famine, or food shortages. Although konzo is attributed to the effect of acute toxicity of cyanide, the lesions produced by acute toxicity of cyanide, in subjects who attempted suicide with cyanide compounds, were predominantly in the basal ganglia, in contradistinction to the clinical site of the lesions in konzo.

Amblyopia

The association of amblyopia and intake of cassava foods was suspected in the 1930s during an epidemic of amblyopia in adolescent school children in southern and eastern Nigeria (Moore, 1930, 1939). The epidemic subsided following addition of vitamin supplements to the diet (Moore, 1934). Subsequent epidemics in Nigeria and other parts of Africa affected adolescents predominantly (Monekosso and Ashby, 1963; Plant et al., 1997). The recent epidemic of optic atrophy, which has occurred in Tanzania since 1988, affected adolescents and young adults predominantly (Bourne et al., 1998; Plant et al., 1997). The features are bilateral painless visual loss, which is progressive over two to 12 weeks (Plant et al., 1997). Central or ceco-central scotomas are found (Plant et al., 1997). No association was found with exposure to cyanide from cassava foods (Dolin et al., 1998; Plant et al., 1997).

Optic atrophy occurring alone or in association with sensory polyneuropathy occurred in epidemics in Cuba between 1992 and 1994 (Ordunez-Garcia et al., 1996; Roman, 1998b). The major features were decreased visual acuity, decreased color vision, central and ceco-central scotomata, and loss of papillomacular bundles (Hedges et al., 1997). Subjects with optic atrophy alone were usually less than 40 years of age, while subjects with optic atrophy and sensory polyneuropathy were 45 to 65 years. Males were more likely to have optic atrophy alone, while females were more likely to have sensory polyneuropathy alone (Hedges et al., 1997). Smoking of cigars (Cuban Neuropathy Field Team, 1995), being female (Rodriguez et al., 1996), and being black (Rodriguez et al., 1996) were risk factors. Exposure to cyanide from cassava foods was not associated (Hedges et al., 1997).

Other medical diseases implicated with the consumption of cassava foods

Diabetes mellitus (Akanji and Famuyiwa, 1993), goiter (Peterson et al., 1995), and mucopolysaccharidosis (Sreeja and Leelamma, 2002) have been associated with the consumption of cassava foods. Although there has been no report of systematic surveys for the occurrence of goiter and diabetes in communities where exposure to cyanide is high in Nigeria, the occurrence of these clinical conditions has not been higher in areas of high exposure to cyanide from cassava foods. Several experimental studies have failed to induce lesions in the pancreas of laboratory animals with cyanide (Mathangi et al., 2000; Soto-Blanco et al., 2001).

Safety of cassava foods

High consumption of cassava foods is not necessarily accompanied by exposure to high levels of cyanide (Chiwona-Karltun et al., 2000). The methods of processing cassava foods in some communities are very effective in reducing the level of cyanogenic compounds in the foods consumed, so that minimal exposure to cyanide ensues. Cassava containing 2000 mg HCN eq./kg dry wt can be processed to foods containing less than 20 mg HCN eq./kg weight (Bainbridge et al., 1998). Employment of very effective methods of processing cassava may be the easiest method to reduce exposure to cyanide in the community.

Storage of some cassava foods for a few weeks before preparation of meals will also reduce the level of cyanogenic compounds (Onabolu et al., 2002).

Reduction of the frequency of consumption of cassava foods will reduce exposure to cyanide. Processing of cassava foods in flour or granular forms with boiling water or heat will reduce the levels of cyanogenic compounds (Onabolu *et al.*, 2002). There is no evidence, so far, that low cyanogenic cultivars will replace high cyanogenic cultivars in farming systems in the tropics. Thus, effective processing of cassava roots may be the most important public health tool to reduce exposure to cyanide from cassava foods.

References

Akanji, A. and Famuyiwa, O. (1993) The effects of chronic cassava consumption, cyanide intoxication and protein malnutrition on glucose tolerance in growing rats, *British Journal of Nutrition*, **69**, 269–276.

Akintowa, A., Tunwashe, O., and Onifade, A. (1994) Fatal and non-fatal acute poisoning attributed to cassava-based meal, *Acta Horticulturae*, **375**, 285–288.

Allem, A. (1994) The origin of *Mannihot esculenta* Crantz (Euphorbiaceae), *Genetic Resources and Crop Evolution*, **41**, 133–150.

Ampe, F. and Brauman, A. (1995) Origin of enzymes involved in detoxification and root softening during cassava retting, *World Journal of Microbiology and Biotechnology*, **11**, 178–182.

Arlandson, M., Decker, T., Roongta, V.A., Bonilla, L., Moyo, K.H., MacPherson, J.C., Hazen, S.L., and Slungaard, A. (2001) Eosinophil peroxidase oxidation of thiocyanate, *Journal of Biological Chemistry*, **276**, 215–224.

Ayernor, G. (1985) Effects of the retting of cassava on product yield and cyanide detoxification, *Journal of Food Technology*, **20**, 89–96.

Bainbridge, Z., Harding, S., French, L., Kapinga, R., and Westby, A. (1998) A study of the role of tissue disruption in the removal of cyanogens during cassava root processing, *Food Chemistry*, **62**, 291–297.

Banea, M., Poulter, N., and Rosling, H. (1992) Shortcuts in cassava processing and risk of dietary cyanide exposure in Zaire, *Food and Nutrition Bulletin*, **14**, 137–143.

Banea, M., Tylleskär, T., Nahimana, G., Nunga, M., Gebre-Medhin, M., and Rosling, H. (1997) Geographical and seasonal association between linamarin and cyanide exposure from cassava and the upper motor neuron disease konzo in Zaire, *Tropical Medicine and International Health*, **2**, 1143–1151.

Bitner, R.S., Kanthasamy, A., Isom, G.E., and Yim, G.K.W. (1995) Seizures and selective CA-1 hippocampal lesions induced by an excitotoxic cyanide metabolite, 2-iminothiazolidine-4-carboxylic acid, *Neurotoxicology*, **16**, 115–122.

Bokanga, M. (1994a) In *Root Crops and Food Security in Africa* (ed. Akoroda, M.O.), Ibadan, Nigeria and Uganda: IITA.

Bokanga, M. (1994b) Distribution of cyanogenic potential in the cassava germplasm, *Acta Horticulturae*, **375**, 117–123.

Bokanga, M. (1994c) Processing of cassava leaves for human consumption, *Acta Horticuticurae*, **375**, 203–207.

Bokanga, M. (1995) Biotechnology and cassava processing in Africa, *Food Technology*, **49**, 86–90.

Bolhius, G. (1954) The toxicity of cassava roots, *Netherlands Journal of Agricultural Science*, **2**, 176–185.

Bourne, R., Dolin, P., Mtanda, A., Plant, G., and Mohammed, A. (1998) Epidemic optic neuropathy in primary school children in Dar es Salaam, Tanzania, *British Journal of Ophthalmology*, **82**, 232–234.

Brimer, L. (1988) In *Cyanide Compounds in Biology* (eds Evered, D. and Harnett, S.), pp. 177–200. New York: Wiley.

Carella, F., Grassi, M., Savoiardo, M., Contri, P., Rapuzzi, B., and Magnoni, A. (1988) Dystonic-Parkinsonian syndrome after cyanide poisoning: clinical and MRI findings, *Journal of Neurology, Neurosurgery, and Psychiatry*, **51**, 1345–1348.

Chiwona-Karltun, L., Tylleskär, T., Mukumbira, J., Gebre-Medhin, M., and Rosling, H. (2000) Low dietary cyanogen exposure from frequent consumption of potentially toxic cassava in Malawi, *International Journal of Food Science and Nutrition*, **51**, 33–43.

Clark, A. (1935) Aetiology of pellagra and allied nutritional diseases, *West African Medical Journal*, **8**, 7–9.

Cliff, J., Lundquist, P., Mårtensson, J., Rosling, H., and Sörbo, B. (1985) Association of high cyanide and low sulphur intake in cassava-induced spastic paraparesis, *Lancet*, **ii**, 1211–1213.

Cock, J.H. (1982) Cassava: a basic energy source in the tropics, *Science*, **218**, 755–762.

Cock, J.H. (1985) *Cassava – New Potentials for a Neglected Crop*. Westport, CT: Praeger.

Cockerell, O. and Ormerod, I. (1993) Strachan's syndrome: variation on a theme, *Journal of Neurology*, **240**, 315–318.

Conn, E. (1969) Cyanogenic glycosides, *Journal of Agricultural and Food Chemistry*, **17**, 519–526.

Conn, E. (1994) Cyanogenesis – a personal perspective, *Acta Horticulturae*, **375**, 31–43.

Cooke, R.D. and Coursey, D.G. (1981) In *Cyanide in Biology* (eds Vennesland, B., Conn, E., Knowles, C., Westley, J., and Wissing, F.), pp. 93–114. London: Academic Press.

Cooke, R.D. and Maduagwu, E.N. (1978) The effect of simple processing on the cyanide content of cassava chips, *Journal of Food Technology*, **13**, 299–306.

Coursey, D.G. (1973) In *Chronic Cassava Toxicity* (eds Nestle, B. and MacIntyre, R.), IDRC monograph 010e. Ottawa: International Development Research Centre.

Coursey, D. and Haynes, P.H. (1970) Root crops and their potential as food in the tropics, *World Crops*, 261.

Cuban Neuropathy Field Team (1995) Epidemic optic neuropathy in Cuba – clinical characterization and risk factors, *New England Journal of Medicine*, **333**, 1176–1182.

Dalakas, M. (1986) Chronic idiopathic ataxic polyneuropathy, *Annals of Neurology*, **19**, 545–554.

Davis, R., Elzubeir, E., and Craston, J. (1988) In Cyanide Compounds in Biology (eds Evered, D. and Harnett, S.), pp. 219–231. New York: Wiley.

De Bruijn, G. (1973) In *Chronic Cassava Toxicity* (eds Nestle, B. and MacIntyre, R.), IDRC monograph 010e, pp. 43–48. Ottawa: International Development Research Centre.

Dolin, P., Mohammed, A., and Plant, G. (1998) Epidemic of bilateral optic neuropathy in Dar es Salaam, Tanzania, *New England Journal of Medicine*, **338**, 1547–1548.

Dufour, D. (1989) Effectiveness of cassava detoxification techniques used by indigenous peoples in NW Amazonia, *Interciencia*, **14**, 86–91.

Dufour, D. (1994) Cassava in Amazonia: lessons in utilisation and safety from native peoples, *Acta Horticulturae*, **375**, 175–182.

El Tinay, A., Bureng, P., and Yas, E. (1984) Hydrocyanic acid levels in fermented cassava, *Journal of Food Technology*, **19**, 197–202.

Ellison, D. and Love, S. (1997) *Neuropathology*. London: Mosby.

Ernesto, M., Cardoso, A., Cliff, J., and Bradbury, J. (2000) Cyanogens in cassava flour and roots and urinary thiocyanate concentration in Mozambique, *Journal of Food Composition and Analysis*, **13**, 1–12.

Essers, A.J.A., Alsén, P., and Rosling, H. (1992) Insufficient processing of cassava induced acute intoxications and the paralytic disease konzo in a rural area of Mozambique, *Ecology of Food and Nutrition*, **27**, 17–27.

Essers, A.J., Ebong, C., van der Grift, R.M., Nout, M.J., Otim-Nape, W., and Rosling, H. (1995a) Reducing cassava toxicity by heap-fermentation in Uganda, *International Journal of Food Science and Nutrition*, **46**, 125–136.

Essers, A., Jurgens, C., and Nout, M. (1995b) Contribution of selected fungi to the reduction of cyanogen levels during solid-substrate fermentation of cassava, *International Journal of Food Microbiology*, **26**, 251–257.

FAO (2002) FAOSTAT Agricultural Data.

FAO/IFAD The World Cassava Economy: Facts, Trends and Outlook (2000) pp. 1–46.

Fomunyam, R.T., Adegbola, A.A., and Oke, O.L. (1984) Hydrolysis of linamarin by intestinal bacteria, *Canadian Journal of Microbiology*, **30**, 1530–1531.

Fomunyam, R.T., Adegbola, A.A., and Oke, O.L. (1985) The stability of cyanohydrins, *Food Chemistry*, **17**, 221–225.

Foss, O.P. and Lund-Larsen, P.G. (1986) Serum thiocyanate and smoking: interpretation of serum thiocyanate levels observed in a large health study, *Scandinavian Journal of Clinical Laboratory Investigation*, **46**, 245–251.

Friederich, J.A. and Butterworth, J.F. (1995) Sodium nitroprusside: twenty years and counting, *Anesthetics and Analgesics*, **81**, 152–162.

Galanti, L.M. (1997) Specificity of salivary thiocyanate as marker of cigarette smoking is not affected by alimentary sources, *Clinical Chemistry*, **43**, 184–185.

Gidamis, A., O'Brien, G., and Poulter, N. (1993) Cassava detoxification of traditional Tanzanian cassava foods, *International Journal of Food Science and Technology*, **28**, 211–218.

Graham, D. (1992) In *Greenfield's Neuropathology* (eds Adams, J. and Duchen, L.), pp. 153–268. London: Edward Arnold.

Grandas, F., Artieda, J., and Obeso, J. (1989) Clinical and CT scan findings in a severe case of cyanide intoxication, *Movement Disorders*, **4**, 188–193.

Hahn, S.K. (1989) An overview of African traditional cassava processing and utilization, *Outlook on Agriculture*, **18**, 110–118.

Hedges, R., Hirano, M., Tucker, K., and Caballero, B. (1997) Epidemic optic and peripheral neuropathy in Cuba: a unique geopolitical public health problem, *Surveys in Ophthalmology*, **41**, 341–353.

Howlett, W.P., Brubaker, G.R., Mlingi, N., and Rosling, H. (1990) Konzo, an epidemic upper motor neuron disease studied in Tanzania, *Brain*, **113**, 223–235.

Howlett, W., Brubaker, G., Mlingi, N., and Rosling, H. (1992) A geographical cluster of konzo in Tanzania, *Journal of Tropical and Geographical Neurology*, **2**, 102–108.

Isom, G. and Baskin, S. (1998) In *Comprehensive Toxicology*, Vol. 3 (ed. Guengerich, F.) pp. 477–488. Oxford: Pergamon.

Jones, D., Trim, D., Bainbridge, Z., and French, L. (1994) Influence of selected process variables on the elimination of cyanide from cassava, *Journal of the Science of Food and Agriculture*, **66**, 535–542.

Kakes, P. (1990) Properties and functions of the cyanogenic system in higher plants, *Euphytica*, **48**, 25–43.

Kanthasamy, A., Rathinavelu, A., Borowitz, J.L., and Isom, G.E. (1994) Interaction of cyanide with a dopamine metabolite: formation of a cyanohydrin adduct and its implications for cyanide-induced neurotoxicity, *Neurotoxicology*, **15**, 887–896.

Kayode, G. (1983) Effects of various planting and harvesting times on the yield, HCN, dry matter accumulation and starch content of four cassava varieties in a tropical rain forest region, *Journal of Agricultural Sciences*, **101**, 633–636.

Kazim, R. and Sun, L.S. (1996) Sodium nitroprusside metabolism in children, *Anesthetics and Analgesics*, **82**, 1301–1302.

Klassen, C. (1996) In *Goodman & Gilman's The Pharmacological Basis of Therapeutics* (eds Hardman, J., Limbird, L., Molinoff, P., Ruddon, R., and Gilman, A.), pp. 1673–1696. New York: McGraw-Hill.

Lakshmy, R. and Srinivasarao, P. (1997) Effect of thiocyanate on microtubule assembly in rat brain during postnatal development, *International Journal of Developmental Neuroscience*, **15**, 87–94.

Lancaster, P. and Brooks, J. (1983) Cassava leaves as human food, *Economic Botany*, **37**, 331–348.

Lancaster, P.A., Ingram, J.S., Lim, M.Y., and Coursey, D.G. (1982) Traditional cassava-based foods: survey of processing techniques, *Economic Botany*, **36**, 12–45.

Lundquist, P., Nilsson, L., and Rosling, H. (1995) Analysis of cyanide metabolite 2-aminothiazolidine-4-carboxylic acid in urine by high-performance liquid chromatography, *Analytic Biochemistry*, **228**, 27–34.

Lundquist, P., Rosling, H., Sörbo, B., and Tibbling, L. (1987) Cyanide concentrations in blood after cigarette smoking, as determined by a sensitive fluorimetric method, *Clinical Chemistry*, **33**, 1228–1230.

McKey, D. and Beckerman, S. (1993) In *Tropical Forests, People and Food. Biocultural Interactions and Applications to Development*, vol. 13 (eds Hladik, C., Hladik, A., Linares, O., Pagezy, H., Semple, A., and Hadley, M.), pp. 83–112. Paris: UNESCO and Parthenon.

McMahon, J., White, W., and Sayre, R. (1995) Cyanogenesis in cassava (*Manihot esculenta Crantz*), *Journal of Experimental Botany*, **46**, 731–741.

Maduagwu, E. (1983) Differential effects on the cyanogenic glucoside content of fermenting cassava root pulp by ß-glucosidase and microbial activities, *Toxicology Letters*, **15**, 335–339.

Mahungu, N., Yamguchi, Y., Almazan, A., and Hahn, S. (1987) Reduction of cyanide during processing of cassava into some traditional African foods, *Journal of Food and Agriculture*, **1**, 11–15.

Mathangi, D., Deepa, R., Mohan, V., Govindarajan, M., and Namasivayam, A. (2000) Long-term ingestion of cassava (tapioca) does not produce diabetes or pancreatitis in the rat model, *International Journal of Pancreatology*, **27**, 203–208.

Ministry of Health Mozambique (1984a) Mantakassa: an epidemic of spastic paraparesis associated with chronic cyanide intoxication in a cassava staple area in Mozambique. 1. Epidemiology and clinical and laboratory findings in patients, *Bulletin of the World Health Organization*, **62**, 477–484.

Ministry of Health Mozambique (1984b) Mantakassa: an epidemic of spastic paraparesis associated with chronic cyanide intoxication in a cassava staple area in Mozambique. 2. Nutritional factors and hydrocyanic content of cassava products, *Bulletin of the World Health Organization*, **62**, 485–492.

Mkpong, O., Yan, H., Chism, G., and Sayre, R. (1990) Purification, characterization, and localization of linamarase in cassava, *Plant Physiology*, **93**, 176–181.

Monekosso, G.L. and Annan, W.G.T. (1964) Clinical epidemiological observations on an ataxic syndrome in western Nigeria, *Tropical Geography and Medicine*, **4**, 316–323.

Monekosso, G.L., Annan, W.G.T., and Ashby, P. (1964) Therapeutic effect of vitamin B complex on an ataxic syndrome in western Nigeria, *Transactions of the Royal Society, Tropical Medicine and Hygiene*, **58**, 432–436.

Monekosso, G.L. and Ashby, P. (1963) The natural history of an amblyopia syndrome in western Nigeria, *West African Medical Journal*, 226–233.

Monekosso, G.L. and Wilson, J. (1966) Plasma thiocyanate and vitamin B12 in Nigerian patients with degenerative neurological disease, *Lancet*, **i**, 1062–1064.

Money, G.L. (1958) Endemic neuropathies in the Epe district of southern Nigeria, *West African Medical Journal*, **7**, 58–62.

Money, G.L. (1959) Clinical aspects of tropical ataxic neuropathies related to malnutrition, *West African Medical Journal*, 3–17.

Money, G.L. and Smith, A.S. (1955) Nutritional spinal ataxia, *West African Medical Journal*, 117–123.

Montaldo, A. (1973) Vascular streaking of cassava root tubers, *Tropical Science*, **15**, 39–46.

Moore, D.G.F. (1930) Partial loss of central acuity of vision for reading and distance in school-children and its possible association with food deficiency, *West African Medical Journal*, **3**, 46–51.

Moore, D.G.F. (1934) Retrobulbar neuritis and partial optic atrophy as sequelae of avitaminosis, *Annals of Tropical Medicine and Parasitology*, **28**, 295–303.

Moore, D.G.F. (1937) Retrobulbar neuritis cum avitaminosis A followed by a post partial optic atrophy – now shown to be of a pellagrinous nature: its serious incidence and its need for a general investigation, *West African Medical Journal*, **9**, 35–40.

Moore, D.G.F. (1939) Retrobulbar neuritis with pellagra in Nigeria, *Journal of Tropical Medicine and Hygiene*, **42**, 109–114.

Muzanila, Y., Brennan, J., and King, R. (2000) Residual cyanogens, chemical composition and aflatoxins in cassava flour from Tanzanian villages, *Food Chemistry*, **70**, 45–49.

Nagahara, N., Ito, T., and Minami, M. (1999) Mercaptopyruvate sulfurtransferase as a defense against cyanide toxication: molecular properties and mode of detoxification, *Histology and Histopathology*, **14**, 1277–1286.

Nambisan, B. and Sundaresan, S. (1985) Effect of processing on the cyanoglucoside content of cassava, *Journal of the Science of Food and Agriculture*, **36**, 1197–1203.

Nambisan, B. and Sundaresan, S. (1994) Distribution of linamarin and its metabolising enzymes in cassava tissues, *Journal of the Science of Food and Agriculture*, **66**, 503–507.

Nartey, F. (1968) Studies on cassava. *Manihot utilissima Pohl-I*. Cyanogenesis: the biosynthesis of linamarin and lotaustralin in etiolated seedlings, *Phytochemistry*, **7**, 1307–1312.

Nartey, F. (1981) In *Cyanide in Biology* (eds Vennesland, B., Conn, E., Knowles, C., Westley, J., and Wissing, F.), pp. 115–132. London: Academic Press.

Nok, A. and Ikediobi, C. (1990) Purification and some properties of linamarase from cassava (*Manihot esculenta*), *Journal of Food Biochemistry*, **14**, 477–487.

Nweke, F.I. and Bokanga, M. (1994) Importance of cassava processing for production in sub-saharan Africa, *Acta Horticulturae*, **375**, 401–412.

Nweke, F. (1994) Cassava processing in Sub-Saharan Africa: implications for expanding cassava production, *Outlook on Agriculture*, **23**, 197–205.

Nweke, F. and Spencer, D. (1995) Future prospects for cassava root yield in Sub-Saharan Africa, *Outlook on Agriculture*, **24**, 35–42.

Nweke, F., Spencer, D., and Lynam, J. (2002) *The Cassava Transformation: Africa's Best-Kept Secret*. East Lansing: Michigan State University Press.

Oduro, I., Ellis, W.O., Dziedzoave, N.T., and Nimako-Yeboah, K. (2000) Quality of gari from selected processing zones in Ghana, *Food Control*, 11, 297–303.

Ohnishi, A., Peterson, C., and Dyck, P. (1975) Axonal degeneration in sodium cyanate-induced neuropathy, *Archives of Neurology*, 32, 530–534.

Oke, O. (1994) Eliminating cyanogens from cassava through processing: technology and tradition, *Acta Horticulturae*, 375, 163–174.

Olsen, K. and Schaal, B. (1999) Evidence on the origin of cassava: phylogeography of *Manihot esculenta*, *Proceedings of the National Academy of Sciences of the United States of America*, 96, 5586–5591.

Oluwole, O.S.A. (2002) *Endemic ataxic polyneuropathy in Nigeria*, Doctoral thesis, Karolinska Institute.

Oluwole, O.S.A., Onabolu, A.O., Cotgreave, I.A., Rosling, H., Persson, A., and Link, H. (2002a) Low prevalence of ataxic polyneuropathy in a community with high exposure to cyanide from cassava foods, *Journal of Neurology*, 249: 1034–1040.

Oluwole, O.S.A., Onabolu, A.O., Link, H., and Rosling, H. (2000) Persistence of tropical ataxic neuropathy in a Nigerian community, *Journal of Neurology, Neurosurgery, and Psychiatry*, 69, 96–101.

Oluwole, O.S.A., Onabolu, A.O., and Sowunmi, A. (2002b) Exposure to cyanide following a meal of cassava food, *Toxicology Letters*, 135: 19–23.

Onabolu, A.O. (2001) *Cassava processing, consumption, and dietary cyanide exposure*, Doctoral thesis, Karolinska Institute.

Onabolu, A.O., Bokanga, M., and Rosling, H. (1999) Cassava processing in a Nigerian community affected by a neuropathy attributed to dietary cyanide exposure, *Tropical Science*, 39, 129–135.

Onabolu, A.O., Oluwole, O.S.A., and Bokanga, M. (2002) Loss of residual cyanogens in a cassava food during short-term storage, *International Journal of Food Science and Nutrition*, 53, 343–349.

Onabolu, A., Oluwole, O., Bokanga, M., and Rosling, H. (2001a) Ecological variation of intake of cassava food and dietary cyanide load in Nigerian communities, *Public Health Nutrition*, 4, 871–876.

Onabolu, A.O., Tylleskär, T., Bokanga, M., and Rosling, H. (2001b) High cassava production and low dietary cyanide exposure in Mid-West Nigeria, *Public Health Nutrition*, 4, 3–9.

Ordunez-Garcia, P., Nieto, F., Espinosa-Brito, A., and Caballero, B. (1996) Cuban epidemic neuropathy, 1991 to 1994: history repeats itself a century after the "amblyopia of the blockade", *American Journal of Public Health*, 86, 735–743.

Osuntokun, B.O. (1968) An ataxic neuropathy in Nigeria: a clinical, biochemical and electrophysiological study, *Brain*, 91, 215–248.

Osuntokun, B.O. (1970) Electrophysiological studies of neuromuscular function in a nutritional ataxic neuropathy in Nigerians, *West African Medical Journal*, 19, 126–129.

Osuntokun, B.O. (1971) Epidemiology of tropical nutritional neuropathy in Nigerians, *Transactions of the Royal Society, Tropical Medicine and Hygiene*, 65, 454–479.

Osuntokun, B.O. (1981) Cassava diet, chronic cyanide intoxication and neuropathy in the Nigerian Africans, *World Review of Nutrition and Diet*, 36, 141–173.

Osuntokun, B.O., Aladetoyinbo, A., and Adeuja, A.O. (1970a) Free-cyanide levels in tropical ataxic neuropathy, *Lancet*, 2, 372–373.

Osuntokun, B.O., Durowoju, J.E., McFarlane, H., and Wilson, J. (1968) Plasma amino-acids in the Nigerian nutritional ataxic neuropathy, *British Medical Journal*, **3**, 647–649.

Osuntokun, B.O., Langman, M.J., Wilson, J., Adeuja, A.O., and Aladetoyinbo, A. (1974) Controlled trial of combinations of hydroxocobalamin-cystine and riboflavine-cystine, in Nigerian ataxic neuropathy, *Journal of Neurology, Neurosurgery, and Psychiatry*, **37**, 102–104.

Osuntokun, B.O., Langman, M.J., Wilson, J., and Aladetoyinbo, A. (1970b) Controlled trial of hydroxocobalamin and riboflavine in Nigerian ataxic neuropathy, *Journal of Neurology, Neurosurgery, and Psychiatry*, **33**, 663–666.

Osuntokun, B.O. and Monekosso, G.L. (1969) Degenerative tropical neuropathy and diet, *British Medical Journal*, **3**, 178–179.

Osuntokun, B.O. and Osuntokun, O. (1971) Tropical amblyopia in Nigerians, *American Journal of Ophtalmology*, **71**, 708–716.

Osuntokun, B.O., Singh, S.P., and Martinson, F.D. (1970c) Deafness in tropical nutritional ataxic neuropathy, *Tropical and Geographical Medicine*, **22**, 281–288.

Oyewole, O. (1990) Optimization of cassava fermentation for fufu production: effects of single starter cultures, *Journal of Applied Bacteriology*, **68**, 49–54.

Oyewole, O. and Odunfa, S. (1992) Effect of processing variables on cassava fermentation for fufu production, *Tropical Science*, **32**, 231–240.

Pereira, J., Seigler, D., and Splittstoesser, W. (1981) Cyanogenesis in sweet and bitter cultivars of cassava, *Horticulture Science*, **16**, 776–777.

Peterson, S., Rosling, H., Tylleskär, T., Gebre-Medhin, M., and Taube, A. (1995) Endemic goitre in Guinea, *Lancet*, **345**, 513–514 (letter).

Plant, G., Dolin, P., Mohammed, A., and Mlingi, N. (1997) Confirmation that neither cyanide intoxication nor mutations commonly associated with Leber's hereditary optic atrophy are implicated in Tanzanian epidemic optic atrophy, *Journal of Neurological Science*, **152**, 107–108.

Plant, G., Mtanda, A., Arden, G., and Johnson, G. (1997) An epidemic optic of neuropathy in Tanzania: characterisation of the visual disorder and associated peripheral neuropathy, *Journal of Neurological Science*, **145**, 127–140.

Poulton, J. (1990) Cyanogenesis in plants, *Plant Physiology*, **94**, 401–405.

Przybylo, H., Stevenson, G., Schanbacher, P., Backer, C., Dsida, R., and Hall, S. (1995) Sodium nitroprusside metabolism in children during hypothermic cardiopulmonary bypass, *Anesthetics and Analgesics*, **81**, 952–956.

Ravi, S. and Padmaja, G. (1997) Mechanism of cyanogen reduction in cassava roots during cooking, *Journal of the Science of Food and Agriculture*, **75**, 427–432.

Rodriguez, A., Pereira, C., Hernandez, F., Lago, P., Balmaseda, A., and Menendez, R. (1996) Prevalence and factors associated to the epidemic neuropathy in a population assisted by a family doctor in Cuba, *Memorias do Instituto Oswaldo Cruz*, **91**, 543–550.

Roman, G. (1998a) Tropical myeloneuropathies revisited, *Current Opinion in Neurology*, **11**, 539–544.

Roman, G.C. (1998b) Epidemic neuropathy in Cuba: a public health problem related to the Cuban Democracy Act of the United States, *Neuroepidemiology*, **17**, 111–115.

Rosenberg, R., Myers, J., and Martin, W. (1989) Cyanide-induced parkinsonism: clinical, MRI, and 6-fluorodopa PET studies, *Neurology*, **39**, 142–144.

Rosling, H. and Tylleskär, T. (1996) In *Tropical Neurology* (eds Shakir, R., Newman, P., and Poser, C.), pp. 353–364. London: Saunders.

Rosling, H. and Tylleskär, T. (2000) In *Experimental and Clinical Neurotoxicology* (eds Spencer, P.S. and Schaumburg, H.), pp. 338–343. Oxford, New York: Oxford University Press.

Ruangkanchanasetr, S., Wananukul, V., and Suwanjutha, S. (1999) Cyanide poisoning, 2 cases report and treatment review, *Journal of the Medical Association of Thailand*, **82**, S162–S167.

Sanni, M., Sobamiwa, A., Eyinla, M., and Rosling, H. (1994) Safety aspects of processing cassava to gari in Nigeria, *Acta Horticulturae*, **375**, 227–231.

Schulz, V. (1984) Clinical pharmacokinetics of nitroprusside, cyanide, thiosulphate and thiocyanate, *Clinical Pharmacokinetics*, **9**, 239–251.

Sinha, S. and Nair, T. (1968) Studies on the variability of cyanogenic glucoside content in cassava tubers, *Indian Journal of Agricultural Sciences*, **38**, 958–963.

Smith, R. (1996) In *Cassarett and Doull's Toxicology: The Basic Science of Poisons* (ed. Klaassen, C.D.), pp. 335–354. New York: McGraw-Hill.

Soto-Blanco, B., Sousa, A., Manzano, H., Guerra, J., and Gorniak, S. (2001) Does prolonged cyanide exposure have a diabetogenic effect?, *Veterinary and Human Toxicology*, **43**, 106–108.

Spencer, P.S. (1999) Food toxins, AMPA receptors, and motor neuron diseases, *Drug Metabolism Reviews*, **31**, 561–587.

Sreeja, V. and Leelamma, S. (2002) Cassava diet – a cause for mucopolysaccharidosis, *Plant Foods and Human Nutrition*, **57**, 141–150.

Sundaresan, S., Nambisan, B., and Easwari Amma, C. (1987) Bitterness in cassava in relation to cyanoglucoside content, *Indian Journal of Agricultural Sciences*, **57**, 37–40.

Swenne, I., Eriksson, U.J., Christoffersson, R., Kagedal, B., Lundquist, P., Nilsson, L., Tylleskär, T., and Rosling, H. (1996) Cyanide detoxification in rats exposed to acetonitrile and fed a low protein diet, *Fundamentals of Applied Toxicology*, **32**, 66–71.

Tor-Agbidye, J., Palmer, V.S., Lasarev, M.R., Craig, A.M., Blythe, L.L., Sabri, M.I., and Spencer, P.S. (1999) Bioactivation of cyanide to cyanate in sulfur amino acid deficiency: relevance to neurological disease in humans subsisting on cassava, *Toxicological Science*, **50**, 228–235.

Tuboku-Metzger, A. (1969) Diet and neuropathy, *British Medical Journal*, **4**, 239.

Tylleskär, T., Banea, M., Bikangi, N., Cooke, R., Poulter, N., and Rosling, H. (1992) Cassava cyanogens and konzo, an upper motoneuron disease found in Africa, *Lancet*, **339**, 208–211.

Tylleskär, T., Banea, M., Bikangi, N., Fresco, L., Persson, L.A., and Rosling, H. (1991) Epidemiological evidence from Zaire for a dietary etiology of konzo, an upper motor neuron disease, *Bulletion of the World Health Organization*, **69**, 581–589.

Tylleskär, T., Howlett, W., Rwiza, H., Aquilonius, S.-M., Stålberg, E., Lindén, B., Mandahl, A., Larsen, H., Brubaker, G., and Rosling, H. (1993) Konzo: a distinct disease entity with selective upper motoneuron damage, *Journal of Neurology, Neurosurgery, and Psychiatry*, **56**, 638–643.

Tylleskär, T., Légué, F., Peterson, S., Kpizingui, E., and Stecker, P. (1994) Konzo in the Central African Republic, *Neurology*, **44**, 959–961.

Uitti, R., Rajput, A., Ashenhurst, E., and Rozdilsky, B. (1985) Cyanide-induced parkinsonism: a clinicopathologic report, *Neurology*, **35**, 921–925.

Ukhun, M. and Iwenor, D. (1989) Toxic and potentially toxic constituents of gari and beef marketed in Nigerian traditional markets, *Bulletin of Environmental Contamination and Toxicology*, **42**, 553–557.

Van Dalen, C., Whitehouse, M., Winterbourn, C., and Kettle, A. (1997) Thiocyanate and chloride as competing substrates for myeloperoxidase, *Biochemistry Journal*, **327**, 487–492.

Vasconcelos, A., Twiddy, D., Westby, A., and Reilly, P. (1990) Detoxification of cassava during gari preparation, *International Journal of Food Science and Technology*, **25**, 198–203.

Way, J.L. (1984) Cyanide intoxication and its mechanism of antagonism, *Annual Review of Pharmacology and Toxicology*, **24**, 451–481.

Way, J. (1988) In *Cyanide Compounds in Biology* (eds Evered, D. and Harnett, S.), pp. 232–243. New York: Wiley.

Westby, A. (1994) Importance of fermentation in cassava processing, *Acta Horticuticurae*, **380**, 249–255.

Westby, A. and Choo, B. (1994) Cyanogen reduction during lactic acid fermentation of cassava, *Acta Horticulturae*, **375**, 209–215.

Westley, J. (1988) In *Cyanide Compounds in Biology* (eds Evered, D. and Harnett, S.), pp. 201–218. New York: Wiley.

Vetter, J. (2000) Plant cyanogenic glycosides, *Toxicon*, **38**, 11–36.

White, W., Aria-Garzon, D., MacMahon, J., and Sayre, R. (1998) Cyanogenesis in cassava: the role of hydroxynitrile lyase in root cyanide production, *Plant Physiology*, **116**, 1219–1225.

4 Phytoestrogens in the prevention and prognosis of female hormonal cancers

Elisa V. Bandera and Lawrence H. Kushi

Introduction

Phytoestrogens are nonsteroidal plant-derived compounds, structurally similar to endogenous estrogens, but capable of showing both estrogenic and anti-estrogenic effects (Setchell, 1998). Although their effects are not totally understood, it has been postulated that phytoestrogens may exert antiestrogenic effects in high-estrogen environments and have weak estrogenic effects in low-estrogen environments (Messina, 1999). Phytoestrogens are divided into four main groups: isoflavonoids, flavonoids, coumestans, and lignans. While the main food source of isoflavones is the soybean, flavonoids are more widely distributed in vegetables, fruits, berries, herbs, and green tea; coumestrol, the main dietary coumestan, is found in alfalfa sprouts and beans; and lignans precursors are present in fiber-rich foods, such as flaxseed and unrefined grain products (Strauss et al., 1998).

Because phytoestrogens have some structural similarity with estradiol, they are capable of binding to estrogen receptors while exerting mild estrogenic activity compared to that of endogenous estrogens. Their potential effect at the estrogen receptor level, as well as their possible influences in estrogen metabolism, have generated substantial interest in the possible health effects of phytoestrogens, in particular as a "natural" alternative to estrogen replacement therapy (ERT) in postmenopausal women. However, their role in cancer is controversial. While there is some experimental and epidemiologic evidence supporting a protective effect in hormone-dependent cancers, there are also reports that suggest possible detrimental effects, particularly regarding breast and endometrial cancers.

The experimental evidence seems to support a protective role of phytoestrogens on hormone-dependent cancer. Phytoestrogens have been reported *in vitro* to interact with steroid metabolism by inhibiting certain enzymes involved in estrogen and androgen biosynthesis and affect estrogen bioavailability by stimulating the production of sex hormone binding globulin (Strauss et al., 1998). They can compete with endogenous and exogenous estrogens for receptor sites and, therefore, may act as estrogen agonists and antagonists. The effect of phytoestrogens at the receptor level is complex and not well understood. However, the experimental evidence seems to indicate that the isoflavone genistein, when administered at moderate to high concentrations with estradiol, has an anti-estrogenic effect (Davis *et al.*, 1999). This is probably a result of competition for estrogen binding sites with estradiol, a much more potent estrogen. The overall experimental evidence seems to indicate that the molecular and cellular effects of phytoestrogens depend on many factors, including concentration, receptor status, endogenous estrogens environment, and the type of target organ or cell (Setchell, 1998). It should be noted here that phytoestrogens have been found to have greater affinity for estrogen receptor type β (ERβ), while reproductive cells, particularly those of the breast and uterus, are rich in ERα (Anderson *et al.*, 2001).

Comparison of international cancer rates provides indirect evidence for a possible protective effect of phytoestrogens, as it reveals lower incidence of breast, endometrial, and ovarian cancers in Asian populations, which typically consume diets high in soy foods, than in Western populations. However, the differences in rates could also be explained by other factors, such as lower fat intake, lower body mass index, and a different reproductive and exogenous hormone exposure history among Asians. Further support for the possible anticarcinogenic effect of phytoestrogens comes from studies that have reported lower steroid hormone levels in postmenopausal women in Japan, rural Chinese women, and female emigrés from Asian countries, than in Caucasian women, as well as in vegetarian than in nonvegetarian women (Shoff *et al.*, 1998).

Studies evaluating the relationship between dietary phytoestrogens/soy and hormonal levels have been inconsistent, but they have generally found decreased midcycle plasma gonadotropin levels, and a tendency toward increased menstrual cycle length, decreased plasma estrogen, and sex hormone-binding globulin concentrations in premenopausal women (Kurzer, 2002). Studies in postmenopausal women have generally not shown any effects of soy on female hormones (Wu *et al.*, 1998). While the hormonal effects found in some studies among premenopausal women are consistent with a protective effect for cancers of the breast, endometrium, and ovary, the short-term and long-term impact of phytoestrogens/soy in female hormonal levels remains unclear.

Although the interest in phytoestrogens as anticarcinogenic agents is based primarily on their potential hormonal effects, there is increasing evidence that non-hormonal mechanisms may be involved, particularly for soy foods. Several phytoestrogens have been shown *in vitro* to exhibit anticarcinogenic effects, including antiproliferative and antioxidant activity, and to inhibit angiogenesis (Strauss *et al.*, 1988).

In addition to the potential beneficial effects of phytoestrogens, there is a growing body of literature raising concerns about the possible detrimental effects of phytoestrogens on breast and endometrial tissues, in particular from supplement sources (Blair Johnson *et al.*, 2001; This *et al.*, 2001). While this has not been widely investigated, studies in women have not found that dietary soy isoflavones affect the endometrium (Balk *et al.*, 2002; Duncan *et al.*, 1999; Hale *et al.*, 2002), whereas estrogenic effects in breast tissue have been reported in experimental studies (de Lemos, 2001; This *et al.*, 2001) and in short-term interventions with isoflavone supplementation in women (This *et al.*, 2001). The lower rates of breast and endometrial cancers in Asian women provide some reassurance of the safety of soy/phytoestrogens at dietary levels. However, the potential for phytoestrogens to induce breast and endometrial growth, particularly at pharmacologic doses and under certain conditions such as in a low estrogenic environment, is a possibility and needs further evaluation.

The purpose of this chapter is to review and summarize the current epidemiologic evidence evaluating the role of dietary phytoestrogens and food sources of these phytochemicals, especially soy, in cancer of the breast, endometrium, and ovary. To our knowledge, none of these epidemiologic studies have evaluated the role of phytoestrogens from supplements or the combined exposure from food and supplement sources. This is in part because supplemental sources of phytoestrogens have only recently become available. As the use of such supplements increases, it will be important to consider their influence, not only to obtain a better assessment of total phytoestrogen intake, but also to elucidate differential effects by phytoestrogen sources.

Phytoestrogens and cancer prevention

Phytoestrogens and breast cancer

Consumption of phytoestrogens and breast cancer risk

Although there is a large body of literature discussing the potential beneficial and detrimental health effects of phytoestrogens, as well as evaluating these effects *in vitro* and *in vivo*, relatively few epidemiologic studies have examined the role of phytoestrogens in the prevention of breast cancer. The vast majority of these epidemiologic studies have been conducted in Asian populations and focused on the effect of soy foods, mainly tofu intake. Soy products are the most important source of phytoestrogens, but they also contain other compounds with anticarcinogenic properties, such as protease inhibitors and phenolic acids (Martini *et al.*, 1999). Conversely, soy foods are not the only source of phytoestrogens (Horn-Ross *et al.*, 2000; Pillow *et al.*, 1999).

To our knowledge, eight case–control studies of soy intake and breast cancer (Table 4.1) have been published in the peer-reviewed literature. Six of these studies, conducted primarily among Asians (Dai *et al.*, 2001; Hirose *et al.*, 1995; Lee *et al.*, 1991, 1992; Shu *et al.*, 2001), but also among Asian-Americans (Wu *et al.*, 1996), and non-Asians (Witte *et al.*, 1997), found an inverse relationship with consumption of soy. We are aware of three prospective studies examining this association, an earlier one among Japanese women (Hirayama, 1990, in: Key *et al.*, 1999), one among Japanese atomic bomb survivors (Key *et al.*, 1999), and another among participants in the Iowa Women Health Study (Greenstein *et al.*, 1996). While Hirayama (1990, in: Key *et al.*, 1999) found that daily consumers of miso soup experienced a reduction of approximately 50% in breast

Table 4.1 Epidemiologic studies of soy consumption and breast cancer risk

Study	Population	Menopausal status (cases)	Dietary factor	Comparison	Adjusted risk estimates (95% confidence intervals)
CASE–CONTROL STUDIES					
Lee et al. (1991, 1992)	Chinese	Premenopausal (109)	Soy protein	<20.3 g/day 20.3–54.9 g/day 55+ g/day	1.0 0.6 (0.3–1.2) 0.4 (0.2–0.9)
		Postmenopausal (91)		<20.3 g/day 20.3–54.9 g/day 55+ g/day	1.0 0.9 (0.4–1.9) 1.1 (0.5–2.3)
Yuan et al. (1995)	Chinese	Combined (834)	Soy protein	Per 18 g/day	1.0 (0.7–1.4)
Hirose et al. (1995)	Japanese	Premenopausal (607)	Bean curd Miso	≥3/week vs less Daily vs less	0.78 (0.60–1.00) 1.16 (0.98–1.37)
		Postmenopausal (445)	Bean curd Miso	≥3/week vs less Daily vs less	0.96 (0.70–1.31) 0.96 (0.78–1.17)
Wu et al. (1996)	Asian-Americans (Chinese, Japanese, or Filipino descent) (597:966)	Combined* (596)	Tofu	Per 1 time/wk 55+ vs ≤12 times/year	0.83 (0.72–0.95) 0.67 (not shown)
Witte et al. (1997)	Non-Asians (Los Angeles, Connecticut, Quebec)	Premenopausal (140)	Tofu	1/wk vs less	0.5 (0.2–1.1)

Study	Population		Intake	Comparison	OR (95% CI)
Horn-Ross et al. (2001) (Bay Area Breast Cancer Study)	Non-Asians	Combined* (1326)	Tofu Soy milk Miso Soy burgers Total isoflavones	≥1/month vs none Any vs none ≥1/mo vs none ≥1/mo vs none Q4 vs Q1	0.89 (0.70–1.10) 0.57 (0.38–0.85) 1.10 (0.81–1.50) 0.74 (0.55–0.99) 1.00 (0.79–1.30)
Dai et al. (2001) (Shanghai Breast Cancer Study)	Chinese	Combined* (1459)	Soy protein intake	Q4 for weekly consumers vs <1 time/week	0.56 (0.32–1.00) ER+/PR+ status: 0.28 (0.13–0.57) BMI ≥25: 0.21 (0.06–0.77)
Shu et al. (2001) (Shanghai Breast Cancer Study)	Chinese	Combined* (1459)	Soy protein intake during adolescence	Q5 vs Q1 (≥11 g/day vs <0.44 g/day)	0.51 (0.40–0.65)
COHORT STUDIES					
Hirayama (1990, in: Key et al., 1999)	Japanese	Aged >40 years	Miso soup	Daily vs less	0.85 (0.68–1.06)
Greenstein et al. (1996) (Iowa Women's Health Study)	Non-Asian	Postmenopausal (1018)	Soy/tofu intake	Consumer vs nonconsumer	0.76 (0.50–1.18)
Key et al. (1999)	Japanese atomic bomb survivors	Combined* (427)	Tofu Miso soup	≥5/week vs ≤1/week	1.07 (0.78–1.47) 0.87 (0.68–1.12)

Abbreviations: BMI, body mass index; ER, estrogen receptor; PR, progesterone receptor; Q, quartile or quintile.
*Similar results in analyses by menopausal status.

cancer risk, the other two prospective studies have offered weak support for an association. Possible reasons for this discrepancy are discussed below.

Earlier studies of phytoestrogens/soy consumption and breast cancer were not specifically designed to test this hypothesis. Consequently, the dietary assessment tool used was typically limited and had not been validated (Wu et al., 1998). A detailed assessment of consumption of phytoestrogens and/or soy foods was conducted in three recent case–control studies (Dai et al., 2001; Horn-Ross et al., 2001; Shu et al., 2001). Horn-Ross et al. (2001) examined the effect of total phytoestrogen intake, individual phytoestrogens and soy foods, and even "hidden sources" of soy, in non-Asians in the San Francisco Bay area, among whom soy consumption was low and infrequent. For example, the highest quartile of phytoestrogen consumption was only about 3 mg/day (less than a serving of tofu per week). They did not find an inverse association at these levels of consumption with any of the phytoestrogens or soy foods evaluated, except with soy milk and soy burgers. Consumers of soy milk had an odds ratio of 0.57 (95% confidence interval (CI): 0.38–0.85) compared to non-consumers after adjusting for relevant confounding factors. The risk by level of consumption could not be evaluated, as only 3% of the cases and 5% of the controls consumed this beverage. It is possible that, in this population, consumption of soy milk acted as a marker of a healthier dietary pattern or lifestyle variable, unaccounted for in their analysis. It should be noted that in this study there was a suggestion of an increased risk of breast cancer for women in the highest quartile of certain types of phytoestrogens, coumestrol (odds ratio (OR): 1.4; 95% CI: 1.1, 1.7) and total lignans (OR: 1.3; 95% CI: 1.0, 1.6). To our knowledge this has not been previously reported.

In the Western New York Diet Study (McCann et al., 2002), in contrast, there was an inverse relationship between lignan intake and breast cancer, particularly among premenopausal women (OR: 0.45; 95% CI: 0.20–1.01). These investigators also found that a CYP17 polymorphism modified this association, with a stronger effect observed for women with at least one A2 allele. CYP17 is a hormone-metabolizing gene, and women, both premenopausal and postmenopausal, with the A2 allele were found to have elevated circulating estrogen levels (Hankinson and Hunter, 2002). These findings confirm the earlier suggestion that phytoestrogens may have anticarcinogenic effects in high estrogen environments.

Strong support for a protective effect of soy on breast cancer was provided by two recent reports from the Shanghai Breast Cancer Study (Dai et al., 2001; Shu et al., 2001). This study is a large population-based case–control study among Chinese women, specifically designed to evaluate soy and breast cancer risk. It used a validated food frequency questionnaire that included over 90% of all common soy foods consumed by Shanghai residents. They found that weekly consumers in the highest quartile of soy protein consumption had a reduced risk of breast cancer compared to those consuming soy less than once a week (OR: 0.56; 95% CI: 0.32–1.00). Earlier studies of soy and breast cancer suggested that the protective effect was limited to premenopausal women (Hirose et al., 1995;

Lee *et al.*, 1991, 1992). In contrast, Wu *et al.* (1996) and Dai *et al.* (2001) found an inverse association for both premenopausal and postmenopausal women. In the Shanghai Breast Cancer Study, the inverse association with soy appeared to be stronger for breast cancers expressing estrogen receptors (ER+/PR+) and those with high BMI, confirming the predicted hormonal activity of soy.

There is increasing evidence that early dietary exposures may be relevant in breast cancer etiology. In female rats, pre-pubertal administration of genistein enhanced cell differentiation in the mammary gland and perinatal exposure to physiologic concentrations of genistein seem to exert a permanent protective effect against breast cancer (Lamartiniere, 2000). To our knowledge the role of early exposure to soy and breast cancer risk has been evaluated in only one epidemiologic study, the Shanghai Breast Cancer Study (Shu *et al.*, 2001). In this case–control study, soy consumption during adolescence was inversely related to breast cancer risk in premenopausal and postmenopausal women. Compared to the lowest quintile, those in the highest quintile of soy protein intake during adolescence had an odds ratio of 0.51 (95% CI: 0.40–0.65; *p* for trend < 0.01). This relationship was independent of adult soy intake. Because reports of adolescent intake rely heavily on memory, there is a large potential for misclassification. Taking this issue into consideration, Shu *et al.* (2001) interviewed participants' biological mothers about their daughters' soy intake during adolescence. They also found an inverse association with adolescent soy intake as reported by the mothers, and the correlations between the two reports of soy intake were 0.29 for cases and 0.30 for controls. Because the correlation coefficients were of similar magnitude for cases and controls and the possible protective role of soy on cancer is not a widespread hypothesis in China, the potential misclassification of exposure is likely to be random, i.e. affecting equally cases and controls. This type of misclassification tends to underestimate the true association.

In addition to the above case–control studies, we are aware of three prospective studies evaluating this association. Although cohort studies avoid certain kinds of bias, such as recall bias, the results of these three studies cannot be considered conclusive, given their limited assessment and/or range of soy consumption. Hirayama (1990, in: Key *et al.*, 1999) found a reduced breast cancer risk for daily miso soup consumers (RR: 0.85; 95% CI: 0.68–1.06) compared to those consuming miso soup less often. There was also a suggestion of an inverse association with soy or tofu intake among participants in the Iowa Women's Health Study (Greenstein *et al.*, 1996). The RR for consumers of soy/tofu was 0.76 (95% CI: 0.50–1.18) compared to non-consumers, but only 2.9% of participants reported consuming soy. As in other studies conducted in Western populations, the level of soy intake was too low to evaluate this hypothesis properly. The third prospective study (Key *et al.*, 1999) failed to find an association with tofu or miso soup among Japanese women, a large proportion of whom had been exposed to high levels of ionizing radiation. Furthermore, this study used a limited food frequency questionnaire to assess soy consumption, which had not been validated. Thus, non-differential misclassification may have operated in this study in biasing the risk estimates towards the null value.

Besides soy foods, other sources of phytoestrogens could modify breast cancer risk, but there is weak epidemiologic evidence for an association with fruits and vegetables (Willett, 2001), pulses and legumes (WCRF/AICR, 1997), or whole grains (Nicodemos *et al.*, 2001). Three case–control studies in Italy (Levi *et al.*, 1993b), France (Challier *et al.*, 1998), and Mexico (Torres-Sánchez *et al.*, 2000) reported a strong inverse relationship with onions. In contrast, no association was found in the Netherlands Cohort Study (Dorant *et al.*, 1995). Onions are rich in the flavonoid quercetin, which has been shown to have antiproliferative and potent antioxidant activity and is able to bind with type II estrogen receptors (Torres-Sánchez *et al.*, 2000).

Biological markers of phytoestrogen intake and breast cancer risk

To avoid the well-known inaccuracies in the assessment of dietary intake, some investigators have relied on biological markers of phytoestrogen intake, such as urinary or serum levels of isoflavones and/or lignans. A small study by Adlercreutz *et al.* (1982) was the first to report lower urinary levels of enterolactone, enterodiol, and equol in postmenopausal breast cancer patients ($n = 7$), compared to healthy postmenopausal omnivorous ($n = 10$) and vegetarians ($n = 10$). Since then, a number of studies, summarized in Table 4.2, have examined the role of phytoestrogen biomarkers on breast cancer risk. Two recent case–control studies conducted in Australia (Ingram *et al.*, 1997) and China (Zheng *et al.*, 1999) tended to support an inverse association between urinary excretion of phytoestrogens and breast cancer. A limitation of these two studies is that urinary specimens were collected after cancer diagnosis. Although the investigators collected urinary samples immediately after diagnosis, it is possible that the disease had affected metabolic processes at the time of urinary collection and/or the cases had changed their dietary intake during that stressful time.

Additional support for a protective effect comes from a case–control study among Finnish women (Pietinen *et al.*, 2001). It found a strong inverse relationship between serum enterolactone, a lignan, and breast cancer risk. In this study, the cases were women with a suspected breast lump or breast symptom who were referred for diagnosis. Although serum samples in this study were collected before the breast cancer diagnosis, cases already had the symptoms of the disease. Further, their concern with the disease may have affected their dietary intake at the time of specimen collection. Pietinen *et al.* discarded this possibility by noting that serum enterolactone levels do not decrease rapidly and the low likelihood of women concerned about a possible cancer diagnosis turning to a lignan-free diet. Although overall these three case–control studies (Ingram *et al.*, 1997; Pietinen *et al.*, 2001; Zheng *et al.*, 1999) tend to support an inverse association between phytoestrogens and breast cancer, their retrospective nature hampers our ability to establish causality. The collection of biological samples around the time of or after diagnosis is a major limitation of these studies.

Table 4.2 Epidemiologic studies of biologic markers of phytoestrogens and breast cancer risk

Study	Population (cases:controls)	Menopausal status	Biological marker		Adjusted risk estimates and 95% confidence intervals
Ingram et al. (1997)	Australian (144:144)	Combined*	Urinary phytoestrogens	Isoflavones:	(Q4 vs Q1)
				Daidzein	0.47 (0.17, 1.33)
				Equol	0.27 (0.10, 0.69)
				Lignans:	
				Enterodiol	0.73 (0.33, 1.64)
				Enterolactone	0.36 (0.15, 0.86)
Zheng et al. (1999)	Chinese (60:60)	Combined	Urinary isoflavones		(T3 vs T1)
				Total	0.50 (0.19, 1.31)
				Daidzein	0.54 (0.22, 1.32)
				Genistein	0.70 (0.27, 1.84)
				Glycitein	0.41 (0.15, 1.11)
Murkies et al. (2000)	Australian (20:20)	Postmenopausal	Urinary phytoestrogens	Significant lower daidzein and genistein in breast cancer patients compared to controls	
Den Tonkelaar et al. (2001)	Dutch (88:268) (Nested case-control study)	Postmenopausal	Urinary phytoestrogens		(T3 vs T1)
				Genistein/creatinine	0.83 (0.46, 1.51)
				Enterolactone/creatinine	1.43 (0.79, 2.59)
Pietinen et al. (2001)	Finnish (194:208)	Combined*	Serum enterolactone	Serum enterolactone	(Q4 vs Q1)
					0.38 (0.18, 0.77)

*Similar results in analyses by menopausal status.

To our knowledge, only one prospective study (den Tonkelaar *et al.*, 2001) has evaluated the relationship between biological markers of phytoestrogens and breast cancer risk. In this study urinary genistein and enterolactone were not associated with breast cancer risk among postmenopausal women participating in a breast cancer screening program in the Netherlands. Although the levels of urinary enterolactone among participants were comparable to those in the Australian study (Ingram *et al.*, 1997) discussed earlier, the levels of urinary isoflavones were considerably lower than those found in the Shanghai Breast Cancer Study (Zheng *et al.*, 1999). Therefore, the study by Den Tonkelaar *et al.* (2001) does not rule out an effect among populations with a different distribution of phytoestrogen intake (e.g. higher levels of isoflavones) or among premenopausal women.

Soy intake and mammographic density

There is a growing interest in mammographic density as a marker or precursor of breast cancer, as it has consistently been associated with breast cancer risk (Atkinson and Bingham, 2002). At the same time, breast density has been shown to reflect the estrogen environment, with tamoxifen and low fat diets decreasing it and hormone replacement therapy increasing it (Messina and Loprinzi, 2001). Consequently, the evaluation of mammographic patterns may be relevant in understanding the role of phytoestrogens in breast cancer risk. This is a new area that has received little attention in epidemiology. Two recent cross-sectional studies (Jakes *et al.*, 2001; Maskarinec and Meng, 2001) exploring the association between soy intake and breast density reported somewhat conflicting results. Maskarinec and Meng (2001) found a positive relationship between soy intake and percent mammographic densities in a multiethnic population in Hawaii. However, there was an inverse relationship between soy intake and the size of the breast, in particular of the non-dense area (i.e. the fatty part of the breast) after adjusting for BMI, age, and parity. They postulated that the size of the non-dense area may be an important predictor of breast cancer risk and that this may be determined by soy intake during developmental years. The findings were stronger for postmenopausal women. The other study by Jakes *et al.* (2001) in Chinese women found an inverse relationship between soy intake and mammographic dense patterns known to be associated with breast cancer after taking into account BMI, age, parity, and energy intake. The relationship was stronger after further adjusting for total fat intake. Similar results were obtained when analyses were limited to postmenopausal women not using HRT. Although not definitive, these studies tend to support the notion that soy intake may decrease breast cancer risk.

Phytoestrogens and breast cancer prevention: summary

Although the current epidemiologic evidence of a relationship between phytoestrogen intake and breast cancer risk is inconclusive, it tends to suggest a possible inverse association. The fairly consistent finding of decreased breast cancer risk with soy intake in Asian populations in case–control studies is intriguing and warrants further evaluation in prospective studies using both comprehensive dietary assessment and biological markers of phytoestrogen intake that are collected before diagnosis. There is growing evidence suggesting a beneficial role of soy on breast cancer only if consumed over a lifetime, particularly before and during adolescence. The preliminary findings of proliferative effects on breast tissue need further examination and their implications for recommendations related to soy intake are unclear. However, they may warrant caution in the use of soy products, particularly for some women, such as postmenopausal women not using hormone replacement therapy, for whom estrogenic effects of phytoestrogens would be anticipated. Further insight into the role of soy isoflavones in breast cancer chemoprevention might be provided by an ongoing phase I clinical trial being conducted at the US National Cancer Institute (Greenwald *et al.*, 2001).

Phytoestrogens and endometrial cancer

Despite the strong and well-established link between unopposed estrogens and endometrial cancer risk, the role of phytoestrogens on the etiology of this disease has received little attention. In four intervention studies among postmenopausal women and one in premenopausal and perimenopausal women, a diet high in isoflavones or isoflavone supplementation did not increase endometrial thickness (Hale *et al.*, 2002). To our knowledge, only one epidemiologic study has specifically evaluated the role of phytoestrogen-containing foods in endometrial cancer risk (Goodman *et al.*, 1997). This study reported decreased risk of endometrial cancer for legumes, particularly for tofu and other soy products, wholegrain foods, vegetables, fruits, and seaweed. These results, as well as those of other studies that examined the risk associated with the major food sources of phytoestrogens, are summarized in Table 4.3. Overall, they tend to support the hypothesis that phytoestrogens are associated with reduced risk of endometrial cancer.

Beans and legumes

In a case–control study conducted in Hawaii, Goodman *et al.* (1997) reported an inverse relationship for all legumes. Further analyses revealed that this effect was stronger for tofu and other soy products, with an odds ratio of 0.46 (95% CI: 0.26–0.83) and a *p* for trend of 0.01, whereas consumption of other peas and beans was weakly and nonsignificantly related to endometrial cancer. Other case–control studies have reported no association with beans (Jain *et al.*, 2000) or legumes (Shu *et al.*, 1993) or an increased risk for peas and beans (Levi *et al.*, 1993b) and pulses and nuts (Tzonou *et al.*, 1996). To our knowledge the study by Goodman *et al.* (1997) is the only study evaluating the role of soybeans in endometrial cancer risk.

Table 4.3 Epidemiologic studies evaluating phytoestrogen-containing foods and endometrial cancer risk

Dietary Factors/Study	Study size/type*	Comparison	Results	Confounders considered
BEANS AND LEGUMES				
Tofu				
Goodman et al., 1997	332:511/cc	Q4 vs Q1	0.5 (0.3–0.9) *p for trend: 0.04*	Pregnancy history, OC, ERT, diabetes, BMI, total calories
Tofu and other soy products				
Goodman et al., 1997	332:511/cc	Q4 vs Q1	0.5 (0.3–0.8) *p for trend: 0.01*	Pregnancy history, OC, ERT, diabetes, BMI, total calories
Other peas and beans				
Levi et al., 1993a	274:572/cc	T3 vs T1	1.98 (–) *p for trend: <0.01*	Age, study center, and total energy intake
Goodman et al., 1997	332:511/cc	Q4 vs Q1	0.7 (0.4–1.2) *p for trend: 0.21*	Pregnancy history, OC, ERT, diabetes, BMI, total calories
Beans				
Jain et al., 2000	552:562/cc	Q4 vs Q1	1.05 (0.7–1.5) *p for trend: 0.90*	Total energy, age, weight, smoking, diabetes, OC, ERT, education, live births (y/n), age at menarche
Legumes				
Shu et al., 1993	268:268/cc	Q4 vs Q1	1.4 (NS) *p for trend: 0.25*	Age, number of pregnancies, BMI, total calories
Goodman et al., 1997	332:511/cc	T3 vs T1	0.6 (0.4–0.9) *p for trend: 0.009*	Pregnancy history, OC, ERT, diabetes, BMI, total calories
Pulses and nuts				
Tzonou et al., 1996	145:298/cc	Quartile increase of intake	1.4 (1.2–1.8) *p for trend: 0.001*	Age, schooling, age at menopause and menarche, OC, ERT, smoking, alcohol, BMI, energy intake, other

WHOLE GRAINS

Wholegrain cereal

Study	Cases:controls	Comparison	OR (CI) / p for trend	Adjusted for
La Vecchia et al., 1986	206:206/cc	Frequently vs occasionally	0.6 (0.3–1.2) p for trend: 0.28	Age, BMI, OC, ERT, age at menarche, age at menopause, and other variables
Goodman et al., 1997	332:511/cc	Q4 vs Q1	0.5 (0.3–0.8) p for trend: 0.009	Pregnancy history, OC, ERT, diabetes, BMI, total calories

Wholegrain bread and pasta

Study	Cases:controls	Comparison	OR (CI) / p for trend	Adjusted for
Levi et al., 1993a	274:572/cc	T3 vs T1	0.4 (–) p for trend: <0.01	Age, study center, and total energy intake
Kasum et al., 2001	382:23,014/c	Q5 vs Q1	0.89 (0.61–1.29) p for trend: 0.24 Never users of HRT: 0.63 (0.39–1.01)	Age, kilocalories, education, BMI, smoking, vitamin use, intake of fruits and vegetables, red meat, refined grains, total fat, and saturated fat, age at menarche, age at menopause, number of live births, and HRT use

VEGETABLES AND FRUITS

Vegetables

Study	Cases:controls	Comparison	OR (CI) / p for trend	Adjusted for
Levi et al., 1993a	274:572/cc	T3 vs T1	0.4 (–) p for trend: <0.01	Age, study center, and total energy intake
Shu et al., 1993	268:268/cc	Q4 vs Q1	1.4 (NS) p for trend: 0.39	Age, number of pregnancies, BMI, total calories
Potischman et al., 1993	399:296/cc	Q4 vs Q1	1.0 (0.6–1.6) p for trend: –	Age, BMI, ever estrogen use, ever OC use, number of births, current smoking, education, total calories
Tzonou et al., 1996	145:298/cc	Quartile increase of intake	0.8 (0.7–1.1) p for trend: 0.24	Age, schooling, age at menopause, age at menarche, OC, ERT, smoking, alcohol, BMI, energy intake, other variables
Goodman et al., 1997	332:511/cc	Q4 vs Q1	0.5 (0.3–0.9) p for trend: 0.03	Pregnancy history, OC, ERT, diabetes, BMI, total calories
Jain et al., 2000	552:562/cc	Q4 vs Q1	0.6 (0.4–0.96) p for trend: 0.04	Total energy, age, weight, smoking (yes/no), diabetes, OC, ERT, education, live births (y/n), age at menarche

Table 4.3 (con'd)

Dietary Factors/Study	Study size/type*	Comparison	Results	Confounders considered
VEGETABLES AND FRUITS				
Green vegetables				
La Vecchia et al., 1986	206:206/cc	≥8 portions/w vs less	0.2 (0.1–0.4) *p for trend:* –	Age, BMI, OC, ERT, age at menarche, age at menopause, and other variables
Jain et al., 2000	552:562/cc	Q4 vs Q1	0.7 (0.5–1.04) *p for trend:* 0.03	Total energy, age, weight, smoking (yes/no), diabetes, OC, ERT, education, live births (y/n), age at menarche
Plant foods				
Zheng et al., 1995	216:23 000/c	High tertile vs low	0.5 (0.3–0.9) *p for trend:* 0.03	Age, age at menopause, parity, postmenopausal hormone use, energy from animal foods
Seaweed				
Goodman et al., 1997	332:551/cc	Q4 vs Q1	0.5 (0.3–0.8) *p for trend:* 0.03	Pregnancy history, OC, ERT, diabetes, BMI, total calories
Fruits				
La Vecchia et al., 1986	206:206/cc	≥14 portions/w vs less	0.6 (0.3–0.9) *p for trend:* –	Age, BMI, OC, ERT, age at menarche, age at menopause, and other variables
Levi et al., 1993a	274:572/cc	T3 vs T1	0.4 (–) *p for trend:* <0.01	Age, study center, and total energy intake
Shu et al., 1993	268:268/cc	Q4 vs Q1	0.7 (NS) *p for trend:* 0.25	Age, number of pregnancies, BMI, total calories
Potischman et al., 1993	399:296/cc	Q4 vs Q1	1.1 (0.6–1.9) *p for trend:* –	Age, BMI, ever estrogen use, ever OC use, number of births, current smoking, education, total calories
Tzonou et al., 1996	145:298/cc	Quartile increase of intake	0.96 (0.8–1.2) *p for trend:* 0.001	Age, schooling, age at menopause, age at menarche, OC, ERT, smoking, alcohol, BMI, energy intake, other variables
Goodman et al., 1997	332:511/cc	Q4 vs Q1	0.5 (0.3–0.8) *p for trend:* 0.004	Pregnancy history, OC, ERT, diabetes, BMI, total calories
Jain et al., 2000	552:562/cc	Q4 vs Q1	1.3 (0.9–1.9) *p for trend:* 0.41	Total energy, age, weight, smoking (yes/no), diabetes, OC, ERT, education, live births (y/n), age at menarche

*cc, case-control; c, cohort. Other abbreviations: OC, oral contraceptive; ERT, estrogen replacement therapy; BMI, body mass index; NS, not statistically significant; (–), 95% confidence intervals not presented; Q, quartile or quantile of intake; T, tertile of intake.

Whole grains

Whole grains, a major source of lignan phytoestrogens, were reported to reduce endometrial cancer risk in two case–control studies, conducted in Switzerland and Italy (Levi *et al.*, 1993b) and Hawaii (Goodman *et al.*, 1997). In an additional case–control study conducted in Italy, the risk of endometrial cancer was lower for women who reported consuming wholegrain cereals frequently compared to those consuming them only occasionally, but risk estimates were not statistically significant (La Vecchia *et al.*, 1986). Nevertheless, a meta-analysis combining these three studies reported a pooled odds ratio for endometrial cancer of 0.55 (95% CI: 0.41–0.69) for high vs low intake of whole grains (Jacobs *et al.*, 1998). In the Iowa Women's Health Study, the only prospective study testing this hypothesis, there was an inverse association between whole grain consumption and endometrial cancer risk only among never-users of hormone replacement therapy (Kasum *et al.*, 2001).

Vegetables and fruits

As shown in Table 4.3, studies have generally found an inverse association with fruit and vegetable consumption after adjusting for relevant confounders. A panel of experts commissioned by the World Cancer Research Fund and the American Institute for Cancer Research (WCRF/AICR, 1997), after reviewing the epidemiologic evidence, concluded in 1997 that diets high in vegetables and fruits might "possibly" decrease the risk of endometrial cancer. However, because the phytoestrogen content of vegetables and fruits is quite variable and they include other phytochemicals with anticarcinogenic properties (Cline and Hughes, 1998), we cannot be certain whether, or the extent to which, phytoestrogens contribute to this potential protective effect.

Possible interactions with other factors

Given the potential antiestrogenic and estrogenic effects of phytoestrogens, it is reasonable to expect an interaction with other factors that have been reported to affect estrogen levels, such as ERT use, obesity, smoking, alcohol, fat intake, reproductive history, and certain polymorphisms in genes involved in estrogen metabolism. Goodman *et al.* (1997) reported an interaction of soy intake with pregnancy history and estrogen use. Stratified analyses revealed that the inverse association observed for soy intake was limited to never-pregnant women and never-users of unopposed estrogens. These findings are in agreement with the inverse association for wholegrain intake found in the Iowa Women's Health Study only among never-users of HRT (Kasum *et al.*, 2001). No other study, to our knowledge, has evaluated these potential interactions.

Phytoestrogens and endometrial cancer: summary

Despite the growing interest in phytoestrogens, there have been few studies investigating their effects on endometrial cancer risk. The experimental and limited epidemiologic evidence accumulated thus far, however, seems to indicate that a diet high in phytoestrogens or soy may reduce the risk of this cancer, particularly in women exposed to high levels of unopposed estrogens. Thus, there is a clear need to examine further the role of phytoestrogens at different levels of estrogen exposure to elucidate their role in endometrial carcinogenesis.

Phytoestrogens and epithelial ovarian cancer

The interest in phytoestrogens with regard to cancer etiology has largely focused on breast cancer. The possibility that phytoestrogens may play a role in the prevention or treatment of ovarian cancer has received little attention. However, one of the reasons most frequently mentioned to support a role of phytoestrogens or soy intake in breast cancer etiology, the lower breast cancer rates in Asian countries and the increased rates experienced by Asian women migrating to Western countries, also applies to ovarian cancer. Although epithelial ovarian cancer has a different etiologic background than breast cancer, based on the current leading theories in ovarian cancer etiology, it is certainly possible that phytoestrogens may affect ovarian carcinogenesis. Moreover, these two types of cancer share relevant etiologic characteristics: they are both hormone-sensitive and express hormonal receptors (estrogens and progesterone) in similar proportions (Perez-Gracia and Carrasco, 2002). Aproximately 63% of ovarian cancers are estrogen-receptor positive (Chen and Anderson, 2001).

While the etiology of ovarian cancer is not well understood, a protective effect of oral contraceptive use and higher parity is widely accepted (Gertig and Hunter, 2002). The main theories proposed to explain ovarian pathogenesis are "incessant ovulation" proposed by Fathalla (1971) and excessive gonadotropin stimulation of the ovarian epithelium proposed by Stadel (1975). Proponents of the former theory argue that ovulation results in minor trauma to the ovarian epithelium leading to rapid proliferation to repair the ovulatory wound. Abnormal proliferation or malignant transformation may result from excess stimulation by hormonal factors, such as estrogen-rich follicular fluid after ovulation or excessive gonadotropin levels leading to stimulation by estrogens or estrogen precursors (Risch, 1998). Based on these theories and what we know about ovarian cancer etiology, factors affecting gonadotropins or estrogens, including their levels, metabolism, actions, or regulation, can potentially affect ovarian cancer risk.

In rats, the phytoestrogen coumestrol has been shown to induce anovulation (Whitten et al., 1993) and a failure to activate luteinizing hormone (LH) production under stimulation with estradiol (Whitten et al., 1993) or gonadotropin-releasing hormone (GnRH) (McGarvey *et al.*, 2001). These results suggest that phytoestrogens, or at least coumestrol, may inhibit gonadotropin secretion by acting at the hypothalamus and pituitary gland. Soy consumption has also been associated with a significant reduction of midcycle gonadotropin levels, both LH and FSH, in humans (Kurzer, 2002). The results for estrogen levels are inconsistent, but have tended to suggest decreased levels with soy consumption (Kurzer, 2002). In addition to hormonal effects, there are other possible mechanisms by which phytoestrogens may potentially decrease ovarian cancer risk, including the antioxidant, antiproliferative and antiangiogenesis effects previously mentioned. Isoflavones, at physiological levels attainable by dietary intakes common among Japanese adults, were shown to inhibit proliferation in ER-positive ovarian cancer cells (Chen and Anderson, 2001). Overall, these findings support a possible role of phytoestrogens on ovarian cancer etiology.

The relatively few studies examining the association between diet and ovarian cancer, although not specifically designed to evaluate the role of phytoestrogens, tend to suggest a protective effect. To our knowledge, the only study evaluating the effect of soy intake, a case–control study in China, found a strong inverse dose–response relationship with "soybean products" (Zhang *et al.*, 2002). The odds ratio for the highest quartile of intake (≥ 30 kg/year) compared to the lowest was 0.4 (95% CI: 0.2–0.7; p for trend: <0.01). This odds ratio was adjusted for age, education, oral contraceptive use, parity, tubal ligation, physical activity, smoking, alcohol, tea drinking, total energy intake, animal fat, fruit and vegetable intake, and other variables.

Epidemiologic studies evaluating other sources or phytoestrogens also tended to support a protective effect. Consumption of wholegrain bread and pasta was inversely related to ovarian cancer in a case–control study conducted in Italy (La Vecchia, 1987). Pulses appear to decrease risk in two other case–control studies in China (Shu *et al.*, 1989) and Italy (Bosetti *et al.*, 2001). Consumption of legumes was also associated with a decreased risk of ovarian cancer in a case–control study in China (Zhang *et al.*, 2002). In contrast, there was no association for legumes (comprising tofu, beans and peas) in the Nurses Health Study (Fairfield *et al.*, 2001), but consumption levels were very low (≥ 0.5 servings per week was the highest category). Total fruit and vegetable intake (Kushi *et al.*, 1999; McCann *et al.*, 2001b; Zhang *et al.*, 2002) and green leafy vegetables (Kushi *et al.*, 1999) have also been found to be associated with decreased risk of ovarian cancer. In the Nurses Health Study (Fairfield *et al.*, 2001) only adolescent fruit and vegetables consumption was associated with decreased risk, suggesting that perhaps, as in breast cancer, early dietary exposure may be relevant.

In conclusion, based on our current knowledge of the epidemiology of ovarian cancer, it is biologically plausible that phytoestrogens may affect its etiology and perhaps its progression. Only a few studies have been conducted in this area, but both the experimental and epidemiologic data tend to support a protective effect and certainly warrant further evaluation of phytoestrogens in ovarian carcinogenesis.

Phytoestrogens and cancer survival

The controversy surrounding the role of phytoestrogens in cancer prevention previously discussed is exacerbated when dealing with cancer survival issues. The scientific evidence for a role of soy in breast cancer survivors was recently reviewed by Messina and Loprinzi (2001). A recent study showed that women with breast cancer, in particular those on tamoxifen, were more likely to have menopausal symptoms and to use alternative therapies to alleviate these symptoms than women without the disease (Harris *et al.*, 2002). One of the most common alternative therapies used was soy. Given these facts, there are two main clinical and research issues for cancer survivors that need immediate attention:

1. **Possible detrimental effects of phytoestrogens.** *Are phytoestrogens a safe alternative to HRT? Do they increase the likelihood of developing other cancers, particularly in the breast or endometrium? Do they affect the efficacy of tamoxifen or other anticancer agents? Is it possible that their potentially estrogenic effects actually decrease survival?*

Unfortunately, there are no clear answers to these questions at the present time. The current scientific evidence is heavily based on research on cell lines or experimental animals, and directly extrapolating it to women may not be appropriate. This is particularly true in the case of phytoestrogens, as they can potentially act in opposite directions (i.e. estrogen agonist or antagonist) depending on many factors, including the dose and the endogenous estrogen environment. As previously mentioned, experimental studies have fairly consistently shown estrogenic and proliferative activity in low estrogen environments and antiproliferative and antiestrogenic effects in high estrogen environments (Messina and Loprinzi, 2001). Based on these findings, estrogenic activity might be expected in postmenopausal breast cancer patients, who are the ones that may be more likely to turn to phytoestrogen or isoflavone supplements as natural alternatives to HRT to alleviate their menopausal symptoms. To our knowledge no epidemiologic study has specifically evaluated possible estrogenic effects of phytoestrogens on tumor promotion or progression among breast cancer survivors. However, it should be noted that two studies showed estrogenic or proliferative effects on normal breast tissue after short-term interventions with isoflavones in premenopausal women (Hargreaves *et al.*, 1999; McMichael-Phillips *et al.*, 1998).

The complexity of action of phytoestrogens is aggravated when tamoxifen is thrown into the equation. Then, we have a mix of compounds capable of acting as estrogen antagonist and weak agonist (phytoestrogens) and an antagonist (tamoxifen). An interaction of phytoestrogen and tamoxifen effects has been demonstrated in *in vitro* and *in vivo* studies (Messina and Loprinzi, 2001; This *et al.*, 2001). Although experimental studies have generally suggested synergistic antiproliferative effects on the breast, these results have not been confirmed in humans. Moreover, two recent studies have reported an inhibitory effect of genistein on the therapeutic effects of tamoxifen in breast cell lines in a low-estrogen environment (Jones *et al.*, 2002) and in the growth of estrogen-dependent breast cancer cells implanted in mice (Ju *et al.*, 2002). Therefore, caution in the simultaneous administration of isoflavones and tamoxifen in breast cancer patients is warranted, in particular to monitor possible effects on the breast tissue and the efficacy of tamoxifen therapy. Interestingly, tamoxifen acts as an agonist in the uterine tissue, and its use among breast cancer patients has been associated with an increased risk of endometrial cancer (Newman *et al.*, 1999). We are not aware of any studies evaluating the possible interaction effects of tamoxifen and phytoestrogens on the endometrium, but such inter-action is certainly possible and needs to be evaluated.

2. **Possible beneficial effects in cancer progression.** *Do phytoestrogens improve the prognosis of cancers of the breast, endometrium, and ovary? Do they improve the efficacy of tamoxifen and other cancer therapies? Do they help to alleviate side-effects from cancer therapies? Can they play a role in the prevention of other malignancies among cancer survivors?*

Again, the answers to these questions are not clear. To our knowledge the effect of phytoestrogen consumption on cancer survival has not been specifically evalu-ated in epidemiologic studies. However, it is a reasonable supposition that the multiple beneficial effects that have been proposed to explain the role of phytoestrogens in cancer prevention, such as antiproliferative, antioxidant, and antiangiogenesis properties, induction of apoptosis, and modulation of steroid hormone metabolism (Anderson *et al.*, 2001), may also improve female hor-monal cancer survival. Moreover, conceivably, they may play a role in preventing secondary malignancies, for example preventing endometrial cancer among breast cancer patients on tamoxifen. However, to our knowledge no studies have evaluated this possibility.

A few studies have evaluated the role of soy phytoestrogens in relieving hot flashes among breast cancer patients, with conflicting results (Van Patten *et al.*, 2002). Further research is needed to examine the possible beneficial effects of long-term phytoestrogen use in alleviating menopausal symptoms and improv-ing quality of life among cancer patients.

While epidemiologic research is urgently needed to assess the possible inter-action of phytoestrogens with other cancer treatments, the available experi-mental evidence seems to suggest beneficial effects. As previously mentioned, genistein has been shown in experimental studies to enhance the antiproliferat-ive effects of tamoxifen on the breast (Messina and Loprinzi, 2001), but the overall evidence is not totally consistent. Also, genistein has been shown to act synergistically with quercetin, a flavonoid (Shen and Weber, 1997), and with tiazofurin, an oncolytic drug (Li and Weber, 1998), in inducing growth inhibi-tion in human ovarian carcinoma cells. The flavonoid quercetin has been shown in *in vitro* studies to regulate ovarian cancer cell growth by interacting with type II estrogen binding sites (Scambia *et al.*, 1990a), and to act synergistically with cisplatin in producing antiproliferative effects (Scambia *et al.*, 1990b).

Conclusions

Although the available experimental and epidemiologic evidence seems to point to a potential beneficial effect of phytoestrogens, particularly soy intake, in the prevention and possibly prognosis of female hormonal cancers, it is still inconclusive. The most consistent epidemiologic evidence comes from case–control studies of soy intake and breast cancer, in which a substantial majority of the studies conducted to date suggest an inverse association. These are supported by three biomarker studies of phytoestrogens and breast cancer risk. Nevertheless, all of these studies are limited by their retrospective nature, and the evidence from prospective studies is limited. The role of phytoestrogens in endometrial and ovarian cancers is uncertain at this time because it has not received much attention. However, the current evidence provides some support for a protective effect and warrants further investigation.

The lower rates of breast, endometrial, and ovarian cancers in Asian countries, where soy intake is high, provide some reassurance that phytoestrogen/soy consumption, as used traditionally in these cultures and as part of a healthy diet, is probably safe. However, the effect of phytoestrogen supplementation at pharmacologic levels is uncertain. Epidemiologic research is urgently needed to elucidate the safety and the possible beneficial effects of phytoestrogens from dietary and supplement sources in the prevention of female hormonal cancers, as well as their possible role – whether beneficial or detrimental – in cancer survival and the quality of life of survivors.

References

Adlercreutz, H., Fotsis, T., Heikkinen, R., Dwyer, J.T., Woods, M., Goldin, B.R., and Gorbach, S.L. (1982) Excretion of the lignans enterolactone and enterodiol and of equol in omnivorous and vegetarian postmenopausal women and in women with breast cancer, *Lancet*, **2**: 1295–1299.

Anderson, J.J.B., Anthony, M.S., Cline, J.M., Washburn, S.A., and Garner, S.C. (2001) Health potential of soy isoflavones for menopausal women, *Public Health Nutrition*, **2**: 489–504.

Atkinson, C. and Bingham, S.A. (2002) Mammographic breast density as a biomarker of effects of isoflavones on the female breast, *Breast Cancer Research*, **4**: 1–4.

Balk, J.L., Whiteside, D.A., Naus, G., DeFerrari, E., and Roberts, J.M. (2002) A pilot study of the effects of phytoestrogen supplementation on postmenopausal endometrium, *Journal of the Society for Gynecologic Investigation*, **9**: 238–242.

Blair Johnson, E., Muto, M.G., Yanushpolsky, E.H., and Mutter, G.L. (2001) Phytoestrogen supplementation and endometrial cancer, *Obstetrics and Gynecology*, **98**: 947–950.

Bosetti, C., Negri, E., Franceschi, S., Pelucchi, C., Talamini, R., Montella, M., Conti, E., and La Vecchia, C. (2001) Diet and ovarian cancer risk: a case–control study in Italy, *International Journal of Cancer*, **93**: 911–915.

Challier, B., Perarnau, J.M., and Viel, J.F. (1998) Garlic, onion, and cereal fibre as protective factors for breast cancer: a French case–control study, *European Journal of Epidemiology*, **14**: 737–747.

Chen, X. and Anderson, J.J.B. (2001) Isoflavones inhibit proliferation of ovarian cancer cells *in vitro* via an estrogen receptor-dependent pathway, *Nutrition and Cancer*, **41**: 165–171.

Cline, J.M. and Hughes, C.L. (1998) Phytochemicals for the prevention of breast and endometrial cancer, *Biological and Hormonal Therapies of Cancer*, **94**: 107–134.

Dai, Q., Shu, X.O., Jin, F., Potter, J.D., Kushi, L.H., Teas, J., Gao, Y.T., and Zheng, W. (2001) Population-based case–control study of soyfood intake and breast cancer risk in Shanghai, *British Journal of Cancer*, **85**: 372–378.

Davis, S.R., Dalais, F.S., Simpson, E.R., and Murkies, A.L. (1999) Phytoestrogens in health and disease, *Recent Progress in Hormone Research*, **54**: 185–211.

De Lemos, M.L. (2001) Effects of soy phytoestrogens genistein and daidzein on breast cancer growth, *The Annals of Pharmacotherapy*, **35**: 1118–1121.

Den Tonkelaar, I., Keinan-Boker, L., Veer, P.V., Arts, C.J., Adlercreutz, H., Thijssen, J.H., and Peeters, P.H. (2001) Urinary phytoestrogens and postmenopausal breast cancer risk, *Cancer Epidemiology Biomarkers and Prevention*, **10**: 223–228.

Dorant, E., van den Brandt, P.A., and Goldbohm, R.A. (1995) Allium vegetable consumption, garlic supplement intake and female breast carcinoma incidence, *Breast Cancer Research and Treatment*, **33**: 163–170.

Duncan, A.M., Underhill, K.E.W., Xu, X., Lavalleur, J., Phipps, W.R., and Kurzer, M.S. (1999) Modest hormonal effects of soy isoflavones in postmenopausal women, *Journal of Clinical Endocrinology and Metabolism*, **84**: 3479–3484.

Fairfield, K.M., Hankinson, S.E., Rosner, B.A., Hunter, D.J., Colditz, G.A., and Willett, W.C. (2001) Risk of ovarian carcinoma and consumption of vitamins A, C, and E and specific carotenoids. A prospective analysis, *Cancer*, **92**: 2318–2326.

Fathalla, M.F. (1971) Incessant ovulation – a factor in ovarian neoplasia?, *Lancet*, **2**: 163.

Gertig, D. and Hunter, D. (2002) Ovarian cancer. In *Textbook of Cancer Epidemiology* (Adami, H.-O., Hunter, D., and Trichopoulos, D. (eds)). New York: Oxford University Press.

Goodman, M.T., Wilkens, L.R., Hankin, J.H., Lyu, L.-C., Wu, A.H., and Kolonel, L.N. (1997) Association of soy and fiber consumption with the risk of endometrial cancer, *American Journal of Epidemiology*, **146**: 294–306.

Greenstein, J., Kushi, L., Zheng, W., Fee, R., Campbell, D., Sellers, T., and Folsom, A. (1996) Risk of breast cancer associated with intake of specific foods and food groups (abstract), *American Journal of Epidemiology*, **143**: S36.

Greenwald, P., Clifford, C.K., and Milner, J.A (2001) Diet and cancer prevention, *European Journal of Cancer*, **37**: 948–965.

Hale, G.E., Hughes, C.L., and Cline, J.M. (2002) Endometrial cancer: hormonal factors, the perimenopausal "window of risk" and isoflavones, *Journal of Clinical Endocrinology and Metabolism*, **87**: 3–15.

Hankinson, S. and Hunter, D. (2002) Breast cancer. In *Textbook of Cancer Epidemiology* (Adami, H.-O., Hunter, D., and Trichopoulos, D. (eds)). New York: Oxford University Press.

Hargreaves, D.F., Potten, C.S., Harding, C., Shaw, L.E., Morton, M.S., Roberts, S.A., Howell, A., and Bundred, N.J. (1999) Two-week dietary supplementation has an estrogenic effect on normal premenopausal breast, *Journal of Clinical Endocrinology and Metabolism*, **84**: 4017–4024.

Harris, P.F., Remington, P.L., Trentham-Dietz, A., Allen, C.I., and Newcomb, P.A. (2002) Prevalence and treatment of menopausal symptoms among breast cancer survivors, *Journal of Pain and Symptom Management*, **23**: 501–509.

Hirose, K., Tajima, K., Hamajima, N., Inoue, M., Takezaki, T., Kuroishi, T., Yoshida, M. and Tokudome, S. (1995) A large-scale hospital-based case–control study of risk factors of breast cancer according to menopausal status, *Japanese Journal of Cancer Research*, **86**: 146–154.

Horn-Ross, P.L., Barnes, S., Lee, M., Coward, L., Mandel, J.E., Koo, J., John, E.M., and Smith, M. (2000) Assessing phytoestrogen exposure in epidemiologic studies: development of a database, *Cancer Causes and Control*, **11**: 289–298.

Horn-Ross, P.L., John, E.M., Lee, M., Stewart, S.L., Koo, J., Sakoda, L.C., Shiau, A.C., Goldstein, J., Davis, P., and Perez-Stable, E.J. (2001) Phytoestrogen consumption and breast cancer risk in a multiethnic population: the Bay Area Breast Cancer Study, *American Journal of Epidemiology*, **154**: 434–441.

Ingram, D., Sanders, K., Kolybaba, M., and Lopez, D. (1997) Case–control study of phyto-oestrogens and breast cancer, *Lancet*, **350**: 990–994.

Jacobs, D.R., Marquart, L., Slavin, J., and Kushi, L.H. (1998) Whole-grain intake and cancer: an expanded review and meta-analysis, *Nutrition and Cancer*, **30**: 85–96.

Jain, M.G., Howe, G.R., and Rohan, T.E. (2000) Nutritional factors and endometrial cancer in Ontario, Canada, *Cancer Control*, **7**: 288–296.

Jakes, R.W., Duffy, S.W., Ng, F.-C., Gao, F., Ng, E.-H., Seow, A., Lee, H.-P., Yu, M.C. (2001) Mammographic parenchymal patterns and self-reported soy intake in Singapore Chinese women, *Cancer Epidemiology Biomarkers and Prevention*, **11**: 608–613.

Jones, J.L., Daley, B.J., Enderson, B.L., Zhou, J.R., and Karistad, M.D. (2002) Genistein inhibits tamoxifen effects on cell proliferation and cell cycle arrest in T47D breast cancer cells, *The American Surgeon*, **68**: 575–578.

Ju, Y.H., Doerge, D.R., Allred, K.F., Allred, C.D., and Helferich, W.G. (2002) Dietary genistein negates the inhibitory effect of tamoxifen on growth of estrogen-dependent human breast cancer (MCF-7) cells implanted in athymic mice, *Cancer Research*, **1**: 2474–2477.

Kasum, C.M., Nicodemus, K., Harnack, L.J., Jacobs, D.R., and Folsom, A.R. (2001) Whole grain intake and incident endometrial cancer: the Iowa Women's Health Study, *Nutrition and Cancer*, **39**: 180–186.

Key, T.J., Sharp, G.B., Appleby, P.N., Beral, V., Goodman, M.T., Soda, M., and Mabuchi, K. (1999) Soya foods and breast cancer risk: a prospective study in Hiroshima and Nagasaki, Japan, *British Journal of Cancer*, **81**: 1248–1256.

Kurzer, M.S. (2002) Hormonal effects of soy in premenopausal women and men, *Journal of Nutrition*, **132**: 570S–573S.

Kushi, L.H., Mink, P.J., Folsom, A.R., Anderson, K.E., Zheng, W., Lazovich, D., and Sellers, T.A. (1999) Prospective study of diet and ovarian cancer, *American Journal of Epidemiology*, **149**: 21–31.

La Vecchia, C., DeCarli, A., Fasoli, M., and Gentile, A. (1986) Nutrition and diet in the etiology of endometrial cancer, *Cancer*, **57**: 1248–1253.

La Vecchia, C., DeCarli, A., Negri, E., Parazzini, F., Gentile, A., Cecchetti, G., Fasoli, M., and Franceschi, S. (1987) Dietary factors and the risk of epithelial ovarian cancer, *Journal of the National Cancer Institute*, **79**: 663–669.

Lamartiniere, C.A. (2000) Protection against breast cancer with genistein: a component of soy, *American Journal of Clinical Nutrition*, **71** (suppl.): 1705S–1707S.

Lee, H.P., Gourley, L., Duffy, S.W., Esteve, J., Lee, J., and Day, N.E. (1991) Dietary effects on breast cancer risk in Singapore, *Lancet*, **331**: 1197–1200.

Lee, H.P., Gourley, L., Duffy, S.W., Esteve, J., Lee, J., and Day, N.E. (1992) Risk factors for breast cancer by age and menopausal status: a case–control study in Singapore, *Cancer Causes and Control*, **3**: 313–322.

Levi, F., Franceschi, S., Negri, E., and La Vecchia, C. (1993a) Dietary factors and the risk of endometrial cancer, *Cancer*, **71**: 3575–3581.

Levi, F., La Vecchia, C., Gulie, C., and Negri, E. (1993b) Dietary factors and breast cancer risk in Vaud, Switzerland, *Nutrition and Cancer*, **19**: 327–335.

Li, W. and Weber, G. (1998) Synergistic action of tiazofurin and genistein in human ovarian carcinoma cells, *Oncology Research*, **10**: 117–122.

McCann, S.E., Moysich, K.B., Freudenheim, J.L., Ambrosone, C.B., and Shields, P.G. (2002) The risk of breast cancer with dietary lignans differs by CYP17 genotype in women. *Journal of Nutrition*, **132**: 3036–3041.

McCann, S.E., Moysich, K.B., and Mettlin, C. (2001b) Intakes of selected nutrients and food groups and risk of ovarian cancer, *Nutrition and Cancer*, **39**: 19–28.

McGarvey, C., Cates, P.S., Brooks, A.N., Swanson, I.A., Milligan, S.R., Coen, C.W., and O'Byrne, K.T. (2001) Phytoestrogens and gonadotropin-releasing hormone pulse generator activity and pituitary luteinizing hormone release in the rat, *Endocrinology*, **142**: 1202–1208.

McMichael-Philips, D.F., Harding, C., Morton, M., Roberts, S.A., Howell, A., Potten, C.S., and Bundred, N.J. (1998) Effects of soy-protein supplementation on epithelial proliferation in the histologically normal human breast, *American Journal of Clinical Nutrition*, **68S**: S1431–S1436.

Martini, M.C., Dancisak, B.B., Haggans, C.J., Thomas, W., and Slavin, J.L. (1999) Effects of soy intake on sex hormone metabolism in premenopausal women, *Nutrition and Cancer*, **34**: 133–139.

Maskarinec, G. and Meng, L. (2001) An investigation of soy intake and mammographic characteristics in Hawaii, *Breast Cancer Research*, **3**: 134–141.

Messina, M.J. (1999) Legumes and soybeans: overview of their nutritional profiles and health effects, *American Journal of Clinical Nutrition*, **70** (suppl.): 439S–450S.

Messina, M.J. and Loprinzi, C.L. (2001) Soy for breast cancer survivors: a critical review of the literature, *Journal of Nutrition*, **131**: 3095S–3108S.

Murkies, A., Dalais, F.S., Briganti, E.M., Burger, H.G., Healy, D.L., Wahlqvist, M.L., and Davis, S.R. (2000) Phytoestrogens and breast cancer in postmenopausal women: a case control study, *Menopause*, **7**: 289–296.

Newman, L.A., Kuerer, H.M., Harper, T., Hunt, K.K., Laronga, C., Breslin, T., and Singletary, S.E. (1999) Special considerations in breast cancer risk and survival, *Journal of Surgical Oncology*, **71**: 250–260.

Nicodemus, K.K., Jacobs, D.R., and Folsom, A.R. (2001) Whole and refined grain intake and risk of incident postmenopausal breast cancer, *Cancer Causes and Control*, **12**: 917–925.

Perez Gracia, J.L. and Carrasco, E.M. (2002) Tamoxifen therapy for ovarian cancer in the adjuvant and advanced settings: systematic review of the literature and implications for future research, *Gynecologic Oncology*, **84**: 201–209.

Pietinen, P., Stumpf, K., Mannisto, S., Kataja, V., Uusitupa, M., and Adlercreutz, H. (2001) Serum enterolactone and risk of breast cancer: a case–control study in Eastern Finland, *Cancer Epidemiology Biomarkers and Prevention*, **10**: 339–344.

Pillow, P.C., Duphorne, M., Change, S., Contois, J.H., Strom, S.S., Spitz, M.R., and Hursting, S.D. (1999) Development of a database for assessing phytoestrogen intake, *Nutrition and Cancer*, **33**: 3–19.

Potischman, N., Swanson, C.A., Brinton, L.A., McAdams, M., Barrett, R.J., Berman, M.L., Mortel, R., Twiggs, L.B., Wilbanks, G.D., and Hoover, R.N. (1993) Dietary associations in a case-control study of endometrial cancer, *Cancer Causes and Control*, **4**: 239–250.

Risch, H.A. (1998) Hormonal etiology of epithelial ovarian cancer, with a hypothesis concerning the role of androgens and progesterone, *Journal of the National Cancer Institute*, **90**: 1774–1786.

Scambia, G., Ranelletti, F.O., Benedetti Panici, P., Piantelli, M., Bonanno, G., De Vicenzo, R., Ferrandina, G., Rumi, C., Larocca, L.M., and Mancuso S. (1990a) Inhibitory effect of quercetin on OVCA 433 cells and presence of type II oestrogen binding sites in primary ovarian tumours and cultured cells, *British Journal of Cancer*, **62**: 942–946.

Scambia, G., Ranelletti, F.O., Benedetti Panici, P., Bonanno, G., De Vicenzo, R., Piantelli, M., and Mancuso, S. (1990b) Synergistic antiproliferative activity of quercetin and cisplastin on ovarian cancer cell growth, *Anticancer Drugs*, **1**: 45–48.

Setchell, K.D.R. (1998) Phytoestrogens: the biochemistry, physiology, and implications for human health of soy isoflavones, *American Journal of Clinical Nutrition*, **68** (suppl.): 1333S–1346S.

Shen, F. and Weber, G. (1997) Synergistic action of quercitin and genistein in human ovarian carcinoma cells, *Oncology Research*, **9**: 597–602.

Shoff, S.M., Newcomb, P.A., Mares-Perlman, J.A., Klein, B.E.K., Haffner, S.M., Storer, B.E., and Klein, R. (1998) Usual consumption of plant food containing phytoestrogens and sex hormone levels in postmenopausal women in Wisconsin, *Nutrition and Cancer*, **30**: 207–212.

Shu, X.O., Gao, Y.T., Yuan, J.M., Ziegler, R.G., and Brinton, L.A. (1989) Dietary factors and epithelial ovarian cancer, *British Journal of Cancer*, **59**: 92–96.

Shu, X.O., Jin, F., Dai, Q., Wen, W., Potter, J.D., Kushi, L.H., Ruan, Z., Gao, Y.T., and Zheng, W. (2001) Soyfood intake during adolescence and subsequent risk of breast cancer among Chinese women, *Cancer Epidemiology, Biomarkers and Prevention*, **10**: 483–488.

Shu, X.O., Zheng, W., Potischman, N., Brinton, L.A., Hatch, M.C., Gao, Y.-T., and Fraumeni, J.F., Jr (1993) A population-based case–control study of dietary factors and endometrial cancer in Shanghai, People's Republic of China, *American Journal of Epidemiology*, **137**: 155–165.

Smith-Warner, S.A., Spiegelman, D., Yaun, S.S., Adami, H.O., Beeson, W.L., van den Brandt, P.A., Folsom, A.R., Fraser, G.E., Freudenheim, J.L., Goldbohm, R.A., Graham, S., Miller, A.B., Potter, J.D., Rohan, T.E., Speizer, F.E., Toniolo, P., Willett, W.C., Wolk, A., Zeleniuch-Jacquotte, A., and Hunter, D.J. (2001) Intake of fruits and vegetables and risk of breast cancer: a pooled analysis of cohort studies, *Journal of the American Medical Association*, **285**: 769–776.

Stadel, B.V. (1975) The etiology and prevention of ovarian cancer (letter), *American Journal of Obstetrics and Gynecology*, **123**: 772–773.

Strauss, L., Santti, R., Saarinen, N., Streng, T., Joshi, S., and Makela, S. (1998) Dietary phytoestrogens and their role in hormonally dependent disease, *Toxicology Letters*, **102–103**: 349–354.

This, P., De la Rochefordiere, A., Clough, K., Fourquet, A., Magdelenat, H., and The Breast Cancer Group of the Institut Curie (2001) Phytoestrogens after breast cancer, *Endocrine-Related Cancer*, **8**: 129–134.

Torres-Sánchez, L., López-Carrillo, L., López-Cervantes, M., Rueda-Neria, C., and Wolff, M.S. (2000) Food sources of phytoestrogens and breast cancer risk in Mexican women, *Nutrition and Cancer*, **37**: 134–139.

Tzonou, A., Lipworth, L., Kalandidi, A., Trichopoulou, A., Gamatsi, I., Hsieh, C.-C., Notara, V., and Trichopoulos, D. (1996) Dietary factors and the risk of endometrial cancer: a case–control study in Greece, *British Journal of Cancer*, **73**: 1284–1290.

Van Patten, C.L., Olivotto, I.A., Chambers, G.K., Gelmon, K.A., Hislop, T.G., Templeton, E., Wattie, A., and Prior, J.C. (2002) Effect of soy phytoestrogens on hot flashes in postmenopausal women with breast cancer: a randomized, controlled clinical trial, *Journal of Clinical Oncology*, **20**: 1449–1455.

Whitten, P.L., Lewis, C., and Naftolin, F. (1993) A phytoestrogen diet induces the premature anovulatory syndrome in lactationally exposed female rats, *Biology of Reproduction*, **49**: 1117–1121.

Willett, W.C. (2001) Diet and breast cancer, *Journal of Internal Medicine*, **249**: 395–411.

Witte, J.S., Ursin, G., Siemiatycki, J., Thompson, W.D., Paginini-Hill, A., Haile, R.W. (1997) Diet and premenopausal bilateral breast cancer: a case–control study, *Breast Cancer Research and Treatment*, **42**: 243–251.

World Cancer Research Fund/American Institute for Cancer Research (1997) *Food, Nutrition, and the Prevention of Cancer: a Global Perspective*. Washington, DC: American Institute of Cancer Research.

Wu, A.H., Ziegler, R.G., Horn-Ross, P.L., Nomura, A.M., West, D.W., Kolonel, L.N., Rosenthal, J.F., Hoover, R.N., and Pike, M.C. (1996) Tofu and risk of breast cancer in Asian-Americans, *Cancer Epidemiology, Biomarkers and Prevention*, **5**: 901–906.

Wu, A.H., Ziegler, R.G., Nomura, A.M., West, D.W., Kolonel, L.N., Horn-Ross, P.L., Hoover, R.N., and Pike, M.C. (1998) Soy intake and risk of breast cancer in Asians and Asian Americans, *American Journal of Clinical Nutrition*, **68** (6 suppl.): 1437S–1443S.

Yuan, J.M., Wang, Q.S., Ross, R.K., Henderson, B.E., and Yu, M.C. (1995) Diet and breast cancer in Shanghai and Tianjin, China, *British Journal of Cancer*, **71**: 1353–1358.

Yuan, J.-M., Yu, M.C., Ross, R.K., Henderson, B.E., and Yu, M.C. (1988) Risk factors for breast cancer in Chinese women in Shanghai, *Cancer Research*, **48**: 1949–1953.

Zhang, M., Yang, Z.Y., Binns, C.W., and Lee, A.H. (2002) Diet and ovarian cancer risk: a case–control study in China, *British Journal of Cancer*, **86**: 712–717.

Zheng, W., Kushi, L.H., Potter, J.D., Sellers, T.A., Doyle, T.J., Bostick, R.M., and Folsom, A.R. (1995) Dietary intake of energy and animal foods and endometrial cancer incidence. *The Iowa Women's Health Study*, *American Journal of Epidemiology*, **142**: 388–394.

Zheng, W., Dai, Q., Custer, L.J., Shu, X.O., Wen, W.Q., Jin, F., and Franke, A.A. (1999) Urinary excretion of isoflavonoids and the risk of breast cancer, *Cancer Epidemiology, Biomarkers and Prevention*, **8**: 35–40.

5   Dietary retinol as a toxic substance

R.J. Rosengren and B.J. Bray

General principles

Vitamin A is the generic term for all derivatives of β-ionone (other than the carotenoids) that possess the biological activity of all-*trans*-retinol, while the term retinoids refers to both synthetic and natural forms of retinol regardless of biological activity (Figure 5.1) (Schumann *et al.*, 1997). There are over 1000 synthetic retinoids, but only retinol, retinal and retinyl esters fulfill all vitamin A activities (Biesalski, 1997). Dietary vitamin A is generally obtained either from animal sources in the form of retinyl esters or from plant sources in the

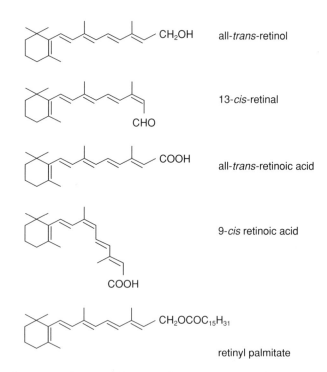

all-*trans*-retinol

13-*cis*-retinal

all-*trans*-retinoic acid

9-*cis* retinoic acid

retinyl palmitate

Figure 5.1 Structures of some of the naturally occurring retinoids.

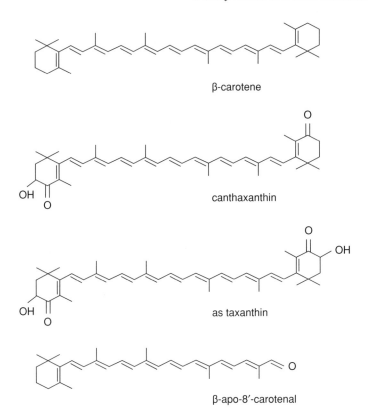

β-carotene

canthaxanthin

as taxanthin

β-apo-8′-carotenal

Figure 5.2 Structures of provitamin A and non-provitamin A carotenoids.

form of the precursor β-carotene (Schumann *et al.*, 1997). β-carotene belongs to a class of naturally occurring carotenoids (over 50 compounds) which, upon metabolic breakdown, exhibit vitamin A activity. However, there also are carotenoids that upon breakdown do not possess vitamin A activity and are termed non-provitamin A carotenoids (Figure 5.2). The ingestion of vitamin supplements can provide an additional source of vitamin A and the absorption of retinoids from these sources is more rapid than from dietary sources (Schumann *et al.*, 1997). The amount of vitamin A ingested by humans or administered to laboratory animals generally is reported in either international units (IU) or retinol equivalents (RE). One international unit of vitamin A is defined as 0.3 µg of all-*trans*-retinol. Retinol equivalent is often used to obtain a single value that represents all dietary sources of carotenoids and vitamin A ingested. Using this nomenclature, 1 µg of all-*trans*-retinol is equivalent to 1 RE and 1 µg of all-*trans*-retinol is assumed to be biologically equivalent to 6 µg of β-carotene (IUPAC-IUB, 1982). Retinyl esters are considered to be as bioavailable as all-*trans*-retinol and therefore, after accounting for the difference in molecular weight, 1.83 µg of retinyl palmitate is equivalent to 1 µg RE.

Retinol uptake, transport and metabolism

Following dietary intake, retinol is converted to retinyl esters by the intestinal enterocyte and transported to the liver in chylomicrons. Plasma levels of retinol are under tight homeostatic control and this process originates in the liver. Excess hepatic retinol is stored in the Ito cells of the liver and in well-nourished individuals, over 90% of total body retinol is stored in these fat-storing cells (Maiani *et al.*, 1993). However, in malnourished individuals, 10 to 50% of retinol may be stored in the kidneys and other tissues (Olson, 1987). In the liver, retinyl esters are hydrolyzed and retinol is then complexed (1:1) with retinol-binding protein (RBP) (Figure 5.3). The retinol–RBP complex is released from the liver into the circulation where it binds to the plasma protein

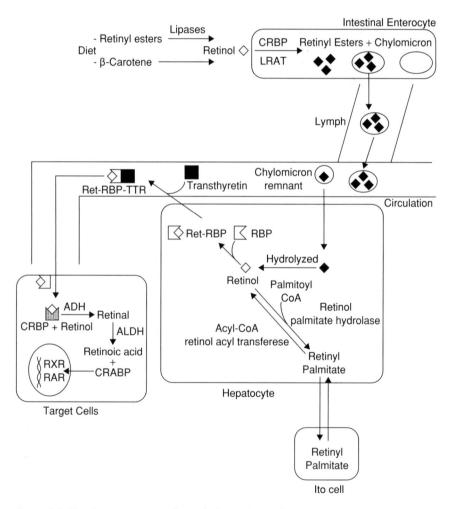

Figure 5.3 Uptake, transport, and metabolism of retinol.

transthyretin (TTR) which prevents the glomerular filtration of RBP. Upon delivery to the target tissues, the TTR dissociates from the retinol–RBP–TTR complex and retinol–RBP is taken up by cell surface receptors. Retinol is further transferred to cellular retinol binding protein (CRBP) at either the cell surface or following internalization. Therefore, one role for CRBP is to deliver retinol to newly synthesized RBP in the endoplasmic reticulum. Once retinol enters the target tissues, metabolism will produce either biologically active retinoids or inactive metabolites. Alcohol dehydrogenase (ADH), especially the isoform ADH-IV, is the main enzyme which catalyzes the reversible interconversion of retinol to the corresponding aldehyde, retinal (Duester, 1996). Retinal can then undergo irreversible oxidative metabolism to retinoic acid by the enzyme aldehyde dehydrogenase (ALDH-1) (Duester, 1996, 1998) or reductive metabolism by retinol dehydrogenase back to retinol, which promotes recycling and storage (Duester, 1996). Cytochrome P450 (CYP450) enzymes, specifically CYP1A1, CYP1A2, CYP1B1 and CYP3A4, are also involved in the conversion of retinal to retinoic acid (Chen *et al.*, 2000). Once retinoic acid is formed it can undergo isomerization to other natural retinoids, namely 13-*cis*-retinoic acid and 9-*cis*-retinoic acid. Retinoic acid can also be further oxidized by CYP2C8 (Leo *et al.*, 1989), or conjugated with glucuronide resulting in polar metabolites which are then secreted in the bile or recycled back into the liver through the process of enterohepatic circulation (Parkinson, 1996).

Role of RXR and RAR

All-*trans*-retinoic acid is the biologically active retinoid which regulates both embryonic development and the maintenance of adult epithelial tissues (Biesalski, 1997). At the cellular level, retinoic acid translocates into the nucleus via binding to cellular retinoic acid binding protein (CRABP) and ultimately produces a biological response through regulation of gene transcription (Figure 5.3). This signaling occurs via nuclear receptors belonging to the superfamily of steroid/thyroid hormone receptors which are characterized by several features including a multiplicity of receptors and ligands, dimer formation, and multiple direct repeats as response elements (van der Saag, 1996). There are two families of retinoic acid receptors termed the retinoic acid receptor (RAR) and the retinoid X receptor (RXR) and each contains three subtypes (α, β, and γ) (Giguere, 1994; van der Saag, 1996). Using either all-*trans*-retinoic acid or the closely related isomer 9-*cis*-retinoic acid, RARs function as ligand-inducible transcriptional regulators which form homodimers or heterodimerize with RXR (Mangelsdorf and Evans, 1995). The RXRs can also homodimerize and act as transcriptional regulators but are solely activated by 9-*cis*-retinoic acid (van der Saag, 1996). Following dimerization, both retinoid receptors bind to retinoic acid response elements (RARE), specific DNA sites located in the 5′ promoter region of responsive genes (Glass *et al.*, 1991). Binding to RARE initiates gene transcription which results in a gene-, ligand- and tissue-specific biological response.

Retinol toxicity

Retinol is generally considered a relatively safe dietary component. However, excessive ingestion can result in a condition referred to clinically as hypervitaminosis A. Generally, children are more susceptible to retinol-induced toxicity. However, this is due to a smaller body mass rather than age-specific physiological differences in retinol metabolism (Bendich and Langseth, 1989). The prevalence of hypervitaminosis A has increased since the introduction of purified vitamin A supplements. Prior to the popularization of supplementation, case reports of hypervitaminosis A were limited to the rare occasions when excess quantities of liver, particularly from carnivorous animals, had been consumed. Conversely, consumption of foods containing the retinol precursor β-carotene has very rarely led to the development of hypervitaminosis A.

Retinol toxicity occurs following the saturation of the retinol binding protein. This results in an increase in the non-specific binding of retinol to plasma lipoproteins and often an increase in the concentration of free retinol in the plasma. Additionally, an increase in circulating retinyl esters occurs which may be a more specific marker for predicting hypervitaminosis A, as plasma retinol levels do not reliably predict clinical symptomatology (Krasinski *et al.*, 1989). Nonetheless, the rise in free retinol causes a disruption of controlled receptor-mediated cell interactions and a perturbation of cellular membranes resulting in an alteration of cell function (Goodman, 1988). Since retinol not bound to RBP is easily oxidized, further damage may occur through retinol-induced pro-oxidant effects elicited by the products of spontaneous oxidation (Dal-Pizzol *et al.*, 2001).

In vitro experiments have examined the pro-oxidant effects elicited by retinol. Specifically, when Sertoli cells isolated from 15 day old Wistar rats were incubated with retinol (7 μM) for 24 h, glutathione peroxidase, catalase and superoxide dismutase were all significantly increased (Dal-Pizzol *et al.*, 2001). These results correlated with other *in vitro* experiments which demonstrated that superoxides were generated in a dose-dependent manner in HL-60 leukemia cells following incubation with retinol (0.5 to 5 μM) (Murata and Kawanishi, 2000). The pro-oxidant effects were sufficient to produce oxidative damage to DNA in both cell types. However, in HP100 cells (an H_2O_2-resistant clone of HL-60 cells), retinol did not induce DNA damage (Murata and Kawanishi, 2000). These results indicated that the superoxide generated by autoxidation of retinol was dismutated to H_2O_2 and this was responsible for the DNA damage. Further research in Sertoli cells demonstrated that metal ions were involved, as iron chelators inhibited many aspects of retinol-induced DNA damage such as chromatin sensitivity to DNAse I (Moreira *et al.*, 1997), increases in thymidine incorporation into DNA (Moreira *et al.*, 1996) and nuclear protein phosphorylation (Moreira *et al.*, 2000). These *in vitro* effects are not likely to be relevant to low doses of retinol *in vivo* as retinol is bound to CRABP. However, they may be causally linked to the toxic effects of retinol at high doses.

Acute toxicity

The acute toxicity of retinol was first described in Arctic explorers and fisherman who had consumed vast quantities of liver from species such as polar bears and seals (Rodahl, 1943). More recently it has been associated with the excessive intake of vitamin supplements, either accidentally or under the mistaken notion that more is better. Symptoms of acute retinol toxicity occur following very high doses (in excess of 1 000 000 IU/day); however, as they often resolve within 24–48 h, death rarely occurs. In most cases, acute hypervitaminosis A is characterized by abdominal pain, nausea, vomiting, fatigue, muscle weakness, headaches, increased intracranial pressure (adults) and bulging fontanels (children), papilledema, skin desquamation, hypocalcemia, blurred vision and photophobia (Bendich and Langseth, 1989; Hathcock *et al.*, 1990; Meyers *et al.*, 1996). Only one death from an acute retinol exposure has been reported (Bush and Dahms, 1984). In this case, a neonate accidentally received a daily dose of approximately 90 000 IU of Aquasol A (a liquid formulation of all-*trans*-retinol) for 11 days. The neonate displayed typical characteristics of retinol toxicity, such as elevated hepatic enzymes, hypocalcemia, hyperphosphatemia, a bleeding disorder and pulmonary insufficiency (Bush and Dahms, 1984). Postmortem examination revealed extensive calcification of the lungs and metastatic calcification of the kidneys, stomach, soft tissue and skin.

Recently it has been suggested that retinol supplementation in Indian children resulted in both retinol-induced toxicity and death (Mudur, 2001). In a pulse campaign designed to reduce hypovitaminosis A related disease in the Assam province of India, health workers may have overdosed approximately three million children with retinol (Mudur, 2001). Within one week of receiving the supplementation, 15 000 children suffered side-effects, 750 exhibited symptoms of retinol toxicity and 14 deaths were reported. However, whether or not an overdose was given is disputed as it would be expected that in a large population some children would present with toxic symptoms (at an incidence rate of just 1%, 30 000 children would be expected to demonstrate adverse effects). Furthermore, the number of deaths was within the expected mortality rates for the region. However, as this occurred in a 2001 program, the results of the investigative report have yet to be published (West and Sommer, 2002).

Chronic toxicity

The majority of cases of hypervitaminosis A occur in individuals chronically exposed to retinol either through the diet or via supplementation. While there is no definitive dose at which symptoms of hypervitaminosis A occur, it is generally agreed that doses of 100 000 IU/day for six months or more are likely to result in clinical symptomatology (Bendich and Langseth, 1989). Chronic hypervitaminosis A is characterized by anorexia, dry itchy skin, desquamation, cheilitis, facial dermatitis, alopecia, increased intracranial pressure, papilledema, hepatomegaly, splenomegaly, fatigue, bone and joint pain, depression and elevated

Table 5.1 Symptoms of chronic hypervitaminosis A (prevalence, as determined from analysis of 200 cases, is indicated in parentheses)

Gastro-intestinal, hepatic
Nausea, vomiting (34%), anorexia (23%), hepatomegaly (16%)

Neurological
Headache (28%), bulging fontanel (26%), irritability (18%), elevated intracranial pressure (16%)

Generalized
Elevated serum retinol concentration (25%), fatigue (32%), ataxia (17%), visual symptoms (14%), hemorrhage (12%)

Effects on skin and mucosal membranes
Cheilitis, mouth or lip fissures (20%), dry skin (17%), alopecia (16%), pruritus (15%)

Bone and muscle
Muscle pain (16%), joint pain (12%)

Hepatic histopathology
Ito cell hypertrophy and hyperplasia, accumulation of perisinusoids, sinusoidal congestion and dilation, sclerosis of central veins, collagenization of the space of Disse, fibrosis, cirrhosis

---

Adapted from Meyers *et al.* (1996).

triglyceride levels (Table 5.1) (Bendich and Langseth, 1989; Hathcock *et al.*, 1990; Meyers *et al.*, 1996; Olson, 1987). Changes in the liver are the most pronounced, particularly on histopathologic examination. Hypertrophy of the Ito cells occurs leading to reversible portal hypertension with ascites, accumulation of perisinusoidal lipocytes, sinusoidal congestion, sclerosis of central veins of the liver and atrophy of hepatocytes (Meyers *et al.*, 1996). These hepatic changes can ultimately lead to hepatic cirrhosis (Hathcock *et al.*, 1990; Meyers *et al.*, 1996). Due to the long half-life of vitamin A it has been concluded that the total cumulative dose over time is the critical factor in determining the extent of hepatic damage (Meyers *et al.*, 1996).

The clinical presentation of hypervitaminosis A is variable and the amount required to produce this disease is dependent on the individual. For example, a 45-year-old woman presented with jaundice, anorexia, weight loss and diffuse pruritus following retinol intake of 25 000 IU/day for six years (Kowalski *et al.*, 1994). Her transaminase levels were slightly increased and a liver biopsy revealed severe damage of the hepatic architecture with Ito cell hyperplasia and collagenization of the space of Disse. It is quite rare for toxic symptoms to be produced from such low doses of retinol. In other cases that report toxicity at low supplementation levels, often there has been a concurrent ingestion of vitamin A supplements and high dietary retinol equivalents. A typical case is exemplified in a 33-year-old male who was taking 20 000 IU/day of retinol supplements for seven years in addition to a diet high in legumes and vegetables (Minuk *et al.*, 1988). The patient sought medical advice for persistent nausea, vomiting and headaches and examination revealed a mild elevation of transaminase levels. As expected, when the retinol supplementation was discontinued the symptoms resolved (Minuk *et al.*, 1988). Clinical presentation of hypervitaminosis A at such low doses is the exception and a survey of 579 cases by Bauernfiend (1980) concluded that chronic vitamin A toxicity occurs following the ingestion of 2500 to 50 000 IU/kg body weight. However, these guidelines may be confounded by the preparation of vitamin A taken. For example, water-based preparations are absorbed more readily than oil-based preparations (Grolier *et al.*, 1995). It has also been reported that the supplement form of retinol may have a greater bioavailability than liver-based sources, thus increasing the risk of toxic symptoms following supplementation (Buss *et al.*, 1994).

Modulation of hypervitaminosis A

Both chemical exposure and the presence of disease can change the threshold level at which retinol-induced hypervitaminosis A occurs. Since the toxic effects of retinol generally occur following the saturation of RBP, diseases that alter the formation of RBP increase the toxicity of retinol. Contraction of hepatitis B falls into this category and can result in retinol toxicity at doses which otherwise would be considered safe (Hatoff *et al.*, 1982). Specifically, a man taking vitamin A supplements (25 000 IU/day) while on a diet high in carrots and green leafy vegetables was admitted to hospital with symptoms of hypervitaminosis A. He had also contracted hepatitis B and one aspect of this disease is a decrease in protein synthesis, which resulted in a decrease in the formation of RBP and ultimately caused the retinol toxicity (Hatoff *et al.*, 1982). A diet chronically containing both low protein and a quantity of retinoids that normally would not be considered toxic can also result in hypervitaminosis A (Weber *et al.*, 1982). This situation occurred in a patient on both vitamin A supplements (50 000 IU/day) and a protein-restricted diet for seven years. Three months after being placed on a diet of increased protein and decreased supplements the patient's symptoms cleared (Weber *et al.*, 1982).

Other disease states that do not necessarily involve changes in protein synthesis can still increase the levels of circulating retinol. In particular, both severe hypertriglyceridemia and renal disease have been associated with an increased risk of developing hypervitaminosis A due to changes in retinol distribution and clearance. Specifically, a 28-year-old woman who had been on dialysis for six years and vitamin A supplementation (5000 IU/day for two years) exhibited hypervitaminosis A-induced alopecia (Schmunes, 1979). This response was purported to be due to kidney failure and the subsequent inability to clear retinol from the plasma (Schmunes, 1979). Similarly, in a patient with severe hypertriglyceridemia, retinol ingestion (60 000 IU/day for seven months) resulted in toxic manifestations (Ellis *et al.*, 1986). In addition, nine patients with type V hyperlipoproteinemia demonstrated a significant increase in plasma retinyl esters. All but one demonstrated the presence of retinol in both the VLDL and chylomicron fractions whereas all control subjects were negative for retinol in these fractions. The authors concluded that the increased VLDL and chylomicron fractions act to prevent the normal binding of retinol to RBP. This resulted in symptoms of hypervitaminosis A by increasing the fraction of unbound retinol in the plasma and decreasing controlled vitamin A cellular signaling (Ellis et al., 1986).

Zinc may protect against some of the toxic consequences of high retinol intake by decreasing the effects of unbound retinol on cellular membranes. The exposure of lymphoblastoid cells to 10 µM retinol for 90 min resulted in a 90% decrease in viability (Pasantes-Morales et al., 1984). When 100 µM zinc chloride was added to the culture media, cell viability increased to 20% and this effect was further augmented by the simultaneous administration of vitamin E (200 µM). Epidemiological evidence suggests further links between vitamin A and zinc intake. Zinc deficiency is often associated with a concurrent vitamin A deficiency, possibly due to retinol sequestering in the liver. Zinc deficiency is associated with the decreased synthesis of RBP (Smith et al., 1974). Specifically, in rats fed a zinc-deficient diet (1.3 mg/kg diet) for three weeks a 39% decrease in RBP was observed as compared to pair fed zinc-sufficient (60 mg/kg diet) controls (Smith et al., 1974). This decrease in RBP may result in an increase in the toxicity of retinol due to pro-oxidant damage although recent studies have suggested that hepatic CRBP is increased in zinc deficiency (Satre et al., 2001), resulting in the hepatic sequestering of retinol rather than generalized symptoms of toxicity. This conclusion is strengthened by studies by Boron et al. (1988) which demonstrated that animals fed a zinc deficient diet (2.3 mg/kg diet) had reduced ADH activity (83% of control) and increased retinal oxidase activity (127% of control), accompanied by an increase in total hepatic vitamin A. Therefore, the interaction between zinc and vitamin A is complex. If hypervitaminosis A and zinc deficiency were to occur simultaneously then an increase in the toxicity of retinol might be observed due to the decreases in RBP levels. However, it is more common for a zinc deficiency to correlate with decreased plasma retinol concentrations due to the sequestering of vitamin A in the liver.

The toxicity of retinol may also be altered by genetic susceptibility. Particularly, individuals with genetic polymorphisms of ADH and/or ALDH may be more susceptible to retinol toxicity due to a decrease in the activity of these enzymes (Carpenter et al., 1987). However, the proportion of the population that is truly at risk due to such polymorphisms has not been thoroughly investigated.

Teratogenicity

Vitamin A intake is essential for proper health throughout life including the embryonic and fetal stages. However, both deficient and excessive vitamin A can result in congenital abnormalities. Deficiency of vitamin A is well established to be a cause of birth defects in various animal models such as the pig, rat and rabbit (Hurley, 1977). However, most teratology studies have concentrated on the excessive administration of the normal metabolites of retinol, all-*trans*-retinoic acid (tretinoin) and 13-*cis*-retinoic acid (isotretinoin), as well as the long-acting synthetic retinoid (etretinate). All of these compounds are used as drug treatments in humans and are teratogenic in the rat, mouse, hamster, guinea pig, rabbit and primate (Birnbaum *et al.*, 1989; Hathcock *et al.*, 1990; Hummler *et al.*, 1990; Rosa *et al.*, 1986; Wiegand *et al.*, 1998). Of these models, rabbits and primates are thought to resemble most closely human exposure due to the similarities in retinol metabolism and kinetics (Dolk *et al.*, 1999). However, isotretinoin and etretinate are teratogenic in humans at doses that are approximately 10-fold lower than the most sensitive species of laboratory animal (Hummler *et al.*, 1990; Teratology Society, 1987). Specifically, isotretinoin has resulted in teratogenicity following 0.4–1.5 mg/kg per day on days 14–49 in humans compared to 140 mg/kg per day in the rat and 10 mg/kg per day in the rabbit (Rosa *et al.*, 1986). Since humans are the most sensitive species, it is difficult to use laboratory animals to predict the ultimate outcome in humans. However, case studies and epidemiological evidence are used to strengthen these findings.

Case reports have demonstrated a correlation between the ingestion of high doses of vitamin A supplements and birth defects in humans (Rosa, 1993). As expected, the incidence rate and specific type of malformation depend on the timing of exposure and the greatest risk for humans occurs during the first trimester. Malformations occur in almost all organ systems and the typical teratogenic response to retinoic acid is termed retinoic acid embryopathology. Specifically, retinoic acid causes malformations of craniofacial, cardiac, thymic and central nervous system structures (Table 5.2). These effects may be due to

Table 5.2 Teratogenicity of retinoic acid (prevalence, as determined from analysis of 339 cases, is indicated in parentheses)

Musculoskeletal; urogenital (29%)
Limb reduction deformities, clubfoot, polydactyly, bony defects of shoulder, forearm, wrist or hand; renal agenesis, congenital hydronephrosis, kidney defects, anomalies of external genitalia, hypospadias

Cranio-facial; central nervous system; thymus (20%)
Cleft palate, micro ears/canals, low-set ears, micrognathia, microphthalmia; hydrocephaly, microcephaly, posterior fossa cyst, cortical blindness, facial nerve palsy; thymic hypoplasia

Neural tube (14%)
Spina bifida, anencephaly, encephalocele

Cardiovascular (15%)
Transposition, hypoplastic aorta, VSD

Other (21%)
Gastrointestinal: tracheoesophageal fistula, congenital hypertrophic pyloric stenosis, atresia or stenosis of intestines; *non-gastrointestinal*: agenesis or hypoplasia of lungs, single umbilical cord artery, anomalies of the spleen, cystic hygroma

---

Adapted from Rosa *et al.* (1986), Rothman *et al.* (1995).

an effect on cephalic neural-crest cells and their derivatives or may be due to the differential expression of different isoforms of ALDH within the brain (Niederreither *et al.*, 2000; Rosa *et al.*, 1986; Rothman *et al.*, 1995). In a study of 339 cases by Rothman *et al.* (1995), 121 infants were born with birth defects that were of cranial-neural-crest origin. When this was correlated to total retinoid intake (from food and supplements) the risk of deformities increased with increased exposure. Specifically, 1% of babies born to women who ingested less than 500 IU/day of retinol exhibited embryopathology. This rate increased to 3% when retinol was ingested at doses greater than 15 000 IU/day. A separate examination of 24 cases demonstrated that ingestion of retinol at doses of 25 000 IU or more during the first trimester led to birth defects in all but one case (Dolk *et al.*, 1999). Additionally, an increased risk was associated with pure vitamin A supplements but not with vitamin A ingested as a multivitamin supplement (Martinez-Frias and Salvador, 1990; Werler *et al.*, 1990).

Analysis of data from a wide range of epidemiological studies has not provided a definitive lowest adverse effect level for the teratogenicity of vitamin A. However, recommendations from the International Vitamin A Consultative Group state that 10 000 IU/day of vitamin A can be safely ingested throughout pregnancy. In developing countries, where hypovitaminosis A is endemic, weekly supplementation of as much as 25 000 IU can be safely used as an alternative to daily supplementation (Underwood, 1998). Furthermore, pharmacokinetic data has demonstrated that following administration of 30 000 IU/day of vitamin A, plasma levels of retinoids did not exceed those found in pregnant women who delivered healthy babies (Miller *et al.*, 1998; Wiegand *et al.*, 1998). Additionally, a study which examined 935 cases of periconceptional vitamin A supplementation found no association between vitamin A supplementation (8000–25 000 IU/day) and neural tube defects or other major malformations (Mills *et al.*, 1997). While this data suggests that vitamin A rich foods such as animal liver can be consumed occasionally during pregnancy and lactation without risk of teratogenic effects (Buss *et al.*, 1994), others have recommended that liver and liver products be avoided during pregnancy (Dolk *et al.*, 1999) and a cautious approach may be prudent in well-nourished individuals.

β-Carotene toxicity

β-carotene is substantially less toxic than retinol and there is no teratogenic risk associated with prolonged consumption of natural sources or supplements containing provitamin A carotenoids (Hathcock *et al.*, 1990; Heywood *et al.*, 1985). Clinical trials have shown β-carotene to be safe at doses up to 180 mg/day for 15 years (Meyers *et al.*, 1996) and it is postulated to be a possible replacement for retinol in supplementation therapy (Hathcock *et al.*, 1990; Mathas-Vliegen and Tytgat, 1983). Due to the limited absorption of β-carotene from the gut and the poor conversion of this precursor to retinol in the intestine, the ingestion of β-carotene rarely results in symptoms of hypervitaminosis A (Grolier *et al.*, 1995; Sharman, 1985). There has been only one reported case of high β-carotene ingestion resulting in hypervitaminosis A and once the patient's diet was properly adjusted the symptoms resolved (Nagai *et al.*, 1999).

More commonly, excessive ingestion of carotenoids leads to hypercarotenemia (Sharman, 1985). This disease is characterized by the yellowing of the skin, particularly in nasolabial folds, the fat pads of the hands and the soles of the feet (Meyers *et al.*, 1996). It is distinguishable from jaundice as the sclera remain white, instead of turning yellow (Olson, 1987). However, these symptoms generally resolve after the carotene intake is restricted. Another serious consequence of hypercarotenemia is amenorrhea (Kemmann *et al.*, 1983). In a review of nine women with amenorrhea, diet was identified as a contributing factor. All of these women were on a diet containing large amounts of raw vegetables, particularly carrots. Unlike previous studies where anorexia was linked to the development of amenorrhea, the women in this study were within normal weight ranges. Following dietary counseling, eight of the patients modified their diet and menstruation returned to normal. One patient subsequently returned to the original diet and amenorrhea recurred. In the two patients that did not modify their eating habits amenorrhea continued. Whether the health problems in these patients were due to the β-carotene content of the food has not been conclusively proven. Other components of the food may have triggered these responses (Mathews-Roth, 1983). In fact, one study reports the development of leukopenia in patients consuming large amounts of carrots and upon modification of the diet the leukopenia reversed (Mathews-Roth, 1983). However, when the patients were challenged with a dose of purified β-carotene the symptoms did not recur, which suggests that other compounds in the carrots were responsible for the leukopenia (Mathews-Roth, 1983).

While β-carotene is essentially non-toxic, interactions between smoking and β-carotene have been reported. Two epidemiological studies have demonstrated an increased risk of lung cancer when smokers used β-carotene supplements. Specifically, after 18 months of β-carotene supplementation (20 mg/day) smokers exhibited an elevated lung cancer risk which continued to increase over time (Heionen *et al.*, 1994). Following 7.5 years of supplementation, the incidence of lung cancer was increased 18% in the supplemented group (Heionen *et al.*, 1994). Subsequently, the β-carotene and retinol efficacy trial (CARET) examined the combination of 30 mg β-carotene and 25 000 IU retinyl palmitate in 18 314 individuals with a high risk of developing lung cancer. The results showed an increase in relative risk from 1.28 to 1.53 over a five-year period (Omenn *et al.*, 1996). Animal studies have supported these epidemiological findings. For example, there was an increase in the proliferation of lung tissue in ferrets exposed to β-carotene (2.4 mg/day) and the equivalent of 20 cigarettes a day (Wang *et al.*, 1999). This correlated with an 18–73% decrease in RARβ expression and a 3–4-fold increase in the immediate early genes, c-fos and c-jun (Wang *et al.*, 1999). Retinoid signaling through RARβ has been proposed to inhibit AP-1 activity and therefore result in tumor suppression. The correlation between an increase in critical components in the AP-1 complex, namely c-fos and c-jun levels, and a decrease in RARβ gene expression supports this conclusion. Therefore, a decrease in RARβ protein levels would result in a decreased ability to suppress tumor growth and may be the cause of the increased risk of lung cancer following β-carotene supplementation. Other mechanisms may contribute to this effect as cleavage products of β-carotene upregulate hepatic enzymes (Gradelet *et al.*, 1996b). Therefore, it is also possible that the increased risk of lung cancer will result from an increase in the activation of carcinogens contained in cigarette smoke. However, definitive proof for such an effect has not been demonstrated.

Retinoid-induced modulation of drug-metabolizing enzymes and cofactors

The cytochrome P450 (CYP450) enzyme system is a superfamily of membrane bound mono-oxogenases that have an essential role in phase I biotransformation reactions as they metabolize a diverse range of endogenous and exogenous compounds (Guengerich, 1987; Vermeulen, 1996). While CYP450 enzymes are found in most tissues, their highest concentrations are found in the liver (Parkinson, 1996). Due to the immense spectrum of isoforms in the CYP450 superfamily, they are further categorized into families and subfamilies. Families, designated CYP1, CYP2, etc., exhibit at least 50% amino acid sequence homology within the grouping, while subfamilies, designated CYP1A, CYP2A, etc., exhibit at least 60% sequence homology (Vermeulen, 1996). Individual isoforms have been assigned numbers, CYP1A1, CYP1A2, etc., in the order in which they have been identified (Vermeulen, 1996). Human liver microsomes can contain 15 or more different CYP450s (Guengerich, 1994), but the most clinically relevant families are CYP1, CYP2, and CYP3. This is due to the fact that most of the endogenous chemicals and drugs metabolized by the CYP450 superfamily are metabolized by one of these three families (Parkinson, 1996). An important feature of these enzymes is that their abundance and activity can be induced and/or inhibited by various chemicals (Parkinson, 1996). Additionally, disease states and changes in physiological parameters such as fasting induces the specific CYP450 isoforms CYP2E1 (Ioannides *et al.*, 1996) and CYP2A1 (Imaoka *et al.*, 1990). This can increase the metabolism of drugs/chemicals metabolized by these CYP450 isoforms and, depending on the chemical, ultimately result in altered therapeutic concentrations of drugs and/or increases the generation of toxic metabolites.

Since the modulation of CYP450 enzyme activity is of clinical significance, many investigations have concentrated on retinol's effect on this enzyme system. These examinations have included studies of animals fed both retinoid supplemented and retinoid deficient diets. When hamsters and rats were fed a retinoid deficient diet for 6–10 weeks, a decrease in total hepatic CYP450 was observed (Grolier *et al.*, 1990; Siddik *et al.*, 1980; Ushio *et al.*, 1995). In the guinea pig, a vitamin A deficient diet for nine weeks decreased the catalytic activity of hepatic CYP1A1, CYP2E1, and CYP2A2 (Miranda *et al.*, 1979). Other studies have also shown that levels of CYP2C7 may be regulated by

Table 5.3 Abundance of clinically important CYP450 isoforms in human liver and selective substrates

CYP450 isoform	Abundance (% of total)	Selective substrates
CYP1A2	12.7 ± 6.2	Caffeine, phenacetin, theophylline, R-warfarin
CYP2A6	4.0 ± 3.2	Coumarin, nicotine
CYP2C8,9,18	18.2 ± 6.7	S-warfarin, phenytoin, ibuprofen, diclofenac
CYP2E1	6.6 ± 2.9	Ethanol, acetaminophen, halothane, nitrosamines
CYP3A	28.8 ± 10.4	Testosterone, tamoxifen, erythromycin, prednisone

Adapted from Parkinson (1996), Vermeulen (1996).

retinoic acid concentrations. Specifically, cultured rat hepatocytes maintained in a retinol deficient environment had a decreased expression of CYP2C7 but the levels returned to normal after retinoic acid administration (Westin *et al.*, 1997). This work demonstrates that retinoids are required to maintain constitutive levels of CYP450 enzymes in various species. However, the mechanism by which retinoid deficiency decreases CYP450 has not been elucidated.

Many studies examining retinoid supplementation and drug metabolism have focused on CYP3A activity, due to the clinical relevance of this isoform as it is responsible for the metabolism of more than 70 medications as well as many endogenous compounds (Pichard *et al.*, 1990) and is the most abundant CYP450 isoform in humans (Table 5.3) (Maurel, 1996). Specific results demonstrated a 1.6-fold increase in the polypeptide levels of hepatic CYP3A in rats fed a diet supplemented with retinyl acetate (25 IU/g) for 15 weeks (Murray *et al.*, 1991). Additionally, Badger *et al.* (1998) reported a 132% increase in rat hepatic CYP3A catalytic activity following one day of retinol gavage (75 mg/kg). However, these values returned to within normal limits 48 h following retinol and by 96 h CYP3A catalytic activity had dropped to below control levels (Badger *et al.*, 1998). CYP3A was also increased in rabbits fed a diet containing 250 IU of retinyl palmitate/g for seven weeks (Miranda and Chhabra, 1981). Additionally, CYP3A mRNA levels were increased approximately 8-fold in rat hepatocytes treated with retinoids (Jurima-Romet *et al.*, 1997). The response is species-specific, however, as retinyl palmitate (50 IU/g diet) decreased CYP3A activity 1.4-fold when administered to Syrian hamsters for five weeks (Ushio *et al.*, 1995). Similar results were seen in Balb/c mice where retinol (75 mg/kg per day, 4 days) decreased both the catalytic activity and polypeptide levels of hepatic CYP3A 2-fold (Bray *et al.*, 2001). Interestingly, the catalytic activity and polypeptide levels of CYP3A returned to normal two days after retinol administration had ceased (Bray and Rosengren, 2001). This could indicate that prolonged drug interactions are less likely to occur through changes in this CYP450 isoform as the activity and protein levels return to normal levels soon after the discontinuation of retinol supplementation in both rats and mice.

The second most abundant CYP450 subfamily in humans is CYP2C (Vermeulen, 1996). Changes in the expression and activity of this subfamily are important due to both its abundance and its role in the metabolism of many medications such as tricyclic antidepressants, phenytoin and warfarin (Richardson and Johnson, 1996). In rats, ingestion of a retinyl acetate (25 IU/g) supplemented diet for 15 weeks resulted in a decrease in hepatic CYP2C11 and CYP2C6 (Murray et al., 1991). This effect was supported by Badger et al. (1998), who demonstrated that a single oral dose of all-trans-retinol (75 mg/kg) decreased CYP2C11 by 30% in male rats. Additionally, an interaction between growth hormone, retinoid function and CYP2C7 has been proposed as hepatocytes treated with retinol and retinoic acid increased CYP2C7 mRNA levels (Westin et al., 1997). Following continuous treatment, growth hormone slightly increased CYP2C7 mRNA while the combination of growth hormone and retinol led to an 8-fold induction of CYP2C7 (Westin et al., 1997).

The CYP1A subfamily constitutes 12% of CYP450 levels in humans and is responsible for the metabolism of both drugs and carcinogens (Vermeulen, 1996). Additionally, there has been some evidence that retinoids may be involved in the regulation of the CYP1A gene. Vecchini et al. (1994) demonstrated the presence of a retinoic acid response element on the human CYP1A1 gene from normal human keratinocytes. In vivo studies have produced mixed results as CYP1A1 activity was inhibited 60% and 55% in the Sprague-Dawley rat following four days of retinyl acetate (320 mg/kg per day) and 13-cis-retinoic acid (235 mg/kg per day) administration, respectively (McCarthy et al., 1987). Alternatively, in both the guinea pig and rabbit no significant change in CYP1A1 activity occurred following dietary supplementation with retinyl palmitate (250–500 IU/g diet) (Miranda and Chhabra, 1981). However, inhibition studies have demonstrated that all-trans-retinol, retinal, retinoic acid and retinyl palmitate are all competitive inhibitors of rat CYP1A1 with K_i values that ranged from 0.068 to 2 μM (Inouye et al., 1999). CYP1A1 is also regulated by ligands for the aryl hydrocarbon receptor (AhR), a ligand-inducible nuclear transcription factor that belongs to the same nuclear receptor family as the retinoic acid receptor and initiates a signal transduction pathway (Whitlock, 1990) in a similar manner to the retinoic acid receptor (Mangelsdorf et al., 1994). Additionally, 2,3,7,8-tetrachlorodibenzo-p-dioxin (TCDD), the most potent ligand for the AhR, exhibits responses similar to retinoic acid (teratogenicity and weight loss) (Birnbaum et al., 1989) and TCDD exposure in rodents results in both the depletion of hepatic retinoids (Fletcher et al., 2001) and the alteration of vitamin A metabolism (Thunberg et al., 1980). Therefore, interactions between these receptors may be partly responsible for the decreased transcriptional activity of CYP1A1 following retinoid exposure.

Other CYP450 isoforms with a lower abundance have also been examined following retinoid treatment. Specifically, the CYP2E and CYP2A subfamilies constitute only 6% and 4% of total hepatic CYP450, respectively (Vermeulen, 1996). However, induction of CYP2E1 has significant consequences as overexpression of this isoform can itself result in an increase in reactive oxygen species, thereby eliciting a toxic response in the absence of a toxic stimulus (Nieto *et al.*, 1999; Wu and Cederbaum, 2001). Additionally, CYP2E1 and CYP2A are responsible for the bioactivation of many chemical carcinogens (Raucy *et al.*, 1993) and toxicants (Chang and Waxman, 1996). In guinea pigs and rats, retinol and derivatives induce CYP2E1. Miranda and Chhabra (1981) showed a 2-fold increase in CYP2E1 activity in guinea pigs fed a retinol-supplemented (500 IU retinyl palmitate/g) diet for six weeks. Furthermore, rats gavaged with all-*trans*-retinol (75 mg/kg) induced hepatic CYP2E1 polypeptide levels and catalytic activity (Badger *et al.*, 1996; Wijeweera *et al.*, 1996). However, retinol did not induce CYP2E1 in all species, as CYP2E1 catalytic activity and polypeptide levels remained at control levels following retinol treatment in mice (Bray *et al.*, 2001; Inder *et al.*, 1999) and retinyl palmitate treatment in rabbits (Miranda and Chhabra, 1981). Investigations with the CYP2A sub-family are limited but have shown that hamsters given a supplement of retinyl palmitate (250 IU/g diet for six weeks) had a marked increase in the activity and polypeptide levels of CYP2A1 (Ushio *et al.*, 1995). Additionally, CYP2A1 and CYP2A2 were also increased in rats following retinyl acetate (25 IU/g diet for 15 weeks) (Murray *et al.*, 1991).

A novel CYP450 family CYP26, also termed P450RAI, has been character-ized in zebrafish, humans and rodents (Ray *et al.*, 1997; White *et al.*, 1996). In addition to catalyzing the metabolism of retinoic acid to 4-oxo-retinoic acid, the expression of this family was shown to be upregulated by retinoic acid. The induction of CYP26 occurred in mice administered a single dose of all-*trans*-retinoic acid (100 mg/kg, ip) but remained undetectable in untreated mice (Ray *et al.*, 1997). Further studies confirmed this response in mice and also demonstrated a dose–response relationship as 5 mg/kg of retinoic acid caused a slight induction of CYP26 while 100 mg/kg resulted in strong induction (Yamamoto *et al.*, 2000). Similarly, CYP26 induction was observed in rats as both retinoic acid administration (100 mg/kg) and dietary vitamin A (50 mg retinyl palmitate/kg diet) induced CYP26 (Yamamoto *et al.*, 2000). Further-more, functionality of CYP26 was demonstrated as the induction of hepatic CYP26 mRNA correlated with the formation of the metabolite 4-oxo-retinoic acid in liver microsomes (Yamamoto *et al.*, 2000). Interestingly, an age-specific induction of CYP26 was observed, as CYP26 was barely detectable in the liver of rats supplemented with vitamin A for two to three months but increased with both age (in rats on the control diet) and duration (in rats supplemented for 8–22 months) (Yamamoto *et al.*, 2000). Therefore, there is strong evidence of the induction of CYP26 by retinoic acid as there was an identifiable dose–response relationship and a significant correlation between hepatic CYP26 mRNA content and total liver retinol (Yamamoto *et al.*, 2000).

The mechanism for the modulation of the various CYP450 isoforms has not been conclusively determined. However, RAR and RXR-specific modulation of CYP450 has been shown (Howell *et al.*, 1998). Ligands with RAR activity (e.g. Tretinoin) decreased hepatic CYP450 levels, while those exhibiting pre-dominantly RXR activity (e.g. Targretin) increased CYP450 levels. CYP3A in particular was decreased by RAR-selective retinoids and induced by RXR-selective retinoids (Howell *et al.*, 1998).

The previous studies all analyzed the effects produced by the administration of specific retinoids. However, carotenoids have been analyzed for their effect on various drug metabolizing enzymes and the compounds studied include precursors of vitamin A such as β-carotene and β-apo-8′-carotene as well as canthaxanthin and astaxanthin which are non-provitamin A carotenoids (Figure 5.2). All of these compounds have been examined in both rats and mice at a level of 300 mg/kg diet for 15 days. In rats, β-apo-8′-carotene induced the catalytic activities of CYP1A1 158-fold and CYP2B 9-fold but did not alter CYP2E1 or CYP3A (Gradelet *et al.*, 1996b). Additionally, canthaxanthin induced the catalytic activity of CYP1A1 139-fold and CYP2B 27-fold while astaxanthin only induced CYP1A1 27-fold (Gradelet *et al.*, 1996a). Further-more, the hepatic carotenoid content was 10-fold higher in canthaxanthin treated rats compared to astaxanthin treated rats. This study was supported by work conducted by Jewell and O'Brien (1999) who demonstrated that both canthaxanthin and astaxanthin induced pulmonary CYP1A1 3-fold and renal CYP1A1 11- to 32-fold. In mice, only a modest 3-fold increase in both CYP1A1 and CYP2B was observed following canthaxanthin ingestion while astaxanthin and β-apo-8′-carotene resulted in a 2-fold increase in CYP2B (Astorg *et al.*, 1997). All other CYP450 isoforms remained unchanged in the mouse. Interest-ingly, in both species β-carotene did not induce CYP450 isoforms. Therefore, dietary carotenoids modulated the activity of CYP1A1 and CYP2B but this effect is specific to both the carotenoid and the species examined.

While many studies have focused on retinoid modulation of CYP450 isoforms, work probing the effect of retinoids on conjugation enzymes has also been conducted. Conjugation reactions function to enhance the elimination of both endogenous and exogenous chemicals by forming metabolites with an increased molecular weight and water solubility. Glucuronide conjugation is one of the major pathways in this system and occurs via the enzyme uridine diphos-phoglucuronosyltransferase (UDPGT) and the high energy cofactor uridine diphosphoglucuronic acid (UDPGA). In general this enzymatic family is non-specific with regard to substrate, but is able to conjugate phenolic compounds with high capacity (Parkinson, 1996). In the mouse, retinol gavage (75 mg/kg per day, four days) did not alter the activity of *p*-nitrophenol-UDPGT (Bray *et al.*, 2000). The effect of retinoids on the activity of this enzyme has not been examined in other species. However, carotenoid ingestion (300 mg/kg diet of β-apo-8′-carotene, canthaxanthin or astaxanthin for 15 days) did not alter UDPGT activity in the mouse (Astorg *et al.*, 1997). In contrast, UDPGT activity in-creased 2-fold in the rat following the ingestion of these carotenoids (Gradelet *et al.*, 1996a, 1996b). Hepatic UDPGA concentration is also a critical determin-ant of glucuronide conjugation. However, only one study has examined hepatic UDPGA stores following retinoid administration. The results demonstrated that oral retinol (75 mg/kg per day, four days) reduced hepatic UDPGA levels by 73% (Bray and Rosengren, 2001). This large reduction in hepatic UDPGA stores significantly altered the capacity of glucuronide conjugation in the mouse. Since the activity of UDPGT was increased 2-fold in rats following carotenoid ingestion, and rats have 12.5% lower hepatic UDPGA levels than mice (Wong, 1977), it is possible that retinoid ingestion would also significantly decrease glucuronide conjugation in this species.

A minor but important conjugation pathway is methylation, which uses the enzyme methyltransferase and the cofactor S-adenosylmethionine (SAM) to mask functional groups by adding a methyl group onto the compound (Parkinson, 1996). Glycine N-methyltransferase (GNMT) is one of the key cytosolic enzymes involved in this process. Methyl groups have an important role in health and disease as reduced methylation of DNA can result in hepatocarcinogenesis (Ghoshal and Farber, 1984). This can occur through either a dietary methyl group deficiency or a direct activation of GNMT activity resulting in a depletion of SAM and ultimately a downregulation of SAM-dependent transmethylation reactions (Mason, 1994). Therefore, retinol-mediated changes in the regulation and function of GNMT have been examined. Induction of GNMT by retinoids was demonstrated when rats were administered retinyl palmitate, 13-*cis*-retinoic acid and all-*trans*-retinoic acid (30 μmol/kg per day, 10 days). All-*trans*-retinoic acid was the most potent inducer of hepatic GNMT as activity and protein levels were increased 124%, while 13-*cis*-retinoic acid increased GNMT activity and protein 74% (Rowling *et al.*, 2002). Interestingly, the increase in GNMT was tissue-specific as retinoids did not alter renal or pancreatic GNMT (McMullen *et al.*, 2002). Additionally, female Sprague-Dawley rats were less sensitive to the effects of all-*trans*-retinoic acid, as GNMT activity was increased 59% compared to a 197% increase in males (McMullen *et al.*, 2002). However, in both sexes, the decrease in the availability of methyl groups for SAM-dependent transmethylation reactions proved to be of biological significance as the SAM-dependent synthesis of creatinine was reduced 21% following the administration of all-*trans*-retinoic acid (McMullen *et al.*, 2002).

Since retinol has antioxidant and cancer preventative properties, many studies have investigated the effect of various retinoids and carotenoids on the activity of glutathione S-transferase (GST). This enzyme, and the cofactor glutathione (GSH), conjugate a wide range of electrophilic compounds (Parkinson, 1996). The proper function of this conjugation system is important as it provides an endogenous protective mechanism for the elimination of free radicals and it has been postulated that retinol's antioxidant properties may result in the enhancement of this endogenous system. However, GST activity consistently remained unchanged following the ingestion of different carotenoids and retinoids by both rats and mice (Astorg *et al.*, 1997; Bray *et al.*, 2001; Gradelet *et al.*, 1996a, 1996b; Jewell and O'Brien, 1999; McCarthy *et al.*, 1987). Additionally, glutathione peroxidase was unchanged in chickens fed 240 mg of retinol acetate/kg diet for 20 days (Ozturk-Urek *et al.*, 2001). Analysis of the cofactor GSH in either mice (Bray *et al.*, 2001) or rats (Rowling *et al.*, 2002) also showed no change in total hepatic GSH following treatment with various retinoids, namely retinol, retinyl palmitate, 13-*cis*-retinoic acid and all-*trans*-retinoic acid. Therefore, it is apparent that retinoid supplementation does not alter glutathione conjugation via changes in either enzyme activity or cofactor concentration.

Modulation of toxicity

Potentiation of chemical-induced hepatotoxicity by retinoids

Numerous studies in a variety of rodent species have demonstrated that retinol pretreatment potentiates the hepatotoxicity of a variety of drugs and chemicals. For example, in the Sprague-Dawley rat, retinol potentiates the hepatotoxicity induced by ethanol (Leo and Lieber, 1983), carbon tetrachloride (CCl_4) (Badger *et al.*, 1996; Hooser *et al.*, 1994), allyl alcohol, endotoxin and acetaminophen (El Sisi *et al.*, 1993b). In the mouse, retinol potentiates the hepatotoxicity of allyl alcohol, galactosamine and acetaminophen (Rosengren *et al.*, 1995). In all these cases, the administration of retinol itself did not induce hepatotoxicity as determined by both histological and enzymatic examinations. Instead, retinol altered specific parameters that resulted in mechanistic-specific potentiation of the hepatotoxicity elicited by each of these chemicals.

The interaction between retinol and ethanol has been extensively examined in the areas of both retinol supplementation and deficiency. Leo *et al.* (1982) first described the potentiation of ethanol toxicity by vitamin A. In this study, male Sprague-Dawley rats were fed diets containing 29 000 IU/L of retinyl acetate, Lieber-DeCarli diet (ethanol as 36% of calories) or a combination of the two for eight weeks. Livers from rats fed retinyl acetate appeared normal while minor hepatic changes were observed in the ethanol-fed rats. However, in combination, striking lesions were produced which included the appearance of giant mitochondria with an unusual dense matrix and a large fusiform crystalline inclusion. These morphological changes correlated with a 40–50% decrease in oxygen consumption in isolated mitochondria in state 3 respiration compared to mitochondria from controls (Leo *et al.*, 1982). Similar effects on mitochondria have been reported in humans. For example, the addition of 10 000 IU vitamin A per day for four months to the diet of an alcoholic resulted in a 1000-fold increase in the size of mitochondria, which also contained striking filamentous or crystalline-like inclusions (Leo and Lieber, 1999; Worner *et al.*, 1988). These types of inclusions have been reported in the mitochondria of hypervitaminosis A patients (Minuk *et al.*, 1988), but in these cases the duration and quantity of vitamin A ingested was significantly greater. Therefore, ethanol elicited a profound effect on the toxicity of retinol. This effect was further characterized in a study in which rats were administered the Lieber-DeCarli diet and retinyl acetate for a much longer duration (nine months). Under these conditions, hepatic inflammation and necrosis occurred which correlated with markedly elevated levels of plasma transaminases (ALT and AST enzyme activities) and mitochondrial injury correlated with increases in glutamate dehydrogenase (GDH) activity (Leo and Lieber, 1999). However, less dramatic results were reported when both BN/BiRij and Wag/Rij rats were administered the Lieber-DeCarli diet and retinyl acetate for 16 months. These rats displayed minimal non-specific reactive inflammation and hepatocyte necrosis (Bosma *et al.*, 1991) with slightly elevated ALT, AST and GDH activities (Seifert *et al.*, 1991). Additionally, the liver stores of retinoids were not altered in these rats. The authors speculated that increases in vitamin A hepatotoxicity might be confined to situations in which ethanol causes a disturbance in retinol metabolism, as previous work had demonstrated that ethanol caused a decrease in hepatic retinoid stores in Sprague-Dawley rats, baboons (Sato and Lieber, 1981) and humans (Leo and Lieber, 1982), but not the BN/BiRij or Wag/Rij rats (Seifert *et al.*, 1991). Therefore, the toxicity of the combination of ethanol and retinol appears to be dependent on the genetic background of the test species and, similar to other interactions, species- and strain-dependent responses occur.

While β-carotene does not induce hepatotoxicity, similar toxic interactions have been reported with ethanol. Specifically, in baboons the combination of ethanol and β-carotene caused mitochondrial damage, as determined by increases in plasma GDH activity and hepatic ultrastructural changes (Leo *et al.*, 1992) and this correlated with 4-fold and 10-fold increases in liver and plasma β-carotene, respectively. Similar results have been demonstrated following combination treatment in rats (Leo *et al.*, 1997). It is interesting to note that ethanol causes an increase in the storage of vitamin A's precursor β-carotene, but decreases the storage of vitamin A. However, the increase in hepatic β-carotene did not reduce the oxidative stress induced by ethanol (Leo *et al.*, 1997).

In the rat, retinol's potentiation of CCl_4-induced hepatotoxicity is linked to an increase in the generation of reactive oxygen species and an increase in CYP2E1 catalytic activity. Specifically, one day of all-*trans*-retinol (75 mg/kg) increased plasma ALT activity and the area of necrotic hepatocytes 10-fold compared to CCl_4 (0.2 ml/kg) alone (Badger *et al.*, 1996). The major theory regarding the mechanism of this potentiation is that retinol pretreatment primes Kupffer cells (the macrophage of the liver) which become activated by the damaged hepatocytes (Figure 5.4). Activated Kupffer cells then release reactive oxygen species that potentiate liver injury. Evidence to support this mechanism includes a 50% reduction in the potentiated liver injury when the Kupffer cell inactivator (gadolinium chloride, 10 mg/kg) was administered prior to retinol (Badger *et al.*, 1996). Additionally, Kupffer cells isolated from rats 24 h following a single dose of retinol (75 mg/kg) produced a 2-fold greater amount of superoxide anion following stimulation compared to control Kupffer cells (Badger *et al.*, 1996). Moreover, other studies examining both Kupffer cell inhibitors (methyl palmitate) and scavengers of reactive oxygen species (catalase and superoxide dismutase) demonstrated that each of these treatments reversed retinol's potentiation of CCl_4-induced hepatotoxicity following seven days of retinol (75 mg/kg) pretreatment (El Sisi *et al.*, 1993a). However, other mechanisms cannot be completely excluded as a single dose of retinol elevated CYP2E1 catalytic activity 2.3-fold, while seven days of retinol elevated CYP2E1 activity 1.9-fold (Badger *et al.*, 1996). Since CCl_4 is bioactivated by CYP2E1 to a toxic free radical, an increase in CYP2E1 catalytic activity could also contribute to

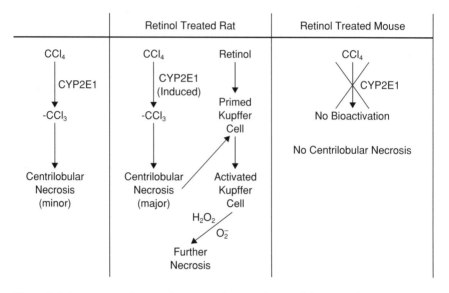

Figure 5.4 Species-specific mechanism of retinol's modulation of CCl₄-induced hepatotoxicity.

the increase in hepatotoxicity. Therefore, the authors concluded that large doses of retinol can influence both the initiation (increase in CYP2E1) of CCl₄-induced hepatotoxicity and its further progression (Kupffer cell activation) and that the dose and duration of retinol treatment has an influence on which effect dominates (Badger *et al.*, 1996). Interestingly, this effect is species-specific as 75 mg/kg of all-*trans*-retinol for three to seven days protected against CCl₄-induced hepatotoxicity in mice (Inder *et al.*, 1999; Rosengren *et al.*, 1995). In this species retinol did not alter constitutive levels of CYP2E1 but instead prevented the bioactivation of CCl₄ by CYP2E1 (Inder *et al.*, 1999). Therefore, species is also a critical factor in determining how retinol modulates the toxicity of CCl₄.

While the interaction between retinol and acetaminophen in the rat has not been defined, the mechanism of this interaction has been elucidated in the mouse. In this species four to seven days of retinol (75 mg/kg) caused a 3-fold increase in the hepatotoxicity induced by acetaminophen as indicated by plasma ALT activity and histological examination of liver sections (Bray and Rosengren, 2001; Rosengren *et al.*, 1995). It was conclusively proven that the mechanism for this effect was due to a 73% depletion of hepatic UDPGA stores 24 hours following retinol treatment (Figure 5.5) (Bray and Rosengren, 2001). This was significant because glucuronide conjugation is the major pathway responsible for the safe elimination of acetaminophen. Therefore, under the conditions of significantly decreased UDPGA most of the acetaminophen administered was bioactivated to N-acetyl *p*-benzoquinoneimine (NAPQI), the toxic metabolite responsible for acetaminophen hepatotoxicity, and thus acetaminophen-induced hepatotoxicity was potentiated. UDPGA was determined to be the limiting

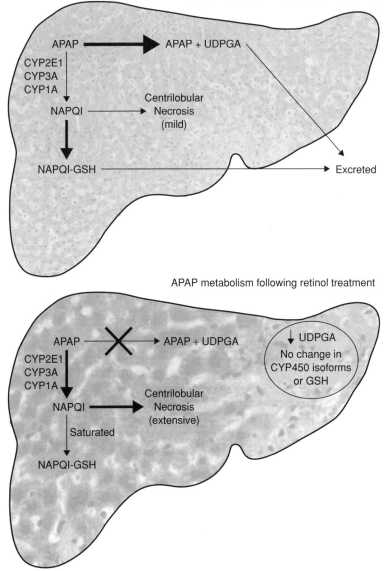

Figure 5.5 Mechanism of retinol's potentiation of acetaminophen (APAP)-induced hepatotoxicity in the mouse.

factor of this conjugation pathway as retinol had no effect on the activity of the enzyme UDPGT (Bray *et al.*, 2000). Additionally, retinol did not alter any of the other pathways responsible for activation or elimination of acetaminophen, namely CYP1A2, CYP2E1, CYP3A and GSH (Bray *et al.*, 2001; Bray and

Rosengren, 2001). Therefore, retinol's depletion of UDPGA was determined to be the mechanism responsible for the potentiated hepatotoxicity. It is worth noting that retinol's depletion of UDPGA could also inhibit the conjugation of other phenolic compounds that undergo extensive glucuronidation and therefore this mechanism defined for acetaminophen and retinol may have wider implications.

Toxic interactions with non-toxic agents

Interestingly, non-toxic concentrations of retinoids have shown toxic responses when concurrently administered with other non-toxic chemicals. Specifically, when retinyl acetate (250 mg/kg diet) and butylated hydroxytoluene (BHT) (5 g/kg diet) were administered to weanling female rats for 27 weeks hepatotoxicity occurred as evidenced by hepatomegaly, periportal fibrosis and bile duct hyperplasia (McCormick et al., 1986). This result was significant, as previous work had shown that both retinyl acetate and BHT at these doses were devoid of hepatotoxicity (McCormick et al., 1984; Moon et al., 1976). The two were administered to determine if the combination would increase their effectiveness as inhibitors of DMBA-induced carcinogenesis. While both compounds increased the magnitude of cancer chemoprevention, the potentiated hepatotoxicity demonstrated that these two compounds could not be used in combination as chemopreventative agents.

Toxic interactions with other vitamins

The excessive consumption of vitamin A can affect both the absorption and physiological functions of other vitamins including D, E, K and C. Specifically, animal studies have demonstrated that vitamin A antagonizes the physiological functions of vitamin D (Metz et al., 1985; Rodahl, 1943; Woodard et al., 1997). Hypervitaminosis A is associated with bone resorption and an increased fracture incidence in both animals (Hough et al., 1988; Wolbach, 1947) and humans (Frame et al., 1974; Gerber et al., 1954; Hathcock et al., 1990). The mechanism of this effect is thought to involve both a direct effect of vitamin A on bone growth and the maintenance and antagonism of the actions of vitamin D. In vitro studies have demonstrated that vitamin A stimulated bone resorption via an increase in osteoclast formation and the stimulation of mature osteoclast activity (Oreffo et al., 1988; Saneshigo et al., 1995). Furthermore, collagen synthesis was inhibited in cultured rat and chick calvarium models (Dickson and Walls, 1985). This is supported by in vivo evidence which reported an 86% decrease in serum bioactive-parathyroid hormone following acute administration of retinyl palmitate (60 mg RE/day for two days) (Frankel et al., 1986). These studies demonstrate both a direct effect of vitamin A on bone resorption and a secondary effect through hormonal activation of osteoclasts. Additionally, in vivo studies have shown that vitamin A antagonizes the effect of vitamin D. In rats, administration of vitamin A (30 000 IU) ameliorated the toxicity of vitamin D (60 000 IU) (Clark and Bassett, 1962). Conversely, addition of vitamin D to a high vitamin A diet in turkey poults reversed the symptoms of hypervitaminosis A (Metz *et al.*, 1985). More recently, Rohde *et al.* (1999) demonstrated that retinyl acetate dose-dependently antagonized the effects of vitamin D. Specifically, when rats were fed increasing doses of retinyl acetate (0–8621 µg/day) there was a progressive decrease in total bone ash and an increase in epiphyseal plate width (Rohde *et al.*, 1999). These effects could be reversed by the addition of vitamin D to the diet. This interaction is thought to be due to competition for RXR, through which both hormones control gene transcription, as vitamin D binds to RXR and modulates gene transcription through vitamin D responsive elements (VDRE) (Munder*et al.*, 1994; Ross *et al.*, 1994). Since 9-*cis*-retinoic acid binds RXR and regulates gene transcription through RARE (Mangelsdorf and Evans, 1995), there is a direct competition between these two vitamins at the receptor level. However, to date most of the evidence for the antagonistic effects of these vitamins has come from animal studies and it has not been definitively proven that this effect occurs in humans. While it has been documented in case studies that hypervitaminosis A results in skeletal changes, a recent epidemiological study failed to demonstrate a link between vitamin A and reduced bone density (Ballew *et al.*, 2001). The evaluation of 5790 participants did not identify a significant relationship between elevated serum retinyl esters ($\geq$10% of total serum vitamin A) and changes in bone mineral density at any of the four sites examined (femoral neck, trochanter, introchanter and total hip). Furthermore, there was no association with an increased risk of osteopenia or osteoporosis (Ballew *et al.*, 2001).

The positive impact of vitamin E on the symptoms of retinol toxicity was first reported in 1941 (Davies and Moore, 1941) and vitamin K_1 may have similar effects. Studies have demonstrated that vitamins E and K_1 act as antioxidants and thus prevent the membrane damage caused by unbound retinol (Lucy and Dingle, 1964; Massey *et al.*, 1982). Furthermore, vitamin E supplementation increased the hepatic storage of retinol (Krasinski *et al.*, 1989; Yang and Desai, 1977). However, this effect has not been examined with vitamin K_1. The accumulation of hepatic retinol may be the result of the inhibition of retinyl palmitate hydrolysis by both of these vitamins. In rat liver preparations, vitamin E (100 µM) and vitamin K_1 (50 µM) non-competitively inhibited retinyl palmitate hydrolysis by 55% and 66%, respectively (Napoli and Beck, 1984; Napoli *et al.*, 1984). The decrease in the hydrolysis of the storage form of retinol to the transportable form results in hepatic sequestering and lower plasma concentrations. Therefore, the combined effect of decreased retinol mobilization and the protective effects at the membrane account for vitamin E's attenuation of retinol toxicity (Jenkins and Mitchell, 1975).

Little has been documented regarding the interactions between vitamin A and vitamin C. However, in guinea pigs hypervitaminosis A is associated with a decrease in both the plasma and hepatic levels of vitamin C (Bendich and Langseth, 1989). In humans, a similar decrease in the storage of vitamin C has been reported (Bendich and Langseth, 1989). Additional findings in guinea pigs demonstrated that vitamin C reduced the toxicity of vitamin A.

Conclusions

Vitamin A has a high degree of therapeutic safety and as such has been examined as a potential chemotherapeutic agent. However, one serious consequence of vitamin A ingestion is that retinoic acid is a known teratogen at low doses. Additionally, overuse of this vitamin, both acutely and chronically, leads to a wide range of toxic side-effects that clinically manifest as hypervitaminosis A. Doses of vitamin A that do not elicit symptoms of hypervitaminosis A impact a wide variety of physiological processes, particularly within the liver. These include alterations in the activity of enzymes such as CYP450 and GNMT and the depletion of the cofactor UDPGA. Through distinct alterations of these processes and others, vitamin A potentiates the hepatotoxicity of ethanol, carbon tetrachloride and acetaminophen in rodents. With the exception of ethanol, the relevance of these effects to humans has not been determined. High levels of vitamin A also interact with the function of a number of other vitamins, namely E, D, K_1 and C. Of particular note is the strong effect of vitamin A on bone growth, an effect that may be due to antagonism of normal vitamin D-mediated responses. However, both vitamins K_1 and E can decrease the toxicity of vitamin A through mechanisms relating to membrane stabilization and enzyme regulation. Overall, there are a multitude of species-specific processes which are either altered by vitamin A or which themselves modulate the toxicity of vitamin A. Therefore, accurately predicting the toxicity of vitamin A in humans is a complex issue.

Acknowledgments

The authors would like to thank M.J. Le Nedelec for generating the figures and Y. Shepard for editorial support.

References

Astorg, P., Gradelet, S., Leclerc, J., and Siess, M.-H. (1997) Effects of provitamin A or non-provitamin A carotenoids on liver xenobiotic-metabolizing enzymes in mice, *Nutrition and Cancer*, **27**: 245–249.

Badger, D., Kraner, J., Fraser, D., Hoglen, N., Halpert, J., and Sipes, I.G. (1998) Reduction of thyroid hormone may participate in the modulation of cytochromes P4502C11 and 3A2 by retinol, *Life Science*, **63**: 367–372.

Badger, D.A., Sauer, J.-M., Hoglen, N.C., Jolley, C.S., and Sipes, I.G. (1996) The role of inflammatory cells and cytochrome P450 in the potentiation of CCl_4-induced liver injury by a single dose of retinol, *Toxicology and Applied Pharmacology*, **141**: 507–519.

Ballew, C., Galuska, D., and Gillespie, C. (2001) High serum retinyl esters are not associated with reduced bone mineral density in the third national health and nutrition examination survey, 1988–1994, *Journal Bone Mineral Research*, **16**: 2306–2312.

Bauernfiend, J.C. (1980) *The Safe Use of Vitamin A: a Report of the International Vitamin A Consultative Group*. Washington, DC: The Nutrition Foundation.

Bendich, A. and Langseth, L. (1989) Safety of vitamin A, *American Journal of Clinical Nutrition*, **49**: 358–371.

Biesalski, H.K. (1997) Bioavailability of vitamin A, *European Journal of Clinical Nutrition*, **51**: S71–S75.

Birnbaum, L.S., Harris, M.W., Stocking, L.M., Clark, A.M., and Morrissey, R.E. (1989) Retinoic acid and 2,3,7,8-tetrachlorodibenzo-p-dioxin selectively enhance teratogenesis in C57BL/6N mice, *Toxicology and Applied Pharmacology*, **98**: 487–500.

Boron, B., Hupert, J., Barch, D.H., Fox, C.C., Friedman, H., Layden, T.J. and Mobarhan, S. (1988) Effect of zinc deficiency on hepatic enzymes and regulating vitamin A status, *Journal of Nutrition*, **118**: 995–1001.

Bosma, A., Seifert, W.F., Wilson, J.H.P., Roholl, P.J.M., Brouwer, A., and Knook, D.L. (1991) Chronic administration of ethanol with high vitamin A supplementation in a liquid diet to rats does not cause liver fibrosis 1. Morphological observations, *Journal of Hepatology*, **13**: 240–248.

Bray, B.J., Goodin, M.G., Inder, R.E., and Rosengren, R.J. (2001) The effect of retinol on hepatic and renal drug-metabolizing enzymes, *Food Chemistry and Toxicology*, **39**: 1–9.

Bray, B.J., Inder, R.E., and Rosengren, R.J. (2000) Retinol-mediated effects on the activation and detoxification pathways of acetaminophen, *Australasian Journal of Ecotoxicology*, **6**: 75–79.

Bray, B.J. and Rosengren, R.J. (2001) Retinol potentiates acetaminophen-induced hepatotoxicity in the mouse: mechanistic studies, *Toxicology and Applied Pharmacology*, **173**: 129–136.

Bush, M.E. and Dahms, B.B. (1984) Fatal hypervitaminosis A in a neonate, *Archives of Pathology and Laboratory Medicine*, **108**: 838–842.

Buss, N.E., Tembe, E.A., Prendergast, B.D., Renwick, A.G., and George, C.F. (1994) The teratogenic metabolites of vitamin A in women following supplements and liver, *Human Experimental Toxicology*, **13**: 33–43.

Carpenter, T.O., Pettifor, J.M., Russell, R.M., Pitha, J., Mobarhan, S., Ossip, M.S., Wainer, S., and Anast, C.S. (1987) Severe hypervitaminosis A in siblings: evidence of variable tolerance to retinol intake, *Journal of Pediatrics*, **111**: 507–512.

Chang, T.K.H. and Waxman, D.J. (1996) The CYP2A subfamily. In *Cytochromes P450: Metabolic and Toxicological Aspects* (ed. C. Ioannides). Boca Raton, FL: CRC Press.

Chen, J., Hosward, W.N., and Juchau, M.R. (2000) Biosynthesis of all-trans-retinoic acid from all-trans-retinol: catalysis of all-trans-retinol oxidation by human P450 cytochromes, *Drug Metabolism and Dispersion*, **28**: 315–322.

Clark, I. and Bassett, C.A.L. (1962) The amelioration of hypervitaminosis D in rats with vitamin A, *Journal of Experimental Medicine*, **115**: 147–155.

Dal-Pizzol, F., Klamt, F., Benfato, M.S., Benard, E.A., and Moreira, J.C.F. (2001) Retinol supplementation induces oxidative stress and modulates antioxidant enzyme activities in rat sertoli cells, *Free Radical Research*, **34**: 395–404.

Davies, A.W. and Moore, T. (1941) Interactions of vitamins A and E, *Nature*, **147**: 794–796.

Dickson, I. and Walls, J. (1985) Vitamin A and bone formation: effects of an excess of retinol on bone collagen synthesis *in vitro*, *Biochemical Journal*, **226**: 789–795.

Dolk, H.M., Nau, H., Hummler, H., and Barlow, S.M. (1999) Dietary vitamin A and teratogenic risk: European Teratology Society discussion paper, *European Journal of Obstetrics and Gynecology*, **83**: 31–36.

Duester, G. (1996) Involvement of alcohol dehydrogenase, short-chain dehydrogenase/reductase, aldehyde dehydrogenase, and cytochrome P450 in the control of retinoid signalling by activation of retinoic acid synthesis, *Biochemistry*, **35**: 12221–12227.

Duester, G. (1998) Alcohol dehydrogenase as a critical mediator of retinoic acid synthesis from vitamin A in the mouse embryo, *Journal of Nutrition*, **128**: 459S–462S.

El Sisi, A.E., Earnest, D.L., and Sipes, I.G. (1993a) Vitamin A potentiation of carbon tetrachloride hepatotoxicity: role of liver macrophages and active oxygen species, *Toxicology and Applied Pharmacology*, **119**: 295–301.

El Sisi, A.E.D., Hall, P., Sim, W.-L.W., Earnest, D.L., and Sipes, I.G. (1993b) Characterization of vitamin A potentiation of carbon tetrachloride-induced liver injury, *Toxicology and Applied Pharmacology*, **119**: 280–288.

Ellis, J.K., Russell, R.M., Makrauer, F.L., and Schaefer, E.J. (1986) Increased risk for vitamin A toxicity in severe hypertriglyceridemia, *Annals of Internal Medicine*, **105**: 877–879.

Fletcher, N., Hanberg, A., and Hakansson, H. (2001) Hepatic vitamin A depletion is a sensitive marker of 2,3,7,8-tetrachlorodibenzo-p-dioxin, *Toxicological Science*, **62**: 166–175.

Frame, B., Jackson, C.E., Reynolds, W.A., and Umphrey, J.E. (1974) Hypercalcaemia and skeletal effects in chronic hypervitaminosis A, *Annals of Internal Medicine*, **80**: 44–48.

Frankel, T.L., Seshadri, M.S., McDowall, D.B., and Cornish, C.J. (1986) Hypervitaminosis A and calcium regulating hormones in the rat, *Journal of Nutrition*, **116**: 578–587.

Gerber, A., Raab, A.P., and Sobel, A.E. (1954) Vitamin A poisoning in adults, *American Journal of Medicine*, **16**: 729–745.

Ghoshal, A.K. and Farber, E. (1984) The induction of liver cancer by dietary deficiency of choline and methionine without added carcinogens, *Carcinogen*, **5**: 1367–1370.

Giguere, V. (1994) Retinoic acid receptors and cellular retinoid binding proteins: complex interplay in retinoid signaling, *Endocrinology Review*, **15**: 61–79.

Glass, C.K., DiRenzo, J., Kurokawa, R., and Han, Z. (1991) Regulation of gene expression by retinoic acid receptors, *DNA and Cell Biology*, **10**: 623–638.

Goodman, D. (1988) Plasma retinol-binding protein. In *The Retinoids* (eds M. Sporn, A. Roberts, and D. Goodman), pp. 41–88. New York: Academic Press.

Gradelet, S., Astorg, P.O., Leclerc, J., Chevalier, J., Vernevaut, M.-F., and Siess, M.-H. (1996a) Effects of canthaxanthin, astaxanthin, lycopene and lutein on liver xenobiotic-metabolizing enzymes in the rat, *Xenobiotica*, **26**: 46–63.

Gradelet, S., Leclerc, J., Siess, M.-H., and Astorg, P.O. (1996b) β-Ao-8′-carotenal, but not β-carotene, is a strong inducer of liver cytochromes P4501A1 and 1A2 in rat, *Xenobiotica*, **26**: 909–919.

Grolier, P., Agoudavi, S., and Azias-Braesco, V. (1995) Comparative bioavailability of diet, oil- and emulsion-based preparations of vitamin A and beta-carotene in rats, *Nutrition Research*, **10**: 1507–1516.

Grolier, P., Antignac, E., Colin, C., and Narbonne, J.F. (1990) Nutrition and membrane function: dietary vitamin A status and drug metabolism enzyme activities interactions, *Food Additives and Contaminants*, **7**: S131–S133.

Guengerich, F.P. (1987) *Mammalian Cytochrome P450*. Boca Raton, FL: CRC Press.

Guengerich, F.P. (1994) Catalytic selectivity of human cytochrome P450 enzymes: relevance to drug metabolism and toxicity, *Toxicology Letters*, **70**: 133–138.

Hathcock, J.N., Hattan, D.G., Jenkins, M.Y., McDonald, J.T., Sundaresan, P.R., and Wilkening, V.L. (1990) Evaluation of vitamin A toxicity, *American Journal of Clinical Nutrition*, **52**: 183–202.

Hatoff, D.E., Gertler, S.L., Miyai, K., Parker, B.A., and Weiss, J.B. (1982) Hypervitaminosis A unmasked by acute viral hepatitis, *Gastroenterology*, **82**: 124–128.

Heionen, O.P. and Albnes, D. (1994) The effect of vitamin E and beta carotene on the incidence of lung cancer and other cancers in male smokers, *New England Journal of Medicine*, **330**: 1029–1035.

Heywood, R., Palmer, A.K., Gregson, R.L., and Hummler, H. (1985) The toxicity of beta-carotene, *Toxicology*, **36**: 91–100.

Hooser, S.B., Rosengren, R.J., Hill, D.A., Mobley, S.A., and Sipes, I.G. (1994) Vitamin A modulation of xenobiotic induced liver injury in rodents, *Environmental Health Perspective*, **102**: 39–43.

Hough, S., Avioli, L.V., Muir, H., Gelderblom, D., Jenkins, G., Kurasi, H., Slatopolsky, E., Bergfeld, M.A., and Teitelbaum, S.L. (1988) Effects of hypervitaminosis A on the bone and mineral metabolism of the rat, *Endocrinology*, **122**: 2933–2939.

Howell, S.R., Shirley, M.A., and Ulm, E.H. (1998) Effects of retinoid treatment of rats on hepatic microsomal metabolism and cytochrome P450. Correlation between retinoic acid receptor/retinoid X receptor selectivity and effects on metabolic enzymes, *Drug Metabolism and Dispersion*, **26**: 234–239.

Hummler, H., Korte, R., and Hendrickx, A. (1990) Induction of malformations in the cynmolgus monkey with 13-cis-retinoic acid, *Teratology*, **42**: 263–272.

Hurley, L.S. (1977) Nutritional deficiencies and excesses. In *Handbook of Teratology. 1. General Principles and Etiology* (eds J.G. Wilson and F.C. Fraser). New York and London: Plenum Press.

Imaoka, S., Terano, Y., and Funae, Y. (1990) Changes in the amount of cytochrome P450s in rat hepatic microsomes with starvation, *Archives of Biochemistry and Biophysics*, **278**: 168–178.

Inder, R.E., Bray, B.J., Sipes, I.G., and Rosengren, R.J. (1999) Role of cytochrome P4502E1 in retinol's attenuation of carbon tetrachloride hepatotoxicity in the mouse, *Toxicological Science*, **52**: 130–139.

Inouye, K., Mae, T., Kondo, S., and Ohkawa, H. (1999) Inhibitory effects of vitamin A and vitamin K on rat cytochrome P4501A1-dependent monoxygenase activity, *Biochemical and Biophysical Research Communications*, **262**: 565–569.

Ioannides, C., Barnett, C., Irizar, A., and Flatt, P. (1996) Expression of cytochrome P450 proteins in disease. In *Cytochromes P450: Metabolic and Toxicological Aspects* (ed. C. Ioannides). Boca Raton, FL: CRC Press.

IUPAC-IUB (1982) Joint Commission of Biochemical Nomenclature. *European Journal of Biochemistry*, **129**: 1–5.

Jenkins, M.Y. and Mitchell, G.V. (1975) Influence of excess vitamin E on vitamin A toxicity in rats, *Journal of Nutrition*, **105**: 1600–1606.

Jewell, C. and O'Brien, N.M. (1999) Effect of dietary supplementation with carotenoids on xenobiotic metabolizing enzymes in the liver, lung, kidney and small intestine of the rat, *British Journal of Nutrition*, **81**: 235–242.

Jurima-Romet, M., Neigh, S., and Casley, W.L. (1997) Induction of cytochrome P4503A by retinoids in rat hepatocyte culture, *Human Experimental Toxicology*, **16**: 198–203.

Kemmann, E., Pasquale, S.A., and Skaf, R. (1983) Amenorrhea associated with carotenemia, *Journal of the American Medical Association*, **249**: 926–929.

Kowalski, T.E., Falestiny, M., Furth, E., and Malet, P.F. (1994) Vitamin A hepatotoxicity: a cautionary note regarding 25 000 IU supplements, *American Journal of Medicine*, **97**: 523–528.

Krasinski, S.D., Russell, R.M., Otradovec, C.L., Sadowski, J.A., Hartz, S.C., Jacob, R.A., and McGandy, R.B. (1989) Relationship of vitamin A and vitamin E intake to fasting plasma retinol, retinol-binding protein, retinyl esters, carotene, alpha-tocopherol, and cholesterol among elderly people and young adults: increased plasma retinyl esters among vitamin A-supplement users, *American Journal of Clinical Nutrition*, **49**: 112–120.

Leo, M.A., Aleynik, S.I., Aleynik, M.K., and Lieber, C.S. (1997) β-carotene beadlets potentiate hepatotoxicity of alcohol, *American Journal of Clinical Nutrition*, **66**: 1461–1469.

Leo, M.A., Arai, M., Sato, M., and Lieber, C.S. (1982) Hepatotoxicity of vitamin A and ethanol in the rat. *Gastroenterology*, **82**: 194–205.

Leo, M.A., Kim, C.I., Lowe, N., and Lieber, C.S. (1992) Interaction of ethanol with β-carotene: delayed blood clearance and enhanced hepatotoxicity, *Journal of Hepatology*, **15**: 883–891.

Leo, M.A., Lasker, J.M., Raucy, J.L., Kim, C., Black, M., and Lieber, C.S. (1989) Metabolism of retinol and retinoic acid by human liver cytochrome P450s, *Archives of Biochemistry and Biophysics*, **269**: 305–312.

Leo, M.A. and Lieber, C.S. (1982) Hepatic vitamin A depletion in alcoholic liver injury, *New England Journal of Medicine*, **307**: 597–601.

Leo, M.A. and Lieber, C.S. (1983) Hepatic fibrosis after long-term administration of ethanol and moderate vitamin A supplementation in the rat, *Journal of Hepatology*, **3**: 1–11.

Leo, M.A. and Lieber, C.S. (1999) Alcohol, vitamin A and β-carotene: adverse interactions, including hepatotoxicity and carcinogenicity, *American Journal of Clinical Nutrition*, **69**: 1071–1085.

Lucy, J.A. and Dingle, J.T. (1964) Fat-soluble vitamins and biological membranes, *Nature*, **204**: 156–160.

McCarthy, D., Lindamood, C., and Hill, D. (1987) Effects of retinoids on metabolizing enzymes and on binding of benzo(a)pyrene to rat tissue DNA, *Cancer Research*, **47**: 5014–5020.

McCormick, D.L., Major, N., and Moon, R.C. (1984) Inhibition of 7,12-dimethylbenz[a]anthracene-induced rat mammary carcinogenesis by concomitant or postcarcinogen antioxidant exposure, *Cancer Research*, **44**: 2858–2863.

McCormick, D.L., May, C.M., Thomas, C.F., and Detrisac, C.J. (1986) Anticarcinogenic and hepatotoxic interactions between retinyl acetate and butylated hydroxytoluene in rats, *Cancer Research*, **46**: 5264–5269.

McMullen, M.H., Rowling, M.J., Ozias, M.K., and Schalinske, K.L. (2002) Activation and induction of glycine N-methyltransferase by retinoids are tissue- and gender-specific, *Archives of Biochemistry and Biophysics*, **401**: 73–80.

Maiani, G., Raguzzini, A., Mobarhan, S., and Ferro-Luzzi, A. (1993) Vitamin A. *International Journal of Vitamin and Nutrition Research*, **63**: 252–257.

Mangelsdorf, D.J. and Evans, R.M. (1995) The RXR heterodimers and orphan receptors, *Cell*, **83**: 841–850.

Mangelsdorf, D.J., Ong, E.S., Dyck, J.A., and Evans, R.M. (1994) The retinoic acid receptor. In *Retinoids: Biology, Chemistry and Medicine* (eds M.B. Sporn, A.B. Roberts, and D.S. Goodman). New York: Raven Press.

Martinez-Frias, M.L. and Salvador, J. (1990) Epidemiological aspects of prenatal exposure to high doses of vitamin A in Spain, *European Journal of Epidemiology*, **6**: 118–123.

Mason, J.B. (1994) Folate and colonic carcinogenesis: searching for a mechanistic understanding, *Journal of Nutrition Biochemistry*, **5**: 170–175.

Massey, J.B., She, H.S., and Pownall, H.J. (1982) Interaction of vitamin E with saturated phospholipid bilayers, *Biochemistry and Biophysics Research Communications*, **106**: 842–847.

Mathas-Vliegen, E.M.H. and Tytgat, G.N.J. (1983) Biological fate of the vitamin A transporting protein complex and beta-carotene after excessive dietary intake, *Digestion*, **27**: 116–122.

Mathews-Roth, M.M. (1983) Amenorrhea associated with carotenemia (letter), *Journal of the American Medical Association*, **250**: 731.

Maurel, P. (1996) The CYP3 family. In *Cytochromes P450: Metabolic and Toxicological Aspects* (ed. C. Ioannides). Boca Raton, FL: CRC Press.

Metz, A.L., Walser, M.M., and Olson, W.G. (1985) The interaction of dietary vitamin A and vitamin D related to skeletal development in the turkey poult, *Journal of Nutrition*, **115**: 929–935.

Meyers, D.G., Maloley, P.A., and Weeks, D. (1996) Safety of antioxidant vitamins, *Archives of Internal Medicine*, **156**: 925–935.

Miller, R.K., Hendrickx, A.G., Mills, J.L., Hummler, H., and Wiegand, U.W. (1998) Periconceptional vitamin A use: how much is teratogenic? *Reproduction and Toxicology*, **12**: 75–88.

Mills, J.L., Simpson, J.L., Cunningham, G.C., Conley, M.R., and Rhoads, G.G. (1997) Vitamin A and birth defects, *American Journal of Obstetrics and Gynecology*, **177**: 31–36.

Minuk, G.Y., Kelly, J.K., and Hwang, W.-S. (1988) Vitamin A hepatotoxicity in multiple family members, *Journal of Hepatology*, **8**: 272–275.

Miranda, C. and Chhabra, R. (1981) Effects of high dietary vitamin A on drug-metabolizing enzyme activities in guinea pig and rabbit, *Drug–Nutrient Interaction*, **1**: 55–61.

Miranda, C., Mukhtar, H., Bend, J., and Chhabra, R. (1979) Effects of vitamin A deficiency on hepatic and extrahepatic mixed-function oxidase and epoxide-metabolizing enzymes in guinea pig and rabbit, *Biochemistry and Pharmacology*, **28**: 2713–2716.

Moon, R.C., Grubbs, C.J., and Sporn, M.B. (1976) Inhibition of 7,12-dimethylbenz[a]anthracene-induced mammary carcinogenesis by retinyl acetate, *Cancer Research*, **36**: 2626–2630.

Moreira, J.C.F., Dal-Pizzol, F., Guma, F.C.R., and Bernard, E.A. (1996) Effects of pretreatment with hydroxiurea on the increase in [methyl-3H] thymidine incorporation induced by retinol treatment in Sertoli cells, *Medical Science Research*, **24**: 383–384.

Moreira, J.C.F., Dal-Pizzol, F., Rocha, A.B., Klamt, F., Ribeiro, N.C., Ferreira, C.J.S., and Bernard, E.A. (2000) Retinol-induced changes in the phosphorylation of histones and high mobility group proteins from Sertoli cells, *Brazilian Journal of Medical and Biological Research*, **33**: 287–293.

Moreira, J.C.F., Dal-Pizzol, F., Von Endt, D., and Bernard, E.A. (1997) Effect of retinol on chromatin structure in Sertoli cells: 1,10-phenanthroline inhibit the increased DNAse I sensitivity induced by retinol, *Medical Science Research*, **25**: 653–658.

Mudur, G. (2001) Deaths trigger fresh controversy over vitamin A programme in India, *British Medical Journal (News)*, **323**: 1206.

Munder, M., Herzberg, I.M., Zierold, C., Moss, V.E., Hanson, K., Clagett-Dame, M., and DeLuca, H.F. (1994) Identification of the porcine intestinal accessory factor that enables DNA sequence recognition by vitamin D receptor, *Proceedings of the National Academy of Science of the USA*, **92**: 2795–2799.

Murata, M. and Kawanishi, S. (2000) Oxidative damage via superoxide generation, *Journal of Biological Chemistry*, **275**: 2003–2008.

Murray, M., Cantrill, E., Martini, R., and Farrell, G.C. (1991) Increased expression of cytochrome P4503A2 in male rat liver after dietary vitamin A supplementation, *Archives of Biochemistry and Biophysics*, **286**: 618–624.

Nagai, K., Hosaka, N., Nakabayashi, T., Amagasaki, Y., and Nakamura, N. (1999) Vitamin A toxicity secondary to excessive intake of yellow-green vegetables, liver and laver, *Journal of Hepatology*, **31**: 142–148.

Napoli, J.L. and Beck, C.D. (1984) Alpha tocopherol and phylloquinone as noncompetitive inhibitors of retinyl ester hydrolysis, *Biochemistry Journal*, **223**: 267–270.

Napoli, J.L., McCormick, A.M., O'Meara, B., and Dratz, E.A. (1984) Vitamin A metabolism: alpha tocopherol modulates tissue retinol levels *in vivo* and retinyl palmitate hydrolysis *in vitro*, *Archives of Biochemistry and Biophysics*, **230**: 194–202.

Niederreither, K., Vermot, J., Schuhbaur, B., Chambon, P., and Dolle, P. (2000) Retinoic acid synthesis and hindbrain patterning in the mouse embryo, *Development Supplement*, **127**(1): 75–85.

Nieto, N., Friedman, S., Greenwel, P., and Cederbaum, A.I. (1999) CYP2E1-mediated oxidative stress induces collagen type I expression in rat hepatic stellate cells, *Journal of Hepatology*, **30**: 987–996.

Olson, J.A. (1987) Recommended dietary intakes (RDI) of vitamin A in humans, *American Journal of Clinical Nutrition*, **45**: 704–716.

Omenn, G.S., Goodman, G.E., Thornquist, M.D., Balmes, J., Cullen, M.R., Glass, A., Keogh, J.P., Meyskens, F.L.J., Valanis, B., Williams, J.H.J., Barnhart, S., Cherniack, M.G., Brodkin, C.A., and Hammar, S. (1996) Risk factors for lung cancer and for intervention effects in CARET, the beta-carotene and retinol efficacy trial, *Journal of the National Cancer Institute*, **88**: 1550–1559.

Oreffo, R.O., Teti, A., Triffitt, J.T., Francis, M.J., Carano, A., and Zallone, A.Z. (1988) Effect of vitamin A on bone resorption: evidence for direct stimulation of isolated chicken osteoclasts by retinol and retinoic acid, *Journal of Bone Mineral Research*, **3**: 203–210.

Ozturk-Urek, R., Bozkaya, L.A., and Tarhan, L. (2001) The effects of some antioxidant vitamin- and trace element-supplemented diets on activities of SOD, CAT, GSH-Px and LPO levels in chicken tissues, *Cell Biochemical Function*, **19**: 125–132.

Parkinson, A. (1996) Biotransformation of xenobiotics. In *Casarett and Doull's Toxicology* (ed. C. Klaassen), pp. 113–186. Maidenhead: McGraw-Hill.

Pasantes-Morales, H., Wright, C.E., and Gaull, G.E. (1984) Protective effects of taurine, zinc and tocopherol on retinol-induced damage in human lymphoblastoid cells, *Journal of Nutrition*, **114**: 2256–2261.

Pichard, L., Fabre, I., Fabre, G., Domergue, J., Aubert, B.S., Mourad, G., and Maurel, P. (1990) Cyclosporin A drug interactions: screening for inducers and inhibitors of cytochrome P-450 (cyclosporin A osidase) in primary cultures of human hepatocytes and in liver microsomes, *Drug Metabolism and Dispersion*, **18**: 595–606.

Raucy, J., Kraner, J., and Lasker, J. (1993) Bioactivation of halogenated hydrocarbons by cytochrome P4502E1, *Critical Review of Toxicology*, **23**: 1–20.

Ray, W.J., Bain, G., Yao, M., and Gottlieb, D.I. (1997) CYP26, a novel mammalian cytochrome P450, is induced by retinoic acid and defines a new family, *Journal of Biological Chemistry*, **272**: 18702–18708.

Richardson, T.H. and Johnson, E.F. (1996) The CYP2C subfamily. In *Cytochromes P450: Metabolic and Toxicological Aspects* (ed. C. Ioannides). Boca Raton, FL: CRC Press.

Rodahl, K. (1943) The vitamin A content and toxicity of bear and seal liver, *Biochemistry Journal*, **37**: 166.

Rohde, C.M., Manatt, M., Clagett-Dame, M., and DeLuca, H.F. (1999) Vitamin A antagonizes the action of vitamin D in rats, *Journal of Nutrition*, **129**: 2246–2250.

Rosa, F.W. (1993) Retinoid embropathy in humans. In *Retinoids in Clinical Practice. The Risk–Benefit Ratio* (ed. G. Koren), pp. 77–109. New York: Marcel Dekker.

Rosa, F.W., Wilk, A.L., and Kelsey, F.O. (1986) Teratogen update: vitamin A congeners, *Teratology*, **33**: 355–364.

Rosengren, R.J., Sauer, J.-M., Hooser, S.B., and Sipes, I.G. (1995) Interactions between retinol and various hepatotoxicants in the Swiss Webster mouse, *Fundamentals of Applied Toxicology*, **25**: 281–292.

Ross, T.K., Darwish, H.M., and DeLuca, H.F. (1994) Molecular biology of vitamin D action, *Vitamins and Hormones*, **49**: 281–327.

Rothman, K.J., Moore, L.L., Singer, M.R., Nguyen, U.D.T., Mannion, S., and Milunsky, A. (1995) Teratogenicity of high vitamin A intake, *New England Journal of Medicine*, **333**: 1369–1373.

Rowling, M.J., McMullen, M.H., and Schalinske, K.L. (2002) Vitamin A and its derivatives induce hepatic glycine N-methyltransferase and hypomethylation of DNA in rats, *Journal of Nutrition*, **132**: 365–369.

Saneshigo, S., Mano, H., Tezuka, K., Mori, Y., Honda, Y., Itabashi, A., Yamada, T., Miyata, K., and Hakeda, Y. (1995) Retinoic acid directly stimulates osteoclastic bone resorption and gene expression of cathepsin K-OC-2, *Biochemistry Journal*, **309**: 721–724.

Sato, M. and Lieber, C.S. (1981) Hepatic vitamin A depletion after chronic ethanol consumption in baboons and rats, *Journal of Nutrition*, **111**: 2015–2023.

Satre, M.A., Jessen, K.A., Clegg, M.S., and Keen, C.L. (2001) Retinol binding protein expression is induced in HepG2 cells by zinc deficiency, *FEBS Letters*, **491**: 266–271.

Schmunes, E. (1979) Hypervitaminosis A in a patient with alopecia receiving renal dialysis, *Archives of Dermatology*, **115**: 882–883.

Schumann, K., Classen, H.G., Hages, M., Prinz-Langenohl, R., Pietrzik, K., and Biesalski, H.K. (1997) Bioavailability of oral vitamins, minerals, and trace elements in perspective, *Arzneim.-Forsch.*, **47**: 369–380.

Seifert, W.F., Bosma, A., Hendriks, H.F.J., Blaner, W.S., van Leeuwen, R.E.W., van Thiel-de Ruiter, G.C.F., Wilson, J.H.P., Knook, D.L., and Brouwer, A. (1991) Chronic administration of ethanol with high vitamin A supplementation in a liquid diet to rats does not cause liver fibrosis 2. Biochemical observations, *Journal of Hepatology*, **13**: 249–255.

Sharman, I.M. (1985) Hypercartotenaemia, *British Medical Journal*, **290**: 95–96.

Siddik, Z., Drew, R., Litterst, C., Mimnaugh, E., Sikic, B., and Gram, T. (1980) Hepatic cytochrome P-450-dependent metabolism and enzyme conjugation of foreign compounds in vitamin A deficient rats, *Pharmacology*, **21**: 383–390.

Smith, J.E., Brown, E.D., and Smith, J.C. (1974) The effect of zinc deficiency on the metabolism of retinol-binding protein in the rat, *Journal of Laboratory and Clinical Medicine*, **84**: 692–697.

Teratology Society (1987) Teratology Society Position Paper, *Teratology*, **35**: 269–275.

Thunberg, T., Ahlborg, U.G., Hakansson, H., Krantz, C., and Monier, M. (1980) Effect of 2,3,7,8-tetrachlorodibenzo-p-dioxin on the hepatic storage of retinol in rats with different dietary supplies of vitamin A (retinol), *Archives of Toxicology*, **45**: 273–285.

Underwood, B.A. (1998) *Safe doses of vitamin A during pregnancy and lactation: a report of the International Vitamin A Consultative Group (IVACG)*.

Ushio, F., Fukuhara, M., Bani, M., and Nabonne, J. (1995) Expression of cytochrome P450 isozymes in syrian hamster after dietary vitamin supplementation and deficiency, *International Journal of Vitamin and Nutrition Research*, **66**: 197–202.

Van der Saag, P.T. (1996) Nuclear retinoid receptors: mediators of retinoid effects, *European Journal of Clinical Nutrition*, **50**: S24–S28.

Vecchini, F., Lenoir-Viale, M., Cathelineau, C., Magdalou, J., Bernard, B., and Shroot, B. (1994) Presence of a retinoid responsive element in the promoter region of the human cytochrome P4501A1 gene, *Biochemistry and Biophysics Research Communications*, **201**: 1205–1212.

Vermeulen, N.P.E. (1996) Role of metabolism in chemical toxicity. In *Cytochromes P450: Metabolic and Toxicological Aspects* (ed. C. Ioannides). Boca Raton, FL: CRC Press.

Wang, X.-D., Liu, C., Bronson, R.T., Smith, D.E., Krinsky, N.I., and Russell, R.M. (1999) Retinoid signalling and activator protein-1 expression in ferrets given beta-carotene supplements and exposed to tobacco smoke, *Journal of the National Cancer Institute*, **91**: 60–66.

Weber, F.L.J., Mitchell, G.E.J., Powell, D.E., Reiser, B.J., and Banwell, J.G. (1982) Reversible hepatotoxicity associated with hepatic vitamin A accumulation in a protein-deficient patient, *Gastroenterology*, **82**: 118–123.

Werler, M.W., Lammer, E.J., Rosenberg, L., and Mitchell, A.A. (1990) Maternal vitamin A supplementation in relation to selected birth defects, *Teratology*, **42**: 497–503.

West, K.P.J. and Sommer, A. (2002) Vitamin A programme in Assam probably caused hysteria (letter), *British Medical Journal*, **324**: 791.

Westin, S., Sonneveld, E., van der Leede, B., van der Saag, P., Gustafsson, J., and Mode, A. (1997) CYP2C7 expression in rat liver and hepatocytes: regulation by retinoids, *Molecular and Cellular Endocrinology*, **129**: 169–179.

White, J.A., Gou, Y.-D., Baetz, K., Beckett-Jones, B., Bonasoro, J., Hsu, K.E., Dilwirth, F.J., Hjones, G., and Petkovich, M. (1996) Identification of the retinoic acid-inducible all-*trans*-retinoic acid 4-hydroxylase, *Journal of Biological Chemistry*, **271**: 29922–29927.

Whitlock, J.P. (1990) Genetic and molecular aspects of 2,3,7,8-tetrachlorodibenzo-p-dioxin action, *Annual Review of Pharmacology and Toxicology*, **30**: 251–277.

Wiegand, U.W., Hartmann, S., and Hummler, H. (1998) Safety of vitamin A: recent results, *International Journal for Vitamin and Nutrition Research*, **68**: 411–416.

Wijeweera, J.B., Gandolfi, A.J., Badger, D.A., Sipes, I.G., and Brendel, K. (1996) Vitamin A potentiation of vinyl chloride hepatotoxicity in rats and precision-cut liver slices, *Fundamental Applied Toxicology*, **34**: 73–83.

Wolbach, B. (1947) Vitamin A deficiency and excess in relation to skeletal growth, *Journal of Bone and Joint Surgery (Britain)*, **29**: 171–192.

Wong, K.P. (1977) Measurement of nanogram quantities of UDP-glucuronic acid in tissues, *Analytical Biochemistry*, **82**: 559–563.

Woodard, J.C., Donovan, G.A., and Fisher, L.W. (1997) Pathogenesis of vitamin (A and D)-induced premature growth-plate closure in calves, *Bone*, **21**: 171–182.

Worner, T.N., Gordon, G., Leo, M.A., and Lieber, C.S. (1988) Vitamin A treatment of sexual dysfunction in male alcoholics, *American Journal of Clinical Nutrition*, **48**: 1431–1435.

Wu, D. and Cederbaum, A.I. (2001) Removal of glutathione produces apoptosis and necrosis in HepG2 cells overexpressing CYP2E1, *Alcoholism: Clinical Experimental Research*, **25**: 619–628.

Yamamoto, Y., Zolfaghari, R., and Ross, A.C. (2000) Regulation of CYP26 (cytochrome P450RAI) mRNA expression and retinoic acid metabolism by retinoids and dietary vitamin A in liver of mice and rats, *FASEB Journal*, **14**: 2119–2127.

Yang, N.Y.J. and Desai, I.D. (1977) Effect of high levels of dietary vitamin E on liver and plasma lipids and fat soluble vitamins in rats, *Journal of Nutrition*, **107**: 1418–1426.

6 Rhabdomyolysis associated with nutritional supplement use*

Daren A. Scroggie, MD

Introduction

The use of alternative medicine in the United States has increased dramatically in the past two decades. Recent estimates reveal that up to 73% of the population may be using some sort of alternative therapy (Ramos-Remus et al., 1999). In particular, the use of nutritional supplements is becoming more prevalent, especially among athletes. Popular sports figures have been touting the benefits of supplements such as androstenedione (Begley and Brant, 1999). From 1990 to 1997 the use of these products increased by over 400%. It is now estimated that Americans spend over $1.5 billion a year on these supplements (Ernst and Chrubasik, 2000).

The supplements are aggressively marketed, not just in herbal shops and health food stores, but also in pharmacies, grocery stores, the Internet, and even gas stations. There remains little or no governmental regulation on these products. Manufacturing practices vary widely from company to company, and there are no standards for purity (Ramos-Remus et al., 1999). As the use of these supplements continues, so does the potential for toxicity.

Reports of serious toxicities from these "natural" substances have also been increasing in recent years. In particular, rhabdomyolysis has been noted with numerous supplements (Donadio et al., 2000; Kamijo et al., 1999; Lee et al., 1999; Martin and Fuller, 1998; Salmon and Nicholson, 1988; Scroggie et al., 2000). In addition, the United States Food and Drug Administration Center for Food Safety and Applied Nutrition Office of Special Nutritionals published a summary of all adverse reactions in 1998. This report contained multiple reports of myalgias, muscle cramps and rhabdomyolysis attributed to various supplements (FDA, 1998). Weight loss products and body building formulas are the most common causes of supplement-induced rhabdomyolysis. The majority of these products contain overlapping combinations of herbs, amino acids, and nutriceuticals. In addition, these supplements are often used to enhance

---

* The views expressed in this article are those of the author and do not reflect the official policy of the Department of Defense or other Departments of the United States Government.

physical stamina and activity, which can also lead to rhabdomyolysis. In order to elucidate the role these supplements may play in the development of rhabdomyolysis, it is useful first to examine normal muscle metabolism, then the disorder itself, and finally the biochemical properties of the various supplements.

Normal muscle metabolism

Normal skeletal muscle uses energy from the oxidation of organic compounds such as glucose. In the mitochondria, the Krebs cycle converts this energy into adenosine triphosphate (ATP). During muscle work, the ATP is broken down into ADP (adenosine diphosphate), releasing phosphate and energy.

Creatine can store energy by binding to phosphate. This phosphate can be readily exchanged with ADP/ATP, allowing creatine to provide a reservoir of high-energy phosphate. Creatine is also needed for the transport of the energy derived from mitochondrial ATP to ATP in the cytosol.

When energy levels fall during muscle work, alternative sources of energy are utilized. These include purines, glycogen, and fatty acids. ATP can be converted into AMP (adenosine monophosphate), which is further metabolized into fumerate, generating ammonia in the process. In the mitochondria, fumerate can enter the Krebs cycle to produce energy. Glycogen is converted to glucose-6-phosphate and can generate ATP via aerobic metabolism (Krebs cycle) or the less efficient anaerobic pathway (leading to lactic acid accumulation). Thus, each of these pathways can lead to the formation of potentially toxic byproducts: ammonia and lactic acid. Fatty acids can also be used to generate ATP. They are transported into the mitochondrial matrix by carnitine, and undergo conversion to acetyl-coenzyme A, which can enter the Krebs cycle to produce energy (Arroyo, 2002).

Rhabdomyolysis

When the normal metabolic pathways are interfered with, muscle injury can result. Massive myocyte injury cause the syndrome known as rhabdomyolysis. Rhabdomyolysis is a heterogeneous group of disorders characterized by increased muscle-specific enzymes (creatine kinase and aldolase) in the serum in combination with increased serum and urine myoglobin as a result of muscle cell injury. Myoglobinuria appears on urinalysis as hematuria in the absence of red blood cells, and can result in pigmented urine. These proteins are released from myocytes after oxidative stresses. These stresses can be a result of direct physical injury from trauma or compression, or due to the toxic effects of drugs, supplements, or altered metabolic activity (see Table 6.1). The mechanisms of toxic or non-traumatic myocyte injury are not as clearly understood as those of direct injury. There appears to be a complex interaction of intracellular ions, metabolic byproducts and adenosine triphosphate (ATP) levels which leads to the activation of destructive enzymes, cell death and the release of cellular contents (Visweswaran and Guntupalli, 1999).

Table 6.1 Causes of rhabdomyolysis

Metabolic myopathies	*Traumatic*
Genes recognized in more than 10 types	Exertion
Remainder unknown	Seizure
Metabolic derangement	Compartment syndrome
Hypokalemia	High-voltage electric shock
Hypophospatemia	Lightning strike
Hypomagnesemia	Prolonged myoclonus
Severe hyponatremia	Crush syndrome
Diabetic ketoacidosis	Prolong immobilization
Nonketotic hyperosmolar coma	Burns
Hypo/hyperthyroidism	Near drowning
Sickle cell trait hyperthermia/hypothermia	Prolonged CPR[1]
Medical conditions	Snake bites
Stem cell transplant	Ischemia
Inflammatory muscle disease	Malignant hyperthermia
Addisonian crisis	Infections
Pancreatitis	HIV,[2] hepatitis, CMV,[3]
Status asthmaticus	EBV,[4] influenza, Coxsackie,
Muscular dystrophies	adenovirus, *Streptococcus*
Toxins	*pneumonia*, *Salmonella*,
Alcohol	*Shigella*, *Legionella*, Rocky
Cocaine, heroin	Mountain spotted fever,
Drugs (over 150 known associations)	leptospirosis, trichonosis,
Sympathomimetics, antipsychotics,	tetanus, gas gangrene
general anesthetics, HMG-CoA inhibitors	

Notes:
1 Cardiopulmonary resuscitation.
2 Human immunodeficiency virus.
3 Cytomegalovirus.
4 Epstein-Barr virus.

This leakage of cellular material leads to both local effects (muscle pain and edema) and systemic problems. Muscle cell injury releases high levels of potassium, which can lead to cardiac arrthymias. In addition, elevated levels of uric acid (from muscle necrosis) and lactate (from anaerobic metabolic) result in an anion gap metabolic acidosis (Farmer, 1997). However, the major toxicity occurs when myoglobin deposits in the kidneys. Normally, myoglobin is rapidly broken down in its component amino acids and iron, which is then complexed with ferritin. In rhabdomyolysis, the renal tubular cells are unable to metabolize the excess iron, resulting in the generation of toxic free radicals. These free radicals cause direct damage to the kidney, resulting in acute tubular necrosis and potentially leading to renal failure (Visweswaran and Guntupalli, 1999). In addition, in many cases of rhabdomyolysis, there are coexisting renal stresses such as hypovolumenia, hypertension, and renal vasoconstriction. Substances that affect any of the normal processes of muscle metabolism or increase the oxidative stresses on the kidneys are more likely to cause rhabdomyolysis.

Table 6.2 Nutritional supplements associated with rhabdomyolysis

Substance	Found in	Notes
Probable link (*these substances have been reported to cause rhabdomyolysis alone or in combination and have a likely mechanism*)		
• *Guarana* extracts	Diet pills	22% caffeine
• Cola nut extracts	Diet pills	Caffeine
• Ephedra	Ma huang, herbal ecstasy	Sympathetic agonist
• L-carnitine	Diet pills, protein supplements, weight loss formulas	
• Picolinate	Weight loss formulas	Picolinate is a tryptophan derivative
• Chromium picolinate	Weight loss formulas	
• Hydroxycitric acid	*Garcinia cambogia* extracts, weight loss formulas	
• Creatine	Muscle building formulas	Very commonly used
• Methylenedioxymethamphetamine	Ecstasy	
• Chinese herbs	Many different names and formulations	
Possible link (*these substances have been reported to cause rhabdomyolysis in combination with the above agents and have a less clear mechanism*)		
• Amino acids (glutamine, taurine, methionine, phenylalanine, lysine)	Muscle building formulas	Common ingredient in many supplements
• Inositol	Weight loss formulas	
• Psyllium seed	Diet pills	
• Choline	Muscle building formulas	
• Kava root	Anti-anxiety; sleeping pills	
Unlikely to be linked (*these substances have been reported to cause rhabdomyolysis in combination with above agents and do not have a likely mechanism*)		
• Trace elements	Most formulations	Zinc, calcium, magnesium, manganese
• Ribonucleic acids (RNA)		
• Inert ingredients		Maltodextrin, dyes

Note that most agents are taken in combination. For example, Diet Fuel® contains ma huang, *Guarana* extract, *Garcina cambogia* extract, chromium picolinate, L-carnitine, potassium phosphate, and magnesium phosphate. In this table, "diet pills" refers to appetite suppressants and "weight loss formulas" refers to products claiming to "burn fat" via thermogenesis.

Biochemistry of nutritional supplements

Dietary supplements are becoming increasingly recognized as potential triggers of rhabdomyolysis (see Table 6.2). In particular, most reports implicate diet aids and body building formulas. While many different brands names are found, there are a handful of ingredients, either alone or in combination, which occur commonly. Among these are ma huang (ephedra), *Garcina cambogia* (hydroxycitric acid), L-carnitine, caffeine (*Guarana*), chromium picolinate, and various amino acids.

Ma huang is a Chinese herb extracted from the *Ephedra sinica* plant. The active ingredient is ephedra, which is a mixture of ephedrine and pseudoephedrine. Ephedrine itself is an alpha and beta agonist, and also causes the release of norepinephrine, which has potent vasoconstrictive effects. Initially, stimulation from these sympathomimetics causes increased metabolic demands on the muscle cells. They may also decrease the supply of nutrients by vasoconstriction. In theory, with longer stimulation, the normal processing of ATP is interrupted as substrates are used up. As a result, the energy produced cannot be released as ATP, but instead is lost as heat. This heat can be directly toxic to the myocytes. Additionally, as ATP levels fall the pumps maintaining electrolyte balance cannot function. The normal electrolyte gradients and osmotic stability are lost, which can also result in myonecrosis. The shift to anaerobic metabolism causes byproducts, such as lactic acid and ammonia, to build up in the muscle cells. These byproducts can cause additional muscle damage (Kirk and Pace, 1997). Without ATP, the calcium ATPase is unable to remove calcium from the cell or store it in intracellular sites. As the concentration of calcium within the cytoplasm rises, degradative enzymes, such as neutral proteases (i.e. calpain) and phospholipases, are activated (Visweswaran and Guntupalli, 1999).

The action of hydroxycitric acid on muscle cells is theoretical and has not been extensively evaluated in the scientific literature. Proponents claim that it acts by inhibiting the formation of fatty acids (Wheeler, 1999). Fatty acids are a major source of energy for muscle cells during prolonged exercise (Turcotte, 1999). Inhibition of fatty acid formation could theoretically deprive overstimulated muscles of an alternative fuel source. This interruption in metabolism may also increase thermogenesis and therefore heat-related muscle damage (Wheeler, 1999).

L-carnitine increases the oxidation of fatty acids and the metabolism of carbohydrates. In addition, it increases the rate of oxidative phophorylation. Of particular note is the effect of the D-isomer of carnitine. Ingestion of the D-isomer can result in a myasthenia gravis-like syndrome (Marcus and Coulston, 1990). The manufacturers claim that it increases the overall muscle metabolism and allows greater muscle power. This overutilization of fatty acids could rapidly deplete the energy reserves of muscle cells, resulting in damage. It is also possible that impurities, such as the D-isomer, could also result in muscle damage.

Guarana extract contains about 22% caffeine. Caffeine increases skeletal muscle contractility and decreases muscle fatigue. In addition, caffeine results in anxiety, restlessness, tremors, insomnia, hyperesthesia, and diuresis (Rall, 1990). In theory, the combination of increased muscle utilization (less fatigue), volume depletion and the psychomotor agitation could lead to overexertion and significant metabolic stress.

Chromium is thought to increase muscle intake and metabolism of glucose (Blumenthal *et al.*, 1998). This may further increase the consumption of limited nutritional resources. In addition, picolinate (the chelator commonly used to bind chromium) is a derivative of tryptophan, impurities of which are known to be toxic (Coleman, 1997; George and Pourmand, 1997; Greenberg *et al.*, 1996).

Amino acids alone are unlikely to be directly pathologic. However, supraphysiologic levels can lead to toxicity. For example, taurine (commonly found in supplements) is involved in osmotic regulation and homeostasis (Finberg, 2000), modulation of voltage induced excitation and contraction (Deluca *et al.*, 1996), and is also thought to increase the action of insulin on muscle cells, increasing glucose uptake and usage (Coleman, 2000). In theory, the net result of excessive taurine supplementation would be increased muscle metabolism. This would increase muscle demand for energy, which may exceed the body's ability to provide that energy, resulting in muscle injury.

Creatine is made from combining arginine, glycine and methionine. It is normally involved in the conversion of ADP to ATP, allowing for more efficient energy production. Its reported side-effects include bloating and dehydration. Many consumers use this supplement for strength training, using high doses in combination with escalating weight lifting (Metzl, 1999). This type of training could easily lead to muscle damage and even rhabdomyolysis.

Since none of the manufacturers of these products are required to adhere to governmental regulations regarding purity or safety, there is a potential for contamination of the supplements. In the past, toxic byproducts have resulted in significant toxicity (George and Pourmand, 1997; Greenberg *et al.*, 1996).

Another potential explanation for the link between these supplements and rhabdomyolysis lies in their psychological effects. The consumer may think that the supplement will protect him or her from injury. He or she may then increase his workout duration or load (Metzl, 1999). This increased exertion alone can lead to rhabdomyolysis (Prendergast and George, 1993).

Conclusion

The recent emphasis on fitness and the American obsession with the "perfect" body has increasingly led to the use of agents to augment performance. Supplements are being used more and more, not just by the professional athlete, but also by the "weekend warrior" hoping for a short cut. As this use becomes more widespread, adverse events such as rhabdomyolysis will become more commonplace. Physicians need to be aware of these potential problems; not just for treating them, but also to counsel patients on the dangers that supplements can pose.

References

Arroyo, R.A. (2002) In *Rheumatology Secrets* (ed. West, S.G.), pp. 507–514. Philadelphia, PA: Hanley and Belfus.

Begley, S. and Brant, M. (1999) The real scandal, *Newsweek*, 15 Feb 1999 48–54.

Blumenthal, M., Busse, W., and Goldberg, A. (1998) *Chromium*. Austin, TX: American Botanical Council.

Coleman, E. (1997) The chromium picolinate weight loss scam, *Sports Medicine Digest*, **19**: 6–7.

Coleman, E. (2000) Vol. 2002 *Heath care reality check*. Online. Available HTTP: <http://www.hcrc.org/faqs/taurine.html> (accessed 9 Jan 2003).

Deluca, A., Pierna, S., and Camerino, D. (1996) Effect of taurine depletion on the excitation–contraction coupling and Cl^- conductance of rat skeletal muscle, *European Journal of Pharmacology*, **296**: 215–222.

Donadio, V., Bonsi, P., Zele, I., Monari, L., Liguori, R., Vetrugno, R., Albani, F., and Montagna, P. (2000) Myoglobinuria after ingestion of extracts of guarana, Ginkgo biloba and kava, *Neurological Science*, **21**: 124.

Ernst, E. and Chrubasik, S. (2000) Phyto-anti-inflammatories. A systematic review of randomized, placebo-controlled, double-blind trials, *Rheumatic Disease Clinics of North America*, **26**: 13–27, vii.

Farmer, J. (1997) In *Critical Care* (eds Civetta, J., Taylor, R., and Kirby, R.), pp. 2195–2201. Philadelphia, PA: Lippincott-Raven.

FDA (1998) Vol. 2002. Online. <http://www.cfsan.fda.gov/~dms/aems.html> (accessed 25 Jan 2002; site closed 29 Aug 2002).

Finberg, L. (2000) Prevention and treatment of diabetes in children, *Journal of Clinical Endocrinology and Metabolism*, **85**: 508–509.

George, K.K. and Pourmand, R. (1997) Toxic myopathies, *Neurology Clinics*, **15**: 711–730.

Greenberg, A.S., Takagi, H., Hill, R.H., Hasan, A., Murata, H., and Falanga, V. (1996) Delayed onset of skin fibrosis after the ingestion of eosinophilia – myalgia syndrome-associated L-tryptophan, *Journal of the American Academy of Dermatology*, **35**: 264–266.

Kamijo, Y., Soma, K., Asari, Y., and Ohwada, T. (1999) Severe rhabdomyolysis following massive ingestion of oolong tea: caffeine intoxication with coexisting hyponatremia, *Veterinary and Human Toxicology*, **41**: 381–383.

Kirk, M. and Pace, S. (1997) Pearls, pitfalls, and updates in toxicology, *Emergency Medical Clinics of North America*, **15**: 427–449.

Lee, C.T., Wu, M.S., Lu, K., and Hsu, K.T. (1999) Renal tubular acidosis, hypokalemic paralysis, rhabdomyolysis, and acute renal failure – a rare presentation of Chinese herbal nephropathy, *Renal Failure*, **21**: 227–230.

Marcus, R. and Coulston, A. (1990) In *Goodman and Gillman's The Pharmacologic Basis of Therapeutics* (eds Goodman, A., Rall, T., Nies, A., and Palmer, T.), pp. 1530–1552. New York: Pergamon Press.

Martin, W.R. and Fuller, R.E. (1998) Suspected chromium picolinate-induced rhabdomyolysis, *Pharmacotherapy*, **18**: 860–862.

Metzl, J.D. (1999) Strength training and nutritional supplement use in adolescents, *Current Opinion in Pediatrics*, **11**: 292–296.

Prendergast, B.D. and George, C.F. (1993) Drug-induced rhabdomyolysis – mechanisms and management, *Postgraduate Medical Journal*, **69**: 333–336.

Rall, T. (1990) In *Goodman and Gillman's The Pharmacological Basis of Therapeutics* (eds Goodman, A., Rall, T., Nies, A., and Palmer, T.), pp. 618–637. New York: Pergamon Press.

Ramos-Remus, C., Gutierrez-Urena, S., and Davis, P. (1999) Epidemiology of complementary and alternative practices in rheumatology, *Rheumatic Disease Clinics of North America*, **25**: 789–804.

Salmon, J. and Nicholson, D. (1988) DIC and rhabdomyolysis following pseudoephedrine overdose, *American Journal of Emergency Medicine*, **6**: 545–546.

Scroggie, D.A., Harris, M.D., and Sakai, L.M. (2000) Rhabdomyolysis associated with nutritional supplement use, *Journal of Clinical Rheumatology*, **6**: 328–332.

Turcotte, L.P. (1999) Role of fats in exercise. Types and quality, *Clinics in Sports Medicine*, **18**: 485–498.

Visweswaran, P. and Guntupalli, J. (1999) Rhabdomyolysis, *Critical Care Clinics*, **15**: 415–428, ix–x.

Wheeler, T. (1999) Vol. 2002 *Health care reality check*. Online. Available HTTP: <http://www.hcrc.org/contrib/wheeler/hydroxyc.html> (accessed 9 Jan 2003; last update July 1999).

7   Allergens in food

S.H. Arshad and C. Venter

Adverse reactions to food have been reported for the past 2000 years. Writings from ancient Rome indicate that the Romans understood that foods consumed safely by most people could provoke adverse reactions in others (Sampson, 1998). Prausnitz and Kustner were the first to discover that the "substance", now known as IgE, responsible for Kustner's allergic reaction to fish was present in his blood serum (Prausnitz and Kustner, 1921).

Background

Food allergy/intolerance is a common medical problem, but epidemiological data is scarce. Food allergy is believed to affect 1.5% of adults and 6–8% of children (Arshad, 2002; Fuglsang et al., 1994). The main UK prevalence data quoted widely is that of the High Wycombe study conducted in the late 1980s which reported a population prevalence rate of 1.4–1.8%, looking at eight different food allergens (Young et al., 1994).

Definitions

"Adverse food reaction" is the umbrella term referring to any untoward reaction following the ingestion of a food (or additive). Adverse reactions to food can be divided into toxic and non-toxic reactions. Toxic reactions are dose-related and can affect any individual due to exposure to compounds which may be naturally occurring in foods or added during food preparation, e.g. scromboid fish poisoning or aflatoxins in peanuts (COT Report, 2000).

Non-toxic reactions can be divided into food allergy (immune mediated), food intolerance (non-immune mediated) and unknown mechanisms. The Committee on Toxicology and Chemicals in Food (COT) report uses the categorization and classification (Figure 7.1) of the European Academy Allergy and Clinical Immunology with the addition of an "unknown" category. The reason for this addition is the fact that in the clinical practice of allergy it quite often happens that we do not know whether we are dealing with an allergy or intolerance due to the time delay between ingestion and symptoms as well as insufficient diagnostic tools (COT Report, 2000; Ortolani et al., 1999). The popular practice

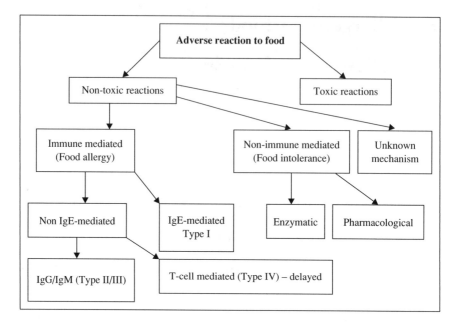

Figure 7.1 Classification of adverse reactions to food.

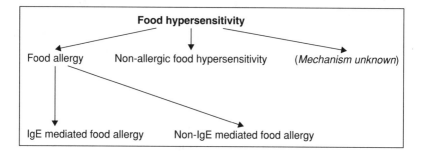

Figure 7.2 Proposed nomenclature for "adverse reactions to food".

of calling all adverse reactions "allergies" is therefore inaccurate and the cause and effect of confusion to both the general public and health professionals.

A recent proposal regarding the nomenclature used in asthma and allergy advised that an adverse reaction to food should be called food hypersensitivity (Figure 7.2). When immunological mechanisms have been demonstrated, the appropriate term is "food allergy" and, if the role of IgE is highlighted, the term is "IgE-mediated food allergy". All other reactions, previously sometimes referred to as "food intolerance", should be referred to as "nonallergic food hypersensitivity". Severe, generalized allergic reactions to food can be classified as anaphylaxis (Johansson *et al.*, 2001).

To this nomenclature, we suggest the addition of another category, namely 'mechanism unknown'.

For the purpose of this chapter the mechanisms and factors involved in food allergy will be discussed, i.e. IgE mediated food allergy or non-IgE mediated food allergy.

Mechanisms involved in food allergy

Four distinct types of hypersensitivity reactions (types I, II, III, IV) are recognized and each type involves different components of the immune system. Food proteins are broken down into small peptides and amino acids by digestive enzymes and are then absorbed to be used for growth, tissue repair or energy. The type I (IgE mediated) response is the classical allergic response; the type II response is the immune complex mediated response and rarely involved in allergic disease. Type III is the IgG mediated response, of which an exaggerated response can cause allergic symptoms. The type IV response is the delayed hypersensitivity response caused by the T-cells (Arshad, 2002; Sampson, 1998).

Manifestations of food allergy

Allergic reactions to food may affect different organs and systems. The clinical manifestations of adverse reactions to food include:

- systemic – anaphylaxis
- gastrointestinal – vomiting, diarrhea, abdominal pain, chronic constipation
- malabsorptive – enteropathy, celiac disease, eosinophilic gastroenteritis
- respiratory – rhinitis, asthma, pneumonitis
- cutaneous – urticaria, eczema, atopic dermatitis, pruritis (Sampson, 1998).

Diagnosis of food allergy/intolerance

There is a substantial gap between perceived and proven food allergy. In an American study, parents of 23% of children reported previous adverse reactions to food, but only 8% of these children (1–3 years old) showed reproducible symptoms of food allergy/intolerance (Bock, 1987).

The importance of correct diagnosis of food allergy should never be underestimated, as over-diagnosis of food allergy has led to malnutrition, eating disorders, psychosocial problems and family disruption. Under-diagnosis, on the other hand, may result in growth failure and permanent physical impairments. Missed diagnosis of serious disease can lead to inappropriate treatment (Ortolani *et al.*, 1999; Sampson, 1998).

Careful history taking and physical examination remains the cornerstone of diagnosis of food allergy. Current accepted tests for diagnosing food allergy include skin prick tests (SPTs), prick to prick test, patch test, specific IgE test and elimination diets followed by food challenges. Food diaries may also assist in the diagnosis of food allergy, especially in immediate type allergy where symptoms appear within 2 h after food consumption.

Basophil histamine release tests, intestinal mast cell histamine release, gastrointestinal permeability tests and endoscopic mucosal biopsy following direct application of food antigen may be used as research tools. This direct application of antigen to the mucosa does not seem to be any safer than a food challenge (Sampson, 1998). Tests such as basophil stimulation are currently being evaluated (Crockard and Ennis, 2001).

There is at present no scientific evidence for the use of food-specific IgG or IgG4 antibody levels, lymphocyte activation, sublingual or intracutaneous activation or tests such as Vegatesting and Kinesiology (Krop *et al.*, 1997; Sampson, 1998).

Food challenging is an integral part of the management of food allergy. Food challenges can be done as open challenges, single-blind challenges or double-blind, placebo-controlled food challenges (DBPCFCs). The DBPCFC is internationally recommended as the "gold standard" for both research and clinical diagnostic evaluations (Bock *et al.*, 1988; Pastorello *et al.*, 1991; Sampson and Ho, 1997). Elimination diets of the suspected food should be followed for a minimum of two weeks or until the symptoms clear up (could be up to 12 weeks in gastrointestinal disease) before one proceeds to a DBPCFC (Sampson, 1998).

Common food allergens

Foods are composed of proteins, carbohydrates, and lipids. The ability of proteins to cause allergic disease has long been established. In general, the major food allergens that have been identified are water-soluble glycoproteins that have molecular weights ranging from 10 to 60 kD and are stable to treatment with heat, acid and proteases (Pittard and Bill, 1979).

Examples of four of the structural protein families that are particularly important in food allergy are as follows:

1   alpha-helical proteins – napkins (=2S albumins from seeds) and non-lipid transfer proteins
2   largely beta-sheet proteins with a prominent helix in close contact – lipocalins, profilins and Bet v 1-related proteins
3   (alpha+beta)-structures, in which the alpha and beta-structural elements are not intimately associated, e.g. lactalbumin
4   serpins (serine protease inhibitors), ovalbumin – Ovalbumin is not itself a protease inhibitor, but is structurally related to this family of rather complex proteins.

In addition to the 3D-structures of intact proteins, the structure of the sugar side-chain that is responsible for cross-reactions among foods from vegetable and invertebrate origin is of interest, but falls beyond the scope of this chapter

(Aalberse and Stapel, 2001). Other physiological and chemical properties that account for their allergenicity are as yet poorly understood.

It is important to realize that only a small proportion of those exposed to a protein allergen will become sensitized, susceptibility being determined by both genetic predisposition and environmental factors.

Codex Guidelines on Nutrition Labelling play an important role in providing guidance to member countries when they wish to develop or update their national regulations and in encouraging harmonization of national standards with international standards. The list of food allergens considered by the Codex Alimentarius Committee on Food Labelling includes:

1   barley, oats, wheat, triticale, and products of these
2   crustaceans and other shellfish and products of these
3   egg and egg products
4   fish and fish products
5   legumes, peas, peanuts, soybeans, and products of these
6   milk and milk products (lactose included)
7   sulfite concentrations of 10 mg/kg or more
8   tree nuts, poppy seeds, sesame seeds and products of these (Bousquet et al., 1998).

The most common food allergens include cow's milk, egg, nuts (tree nuts and peanuts), fish, wheat, and soya. Other less common food allergens include cereals, fruit, and vegetables. Practically all food containing traces of protein is able to sensitize some people, which can lead to allergic disease.

Cow's milk allergy

Prevalence

In the UK it is estimated that 2–3% of children develop cow's milk allergy (Arshad, 2002; Hide, 1994). Internationally it is considered that 80% of children with cow's milk allergy outgrow this allergy by the age of five (Host et al., 1995).

Mechanisms

Adverse reactions to cow's milk ingestion could be due to immunological, metabolic, infective or other causes (Arshad, 2002; Host et al., 1995; Host and Halken, 1990). Cow's milk protein allergy/intolerance may be due to the interaction between one or more milk proteins and involve one or more immune mechanisms, possibly any of the four basic types of immune reactions. Immunologically mediated reactions are defined as cow's milk protein allergy (CMPA). Most CMPA is caused by IgE-mediated (type I) reactions. Type IV (cell-mediated reactions) have also been demonstrated and reviewed (Host et al., 1995). Non-immunological reactions against cow's milk proteins are defined as cow's milk protein intolerance (CMPI). In most cases, extensive diagnostic tests for the type II or III or IV reactions cannot be performed. CMPA and CMPI cannot be differentiated on the basis of clinical symptoms alone, and this makes accurate diagnostic labeling difficult. Cow's milk challenges followed by a lactose challenge can rule out the difference between lactose intolerance and other forms of cow's milk allergy/intolerance, but do not necessarily define the mechanism involved (Host *et al.*, 1995).

Symptoms most commonly associated with cow's milk allergy

- Eczema/Erythemous rash, oropharyngeal edema, cough, wheezing, whistling in chest, rhinitis, urticaria, vomiting, diarrhea (Baehler *et al.*, 1996)
- Constipation (Daher *et al.*, 2001)
- Severe abdominal distension, colic (Hill *et al.*, 1993; Host *et al.*, 1995; Host and Halken, 1990; Majamaa *et al.*, 1999)

Development of sensitization

It seems that giving cow's milk formula as a first feed to infants with a family history of atopy could lead to the development of cow's milk allergy, and these mothers should probably be advised accordingly (Oliveira *et al.*, 2002).

Development of tolerance

Cow's milk allergy is usually a transient condition of early childhood, but can persist to adult life in a few cases.

The best method to ascertain clinical tolerance appears to be the food challenge rather than *in vitro* and *in vivo* tests (Sampaio *et al.*, 2002). Interestingly, high total IgE and milk-specific IgE plus immediate symptoms at the onset of cow's milk allergy are associated with persistent allergy. However, delayed, often gastrointestinal symptoms in milk allergy, low total IgE and low specific IgE at the onset of cow's milk allergy seems to favor tolerance (Vanto *et al.*, 2002).

Allergens in milk

Cow's milk contains at least 30 protein components that may provoke an antibody response in humans (Bleumink and Young, 1968; Wal, 2001).

The protein fractions in milk include whey and casein. Casein appears to be the most potent allergen in skin tests and β-lactoglobulin in oral challenges (Docena *et al.*, 1996; Goidman *et al.*, 1963a, 1963b).

WHEY

The whey fraction of cow's milk comprises β-lactoglobulin, α-lactoglobulin, bovine immunoglobulins, and bovine serum albumin. Minute quantities of other proteins such as lactoferrin, transferrin, lipases, and esterases are also present. Both β-lactoglobulin and α-lactoglobulin are considered major allergens in cow's milk (Rolfsen *et al.*, 1987). Heat denatures all the whey fractions. However, β-lactoglobulin is resistant to pasteurization and the allergenicity of this protein may even be enhanced by pasteurization (Bleumink and Young, 1968).

Specific IgE antibodies to β-lactoglobulin are found in the sera of cow's milk allergic patients (Ball *et al.*, 1994; Rolfsen *et al.*, 1987).

CASEIN

Casein is a major allergen of cow's milk. It makes up about 75–86% (Swaisgood, 1982) of all milk proteins and is the main constituent in cheese. The casein fraction of milk comprises proteins that are resistant to heat and acid. Casein is composed of five basic caseins, namely α casein, $α_s$ casein, β casein, κ casein, and γ casein. Casein and caseinates are widely used as extenders and tenderizers in sausages, soups, and stews. Casein is also the major protein found in high-protein beverage powders, fortified cereals and infant formulas (Gern *et al.*, 1991).

The whey proteins in cow's milk quite often seem to be contaminated with lactose, whereas caseins have a very low lactose content, but could be contaminated by whey proteins to some degree (Joneja, 1998; Sampson, 1998).

Cocco and colleagues identified eight major and two minor IgE binding epitopes on αs1 casein and also found amino acids (in these epitopes) critical for IgE binding. Their results imply that single amino acid substitutions in critical positions could be used in future immunotherapeutic interventions (Cocco *et al.*, 2002).

Effect of heating and processing

Milk allergens (caseins, alpha-lactalbumin and beta-lactoglobulin) are heat-stable, but food processing such as heat treatment and enzymic hydrolysis may cause a loss of allergenicity (Bousquet *et al.*, 1998).

Cross-reactions

Immunoblotting techniques have shown cross-reactivity between milk proteins in cow's milk, goat's milk and sheep's milk and that cow's milk allergic individuals often exhibit IgE to goat's or sheep's milk. The general advice is therefore to avoid goat's milk and ewe's milk when allergic to cow's milk due to the cross-reactivity of the proteins found in these milks (Gjesing *et al.*, 1986). Clinically up to 50% of children with cow's milk allergy can also be allergic to goat's milk (Ellis *et al.*, 1991).

Skin testing to beef is quite often positive in cow's milk allergic patients. However, only a very small number of children may react to raw beef and most can ingest cooked beef without any adverse effects (Werfel *et al.*, 1997).

About 25% of individuals allergic to cow's milk will be allergic to soymilk (Lee and Heiner, 2002).

Docena and colleagues found that both moderately and extensively hydrolyzed infant formulas contain residual peptides that could lead to immunogenic reactions. This could hold implications for clinical treatment and safety of these milks might have to be established first in some highly sensitive individuals (Docena *et al.*, 1996).

Egg allergy

Prevalence and background

Hen's egg is one of the most frequent causes of immediate food allergy in children in the USA and Europe, but also plays a role in allergic reactions in adults (Crespo *et al.*, 1995; Mandallaz *et al.*, 1988). Hen's eggs are slightly more allergenic than duck eggs (Yunginger, 1990).

Hattevig and colleagues found that egg-white sensitivity was a better indicator of atopy than total IgE and egg-white allergy was also an indicator of developing inhalant allergy by the age of seven (Hattevig *et al.*, 1987) and respiratory symptoms by age four years (Tariq *et al.*, 2000).

Mechanisms

Both immediate and delayed allergic reactions play a role in egg allergy (May, 1976).

Symptoms related to egg allergy

* Eczema, pruritis and dermatitis especially in infancy, urticaria, angioedema (Eggesbo *et al.*, 2001)
* Asthma, bronchospasm (Fremont *et al.*, 1997)
* Anaphylaxis, exercise-induced anaphylaxis (Asero *et al.*, 1997)
* Rhinorrhea, irritability, cough, vomiting, rash (Langeland, 1985)
* Contact urticaria (Yamada *et al.*, 2000)

Allergens in egg

Eggs are composed of 56–61% egg white and 27–32% egg yolk. The egg white appears to be slightly more allergenic than the yolk (Anet *et al.*, 1985). Also, mixed/well cooked egg (cake) seems to be better tolerated than whole egg when ingested in the same amounts (Potamianou-Taprantzi *et al.*, 2002).

Commercially prepared food may quite often contain egg or egg white. Leduc and colleagues found that egg white antigens are detectable in sterilized meat by enzyme-linked immunoabsorbent assay (ELISA) techniques. Ingestion of processed food could thus prove to be a problem in patients suffering from severe food allergies (Leduc *et al.*, 1999).

Egg white

54% of egg white is composed of the protein ovalbumin (Gal d2). Other major proteins include ovotransferrin (12%), ovomucoid – Gal d1(11%), ovomucin (3.5%) and lysozyme – Gal d 4 (3.4%). Ovoflavoprotein is found in both egg white and yolk. Onvoinhibitor, avodin (0.5%), ovomacroglobulin, G2 and G3 globulins and cystatin are also proteins found in egg white (Bernhisel-Broadbent *et al.*, 1994; Hoffman, 1983; Holen and Elsayed, 1990; Langeland, 1982).

The allergenicity of ovalbumin, ovotransferrin, ovomucoid and lysozyme has been identified by a number of studies (Bernhisel-Broadbent *et al.*, 1994; Hoffman, 1983; Holen and Elsayed, 1990; Langeland, 1982).

Ovalbumin has a molecular weight of 43 kD and was previously considered to be the most important allergen in egg white, but ovomucoid has now been demonstrated as the dominant allergen (Bernhisel-Broadbent *et al.*, 1994).

Effect of heating or processing on the allergens

Ovomucoid has a molecular weight of 28 kD and is resistant to heat, acid and proteolytic enzymes. However, cooked egg is usually less allergenic than raw egg (Cooke and Sampson, 1997; Yunginger, 1990).

Egg yolk

The proteins found in egg yolk include lipovittelin, phosvitin, egg yolk specific lipoprotein and apovitellin I and IV (Walsh *et al.*, 1987).

It has been suggested that egg allergy in adults may be due to the livetins in egg yolk as opposed to egg white proteins in children (Mandallaz *et al.*, 1988).

Cross-reactivity

IgE antibodies from egg-allergic children have been shown to cross-react with egg proteins of other birds. Many egg-allergic patients have positive SPT or *in vitro* tests to chicken meat, but most can ingest chicken without any adverse reaction (Langeland, 1983).

Egg allergy in adults caused by livetins can be provoked by inhalation of tame bird dander (Mandallaz *et al.*, 1988).

Fish/shellfish

Adverse reactions to fish/shellfish are common and a frequent cause of several types of symptoms, which may begin with oral allergy syndrome and end in anaphylaxis. These reactions are frequently related to asthmatic symptoms (Cunha *et al.*, 2002; Swoboda *et al.*, 2002). Shellfish (crustaceans) include shrimps, crayfish, crabs, and lobsters. Molluscs include bivalves (clams, oysters, mussels and scallops), snails, octopus, squid, and cuttlefish (Bousquet *et al.*, 1998).

The route of exposure can vary between oral ingestion, inhalation and skin contact (Cunha et al., 2002).

Fish

When dealing with allergic reactions to fish, it is important to distinguish between those induced by fish allergy and those induced by non-allergic reactions such as histamine poisoning.

There appear to be some specie differences, but extensive cross-reactivities exist among fish species, such as cod, eel, bass, tuna, sole, and dentex (de Martino et al., 1990).

ALLERGENS IN FISH

The major allergen in cod, allergen M or Gad c1, has been isolated from the myogen fraction of the white meat. It is heat stable and resistant to proteolytic digestion and is composed of 113 amino acids (Elsayed and Bennich, 1975).

Swoboda and colleagues suggested that it may be possible to develop strategies for immunotherapy against fish allergy, using the major cross-reactive fish allergen, carp paralbumin (Swoboda et al., 2002).

EFFECT OF COOKING OR PROCESSING

Cooking appears to reduce the allergenicity of fish, but does not eliminate it. However, some fish-allergic patients seems to tolerate canned tuna and salmon. These findings suggest that at least some of the major fish allergens responsible for IgE mediated reactions are heat labile. However, some fish allergens may still be present in processed fish (Bousquet et al., 1998).

SYMPTOMS ASSOCIATED WITH FISH

Urticaria, respiratory symptoms and gastrointestinal symptoms are common manifestations of allergy to fish (Cunha et al., 2002). Anaphylactic reactions may occur even to very minute quantities found in contaminated oil used for frying (Yunginger et al., 1988).

Crustaceans

Tropomyosin has been identified as the major allergen in crustaceans and is heat stable. Tropomyosin is also thought to be the common allergen responsible for cross-reactivity between crustacean species and even molluscs (Leung et al., 1996; Shanti et al., 1993).

Shrimp was found to cause allergic, even anaphylactic, reactions by DBPCFC in some instances (Bousquet et al., 1998).

Molluscs

Allergic reactions to squid have been demonstrated in the past as well as cross-reactivity between squid and shrimps. However, no cross-reactivity was found between squid and octopus or other molluscs. Limpet (cooked) was also found to cause allergic reaction, including bronchospasm and anaphylaxis in some individuals (Bousquet *et al.*, 1998).

Wheat

Cereals or grains are frequently implicated in food-allergic reactions in children and adults. Cereals account for about 70% of the world's protein intake and include wheat, spelt, barley, oats, rye, rice, corn, sorghum, and millet.

Most varieties of wheat derive from *T. aestivum* (bread wheat). *T. durum* (durum wheat) is a source for Italian pasta, Indian chappatis and Chinese noodles. All varieties of wheat contain soluble and insoluble (gluten) proteins. The softer wheat with the lowest protein content is used for biscuits, cakes and pastry. The harder wheat with higher protein content is used for bread, semolina, couscous, and pasta.

Simonato and colleagues showed that the baking process increases the resistance of the potential allergens of the wheat flour to proteolytic digestion, allowing them to reach the intestinal tract, where they can elicit the immunological response. Therefore, baked bread seems to be potentially more allergenic than flour (Simonato *et al.*, 2001b).

Allergens in wheat

Four major groups of wheat proteins have been identified: water soluble, salt soluble, alcohol soluble, and alcohol insoluble. These are glutenins, globulins, gliadins, and albumins. Sutton and colleagues suggested that the glutenins and globulins were responsible for wheat allergy, gliadins for celiac disease, and the albumins for baker's asthma (Baldo, 1996; Sutton *et al.*, 1982). Varjonen and colleagues found, however, that the strong association between positive oral wheat challenges and positive skin prick tests with the ethanol soluble gliadin is an important allergen in wheat-allergic children with atopic dermatitis (Varjonen *et al.*, 1995).

Symptoms related to wheat allergy

- Atopic dermatitis (Varjonen *et al.*, 1997)
- Anaphylaxis (Vichyanond *et al.*, 1990)
- Exercise induced anaphylaxis (Palosuo *et al.*, 1999)
- Gastrointestinal symptoms (Sampson and Ho, 1997)
- Asthma and baker's asthma (Williams *et al.*, 1987)
- Cough, wheeze, shortness of breath, fever, stuffy nose, skin itching, rash (Manfreda *et al.*, 1986)

- Contact dermatitis (Manfreda *et al.*, 1986)
- Urticaria (Kanny *et al.*, 2001)
- Occular complication (Uchio *et al.*, 1998)
- Ulcerative colitis (Moneret Vautrin *et al.*, 2001)

Simonato and colleagues concluded in their study that Irritable Bowel Syndrome (IBS) could be an IgE mediated hypersensitivity reaction induced by prolamin components that are not detected by current allergy tests, but only by immunoblot. The wheat protein preparation commonly used is of limited value in diagnosing allergy (gut related) to wheat (Simonato *et al.*, 2001a).

Cross-reactivity

There appears to be extensive cross-reactivity between wheat, rye and barley when one looks at skin prick tests, radioallergosorbent test (RAST) and sodium dodecyl sulfate–polyacrylamide gel electrophoresis (SDS-PAGE) immunoblotting. The degree of cross-reactivity closely paraleled their taxonomic relationship and appeared to be in the following order of decreasing closeness: wheat, triticale, rye, barley, oat, rice, and corn. The allergenicity in the rye and wheat extracts was found to be distributed among various fractions of different molecular weights (Baldo *et al.*, 1980; Block *et al.*, 1984). However, clinical cross-reactivity is not often seen, and commonly a positive skin prick test will not be reflected in clinical allergy (Jones and Sampson, 1996). The high number (approximate 80%) of false positive skin and serology tests for wheat is most likely due to the presence of IgE to grass pollen (Bousquet *et al.*, 1998).

SDS-PAGE and immunoblot analysis with patients' sera revealed 27 to 31 protein bands in the region of 7.8 to 66.5 kD for each of the six grains studied (Sampson, 1998). More than half of sera from 32 flour-allergic patients reacted to an allergen of 66 kD in Western blotting (Sandiford *et al.*, 1995).

Inhalation of flour dust can lead to occupational asthma and rhinitis (Thiel and Ulmer, 1980). Interestingly, these patients can ingest cereal grains without any adverse affects. In contrast, patients who suffer from psyllium allergy due to airborne sensitization have suffered anaphylaxis after ingesting cereals containing psyllium (James *et al.*, 1991).

In one interesting study, patients allergic to the water soluble proteins in wheat were found to be sensitive to bromelain, the protein in pineapple (cross-reactivity between bromelain and soluble fraction from wheat; Tanabe *et al.*, 1997).

It is important to notice that the presence of IgA and IgG antibodies to different cereal antigens is a result of natural exposure and in diseases such as atopic dermatitis displays little diagnostic significance, in contrast to anti-gliadin antibody response in dermatitis herpetiformis and celiac disease. Patients with celiac disease do not show IgE antibodies to gluten (Baldo and Wrigley, 1978).

Low-allergen wheat

A so-called hypoallergenic wheat has been produced, and the efficacy of these preparations has been reported in Japanese literature (Ikezawa *et al.*, 1994). Studying the antibodies raised against major food allergens, e.g. 27 kD wheat albumin, makes it possible to select less allergenic or low-allergenic strains.

Soya

Soya causes a significant number of hypersensitivity reactions in infants and young children and is considered to be a classical food allergen (Yunginger, 1990). Soybean is not only a food allergen, but also an occupational aero-allergen inducing asthma (Anto *et al.*, 1989).

Soya is considered the world's most important legume, as soya protein is widely used to increase the protein content of food, more specifically convenience foods.

Various food technologies are applied for their production, e.g. soybean oil, soya lecithin, soya sauce, and texturized or hydrogenated vegetable protein (Franck *et al.*, 2002). The allergenicity of natural soybean may be modified by these treatments.

Symptoms associated with soya allergy

- Anaphylaxis (Foucard and Malmheden, 1999)
- Atopic dermatitis (Burks *et al.*, 1988)
- Rhinitis, conjunctivitis and bronchospasm after inhalation of soybean dust
- Angioedema, abdominal pain, laryngeal edema, respiratory complaints and urticaria
- Infantile colitis, food protein-enterocolitis syndrome (Jenkins *et al.*, 1984; Sicherer *et al.*, 1998)

Allergens in soya

The allergenicity in legumes is mostly related to allergens from their seeds and storage proteins (Pereira *et al.*, 2002). Approximately 10% of the seed proteins are water-soluble albumins and the remainder are salt-soluble globulins (Burks *et al.*, 1988). A number of soy proteins including the Kunitz-type soybean trypsin inhibitor have been identified as allergens (Seppala *et al.*, 2002). The four major protein fractions identified are: 2S (contained in whey fraction), 7S (50% β-conglycinin), 11S (glycinin), and 15S (aggregated glycinin). Cross-reactivity is seen between these three fractions (Shibasaki *et al.*, 1980).

In a study carried out by Burks *et al.* on a small number of children, no difference in the allergenicity of these three fractions was found, although an earlier study suggested that the 2S fraction had the highest allergenic potential (Burks *et al.*, 1988; Shibasaki *et al.*, 1980). Heating increases the allergenicity of 2S globulin, but reduces the allergenicity of the other globulins (Shibasaki *et al.*, 1980).

Seven soya-allergic subjects who ingested up to 8 ml of soybean oil did not show any reaction, even though soybean proteins were found in similar soya fat products such as lecithin, margarine, and oil (Porras *et al.*, 1985). Similarly, Bush and colleagues found soya oil consumption safe for soya allergy sufferers (Bush *et al.*, 1985).

Franck *et al.* (2002) did a very interesting study comparing the allergenicity of native soybean proteins with that of soymilk and texturized protein products. They used soybean flour, soymilk, texturized soy proteins, and two infant formulas, the first containing total proteins and the second containing a soy protein hydrolysate.

The study showed that soybean flour protein and soymilk had a difference in the proportions of the various protein fractions, with a higher concentration of 37 kD protein in flour and 33 kD protein in milk. Infant formula 1 contained proteins with a molecular weight below 28 kD. Immunoblotting revealed a lack of allergenicity in this infant formula. The texturized extract contained high proportions of 31 to 34 and 38 kD proteins. Sera recognizing the 38 and 50 kD proteins in texturized soy protein also recognized the 37 and 49 kD proteins in soybean flour and in soymilk, suggesting a protein glycation by texturization processes. The 30 to 34 kD band in texturized proteins was devoid of any allergenicity. This study seems to indicate that the 30 kD allergen (Gly m Bd 30) disappears during the production of texturized soy protein. They concluded that further studies on texturization might generate modified technologies in order to create hypoallergenic texturized proteins.

Thermal denaturation of soybean extracts does not affect IgE and IgG-specific binding activity. Chemical denaturation appears to reduce minimally the binding of these proteins (Burks *et al.*, 1992).

Cross-reactions

Although legumes show extensive cross-reactivity by *in vitro* methods, e.g. RAST, ELISA, and SDS-PAGE immunoblotting and skin testing, most legume-allergic patients can eat peanuts and vice versa (Belver *et al.*, 2002; Bernhisel-Broadbent and Sampson, 1989; Bernhisel-Broadbent *et al.*, 1989). However, Foucard and Malmheden (1999) showed that patients with severe peanut-allergic reactions may suffer from soybean anaphylaxis.

About 25% of cow's milk allergic patients become allergic to soymilk (Lee and Heiner, 2002). At present, however, soymilk/formula is still regarded as a safe substitute for cow's milk/formula (Zeiger, 1987).

Children with suspected food allergy to soy show frequently positive SPT to soybean and potato. This may be due to cross-reactive IgE antibodies against potato allergens and soya and vice versa (Seppala *et al.*, 2002).

Sesame

Sesame seed allergy is becoming increasingly prevalent and sesame is described as one of the "emerging" allergens, probably because of its use in international fast-food and bakery products (Bousquet *et al.*, 1998; Dutau *et al.*, 1999). However, few studies have focused on the identification of its major allergenic proteins.

Sesame was found to be a major cause of IgE mediated food allergy in Israel. It is second only to cow's milk as a cause of anaphylaxis in that country (Dalal *et al.*, 2002).

In the UK, no prevalence data is available but anecdotal information and experience in allergy clinics points towards a rise in sesame allergy. The Food Standards Agency (FSA) has allocated a research grant to study the prevalence and incidence of sesame sensitization in a birth cohort and a cohort of 6-, 11- and 15-year-old children.

Sporik and Hill (1996) found a sensitization rate to sesame of 531 out of 2789 children that attended the allergy department at the Royal Children's Hospital, Melbourne in 1990–1996.

Symptoms associated with sesame allergy

- Urticaria, angioedema, and wheezing (Levy and Danon, 2001)
- Atopic dermatitis (Eigenmann *et al.*, 1998; Levy and Danon, 2001)
- Occupational asthma, rhinitis and urticaria (Keskinen *et al.*, 1991)

Allergens in sesame

Four proteins are found in sesame seeds (*Sesamum indicum*) of which a 7S vicilin-type globulin, a seed storage protein of sesame (Ses i 3) and a 2S albumin, another seed storage protein of sesame (Ses i 2) were the two major ones (Beyer *et al.*, 2002). Seed storage proteins are known food allergens in peanut, walnut, Brazil nut, and soybean.

Cross-reactivity

Homology between Ses i 3 (a major sesame allergen) and the peanut allergen Ara h 1 were found. In addition, the proteins at 78 and 34 kD were found to be homologous to the embryonic abundant protein and the seed maturation protein of soybeans, respectively (Beyer *et al.*, 2002).

Allergy to poppy seed and/or sesame seed often occurs in patients with simultaneous sensitization to nuts and flour. Common allergenic structures in hazelnut, rye, sesame and poppy seed have also been identified (Vocks *et al.*, 1993).

Sesame oil

Sesame oil is one of the few vegetable oils that can be used without refining, as reflected in the distinctive taste and flavor. The protein content and allergenicity of sesame oil are therefore much higher than for other vegetable oils. Anaphylaxis to sesame oil has also been reported (Hayakawa *et al.*, 1987). Hummus, tahini and halva are other sources of sesame seed increasingly being used worldwide.

Less commonly encountered food allergens

The Prunoideae subfamily (peach, plum, apricot, cherry, almond)

Some evidence exists regarding adverse reactions, even anaphylaxis, to these fruits (Escribano *et al.*, 1996; Ortolani *et al.*, 1993). However, the evidence for including the Prunoideae subfamily in a list of food allergens is still insufficient.

Celery, rice, and buckwheat

Although some evidence exists regarding the allergenicity of these three foods, they do not yet fulfill the criteria for addition to the list of commonly known food allergens and do not need to be identified on labeling (Bousquet *et al.*, 1998).

Beef

Beef allergy can cause symptoms such as vomiting, diarrhea, wheeze, and atopic dermatitis. Han and colleagues found that the (approximately) 200 kDa, 67 kDa and 60 kDa components in the beef extract had strong allergenicity (Han *et al.*, 2000).

Citrus fruits

Fruits in this family include orange, satsuma, lemon, lime, grapefruit, tangerine and clementine. Oranges and other citrus fruits are known to cause symptoms of atopic dermatitis (Steinman and Potter, 1994) as well as rhinitis, urticaria, angioedema, bronchospasm, and contact dermatitis to the orange peel (Cardullo *et al.*, 1989).

Foods involved in oral allergy syndrome

The oral allergy syndrome (OAS) is a common adverse reaction to the ingestion of certain "trigger" foods and is especially prevalent in atopic individuals. OAS is rarely dangerous, but the symptoms may concern patients. Severe forms of OAS may precede food-induced anaphylaxis. Food allergens frequently implicated to cross-react with birch pollen are hazelnut, peach, apple, apricot, plum, cherry, pear, peanut, maize, carrot, new potato, chickpea, and lettuce. Interestingly, most patients can tolerate these foods in a cooked form, even though they may not be able to tolerate the raw fruit or vegetable (Sloane and Sheffer, 2001).

Foods cross-reacting with latex

There is little exact epidemiological data on the prevalence and incidence of latex allergy. On the basis of present data, latex allergy in normal population is low, under 1%. Studies have found cross-reactivity between the plant pathogenesis-related and storage proteins in fruit and vegetables such as avocado, melon, banana, chestnut, apricot, cherry, grape, kiwi, papaya, passion fruit, peach, pineapple, fig, and pepper and the proteins found in latex. However, despite positive skin prick tests, only about half of latex allergic subjects have clinical symptoms after eating cross-reacting foods (Turjanmaa and Makinen-Kiljunen, 2002).

Spices

Food allergy to spices is infrequent. At present, it is found only in adults and accounts for 6.4% of food allergies in adults (Moneret-Vautrin *et al.*, 2002).

The threshold dose for allergens

Those dealing with food-allergic patients know that very small quantities of food can possibly lead to severe reactions in highly sensitive individuals suffering from IgE-mediated allergic reactions. The threshold dose for provocation of allergic reactions is therefore often considered to be zero. Such a threshold dose, however, creates substantial problems for the food industry (Hefle and Taylor, 2002).

Madsen (2001) recommended the use of the elements of chemical risk assessment, namely hazard identification, dose–response assessment, exposure assessment and risk characterization in food allergy risk assessment. This will enable us to avoid labeling such as "may contain traces", as in the long run unjustified warnings will not help the allergic consumer and will create more confusion than guidance.

A Food Standards Agency (FSA) commissioned report, produced by the Anaphylaxis Campaign (AC), claims that the labeling of products that may contain nuts is both inconsistent and confusing to the consumer. According to the survey, 56% of products in an average shopping basket contained labeling to suggest that they may contain nuts; of these products, 11% provided allergen information in a separate place to the ingredients listing. The task group also found that it took 25 min longer to buy a list of 16 items without a "may contain" warning compared to the control group (any suitable products). The average cost of the shopping list with "may contain" labeling was also 11% higher (FSA and AC, 2002).

Food becomes contaminated with other food products from harvesting, transportation, storage, and preparation. This means that equipment handling food known to cause food allergies has to be cleaned before being used for other products. But just how clean should this equipment be to prevent cross-contamination? Does this mean that all foods that may be contaminated with food allergens should carry a "may contain traces" warning (Taylor *et al.*, 2002)?

A safe threshold dose can be defined as the lowest amount of the offending food that would elicit mild objective symptoms (e.g. mild urticaria, erythema and oral angioedema) in the most sensitive individuals. The problem arises here that individuals react to different amounts of the offending foods (Hourihane *et al.*, 1997) which can only partly be explained by the mechanisms involved. Inter- and intra-individual differences exist because of confounding factors, and the threshold doses for different foods are not equal (Taylor *et al.*, 2002).

Evidence regarding a threshold dose

At the moment mostly anecdotal evidence is available regarding the threshold dose eliciting an allergic reaction. Numerous studies reported reactions after ingestion of minute amounts of allergenic foods (as little as 200 µg whey protein), but the reliability of the analytical results should be questioned because validated and standardized methods are not yet available.

Current information on the threshold dose for foods is reported by Taylor *et al.* (2002):

- 1 mg of peanut
- 1 mg of liquid egg
- 0.02 ml of cow's milk
- 5 mg of cod or herring (fish)
- 1 mg of ground mustard.

Hourihane and colleagues (1997) determined that the no effect level/lowest effect level provoking subjective reactions to peanut were 50 µg and 100 µg respectively.

To apply this in the context of a typical serving of food containing undeclared residues of an allergenic food, 1 mg of an allergenic food in a typical 50 g serving would be equivalent to 20 mg of allergenic food per kilogram ingested food product, thus 20 ppm (Taylor *et al.*, 2002).

From the above description, one can see that the threshold doses for allergenic foods are measurable and above zero. One problem is that if a patient reacts to the smallest dose given, it is not necessarily the threshold dose: the threshold dose can lie somewhere between the smallest dose given and zero.

The authors of this paper concluded, however, that because this data was obtained by different protocols, the estimation of a threshold dose was very difficult. Development of a standardized protocol for clinical experiments to allow determination of a threshold dose is needed.

Biotechnology and food allergens

A number of advances in the scientific knowledge concerning adverse food reactions to food have been made in the past few years. This includes understanding about the nature of the food allergen itself, the molecular characterization of the epitopes on these allergens, the pathophysiology of the clinical reaction, and the diagnostic methods (Burks *et al.*, 2001).

The increase in the world population put increasing pressure on agriculture to provide enough food for everyone. This led to developments in agricultural biotechnology which aim to provide foods with a better quality, improved nutritional content and health attributes, resistance to spoilage, and could even lead to foods with reduced levels of allergenicity (IFT Expert Report, 2000). Planting of insect resistant corn and herbicide resistant soya began in the mid-1990s and has reached 30–50% of the crops in North America (Taylor and Hefle, 2001).

These new developments have increased the significance of the toxicology of proteins. The central issue is that of defining and characterizing the allergenic potential of the protein involved (Kimber *et al.*, 1997; Nestle, 1996). Not all proteins display allergenic potential, despite being immunogenic. The bases for these differences are unclear.

Genetic modification of a food ultimately results in the introduction of new proteins into the plant. In the USA, a wide range of genetically modified (GM) foods is available, but in Europe very few GM products have been approved for marketing as foods, partly due to the widespread public concern about their safety and impact on the environment. The safety, including the potential allergenicity of the protein in terms of the ability to induce allergenic sensitization and the likelihood of this happening, must therefore be assessed (Taylor and Hefle, 2001; Cockburn, 2002).

There are two issues that need to be addressed: firstly, the transfer of a known allergen may occur from a crop into a non-allergenic target crop; secondly, the creation of a neo-allergen where *de novo* sensitization can occur (Lack, 2002). Nearly 10 years after the introduction of GM food crops, only limited evidence is still available about their safety. However, the lack of any adverse effects resulting from the production and consumption of GM crops grown on more than 300 million cumulative acres over the past five years and no evidence that the technology used for the production of GM foods poses an allergic threat, supports the safety issue of using these foods (Cockburn, 2002). This does not rule out the need for sufficient investigations. Worldwide agreement by regulatory bodies regarding foods processed through biotechnology is needed, to ensure safe clinical practice and evidence-based advice to our patients.

The International Food Biotechnology Council (IFBC) and the International Life Sciences Institute (ILSI) addressed the issue of the allergenicity of genetically modified foods (Figure 7.3). The recommended first step in determining the safety of using a protein is to consider the source of the protein and whether it is derived from an allergenic food. The IFBC/ILSI report contains an extensive list of 160 food-related substances that have been associated with allergic reactions in individuals at some point (Taylor and Hefle, 2001). The protein in question is tested with the sera of at least 14 people allergic to the food by *in vitro* methods. If no reaction occurs, it is assumed that there is a very high

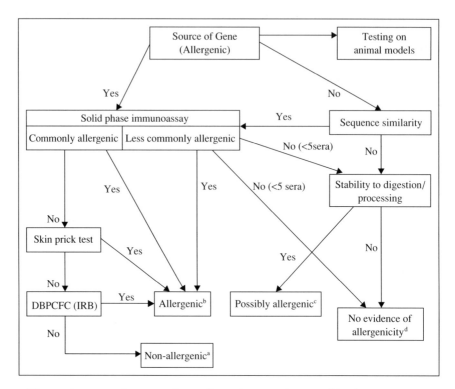

^a The combination of tests involving allergic human subjects or blood serum from such subjects would provide a high level of confidence that no major allergens were transferred. The only remaining uncertainty would be the likelihood of a minor allergen affecting a small percentage of the population allergic to the source material.

^b Any positive results obtained in tests involving allergic human subjects or blood serum from such subjects would provide a high level of confidence that the novel protein was a potential allergen. Foods containing such novel proteins would need to be labeled to protect allergic consumers.

^c A novel protein with either no sequence similarity to known allergens or derived from a less commonly allergenic source with no evidence of binding to IgE from the blood serum of few allergic individuals (n < 5) but that is stable to digestion and processing should be considered as possible allergens. Further evaluation would be necessary to address this uncertainty. The nature of the tests would be determined on a case-by-case basis.

^d A novel protein with no sequence similarity to known allergens and that was not stable to digestion and processing would have no evidence of allergenicity. Similarly, a novel protein expressed by a gene obtained from a less commonly allergenic source and demonstrated to have no binding with IgE from the blood serum of a small number of allergic individuals (n = >5 but, <14) provides no evidence of allergenicity. Stability testing may be included in these cases. However, the level of confidence based on only two decision criteria is modest. It is suggested that other criteria should be considered, such as the expression of the novel protein. (Adapted from Taylor and Hefle, 2001.)

Figure 7.3 Assessment of the allergenic potential of foods derived from genetically modified crop plants.

probability that the protein does not represent an important food allergen (Kimber *et al.*, 1997).

The potential allergenicity of the introduced proteins can also be evaluated by looking at the sequence homology of the newly introduced protein to known allergens by comparing the amino acid sequences of the novel protein to those of known allergens, the expressions level of the novel protein in the modified crop, the functional classification of the novel protein and other physiochemical properties of the protein such as heat stability and digestive stability (Oehlschlager *et al.*, 2001). Additionally, Th-2 cell stimulation, the production of IL-4 and IgE antibody production in animals may help to evaluate the potential allergenicity of a protein (Lehrer *et al.*, 1996). Applying these criteria gives reasonable assurance that genetically modified foods will not become allergenic. Reduced allergen content of biotechnologically altered rice was shown. In contrast, increased allergenicity of soya bean was seen when protein from Brazil nut was transferred to the soybean, but these products were never brought to the market (Nestle, 1996; Nordlee *et al.*, 1996).

Taking all of this into account, the European Parliament has recently voted that animal feeds and human foods containing genetically modified organisms should be labeled as such. Additionally, the Commission has declared that there will not be a "genetically modified free" label, but that a product must be labeled as "containing genetically modified ingredients" unless it contains less than 0.5% genetically modified material. According to a spokesman from the European biotech industry group EuropaBio, this 0.5% threshold is unattainable due to cross-pollination and/or contamination during storage, distribution, and processing (Editorial, 2002).

Conclusion

Food allergy has been with us for a long time. Whether prevalence is on the increase is a question that remains to be answered. Good history taking and medical assessments are cornerstones of food allergy diagnosis. The double-blind placebo-controlled food challenge is considered the gold standard for food allergy diagnosis at present, but controlled research to test the validity and necessity of this procedure is needed. Cow's milk, egg, fish/shellfish, soya, wheat and nuts (tree nuts and peanuts) are considered the main allergens, with new allergens emerging such as sesame seed. The threshold level for different foods has not been established yet, an issue that needs to be addressed as this will clear a lot of confusion, especially regarding labeling issues. Genetically modified foods need proper assessment regarding allergenicity and safety before being released on the market.

References

Aalberse, R.C. and Stapel, S.O. (2001) Structure of food allergens in relation to allergenicity, *Pediatric Allergy and Immunology*, **12**: 10–14.

Anet, J., Back, J.F., Baker, R.S., Barnett, D., Burley, R.W., and Howden, M.E. (1985) Allergens in the white and yolk of hen's egg. A study of IgE binding by egg proteins, *International Archives of Allergy and Applied Immunology*, **77**: 364–371.

Anto, J.M., Sunyer, J., Rodriguez-Roisin, R., Suarez-Cervera, M., and Vazquez, L. (1989) Community outbreaks of asthma associated with inhalation of soybean dust. Toxicoepidemiological Committee, *New England Journal of Medicine*, **320**: 1097–1102.

Arshad, S.H. (2002) *Allergy: an Illustrated Colour Text*. London: Churchill Livingstone.

Asero, R., Mistrello, G., Roncarolo, D., Antoniotti, P., and Falagiani, P. (1997) Exercise-induced egg anaphylaxis, *Allergy*, **52**: 687–689.

Baehler, P., Chad, Z., Gurbindo, C., Bonin, A.P., Bouthillier, L., and Seidman, E.G. (1996) Distinct patterns of cow's milk allergy in infancy defined by prolonged, two-stage double-blind, placebo-controlled food challenges, *Clinical and Experimental Allergy*, **26**: 254–261.

Baldo, B.A. (1996) Allergies to wheat, yeast and royal jelly: a connection between ingestion and inhalation? *Monographs of Allergy*, **32**: 84–91.

Baldo, B.A., Krilis, S., and Wrigley, C.W. (1980) Hypersensitivity to inhaled flour allergens. Comparison between cereals, *Allergy*, **35**: 45–56.

Baldo, B.A. and Wrigley, C.W. (1978) IgE antibodies to wheat flour components. Studies with sera from subjects with baker's asthma or coeliac condition, *Clinical Allergy*, **8**: 109–124.

Ball, G., Shelton, M.J., Walsh, B.J., Hill, D.J., Hosking, C.S., and Howden, M.E. (1994) A major continuous allergenic epitope of bovine beta-lactoglobulin recognized by human IgE binding, *Clinical and Experimental Allergy*, **24**: 758–764.

Belver, M.T., Pascual, C., Pereira, M.J., Valls, A., Garcia Ara, M.C., Boyano, T., and Martin Esteban, M. (2002) Cross-reactivity between lentils and chickpeas towards peanuts and soy, in a Spanish children population, *Allergy*, **57**: 84S.

Bernhisel-Broadbent, J., Dintzis, H.M., Dintzis, R.Z., and Sampson, H.A. (1994) Allergenicity and antigenicity of chicken egg ovomucoid (Gal d III) compared with ovalbumin (Gal d I) in children with egg allergy and in mice, *Journal of Allergy Clinical Immunology*, **93**: 1047–1059.

Bernhisel-Broadbent, J. and Sampson, H.A. (1989) Cross-allergenicity in the legume botanical family in children with food hypersensitivity, *Journal of Allergy and Clinical Immunology*, **83**: 435–440.

Bernhisel-Broadbent, J., Taylor, S., and Sampson, H.A. (1989) Cross-allergenicity in the legume botanical family in children with food hypersensitivity. II. Laboratory correlates, *Journal of Allergy and Clinical Immunology*, **84**: 701–709.

Beyer, K., Bardina, L., Grishina, G., and Sampson, H.A. (2002) Identification of sesame seed allergens by 2-dimensional proteomics and Edman sequencing: seed storage proteins as common food allergens, *Journal of Allergy and Clinical Immunology*, **110**: 154–159.

Bleumink, E. and Young, E. (1968) Identification of the atopic allergen in cow's milk, *International Archives of Allergy and Applied Immunology*, **34**: 521–543.

Block, G., Tse, K.S., Kijek, K., Chan, H., and Chan-Yeung, M. (1984) Baker's asthma. Studies of the cross-antigenicity between different cereal grains, *Clinical Allergy*, **14**: 177–185.

Bock, S.A. (1987) Prospective appraisal of complaints of adverse reactions to foods in children during the first 3 years of life, *Pediatrics*, **79**: 683–688.

Bock, S.A., Sampson, H.A., Atkins, F.M., Zeiger, R.S., Lehrer, S., Sachs, M., Bush, R.K., and Metcalfe, D.D. (1988) Double-blind, placebo-controlled food challenge (DBPCFC) as an office procedure: a manual, *Journal of Allergy and Clinical Immunology*, **82**: 986–997.

Bousquet, J., Bjorksten, B., Bruijnzeel-Koomen, C.A., Huggett, A., Ortolani, C., Warner, J.O., and Smith, M. (1998) Scientific criteria and the selection of allergenic foods for product labelling, *Allergy*, **53**: 3S–21S.

Burks, A.W. Jr, Brooks, J.R., and Sampson, H.A. (1988) Allergenicity of major component proteins of soybean determined by enzyme-linked immunosorbent assay (ELISA) and immunoblotting in children with atopic dermatitis and positive soy challenges, *Journal of Allergy and Clinical Immunology*, **81**: 1135–1142.

Burks, A.W., Williams, L.W., Thresher, W., Connaughton, C., Cockrell, G., and Helm, R.M. (1992) Allergenicity of peanut and soybean extracts altered by chemical or thermal denaturation in patients with atopic dermatitis and positive food challenges, *Journal of Allergy and Clinical Immunology*, **90**: 889–897.

Burks, W., Helm, R., Stanley, S., and Bannon, G.A. (2001) Food allergens, *Current Opinion in Allergy and Clinical Immunology*, **1**: 243–248.

Bush, R.K., Taylor, S.L., Nordlee, J.A., and Busse, W.W. (1985) Soybean oil is not allergenic to soybean-sensitive individuals, *Journal of Allergy and Clinical Immunology*, **76**: 242–245.

Cardullo, A.C., Ruszkowski, A.M., and DeLeo, V.A. (1989) Allergic contact dermatitis resulting from sensitivity to citrus peel, geraniol, and citral, *Journal of the American Academy of Dermatology*, **21**: 395–397.

Cocco, R.R., Jarvinen, K.M., Beyer, K., and Sampson, H.A. (2002) Mutational analysis of IgE epitopes of bovine alpha-1 casein, a major cow's milk protein, *Allergy*, **57**: 73S.

Cockburn, A. (2002) Assuring the safety of genetically modified (GM) foods: the importance of an holistic, integrative approach, *Journal of Biotechnology*, **98**: 79–106.

Committee on the Toxicity and Chemicals in Food (COT) Report (2000) Adverse Reactions to Food. In *Committee on the Toxicity and Chemicals in Food, Consumer Products and the Environment: Adverse Reactions to Food and Food Ingredients* (eds Woods, H.F. and Aggett, P.F.), pp. 11–14. London: COT Secretariat Food Standards Agency.

Cooke, S.K. and Sampson, H.A. (1997) Allergenic properties of ovomucoid in man, *Journal of Immunology*, **159**: 2026–2032.

Crespo, J.F., Pascual, C., Burks, A.W., Helm, R.M., and Esteban, M.M. (1995) Frequency of food allergy in a pediatric population from Spain, *Pediatric Allergy and Immunology*, **6**: 39–43.

Crockard, A.D. and Ennis, M. (2001) Basophil histamine release tests in the diagnosis of allergy and asthma, *Clinical and Experimental Allergy*, **31**: 345–350.

Cunha, L., Marino, E., Fernandez, R., and Falcao, H. (2002) Clinical characteristics of adverse reactions with fish/shellfish in a paediatric population, *Allergy*, **57**: 87S.

Daher, S., Tahan, S., Sole, D., Naspitz, C.K., Silva Patricio, F.R., Neto, U.F., and De Morais, M.B. (2001) Cow's milk protein intolerance and chronic constipation in children, *Pediatric Allergy and Immunology*, **12**: 339–342.

Dalal, I., Binson, I., Reifen, R., Amitai, Z., Shohat, T., Rahmani, S., Levine, A., Ballin, A., and Somekh, E. (2002) Food allergy is a matter of geography after all: sesame as a major cause of severe IgE mediated food allergic reactions among infants and young children in Israel, *Allergy*, **57**: 362.

De Martino, M., Novembre, E., Galli, L., de Marco, A., Botarelli, P., Marano, E., and Vierucci, A. (1990) Allergy to different fish species in cod-allergic children: *in vivo* and *in vitro* studies, *Journal of Allergy and Clinical Immunology*, **86**: 909–914.

Docena, G.H., Fernandez, R., Chirdo, F.G., and Fossati, C.A. (1996) Identification of casein as the major allergenic and antigenic protein of cow's milk, *Allergy*, **51**: 412–416.

Dutau, G., Rittie, J. L., Rance, F., Juchet, A., and Bremont, F. (1999) New food allergies, *Presse Medicale*, **28**: 1553–1559.

Editorial (2002) Decision to label GM food, *Chemistry and Industry*, **14**: 5.

Eggesbo, M., Botten, G., Halvorsen, R., and Magnus, P. (2001) The prevalence of allergy to egg: a population-based study in young children, *Allergy*, **56**: 403–411.

Eigenmann, P.A., Sicherer, S.H., Borkowski, T.A., Cohen, B.A., and Sampson, H.A. (1998) Prevalence of IgE-mediated food allergy among children with atopic dermatitis, *Pediatrics*, **101**: E8.

Ellis, M.H., Short, J.A., and Heiner, D.C. (1991) Anaphylaxis after ingestion of a recently introduced hydrolyzed whey protein formula, *Journal of Pediatrics*, **118**: 74–77.

Elsayed, S. and Bennich, H. (1975) The primary structure of allergen M from cod, *Scandanavian Journal of Immunology*, **4**: 203–208.

Escribano, M.M., Munoz, F.J., Velazouez, E., Gonzalez, J., and Conde, J. (1996) Anaphylactic reaction caused by cherry ingestion, *Allergy*, **51**: 756–757.

Food Standards Agency (FSA) and Anaphylaxis Campaign (AC) (2002) *May Contain Labelling: the Consumer Perspective*, Dionne Davey (Project officer). London: Food Standards Agency.

Foucard, T. and Malmheden, Y.I. (1999) A study on severe food reactions in Sweden – is soy protein an underestimated cause of food anaphylaxis?, *Allergy*, **54**: 261–265.

Franck, P., Moneret Vautrin, D.A., Dousset, B., Kanny, G., Nabet, P., Guenard Bilbaut, L., and Parisot, L. (2002) The allergenicity of soybean-based products is modified by food technologies, *International Archives Allergy Immunology*, **128**: 212–219.

Fremont, S., Kanny, G., Nicolas, J.P., and Moneret-Vautrin, D.A. (1997) Prevalence of lysozyme sensitization in an egg-allergic population, *Allergy*, **52**: 224–228.

Fuglsang, G., Madsen, G., Halken, S., Jorgensen, S., Ostergaard, P.A., and Osterballe, O. (1994) Adverse reactions to food additives in children with atopic symptoms, *Allergy*, **49**: 31–37.

Gern, J.E., Yang, E., Evrard, H.M., and Sampson, H.A. (1991) Allergic reactions to milk-contaminated "nondairy" products, *New England Journal of Medicine*, **324**: 976–979.

Gjesing, B., Osterballe, O., Schwartz, B., Wahn, U., and Lowenstein, H. (1986) Allergen-specific IgE antibodies against antigenic components in cow milk and milk substitutes, *Allergy*, **41**: 51–56.

Goidman, A., Anderson D., *et al.* (1963a) Milk allergy part I: oral challenge with milk and isolated milk proteins in allergic children, *Pediatrics*, **20**: 400–407.

Goidman, A., Sellars, W.A., Halpern, S.R., *et al.* (1963b) Milk allergy part II: skin testing of allergic and normal children with purified milk proteins, *Pediatrics*, **32**: 572–579.

Han, G.D., Matsuno, M., Ito, G., and Suzuki, A. (2000) Meat allergy: investigation of potential allergenic proteins in beef, *Biosciences Biotechnology and Biochemistry*, **64**: 1887–1895.

Hattevig, G., Kjellman, B., and Bjorksten, B. (1987) Clinical symptoms and IgE responses to common food proteins and inhalants in the first 7 years of life, *Clinical Allergy*, **17**: 571–578.

Hayakawa, R., Matsunaga, K., Suzuki, M., Hosokawa, K., Arima, Y., Shin, C.S., and Yoshida, M. (1987) Is sesamol present in sesame oil?, *Contact Dermatitis*, **17**: 133–135.

Hefle, S.L. and Taylor, S.L. (2002) How much food is too much? Threshold doses for allergenic foods, *Current Allergy and Asthma Report*, **2**: 63–66.

Hide, D.W. (1994) Food allergy in children, *Clinical and Experimental Allergy*, **24**: 1–2.

Hill, D.J., Firer, M.A., Ball, G., and Hosking, C.S. (1993) Natural history of cows' milk allergy in children: immunological outcome over 2 years, *Clinical and Experimental Allergy*, **23**: 124–131.

Hoffman, D.R. (1983) Immunochemical identification of the allergens in egg white, *Journal of Allergy and Clinical Immunology*, **71**: 481–486.

Holen, E. and Elsayed, S. (1990) Characterization of four major allergens of hen egg white by IEF/SDS-PAGE combined with electrophoretic transfer and IgE-immunoautoradiography, *International Archives of Allergy and Applied Immunology*, **91**: 136–141.

Host, A. and Halken, S. (1990) A prospective study of cow milk allergy in Danish infants during the first 3 years of life. Clinical course in relation to clinical and immunological type of hypersensitivity reaction, *Allergy*, **45**: 587–596.

Host, A., Jacobsen, H.P., Halken, S., and Holmenlund, D. (1995) The natural history of cow's milk protein allergy/intolerance, *European Journal of Clinical Nutrition*, **49**: 13S–18S.

Hourihane, J.O.'B., Kilburn, S.A., Nordlee, J.A., Hefle, S.L., Taylor, S.L., and Warner, J.O. (1997) An evaluation of the sensitivity of subjects with peanut allergy to very low doses of peanut protein: a randomized, double-blind, placebo-controlled food challenge study, *Journal of Allergy and Clinical and Immunology*, **100**: 596–600.

IFT Expert Report (2000) IFT expert report on biotechnology and foods. Benefits and concerns associated with recombinant DNA biotechnology-derived foods, *Food Technology*, **54**: 61–80.

Ikezawa, Z., Tsubaki, K., and Yokota, S. (1994) Effect of hypoallergenic wheat (HAW-A1) on atopic dermatitis (AD) with wheat allergy, and its antigenic analysis using sera from patients with AD, *Arerugi*, **43**: 679–688.

James, J.M., Cooke, S.K., Barnett, A., and Sampson, H.A. (1991) Anaphylactic reactions to a psyllium-containing cereal, *Journal of Allergy and Clinicial Immunology*, **88**: 402–408.

Jenkins, H.R., Pincott, J.R., Soothill, J.F., Milla, P.J., and Harries, J.T. (1984) Food allergy: the major cause of infantile colitis, *Archives of Diseases of Childhood*, **59**: 326–329.

Johansson, S.G., Hourihane, J.O., Bousquet, J., Bruijnzeel-Koomen, C., Dreborg, S., Haahtela, T., Kowalski, M.L., Mygind, N., Ring, J., van Cauwenberge, P., Hage-Hamsten, M., and Wuthrich, B. (2001) A revised nomenclature for allergy. An EAACI position statement from the EAACI nomenclature task force, *Allergy*, **56**: 813–824.

Joneja, J. (1998) *Dietary Management of Food Allergies and Intolerances. A Comprehensive Guide*, 2nd edn. Vancouver: J.A. Hall Publications.

Jones, S.M. and Sampson, H.A. (1996) The role of allergens in atopic dermatitis. In *Atopic Dermatitis: from Pathogenesis to Treatment* (ed. D.Y.M. Leung). Georgetown, TX: RG Landes Co.

Kanny, G., Chenuel, B., and Moneret-Vautrin, D.A. (2001) Chronic urticaria to wheat, *Allergy*, **56**: 356–357.

Keskinen, H., Ostman, P., Vaheri, E., Tarvainen, K., Grenquist-Norden, B., Karppinen, O., and Nordman, H. (1991) A case of occupational asthma, rhinitis and urticaria due to sesame seed, *Clinical and Experimental Allergy*, **21**: 623–624.

Kimber, I., Lumley, C.E., and Metcalfe, D.D. (1997) Allergenicity of proteins, *Human Experimental Toxicology*, **16**: 516–518.

Krop, J., Lewith, G.T., Gziut, W., and Radulescu, C. (1997) A double blind, randomized, controlled investigation of electrodermal testing in the diagnosis of allergies, *Journal of Alternative and Complementary Medicine,* **3**: 241–248.

Lack, G. (2002) Clinical risk assessment of GM foods, *Toxicological Letters,* **127**: 337–340.

Langeland, T. (1982) A clinical and immunological study of allergy to hen's egg white. III. Allergens in hen's egg white studied by crossed radio-immunoelectrophoresis (CRIE), *Allergy,* **37**: 521–530.

Langeland, T. (1983) A clinical and immunological study of allergy to hen's egg white. VI. Occurrence of proteins cross-reacting with allergens in hen's egg white as studied in egg white from turkey, duck, goose, seagull, and in hen egg yolk, and hen and chicken sera and flesh, *Allergy,* **38**: 399–412.

Langeland, T. (1985) Allergy to hen's egg white in atopic dermatitis, *Acta Dermatologica et Venereologica Supplement (Stockholm),* **114**: 109–112.

Leduc, V., Demeulemester, C., Polack, B., Guizard, C., Le Guern, L., and Peltre, G. (1999) Immunochemical detection of egg-white antigens and allergens in meat products, *Allergy,* **54**: 464–472.

Lee, E.J. and Heiner, D.C. (2002) Allergy to cow's milk – 1985, *Pediatrics in Review,* **7**: 195–203.

Lehrer, S.B., Horner, W.E., and Reese, G. (1996) Why are some proteins allergenic? Implications for biotechnology, *Critical Reviews in Food Science and Nutrition,* **36**: 553–564.

Leung, P.S., Chow, W.K., Duffey, S., Kwan, H.S., Gershwin, M.E., and Chu, K.H. (1996) IgE reactivity against a cross-reactive allergen in crustacea and mollusca: evidence for tropomyosin as the common allergen, *Journal of Allergy and Clinical Immunology,* **98**: 954–961.

Levy, Y. and Danon, Y.L. (2001) Allergy to sesame seed in infants, *Allergy,* **56**: 193–194.

Madsen, C. (2001) Where are we in risk assessment of food allergens? The regulatory view, *Allergy,* **56**: 91S–93S.

Majamaa, H., Moisio, P., Holm, K., Kautiainen, H., and Turjanmaa, K. (1999) Cow's milk allergy: diagnostic accuracy of skin prick and patch tests and specific IgE, *Allergy,* **54**: 346–351.

Mandallaz, M.M., de Weck, A.L. and Dahinden, C.A. (1988) Bird-egg syndrome. Cross-reactivity between bird antigens and egg-yolk livetins in IgE-mediated hypersensitivity, *International Archives of Allergy and Applied Immunology,* **87**: 143–150.

Manfreda, J., Holford-Strevens, V., Cheang, M., and Warren, C.P. (1986) Acute symptoms following exposure to grain dust in farming, *Environmental Health Perspectives,* **66**: 73–80.

May, C.D. (1976) Objective clinical and laboratory studies of immediate hypersensitivity reactions to foods in asthmatic children, *Journal of Allergy and Clinical Immunology,* **58**: 500–515.

Moneret Vautrin, D.A., Sainte-Laudy, J., and Kanny, G. (2001) Ulcerative colitis possibly due to hypersensitivity to wheat and egg, *Allergy,* **56**: 458–459.

Moneret-Vautrin, D.A., Morisset, M., Lemerdy, P., and Kanny, G. (2002) Food allergy and IgE sensitization caused by spices: CICBAA data, *Allergy and Immunology (Paris),* **34**: 135–140.

Nestle, M. (1996) Allergies to transgenic foods – questions of policy, *New England Journal of Medicine,* **334**: 726–728.

Nordlee, J.A., Taylor, S.L., Townsend, J.A., Thomas, L.A., and Bush, R.K. (1996) Identification of a Brazil-nut allergen in transgenic soybeans, *New England Journal of Medicine*, **334**: 688–692.

Oehlschlager, S., Reece, P., Brown, A., Hughson, E., Hird, H., Chisholm, J., Atkinson, H., Meredith, C., Pumphrey, R., Wilson, P., and Sunderland, J. (2001) Food allergy – towards predictive testing for novel foods, *Food Additives and Contamination*, **18**: 1099–1107.

Oliveira, S., Camara, P., Ornelas, P., and Borges, F.D. (2002) Prospective study on cow's milk allergy (CMA) in newborns, *Allergy*, **57**: 25S–26S.

Ortolani, C., Bruijnzeel-Koomen, C., Bengtsson, U., Bindslev-Jensen, C., Bjorksten, B., Host, A., Ispano, M., Jarish, R., Madsen, C., Nekam, K., Paganelli, R., Poulsen, L.K., and Wuthrich, B. (1999) Controversial aspects of adverse reactions to food. European Academy of Allergology and Clinical Immunology (EAACI) Reactions to Food Subcommittee, *Allergy*, **54**: 27–45.

Ortolani, C., Pastorello, E.A., Farioli, L., Ispano, M., Pravettoni, V., Berti, C., Incorvaia, C., and Zanussi, C. (1993) IgE-mediated allergy from vegetable allergens, *Annals of Allergy*, **71**: 470–476.

Palosuo, K., Alenius, H., Varjonen, E., Koivuluhta, M., Mikkola, J., Keskinen, H., Kalkkinen, N., and Reunala, T. (1999) A novel wheat gliadin as a cause of exercise induced anaphylaxis, *Journal of Allergy and Clinical Immunology*, **103**: 912–917.

Pastorello, E.A., Pravettoni, V., Stocchi, L., Bigi, A., Schilke, M.L., and Zanussi, C. (1991) Are double-blind food challenges necessary before starting an elimination diet?, *Allergy Proceedings*, **12**: 319–325.

Pereira, M.J., Pascual, C.Y., Belver, M.T., Diaz Pena, J.M., Sanchez Monge, R., Gomez Palacios, A., Salcedo, G., and Martin Esteban, M. (2002) Lentil allergen and cross-reactivity with chickpeas, peanuts and soy, *Allergy*, **57**: 84S.

Pittard, W.B., III and Bill, K. (1979) Differentiation of cord blood lymphocytes into IgA-producing cells in response to breast milk stimulatory factor, *Clinical Immunology and Immunopathology*, **13**: 430–434.

Porras, O., Carlsson, B., Fallstrom, S.P., and Hanson, L.A. (1985) Detection of soy protein in soy lecithin, margarine and, occasionally, soy oil, *International Archives of Allergy and Applied Immunology*, **78**: 30–32.

Potamianou-Taprantzi, P., Zanikou, S., Psarros, P., Syrigou, E., Manoussakis, M., and Saxoni-Papageorgiou, P. (2002) Relationship between egg-specific serum IgE concentration and the outcome of specific provocation to egg allergic children, *Allergy*, **57**: 79S.

Prausnitz, C. and Kustner, H. (1921) Studies on supersensitivity, *Centralbl. Bakteriol.*, **86**: 160–169.

Rolfsen, W., Tibell, M., and Yman, L. (1987) Cow's milk proteins as allergens and antigens, *Allergol. Immunol. Clinica (Madrid)*, **2**: 213.

Sampaio, G., Almeida, T., Prates, S., Arede, S., Loureiro, V., Matos, V., Murta, R., Almeida, M.M., and Pinto, J.R. (2002) Persistent cow's milk allergy in children. A follow-up study, *Allergy*, **57**: 25S.

Sampson, H.A. (1998) Adverse reactions to food, in *Allergy: Principles and Practice* (ed. E. Middleton *et al.*), vol. II, 5th edn, pp. 1162–1182. New York: Mosby.

Sampson, H.A. and Ho, D.G. (1997) Relationship between food-specific IgE concentrations and the risk of positive food challenges in children and adolescents, *Journal of Allergy and Clinical Immunology*, **100**: 444–451.

Sandiford, C.P., Tee, R.D., and Newman-Taylor, A.J. (1995) Identification of crossreacting wheat, rye, barley and soya flour allergens using sera from individuals with wheat-induced asthma, *Clinical and Experimental Allergy*, 25: 340–349.

Seppala, U., Majamaa, H., Turjanmaa, K., Vanto, T.T., Kalkkinen, N., Palosuo, K., and Reunala, T. (2002) Frequent skin prick test sensitivity to soy and potato in children: cross-reactivity to structurally allergens?, *Allergy*, 57: 80S.

Shanti, K.N., Martin, B.M., Nagpal, S., Metcalfe, D.D., and Rao, P.V. (1993) Identification of tropomyosin as the major shrimp allergen and characterization of its IgE-binding epitopes, *Journal of Immunology*, 151: 5354–5363.

Shibasaki, M., Suzuki, S., Tajima, S., Nemoto, H., and Kuroume, T. (1980) Allergenicity of major component proteins of soybean, *International Archives of Allergy and Applied Immunology*, 61: 441–448.

Sicherer, S.H., Eigenmann, P.A., and Sampson, H.A. (1998) Clinical features of food protein-induced enterocolitis syndrome, *Journal of Pediatriacs*, 133: 214–219.

Simonato, B., De Lazzari, F., Pasini, G., Polato, F., Giannattasio, M., Gemignani, C., Peruffo, A.D., Santucci, B., Plebani, M., and Curioni, A. (2001a) IgE binding to soluble and insoluble wheat flour proteins in atopic and non-atopic patients suffering from gastrointestinal symptoms after wheat ingestion, *Clinical and Experimental Allergy*, 31: 1771–1778.

Simonato, B., Pasini, G., Giannattasio, M., Peruffo, A.D., De Lazzari, F., and Curioni, A. (2001b) Food allergy to wheat products: the effect of bread baking and *in vitro* digestion on wheat allergenic proteins. A study with bread dough, crumb, and crust, *Journal of Agriculture and Food Chemistry*, 49: 5668–5673.

Sloane, D. and Sheffer, A. (2001) Oral allergy syndrome, *Allergy and Asthma Proceedings*, 22: 321–325.

Sporik, R. and Hill, D. (1996) Allergy to peanut, nuts, and sesame seed in Australian children, *British Medical Journal*, 313: 1477–1478.

Steinman, H.A. and Potter, P.C. (1994) The precipitation of symptoms by common foods in children with atopic dermatitis, *Allergy Proceedings*, 15: 203–210.

Sutton, R., Hill, D.J., Baldo, B.A., and Wrigley, C.W. (1982) Immunoglobulin E antibodies to ingested cereal flour components: studies with sera from subjects with asthma and eczema, *Clinical Allergy*, 12: 63–74.

Swaisgood, H.E. (1982) Chemistry of milk proteins, in *Developments in Diary Chemistry* (ed. P.F. Fox). London: Applied Science Publishers.

Swoboda, I., Bugajska-Schretter, A., Verdino, P., Keller, W., Sperr, W.R., Valenta, P., and Spitzauer, S. (2002) Recombinant carp parvalbumin, the major cross-reactive fish allergen: a tool for diagnosis and therapy for fish allergy, *Allergy*, 57: 80S.

Tanabe, S., Tesaki, S., Watanabe, M., and Yanagihara, Y. (1997) Cross-reactivity between bromelain and soluble fraction from wheat flour, *Arerugi*, 46: 1170–1173.

Tariq, S.M., Matthews, S.M., Hakim, E.A., and Arshad, S.H. (2000) Egg allergy in infancy predicts respiratory allergic disease by 4 years of age, *Pediatric Allergy and Immunology*, 11: 162–167.

Taylor, S.L. and Hefle, S.L. (2001) Will genetically modified foods be allergenic?, *Journal of Allergy and Clinical Immunology*, 107: 765–771.

Taylor, S.L., Hefle, S.L., Bindslev-Jensen, C., Bock, S.A., Burks, A.W. Jr, Christie, L., Hill, D.J., Host, A., Hourihane, J.O., Lack, G., Metcalfe, D.D., Moneret-Vautrin, D.A., Vadas, P.A., Rance, F., Skrypec, D.J., Trautman, T.A., Yman, I.M., and Zeiger, R.S. (2002) Factors affecting the determination of threshold doses for allergenic foods: how much is too much?, *Journal of Allergy and Clinical Immunology*, 109: 24–30.

Thiel, H. and Ulmer, W.T. (1980) Bakers' asthma: development and possibility for treatment, *Chest*, **78**: 400S–405S.

Turjanmaa, K. and Makinen-Kiljunen, S. (2002) Latex allergy: prevalence, risk factors, and cross-reactivity, *Methods*, **21**: 10–14.

Uchio, E., Miyakawa, K., Ikezawa, Z., and Ohno, S. (1998) Systemic and local immuno-logical features of atopic dermatitis patients with ocular complications, *British Journal of Ophthalmology*, **82**: 82–87.

Vanto, T.T., Helppila, S., Juntunen-Backman, K., Kalimo, K., Klemola, T., Korpela, R., Koskinen, P., and Syvanen, P. (2002) Development of tolerance to milk in children with cow's milk hypersensitivity: predictive factors, *Allergy*, **57**: 25S.

Varjonen, E., Vainio, E., and Kalimo, K. (1997) Life-threatening, recurrent anaphylaxis caused by allergy to gliadin and exercise, *Clinical and Experimental Allergy*, **27**: 162–166.

Varjonen, E., Vainio, E., Kalimo, K., Juntunen-Backman, K., and Savolainen, J. (1995) Skin-prick test and RAST responses to cereals in children with atopic dermatitis. Characterization of IgE-binding components in wheat and oats by an immunoblotting method, *Clinical and Experimental Allergy*, **25**: 1100–1107.

Vichyanond, P., Visitsuntorn, N., and Tuchinda, M. (1990) Wheat-induced anaphylaxis, *Asian Pacific Journal of Allergy and Immunology*, **8**: 49–52.

Vocks, E., Borga, A., Szliska, C., Seifert, H.U., Seifert, B., Burow, G., and Borelli, S. (1993) Common allergenic structures in hazelnut, rye grain, sesame seeds, kiwi, and poppy seeds, *Allergy*, **48**: 168–172.

Wal, J.M. (2001) Structure and function of milk allergens, *Allergy*, **56**: 35–38.

Walsh, B.J., Elliott, C., Baker, R.S., Barnett, D., Burley, R.W., Hill, D.J., and Howden, M.E. (1987) Allergenic cross-reactivity of egg-white and egg-yolk proteins. An *in vitro* study, *International Archives of Allergy and Applied Immunology*, **84**: 228–232.

Werfel, S.J., Cooke, S.K., and Sampson, H.A. (1997) Clinical reactivity to beef in children allergic to cow's milk, *Journal of Allergy and Clinical Immunology*, **99**: 293–300.

Williams, A.J., Church, S.E., and Finn, R. (1987) An unsuspected case of wheat induced asthma, *Thorax*, **42**: 205–206.

Yamada, K., Urisu, A., Kakami, M., Koyama, H., Tokuda, R., Wada, E., Kondo, Y., Ando, H., Morita, Y., and Torii, S. (2000) IgE-binding activity to enzyme-digested ovomucoid distinguishes between patients with contact urticaria to egg with and without overt symptoms on ingestion, *Allergy*, **55**: 565–569.

Young, E., Stoneham, M.D., Petruckevitch, A., Barton, J., and Rona, R. (1994) A population study of food intolerance, *Lancet*, **343**: 1127–1130.

Yunginger, J.W. (1990) Classical food allergens, *Allergy Proceedings*, **11**: 7–9.

Yunginger, J.W., Sweeney, K.G., Sturner, W.Q., Giannandrea, L.A., Teigland, J.D., Bray, M., Benson, P.A., York, J.A., Biedrzycki, L., and Squillace, D.L. (1988) Fatal food-induced anaphylaxis, *Journal of the American Medical Association*, **260**: 450–1452.

Zeiger, R.S. (1987) Challenges in the prevention of allergic disease in infancy, *Clinical Reviews of Allergy*, **5**: 349–373.

8 Dietary phosphorus as a nutritional toxin: the influence of age and sex

Leonard Sax

Summary

Several reports have suggested that consumption of cola beverages leads to decreased bone density. Phosphoric acid, an additive found in all cola beverages, may be responsible for this effect. Critics have argued that any apparent negative effect of cola beverages is a result of displacement of other nutrients rather than a direct effect of phosphoric acid. They also point out that the amount of phosphorus in cola beverages is small compared with the total amount of phosphorus consumed in a typical Western European or North American diet. However, inorganic phosphates – such as those found in cola beverages – may be absorbed faster and have a different physiological effect than the protein-bound phosphorus found in meat, nuts, and other natural sources of phosphorus.

There are important sexual dimorphisms in bone physiology, and bone physiology varies as a function of age. Careful analysis of the evidence suggests that while phosphorus may indeed be hazardous to bone in children and young women, it is probably not harmful to bone in older men.

Introduction

Many investigators (Garcia-Contreras *et al.*, 2000; Massey and Strang, 1982; Wyshak, 2000; Wyshak *et al.*, 1989; Wyshak and Frisch, 1994; Petridou *et al.*, 1997) have suggested that consumption of cola beverages may lead to decreased bone density and an increased risk of broken bones. Massey and Strang (1982) were the first to propose that phosphoric acid, an additive found in all cola beverages, may be responsible for this effect; their hypothesis was strengthened and further developed by Calvo and Park (1996), Garcia-Contreras *et al.* (2000), and Sax (2001), among others. Recent critics of this hypothesis (e.g. Adamson, 2001; Allison, 2001; Heaney and Nordin, 2002; Williams, 2001) have raised three objections:

1   the evidence that cola beverages adversely affect bone density derives from survey data and from animal studies rather than from randomized controlled trials in humans

2   any apparent negative effect of cola beverages may be a result of displacement of other nutrients rather than a direct effect of phosphoric acid. For example, children who drink more soda may be drinking less milk, and the decrease in milk consumption may be the proximate cause of their (purported) osteopenia

3   the amount of phosphorus in an eight-ounce cola beverage – between 40 and 60 mg – is small compared with the total amount of phosphorus consumed in a typical Western European or North American diet, i.e. between 1200 and 1500 mg/day.

This chapter will begin by reviewing the theoretical and empirical bases for the claim that phosphoric acid may lead to decreased bone density. Each of the three objections offered by critics of this hypothesis will then be considered.

We shall see that much of the variance in the data can be accounted for if one recognizes the sexual dimorphism in human bone physiology. Females and males build and maintain bone differently. These sex differences in bone physiology, in turn, vary as a function of age. As we shall see, the evidence suggests that dietary phosphates are probably not harmful to adult men, but are likely to be deleterious to young women and girls.

Biochemical considerations

Many investigators have found a significant and sustained rise in serum parathyroid hormone (PTH) in humans who ingest supplemental phosphates (e.g. Calvo *et al.*, 1988, 1990; Reiss *et al.*, 1970; Silverberg *et al.*, 1986, 1989). There are at least three mechanisms whereby phosphoric acid might cause a rise in PTH. One mechanism is loss of free ionized calcium to formation of calcium phosphate complexes in the blood.

$$Ca^{2+} + 2HPO_4^{-1} \leftrightharpoons Ca(HPO_4)_2 \downarrow$$

A second mechanism whereby dietary phosphate might trigger a rise in PTH involves precipitation of calcium (in the form of calcium phosphate) within the gut prior to absorption. In this case, the rise in PTH is due to a decrease in calcium absorption from the gut, rather than a loss of free ionized calcium from the plasma. These two mechanisms are of course not exclusive; both could be in play.

A third mechanism whereby ingestion of phosphates could lead to a rise in PTH involves a drop in 1,25-dihydroxyvitamin D. Portale *et al.* (1986) gave 1500 mg phosphorus per day to six healthy men, for nine days. They then restricted the diet to 500 mg phosphorus per day for 10 days; this restriction resulted in an 80% increase in 1,25-dihydroxyvitamin D. Finally, they increased the daily phosphorus intake to 3000 mg/day for another 10 days, resulting in a rapid drop in 1,25-dihydroxyvitamin D to levels almost 30% below the baseline obtained when the intake was 1500 mg per day. Thus, raising dietary phosphorus lowered levels of 1,25-dihydroxyvitamin D, while lowering dietary phosphorus raised levels of 1,25-dihydroxyvitamin D.

If dietary calcium is plentiful, then calcium lost to the formation of calcium phosphate can be replenished from the diet. And, while a lower level of 1,25-dihydroxyvitamin D would decrease the efficiency with which calcium is absorbed from the gut, a diet rich in calcium can compensate for a drop in 1,25-dihydroxyvitamin D. But if levels of dietary calcium do not keep pace with the levels of phosphate in the diet, then increased consumption of dietary phosphates could lead to a rise in PTH, by any of the following mechanisms:

1   by complexing calcium in the chyme, thereby impairing calcium absorption
2   by lowering the concentration of free ionized calcium in plasma by complexing calcium ion with phosphate ion
3   by reducing the levels of 1,25-dihydroxyvitamin D, thereby decreasing absorption of calcium.

The final common result in each case is an increase in serum PTH, which will promote the mobilization of calcium from bone via bone resorption, maintaining a constant concentration of free ionized calcium in the plasma at the expense of bone density.

Numerous animal studies have demonstrated that diets with low calcium-to-phosphorus ratios give rise to low bone densities (see Calvo (1994) for review). The dietary calcium-to-phosphorus ratio has been shown to predict bone density, independent of the absolute intake of both elements, over a wide range of intakes in laboratory animals (e.g. Shah *et al.*, 1967). The demonstration that parathyroidectomy can prevent the bone loss associated with a high phosphorus diet (Anderson and Draper, 1972) confirms that the final common pathway to bone loss caused by high phosphorus intakes is indeed an elevation in PTH.

Two studies in humans have demonstrated findings which tend to confirm the overall picture derived from animal studies: namely, that the dietary calcium-to-phosphorus ratio correlates significantly, and positively, with bone density. Metz *et al.* (1993), studying 24-to-28-year-old Caucasian women, reported a significant positive correlation between the dietary calcium-to-phosphorus ratio and distal bone mineral content ($p = 0.0068$). A study of 510 perimenopausal women (Brot *et al.*, 1999) reported similar findings: while they found no consistent correlation between phosphorus consumption alone and bone density, and an intermediate positive correlation ($p < 0.01$) between calcium consumption and bone density, the strongest predictor of bone density was the dietary calcium-to-phosphorus (Ca:P) ratio. "The Ca:P ratio proved to be a significant independent predictor of bone mineral content and bone mineral density in all regions ($p < 0.0005$)."

Cola beverages

Phosphate additives are used as flavor stabilizers in all popular cola beverages sold in the United States. (Non-cola carbonated beverages use citric acid rather than phosphates for this purpose.) Several investigators have suggested that consumption of cola beverages, and the associated decline in milk consumption, may decrease bone density, particularly in children and young women. A study from the Harvard School of Public Health (Wyshak, 2000) reported that active teenage girls who drink cola beverages had a fracture risk 4.94 times higher than girls who denied drinking cola beverages, even if those other girls drank non-cola carbonated beverages ($p = 0.002$). This finding appeared to confirm and extend previous findings (Wyshak *et al.*, 1989; Wyshak and Frisch, 1994) indicating that consumption of cola beverages predicted high fracture risk in teenage girls. However, all three of these studies relied on questionnaires and self-report: none included any independent measure of cola beverage consumption or bone density, nor was any attempt made to confirm that girls who believed that they had sustained a broken bone had actually done so.

Another study sought to ascertain the dietary habits of Greek children seen in an emergency department for bone fracture (Petridou *et al.*, 1997). Children with a single uncomplicated fracture were interviewed in case–control fashion, paired with children seen at the same time in the same emergency department with unrelated complaints such as stomach upset or sore throat. In this study, consumption of cola beverages was strongly associated with an increased risk of fracture. Children who drank more than 1.5 cans of cola beverages per day were 4.8 times as likely to sustain a fracture as children who drank no cola beverages ($p = 0.001$). Interestingly, consumption of *non*-cola carbonated beverages was not significantly associated with an increased risk of fracture. Unfortunately, this study did not break down results by gender.

Is cola to blame, or does cola merely displace other nutrients?

Some (e.g. Adamson, 2001; Allison, 2001; Heaney and Nordin, 2002; Williams, 2001) have suggested that the increased risk of fracture associated with consumption of cola beverages is not a result of anything in the beverage itself, but is rather due to the displacement of other foods and beverages such as milk. Garcia-Contreras and associates (2000) paired ovariectomized rats consuming water as their sole beverage with ovariectomized rats consuming cola soft drinks as their sole beverage. Bone density was significantly lower in the group drinking cola beverages ($p < 0.02$), and their levels of activated vitamin D was also significantly lower ($p < 0.0001$). However, the rats drinking the cola beverages ate much less lab chow than did the rats who had only water to drink: 11 g of chow per day in the cola group, vs 18 g per day in the water group ($p < 0.001$). The authors recognized that the reduction in bone density and activated vitamin D in the cola group might be a result of the lower food intake of the rats in the cola group, rather than a direct effect of the cola itself.

Accordingly, Garcia-Contreras and associates reported a second study in the same paper, in which they investigated this possibility. This time, they employed a pair-feeding strategy. Animals were divided into pairs, with one animal in each pair having access to water while the other animal had access to cola beverages. Every day, these investigators measured the amount of lab chow consumed by the animal with access to cola beverages. The next day, the "partner" animal (with access to water) was given only that amount of chow which had been consumed the previous day by the animal with access to cola beverages. Thus, these investigators were able to compare animals consuming the same amount of solid food, the only difference between the groups being that the animals in one group drank only cola beverages while the animals in the other group drank only water.

By the end of this second study, the pair-fed animals with access to water were significantly thinner than the animals with free access to cola beverages. Whereas the animals with access to cola beverages gained an average of 32 g of body weight during the study, the animals with access only to water lost an average of 14 g of body weight ($p < 0.001$). Nevertheless, despite their lower overall weight, the animals with access only to water had much stronger bones, and dramatically higher bone calcium: 1.32 mg/g, vs only 0.85 mg/g in the group with access to cola beverages ($p < 0.001$). These results strongly suggest that the negative effects of cola beverages on bone density are a direct result of the cola beverage itself, and not a consequence of displacement of other nutrients from the diet.

Sexual dimorphism

Numerous animal studies have demonstrated sexual dimorphism in bone physiology (e.g. Oz et al., 2000; Sims et al., 2002). A meticulous study of 500 girls and boys found substantial sex differences in the determinants of bone density in children and adolescents (Boot et al., 1997). In boys, physical activity was strongly associated with bone density: more active boys had higher bone density and higher bone mineral content than less active boys. In girls, this study found no significant association between physical activity and bone density. Another recent study reported a slight positive association between physical activity and bone density in girls; however, even in this study, the least active boy accrued bone mineral at a rate equal to that of the most active girl, while the most active boy accrued bone mineral at a rate far above that of the most active girl (Anderson, 2001). Still another recent study (Carter et al., 2001) confirmed that 13-year-old boys on average have significantly higher total body bone mineral content than 13-year-old girls (1793 g vs 1581 g, $p = 0.005$).

Calvo et al. (1988) studied the effects of a low-calcium, high-phosphorus diet in young women and young men (ages 18 to 25). In both women and men, the diet caused a rise in PTH levels, but this rise was substantially greater in the women than it was in the men. Despite the fact that the women manifested a higher rise in PTH, the women did not maintain a constant serum calcium concentration. Whereas the diet had no effect on serum calcium in the men, the low-calcium, high-phosphorus diet gave rise to a significant decline in serum calcium concentration in women.

There is evidence that the mechanism underlying the age-related decline in bone density may differ between females and males (e.g. Chailurkit *et al.*, 2001). In females, the primary mechanism appears to be an increase in bone resorption, whereas in males, the primary mechanism responsible for the age-related decline in bone density appears to be a decline in bone formation.

The influence of age

Draper and Bell (1979) studied the effects of high dietary phosphate loads on loss of calcium from the skeleton of rats aged six months and 16 months. In the younger rats, a high-phosphate diet had a dramatic effect in promoting calcium loss, an effect which persisted throughout the seven weeks of the study. In older rats, the high-phosphate diet had a much smaller effect, which diminished quickly and was almost gone within four weeks. The lead investigator subsequently concluded that the loss of sensitivity of aging bone to high-phosphorus diets is related to a change in the proportions of trabecular and compact bone: in humans, for example, the proportion of trabecular bone as a fraction of total bone in the human iliac crest decreases from approximately 45% at 20 years of age to just 25% at 85 years of age (Draper and Scythes, 1981).

In adult men, dietary phosphates appear to have little effect on bone density. Spencer *et al.* (1978) studied calcium balance and calcium absorption in middle-aged men (average age of 54 years). They found no effect on calcium balance or calcium absorption in response to an increase in dietary phosphates, over a 25-fold variation in dietary calcium-to-phosphorus ratios (2.5:1 to 1:10). Elmstahl *et al.* (1998) have even shown that low intakes of phosphorus appear to *increase* fracture risk in middle-aged and elderly Swedish men.

In older *women*, the data are mixed. Heaney and Recker (1982) studying middle-aged Roman Catholic nuns, found no net effect of different levels of phosphorus consumption on calcium balance, and another study of older women found no increased risk of osteopenia among women who consumed carbonated beverages (Kim *et al.*, 1997). However, we have already considered a study of 510 perimenopausal women in which the dietary calcium-to-phosphorus ratio was highly predictive of bone density (Brot *et al.*, 1999). We should recall that this study also reported no significant correlation between phosphorus consumption and bone density. The calcium-to-phosphorus ratio may have more significance than phosphorus consumption *per se*, particularly in older women.

Organic and inorganic dietary phosphorus

A spokesman for the soda industry made the following rebuttal to claims that phosphoric acid in cola beverages may adversely affect bone density:

> . . . [M]ilk, cheese, beef, yeast bread, poultry, cereal, eggs, and fish are the major sources of phosphorus in the diet. Soft drinks contribute only about 2% of dietary phosphorus. To be more exact, a 12-oz can of a cola beverage contains between 27 and 62 mg of phosphorus, while the amount of phosphorus consumed per person in unprocessed food is about 1430 to 1520 mg daily . . .
>
> (Adamson, 2001, p. 200)

According to this argument, cola beverages contribute only a small fraction of the total phosphorus in the typical American or European diet, and therefore the amount of phosphorus in cola beverages cannot be clinically significant.

This argument overlooks the fact that the phosphorus in "milk, cheese, beef, yeast bread, poultry, cereal, eggs, and fish" is protein-bound, while the phosphorus in cola beverages is inorganic phosphate. Inorganic phosphate is rapidly absorbed from the gut and enters the bloodstream. Protein-bound phosphorus is absorbed more slowly and may remain protein-bound, making it less available to combine with free calcium ion in the bloodstream.

Consider the analogy to carbohydrates. Starch and sugar are both carbohydrates. Starch is hydrolyzed into simple sugars, but this process takes time. As a result, ingestion of simple sugars has nutritional and physiologic consequences which are distinctly different from ingestion of carbohydrates such as starch, even though starch is ultimately broken down into simple sugars. Likewise, even though protein-bound phosphorus may eventually by released as free phosphate, this process occurs slowly and may not have the hypocalcemic effect of ingestion of simple phosphates in cola beverages.

In any event, the contribution of phosphorus from cola beverages may be more substantial, particularly in children, than is generally recognized. Harnack *et al.* (1999) found that the dietary calcium-to-phosphorus ratio declined monotonically as a function of the amount of carbonated beverages consumed, and this decline was statistically significant (see especially their Table 3).

Public health implications

The risk of fractures in childhood and adolescence appears to have nearly doubled between the 1960s and the 1990s (Johansen *et al.*, 1997). One study reported that by their 15th birthday almost two-thirds (63.7%) of boys and more than one-third (39.1%) of girls now have sustained at least one broken bone. These investigators suggested that today's children may have "a tendency towards fracturing bones at lower levels of trauma" than did children of past eras, but they did not explore possible mechanisms underlying this new tendency (Lyons *et al.*, 1999).

The increase in the risk of fractures in this context suggests that some change in children's nutritional habits may be at least partly responsible for the increased fracture risk. Between 1970 and 1997, per capita consumption of carbonated soft drinks increased 118% while consumption of milk declined 23% (Golden, 2000). The average teenager now drinks 65 gallons of carbonated beverages per year; this figure does not include juice or sports drinks (Summar, 2000). Today, almost one-fourth of adolescents consume more than 26 oz of carbonated beverages every day (Harnack *et al.*, 1999). Roughly 70% of soda beverages consumed by college students contain phosphoric acid (Massey and Stang, 1982); during exam period, consumption of cola beverages increases (Khan, 1980). The rapid increase in the consumption of phosphates in the diet of children, and the general decrease in the calcium-to-phosphorus ratio in the diet, may be playing a role in the changing epidemiology of fractures in childhood and adolescence (Calvo and Park, 1996).

On the other hand, some investigators contend that middle-aged and elderly people may suffer from a deficiency of dietary phosphorus (Heaney and Nordin, 2002). In this age group, it may actually be appropriate to provide dietary supplements containing phosphates, particularly for men.

Conclusion

There is substantial evidence that phosphoric acid in cola beverages may adversely effect bone density, by any of the three mechanisms discussed herein. This effect is most pronounced in children and in young women. In older men (and perhaps older women), phosphates may be less harmful; some have argued that phosphates might actually be beneficial for the elderly. Further research is necessary in order to clarify the nutritional needs of females and males at different stages of the life cycle. It is conceivable that in the future, well-informed doctors will take the cola away from the teenagers and give it to Grandpa instead.

References

Adamson, R.H. (2001) Soft drinks: a safe refreshment, *Archives of Pediatric and Adolescent Medicine*, **155**: 200.

Allison, D.B. (2001) Hold the cola alarm, *Archives of Pediatric and Adolescent Medicine*, **155**: 201–202.

Anderson, G.H. and Draper, H.H. (1972) Effect of dietary phosphorus on calcium metabolism in intact and parathyroidectomized adult rats, *Journal of Nutrition*, **102**: 1123–1132.

Anderson, J.J.B. (2001) Calcium requirement during adolescence to maximize bone health, *Journal of the American College of Nutrition*, **20**: 186S–191S.

Boot, A.M., Ridder, M.A.J., Pols, H.A.P., Krenning, E.P., and Keizer-Schrama, S.M. (1997) Bone mineral density in children and adolescents: relation to puberty, calcium intake, and physical activity. *Journal of Clinical Endocrinology and Metabolism*, **82**: 57–62.

Brot, C., Jorgensen, N., Madsen, O.R., Jensen, L.B., and Sorensen, O.H. (1999) Relationships between bone mineral density, serum vitamin D metabolites and calcium-to-phosphorus intake in healthy perimenopausal women, *Journal of Internal Medicine*, **245**: 509–516.

Calvo, M.S. (1994) The effects of high phosphorus intake on calcium homeostasis. In *Advances in Nutritional Research*, vol. 9, pp. 183–207. New York: Raven.

Calvo, M.S., Kumar, R., and Heath, H. (1988) Elevated secretion and action of serum parathyroid hormone in young adults consuming high phosphorus, low calcium diets assembled from common foods, *Journal of Clinical Endocrinology and Metabolism*, **66**: 823–829.

Calvo, M.S., Kumar, R., and Heath, H. (1990) Persistently elevated parathyroid hormone secretion and action in young women after four weeks of ingesting high phosphorus, low calcium diets, *Journal of Clinical Endocrinology and Metabolism*, **70**: 1334–1340.

Calvo, M.S. and Park, Y.K. (1996) Changing phosphorus content of the U.S. diet: potential for adverse effects on bone, *Journal of Nutrition*, **126**: 1168S–1180S.

Carter, L.M., Whiting, S.J., Drinkwater, D.T., Zello, G.A., Faulkner, R., and Bailey, D.A. (2001) Self-reported calcium intake and bone mineral content in children and adolescents, *Journal of the American College of Nutrition*, **20**: 502–509.

Chailurkit, L., Pongchaiyakul, C., Charoenkiatkul, S., Kosulwat, V., Rojroongwasinkul, N., and Rajatanvin, R. (2001) Different mechanism of bone loss in ageing women and men in Khon Kaen province, *Journal of the Medical Association of Thailand*, **84**: 1175–1182.

Draper, H.H. and Bell, R.R. (1979) Nutrition and osteoporosis. In *Advances in Nutritional Research*, vol. 2 (ed. H.H. Draper), pp. 79–106. New York: Plenum.

Draper, H.H. and Scythes, C.A. (1981) Calcium, phosphorus, and osteoporosis, *Federation Proceedings*, **40**: 2434–2438.

Elmstahl, S., Gullberg, B., Janzon, L., Johnell, O., and Elmstahl, B. (1998) Increased incidence of fractures in middle-aged and elderly men with low intakes of phosphorus and zinc, *Osteoporosis International*, **8**: 333–340.

Garcia-Contreras, F., Paniagua, R., Avila-Diaz, M., Cabrera-Muñoz, L., Martinez-Muñiz, I., Foyo-Niembro, E., and Amato, D. (2000) Cola beverage consumption induces bone mineralization reduction in ovariectomized rats, *Archives of Medical Research*, **31**: 360–365.

Golden, N.H. (2000) Osteoporosis prevention, *Archives of Pediatric and Adolescent Medicine*, **154**: 542–543.

Harnack, L., Stang, J., and Story, M. (1999) Soft drink consumption among US children and adolescents: nutritional consequences, *Journal of the American Dietetic Association*, **99**: 436–441.

Heaney, R.P. and Nordin, B.E. (2002) Calcium effects on phosphorus absorption: implications for the prevention and co-therapy of osteoporosis, *Journal of the American College of Nutrition*, **21**: 239–244.

Heaney, R.P. and Recker, R.R. (1982) Effects of nitrogen, phosphorus, and caffeine on calcium balance in women, *Journal of Laboratory and Clinical Medicine*, **99**: 46–55.

Johansen, A., Evans, R.J., Stone, M., Richmond, P.W., Lo, S., and Woodhouse, K.W. (1997) Fracture incidence in England and Wales: a study based on the population of Cardiff, *Injury*, **28**: 655–660.

Khan, M.A. (1980) Observations on beverage preferences of college students at specific times, *Journal of the American Dietetic Association*, **77**: 56–57.

Kim, S.H., Morton, D.J., and Barrett-Connor, E. (1997) Carbonated beverage consumption and bone mineral density among older women: the Rancho Bernardo Study, *American Journal of Public Health*, **87**: 276–279.

Lyons, R.A., Delahunty, A.M., Kraus, D., Heaven, M., McCabe, M., Allen, H., and Nash, P. (1999) Children's fractures: a population based study, *Injury Prevention*, **5**: 129–132.

Massey, L.K. and Strang, M.M. (1982) Soft drink consumption, phosphorus intake, and osteoporosis, *Journal of the American Diet Association*, **80**: 581–582.

Metz, J.A., Anderson, J.J.B., and Gallagher, P.N. (1993) Intakes of calcium, phosphorus, and protein, and physical activity level are related to radial bone mass in young adult women, *American Journal of Clinical Nutrition*, **58**: 537–542.

Oz, O., Zerwekh, J.E., Fisher, C., Graves, K., Nanu, L., Millsaps, R., and Simpson, E.R. (2000) Bone has a sexually dimorphic response to aromatase deficiency, *Journal of Bone Mineral Research*, **15**: 507–514.

Petridou, E., Karpathios, T., Dessypris, N., Simon, E., and Trichopoulos, D. (1997) The role of dairy products and non alcoholic beverages in bone fractures among schoolage children, *Scandinavian Journal of Socical Medicine*, **25**: 119–125.

Portale, A.A., Halloran, B.P., Murphy, M.M., and Morris, R.C. (1986) Oral intake of phosphorus can determine the serum concentration of 1,25-dihydroxyvitamin D by determining its production rate in humans, *Journal of Clinical Investigation*, **77**: 7–12.

Reiss, E., Canterbury, J.M., Bercovitz, M.A., and Kaplan, E.L. (1970) The role of phosphate in the secretion of parathyroid hormone in man, *Journal of Clinical Investigation*, **49**: 146–149.

Sax, L. (2001) The Institute of Medicine's "Dietary Reference Intake" for phosphorus: a critical perspective, *Journal of the American College of Nutrition*, **20**: 271–278.

Shah, B.G., Krisnato, G.V.G., and Draper, H.H. (1967) The relationship of Ca and P nutrition during adult life and osteoporosis in aged mice, *Journal of Nutrition*, **92**: 30–42.

Silverberg, S.J., Shane, E., Clemens, T.L., Dempster, D.W., Segre, G.V., Lindsay, R., and Bilezikian, J.P. (1986) The effect of oral phosphate administration on major indices of skeletal metabolism in normal subjects, *Journal of Bone Mineral Research*, **1**: 383–388.

Silverberg, S.J., Shane, E., del la Cruz, R.N., Segre, G.V., Clemens, T.L., and Bilezikian, J.P. (1989) Abnormalities in parathyroid hormone secretion and 1,25-dihydroxyvitamin D_3 formation in women with osteoporosis. *New England Journal of Medicine*, **320**: 277–281.

Sims, N.A., Dupont, S., Krust, A., Clement-Lacroix, P., Minet, D., Resche-Rigon, M., Gaillard-Kelly, M., and Baron, R. (2002) Deletion of estrogen receptors reveals a regulatory role for estrogen receptors-ß in bone remodeling in females but not in males, *Bone*, **30**: 18–25.

Spencer, H., Kramer, I., Osis, D., and Norris, C. (1978) Effect of phosphorus on the absorption of calcium and on the calcium balance in man, *Journal of Nutrition*, **108**: 447–457.

Summar, S. (2000) Adolescent eating habits, 1965–1996, *Pediatric Primary Care*, **14**(9): 35–36.

Williams, C.L. (2001) Methodology of concern, *Archives of Pediatric and Adolescent Medicine*, **155**: 201.

Wyshak, G. (2000) Teenaged girls, carbonated beverage consumption, and bone fractures, *Archives of Pediatric and Adolescent Medicine*, **154**: 610–613.

Wyshak, G. and Frisch, R.E. (1994) Carbonated beverages, dietary calcium, the dietary calcium/phosphorus ratio, and bone fractures in girls and boys, *Journal of Adolescent Health*, **15**: 210–215.

Wyshak, G., Frisch, R.E., Albright, T.E., Schiff, I., and Witschi, J. (1989) Nonalcoholic carbonated beverage consumption and bone fractures among women former college athletes, *Journal of Orthopedic Research*, **7**: 91–99.

9 Metals in wine

Maurizio Aceto

Introduction

The metal content of wine is a topic of interest to analytical chemists but has received little attention from enologists and wine producers. This is due to the fact that metals, among the thousands or more of chemical species present in wine, are considered to contribute sparely to its flavor and are seen as something that should better be absent than present. Some metals are known to generate undesired phenomena in wine (Cu and Fe hazes), while others are considered toxic (Cd, Hg, Pb). If we add that metal determination is usually performed by expensive analytical techniques, it is understandable why metals analysis is not popular in the field of wine science.

Nevertheless, there are at least five good reasons to be interested in metals:

1   *the physiological effects on vine growth* – some metals are soil nutrients essential to the healthy growth of vines and hence, after all, to the production of quality wines
2   *the physiological effects on human health* – it is important to value the contribution of wine to the dietary intake of both essential and toxic elements
3   *the influence on organoleptic features* – some metal ions, though present at mg/l concentrations or less, can positively influence wine taste or can cause alterations of organoleptic features of a wine, for example varying its clarity
4   *the legal requirements* – according to legislation (which is different from country to country), some metals need to be kept under minimum values in wine due to their toxicity
5   *the provenance of the wine* – metal distribution can be used in classification studies to determine the geographic provenance of a wine.

The role of metals in wine was reviewed in the fundamental work of Pereira (1988), who considered several aspects throughout the winemaking process.

Mean concentrations of metals in wine are reported in Table 9.1; values are adapted from Eschnauer (1986, 1989b) and Greenough *et al.* (1997).

Much of the present knowledge about metals in wine is due to the pioneering works of Eschnauer (1974, 1982, 1986), who elucidated the content and the

Table 9.1 Concentration ranges of inorganic species in wines

Species	Concentration range	Species	Concentration range
K	300–1500 mg/L	Pb	10–300 μg/L
P[a]	300–800 mg/L	Ti	1–300 μg/L
Ca	50–150 mg/L	Li	10–200 μg/L
Mg	50–150 mg/L	Cr	30–60 μg/L
Na	5–60 mg/L	Ni	30–50 μg/L
Si	1.5–6 mg/L	Ag	5–20 μg/L
Mn	1–6 mg/L	As	3–20 μg/L
B	1–5 mg/L	Co	1–20 μg/L
Fe	1–5 mg/L	Mo	1–10 μg/L
Rb	0.2–4.2 mg/L	Sb	6 μg/L
Zn	0.5–3.5 mg/L	Cs	2–3 μg/L
Sr	0.2–3.5 mg/L	W	0.01–1 μg/L
Cu	0.01–1 mg/L	Cd	0.01–1 μg/L
Al	0.5–1 mg/L	REE[b]	<1 μg/L
Sn	10–700 μg/L	Se	<1 μg/L
V	1–300 μg/L	Hg	<0.1 μg/L
Ba	40–300 μg/L	Tl	<0.1 μg/L

[a] As PO_4^{3-}.
[b] Rare earth elements.

various factors affecting the concentration of the elements in wine, ranging from major to ultra-trace. Of particular interest are some papers published over a period of 20 years, where individual elements were studied, identifying their natural and artificial sources; examples are those concerning Tl (Eschnauer *et al.*, 1984), Se (Eschnauer *et al.*, 1989a), Cd (Eschnauer *et al.*, 1996) and Pb (Eschnauer and Scollary, 1996).

Why determine metals in wine?

For the abovementioned reasons, the matter of metals in wine is an important one. The mineral components of wine, taken as a whole, represent a mere 0.2–0.3% of its total composition. Nevertheless, their effects are wide and can be positive or negative, as a consequence of the ambivalent nature of metals, as outlined below.

Physiological effects on vine growth

A number of metals or semi-metallic elements such as Al, As as As(III), B, Be, Cd, Co, Cr as Cr(VI), Cu, Mo, Ni, Se as Se(IV), and Tl can be harmful to plants. Indeed, an even larger group of metals or semi-metallic elements are also for good vine growth. Being present in soil at trace level concentrations, metals such as Cu, Fe, Mn, and Zn are nutrients playing a physiological role in the growth of plants. As, Cd, Hg and Pb, on the contrary, have no physiological role and should be absent or at ultra-trace concentration in soil; their toxicity can be exerted by forming antimetabolites, by reacting with essential metabolites, or by substituting for other essential ions. Se is known to be essential or toxic as a response to slight changes in its concentrations.

The likely effects of either essentiality or toxicity depend on the metal concentration, the chemical species and the vine's uptake capacity. The mobility of metals from soils to plants is regulated by the physicochemical properties of the soil and plant species, but these can be altered by human or environmental factors. Uptake by vines occurs as free ions or as chelates, the former being associated with the *bioavailable* fraction. While essential metals are absorbed with an active mechanism that implies contribution of metabolic energy, unessential and toxic metals are taken up with a passive mechanism of diffusion through plant tissues.

It is well known that several metals are considered essential for the healthy growth of vines. Treatments of soil, vine and fruit are usually carried on with substances containing metallic oligoelements. An example is the addition of Cr, Mo and W to soil (or as a spray) which increases both grape yield and grape content of important compounds such as sugars, polyphenols and esters. This eventually results in the production of wines with a smoother taste and good bouquet. Mn is another key metal ion in grape treatment: it is known to increase the content of essential amino acids and, therefore, the quality of wines. Other examples are reported by Pereira (1988).

Physiological effects on human health

Beverages may contribute significantly to the daily intake of either essential or toxic trace elements, on the basis of the average daily consumption of liquids that can be estimated as 1.5–2 L/day. It is noteworthy that some elements, Pb among them, are absorbed from the gastrointestinal tract more readily from beverages than from food (Heard *et al.*, 1983). Among beverages, wine has significantly high levels of As, Cr and Pb (Pedersen *et al.*, 1994).

Before discussing the effects on human health of wine consumption from the point of view of its metal content, it is important to state that wine does not constitute a major risk of assumption of undesired or toxic metal ions. This is particularly true if we consider that the content of most toxic metals in wine has decreased noticeably in the past 30 years, due to higher standards of purity in enological processes (Eschnauer, 1982). On the contrary, wine can be considered a source of those elements that are considered essential to human life. This appears to be true for Co, Cr, Cu, Fe, Mn, Mo, Se, Si, Sn, V, and Zn: wine consumption contributes a fraction of total human dietary intake.

The best way to evaluate the effects of metal assimilation through wine consumption is to calculate the contribution of wine to the *dietary intake* for essential elements, or to the *tolerable intake* for toxic elements. It is therefore important to have some reference values to deal with: these are issued and periodically updated by national nutrition boards and international institutions such as the World Health Organization (WHO) and the Food and Agriculture Organization (FAO). For the sake of clarity we will describe essential and toxic

Table 9.2 Physiological role of metals present in wine (elements in bold type are generally considered to be trace elements)

Elements essential to all animals and plants	Ca, **Cu**, **Fe**, K, Mg, **Mn**, Na, P, **Se**, **Zn**
Elements essential to several classes of animals and plants	**Co**, **Mo**, Si, **V**, **W**
Elements essential to a wide variety of species in one class	Cr
Elements essential to one or two species only	**Al**, **Ba**, **Li**, **Ni**, **Sr**
Elements essential according to recent works, but of unknown function	**Rb**, **Sn**
Unessential or toxic elements	**As**, **Cd**, **Hg**, **Pb**

metals separately; however, it must be remembered that some elements recognized as toxic at moderate or high concentrations can become essential for the normal functioning of cell metabolism at trace level. Sometimes, the quantitative difference between essential amounts and toxic concentrations of these elements is very small. According to a well-acknowledged definition, 'an element is already useful to the organism and to the maintenance of health when a measurable deficit in the diet reduces the growth and vitality of humans, animals or plants to a reproducible degree' (Mertz and Cornatzer, 1971).

In Table 9.2 metals present in wine are listed with reference to their physiological role.

In order to assess the physiological effect of metals, either toxic or essential, it is important to emphasize the concept of *speciation*. It is well known that data pertaining to the total concentration of an element does not provide any information on effects on human health (as for all living organisms). Information about its nutritional function, chemical form and availability should be collected by means of understanding its role in speciation studies. Several speciation studies have been carried on wine, mostly concerning copper, iron, and lead species.

Essential metals

According to the previous definition and to more recent studies (Kieffer, 1991), 22 metallic and semi-metallic elements can be considered *essential* to human life when present in proper concentrations: Al, Ba, Ca, Co, Cr, Cu, Fe, K, Li, Mg, Mn, Mo, Na, Ni, P, Rb, Se, Si, Sn, Sr, V, and Zn. Apart from calcium, magnesium, phosphorus, potassium and sodium, which account for approximately 2% of human body weight, the other metals are indeed trace elements which cover a mere 0.012%. Nevertheless, their influence on body functions is extremely great. The main physiological role of essential metals is the correct functioning of enzymatic and metabolic reactions.

Essential metals must be consumed in adequate quantities. The desirable ranges of intake are established by national nutrition boards and are called

Table 9.3 Recommended dietary allowances of essential metals

Element	RDA (mg/day)
Calcium	1000–1300
Phosphorus	700–1250
Magnesium	240–420
Iron	8–27
Zinc	8–12
Manganese	1.9–2.6
Copper	0.700–1.300
Molybdenum	0.034–0.050
Chromium	0.025–0.045
Selenium	0.040–0.070

recommended dietary allowances (RDAs). Table 9.3 reports values of RDAs for adults issued by the Food and Nutrition Board of the USA National Academy of Sciences (Food and Nutrition Information Center, 2002). It is important to note that these values take into account the fact that only a limited fraction of metal ions present in food can be absorbed in the intestine.

We will now deal with the nutritional aspects of single elements.

ALUMINUM

Lopez *et al.* (1998) estimated the contribution of alcoholic beverages to Al dietary intake in Spain, finding that wine provided the greatest part with about 5% of the total diet.

CHROMIUM

Pedersen *et al.* (1994), in their survey on dietary habits in Denmark, found that wine consumption contributed 4% of the total daily intake of Cr in the Danish diet. Cabrera-Vique *et al.* (1997) demonstrated that, with reference to the French population, wine consumption contributes up to 10% of daily total dietary intake of chromium.

IRON

Concerning Fe, several studies reveal that wine and alcoholic beverages are an important source, contributing 10% of dietary intake (Darret *et al.*, 1986).

NICKEL

Pedersen *et al.* (1994) estimated that the contribution of wine to the total Ni intake in the Danish diet was 1.5%. Teissedre *et al.* (1998b) calculated the total Ni daily dietary intake for the French population from wine consumption to be 4.37 µg/day per person, contributing 7% of total dietary intake.

POTASSIUM

The high ratio of K/Na in wine is of interest in nutritional studies of the effect of diet on hypertension (Ough and Amerine, 1988).

VANADIUM

Vanadium levels in French and Californian wines were determined by Teissedre *et al.* (1998a): they estimated that the contribution of wine consumption to daily vanadium dietary intake of the French population was 11 μg/day per person, which seems too high when compared with the total vanadium daily intake estimated by Wennig and Kirsch (1988) and equal to 0.01–0.03 mg/day.

Unessential metals

A widely used parameter in assessing limits for unessential metals in the diet is the *provisional tolerable weekly intake* (PTWI) issued by the Joint FAO/WHO Expert Committee on Food Additives (JECFA), an international scientific committee dealing with contaminants and additives in food. The concept of PTWI was established in 1972 by JECFA. It is an intake value expressed on a weekly basis, presented in μg of contaminant per week per 1 kg of body weight; it emphasizes the importance of long-term exposure that is not expressed by the *provisional maximum tolerable daily intake* (PMTDI), its analog on a daily basis. PTWI values recommended by JECFA are listed in Table 9.4.

Many studies in the past 10 years have demonstrated that wine contributes a significant fraction of the PTWI of toxic metals. However, the PTWIs are established for total metal concentration regardless of its chemical form, though it is well known that in wine (as in many other complex systems) metals can be present as complexes rather than as free ions. Their absorption rate and

Table 9.4 PTWI values recommended by JECFA

Metal	mg/kg of body weight	mg for a 60 kg person
Aluminum	7	420
Arsenic	0.015	0.9
Cadmium	0.007	0.42
Copper	3.5	210
Iron	5.6	336
Lead	0.025[a]	1.5
Mercury	0.005	0.30
Methyl mercury	0.0033	0.198
Nickel	0.035[b]	2.1
Tin	14	840
Zinc	7	420

[a] This value does not apply to infants and children.
[b] Value not issued by JECFA.

physiological effects are therefore strongly dependent on the predominant chemical species. For example, several studies found that Pb exists in wine mainly as a complexed species and only a small fraction exists as Pb^{2+} free ion (Fournier *et al.*, 1998; McKinnon and Scollary, 1997; Szpunar *et al.*, 1998). Information concerning the various forms in which metals can exist in wine is reported in "sources of metals in wine" below under each metal heading.

ARSENIC

Pedersen *et al.* (1994) calculated that wine consumption contributed to 0.4% of the total as daily intake in the Danish diet. Herce-Pagliai *et al.* (2002) analyzed wine samples from the south of Spain and suggested that the consumption of wine makes no significant contribution to the total and inorganic arsenic intake for normal drinkers.

CADMIUM

Pedersen *et al.* (1994), with reference to the Danish population, estimated the contribution of wine consumption to the total Cd intake to be negligible, being equal to 0.075% of PTWI. Mena *et al.* (1996) studied the contribution of alcoholic beverages to cadmium intake in Spain; they found that a toxicological risk was not imminent, but alcoholic beverages could contribute a considerable fraction of the total dietary cadmium intake. Tahvonen (1998), in a survey of beverages consumed in Finland, found that they contribute only a negligible amount of Cd to the average Finnish diet.

LEAD

Due to its toxicological relevance, research on Pb is highly developed. Studies in the late 1980s and initial 1990s reported the relevance of wine consumption to Pb intake. Elinder *et al.* (1988) found that Pb concentrations in blood samples from the Swedish population were higher in patients with high wine consumption. Calculations on the Pb daily intake via food in Sweden showed that a consumption of 0.5 L/day of wine would double the daily oral Pb intake. In a survey on alcoholic beverages sold in the UK, Smart *et al.* (1990) found that Pb intake from wine was equal to the intake from the remainder of the diet. Pedersen *et al.* (1994), in a survey on the Danish market, found that the major source of Pb intake coming from beverages was from wine and estimated that the consumption of half a bottle per day doubled the daily intake of lead and contributed 12% of the PTWI of Pb. De la Torre (1997), using the basis of mean lead content in wines produced in France, Italy, and Spain, calculated that wine contribution to the daily intake of Pb was well below 10% of the tolerable daily intake. Tahvonen (1998), in a survey of beverages consumed in Finland, found that their contribution of Pb to the average Finnish diet was negligible; however, as the total Pb intake is low in Finland (about 12 μg/day), the share of beverages was equal to about a fifth of the total Pb intake. It is noteworthy that uptake of Pb from wine is minimal when consumed with food, as was found by Gulson *et al.* (1998).

MERCURY

Pedersen *et al.* (1994) calculated that beverages contribute only 5% of the daily Hg intake in the Danish diet, with wine accounting for a minor fraction of this value.

Influence on organoleptic features

Metals play an important role in wine's organoleptic features, either positively or negatively. Their influence starts in the winemaking process, where some of them are nutrients for the development of yeasts cells and others can act as poisons to the yeast enzyme systems. It is generally accepted that the quality of a wine depends largely on the presence of inorganic micro-constituents, and that metals can influence stability, color, clarity, and other characteristics.

Beneficial effects on yeast cell reproduction, and increases in alcohol and bio-mass content, are reported to result from must treatment with Cr, Mn, Mo, W, and Zn. Cu has a double role: its content in must influences polyphenoloxidase activity during fermentation, but in the meantime it produces an increase in the formation of hydrogen sulfide. Fe(II) and Mn salts are known as fermentation accelerators. Ni is thought to be effective in increasing acetal levels in finished wine.

On the other hand, high concentrations of Cd, Cr(VI), Hg, Pb, Tl, but also of Co, Cr(III), Cu, V, and Zn, have toxic effects on yeasts by inhibiting fermentation. Ca and K can cause precipitation of tartaric salts in bottled wines. Cu and Fe have been the subject of active enological research for their relevance in causing haze phenomena and discoloration of wine; Al and Sn are also known for pro-ducing similar spoilage events. An increase in the content of Al, Cu, Fe, Si, and Zn can lead to unwanted turbidity and to a conspicuous taste (bitter or metallic); these are the so-called *wine-sensitive* elements. Speciation studies can help us to understand the spoilage processes induced by metals. McKinnon and Scollary (1997) used ultrafiltration to study the distribution in different particle size fractions of some metals associated with wine spoilage processes, or regarded as potentially toxic; the results allowed the individuation of compounds with which metals can interact while forming haze.

Even the taste of wine is influenced by metals (Pereira, 1988): statistical analysis demonstrated that positive correlations exist between wine quality and K, Mn, and Z content in dry white wine or Mg in red wines. Na (saline taste), Sn (weaker aroma), Zn (sour taste) are all known to produce undesirable effects. K gives a pleasant acid taste in the right concentration, in higher concentrations the wine tastes bitter and in lower concentrations it becomes insipid.

The effect of metals on maturing and aging of wines is another field of enological research. As a general rule, aging of wine increases the lability of metals, due to the decrease of organic matter content (Arcos *et al.*, 1993). A low Fe content is generally preferred for aging of red wines, since this element promotes oxidation. Other metals that stimulate auto-oxidation in wines are Be, Co, and Mn, while Mo and Zn seem to have an opposite effect. Ag acts as a protective agent against acetic acid fermentation, thus aiding in the preservation of wine quality.

Legal requirements

Some countries and international organizations have issued regulations containing maximum admissible levels of metals and metalloids in wine. Examples are reported in Tables 9.5 and 9.6 (values taken mostly from Stockley and Lloyd-Davies, 2001). Limits are proposed both for metals considered toxic and for metals that can become undesired or toxic in high concentrations. As can be noted, there is no uniformity as to which metals are controlled and which maximum concentrations are allowed. This can have commercial consequences because wines produced for export need to fulfill more or less severe requisites depending on the countries they are exported to. As a rule, wines produced in a country must first comply with national regulations; nevertheless, importing countries could propose more stringent or additional regulations (i.e. lower limits or different analytes checked) that exported wines must also comply with.

Table 9.5 Legal limits for metals in wines (concentrations expressed in mg/kg)

Country	Ag	Al	B[a]	Ca[b]	Cr	Cu	Fe	Na[c]	Sb	Se	Sn	Ti	Zn
Argentina			0.25			1.0		230					
Australia						5.0			0.15	0.2	50.0		5.0
Canada	0.5[d]						20.0[d]	500[e]	0.02[d]				5.0[d]
Germany		8.0	80.0			2.0					1.0	1.0	5.0
Italy						10.0							5.0
New Zealand						2.0			0.15		40.0		5.0
Russia						5.0	10.0						
South Africa			80.0			1.0	10.0	100		1.0	100.0		5.0
Switzerland			80.0			1.0		60					5.0
USA						0.5							
FAO/WHO[f]													
EU[g]						1.0							
OIV[h]		10.0			0.1	1.0		60	0.20	0.1	5.0		5.0

[a] Expressed as boric acid.
[b] Expressed as Ca oxide.
[c] *Exceeding sodium*, i.e. Na that stoichiometrically exceeds chloride concentration.
[d] Société des Alcools du Quebec.
[e] Liquid Control Board of Ontario.
[f] FAO/WHO, Food and Agriculture Organization/World Health Organization.
[g] EU, European Union.
[h] OIV, Office International de la Vigne et du Vin.

Table 9.6 Legal limits for toxic metals in wines (concentrations expressed in mg/kg)

Country	As	Cd	Hg	Pb
Argentina		0.01		0.20
Australia	0.1	0.05	0.030	0.20
Brazil		0.20		0.50
Canada	0.1[a,b]	0.50[a,b]	0.100[a,b]	0.20[a,b]
Germany	0.1	0.01	0.010	0.25
Italy				0.30
Malta	0.2			0.20
New Zealand	0.2			0.20
Russia	0.2	0.03	0.005	0.30
South Africa	0.2	0.01	0.050	0.20
Switzerland	0.2	0.01		0.10
USA				0.30
FAO/WHO[c]				0.20
EU[d]				0.20
OIV[e]	0.2	0.01	0.020	0.20

[a] Société des Alcools du Quebec.
[b] Liquid Control Board of Ontario.
[c] FAO/WHO, Food and Agriculture Organization/World Health Organization.
[d] EU, European Union.
[e] OIV, Office International de la Vigne et du Vin.

Provenance of wines

In the past 20 or more years, several authors have proposed that the distribution of trace metals in a wine, lanthanides in particular, are indicative of the geographic origin of the wine (Baxter *et al.*, 1997; Greenough *et al.*, 1997). In other words, it is possible that the concentrations of these elements in the final product, i.e. bottled wine, reflect those present in soil, throughout the various winemaking processes. This would enable discrimination between different wines, to *trace back* the provenance of a wine and, consequently, to test its authenticity, a feature particularly appealing for producers of high-quality wines (for example, for *Barbaresco*, *Barolo* and *Brunello di Montalcino* in Italy). Many studies have been published since the first ones by Siegmund and Bachmann (1978) on the classification of German wines, and by Kwan *et al.* (1979) on the discrimination of Pinot Noir samples produced in France and in the USA. Successful classification of the samples analyzed is obtained through the application of multivariate statistical techniques of pattern recognition, either applied to elemental data alone (Baxter *et al.*, 1997; Greenough *et al.*, 1997) or to elemental and other chemical data (Martin *et al.*, 1999; Rebolo *et al.*, 2000). Research in this field has developed mainly in France (McCurdy *et al.*, 1992), but the topic has not been fully worked out because it is unclear whether the various passages involved in the wine production cycle leave metal distribution unchanged or not (Jakubowski *et al.*, 1999). Moreover, it must be considered that the absorption of mineral substances by vines does not reflect indifferently the composition of soil solution, but that it responds to preferential activities that are a consequence of the plant's needs. Finally, the availability of microelements in soil depends upon their solubility, which differs for each of them according to their chemical species (Greenough *et al.*, 1996).

In any case, through the selection of proper variables, there is no doubt that once a reliable procedure has been established, the determination of ultra-trace metals in wine could be a powerful way to detect adulterations and to acknowledge high-quality productions. Traceability studies should use only those elements that best reflect metal distribution in soil, allowing for discrimination of wines produced in different zones. This can be done by considering the different factors that determine metal content in wines:

- availability of mineral substances in the soil in which vineyards are located
- capacity of vines to assume mineral substances from soil; these two factors determine the concentrations of trace elements, such as Ba, Li, Rb, Sr and lanthanides
- contributions from various steps of the production cycle, from grapes to the finished and bottled products – treatments preliminary to grape-harvest, fermentation reactions, additions of compounds with various functions, conservation, bottling, and aging; concentrations of most alkaline, alkali-earth and transition metals, are strongly influenced by these processes.

The final metal distribution is then a sum of factors, a few of which can be out of control or not discriminated. It is possible to distinguish three kinds of variables, on the basis of their discriminating power:

1 metals whose concentration in wine is determined by mineral contribution from soil or metal uptake capacity of grape. Al, Ba, Li, Mn, Mo, Rb, Si, Sr, and Ti should behave this way, apart from possible *illicit* treatments during winemaking
2 metals whose concentration is the sum of several factors, some natural, some deriving from the production cycle; this behaviour is typical of many elements – Na, K, Ca, Mg, Cu, Fe, and Zn, among others
3 metals whose concentration is almost exclusively influenced by artificial sources – Pb, for example, is mostly derived from anthropic activities or pollution phenomena (fungicidal treatments, tinned containers, vehicular traffic); Co, Cr, Ni, and V, present in wines at very low concentrations, most probably derive from interaction of musts and wines with metallic containers rather than from natural sources.

From the above considerations, it is obvious that the variables with higher discriminating power are those in the first group, as they best reflect peculiarities in the soil or in the grape.

A similar and even more powerful approach to traceability is isotope ratio analysis: some authors proposed that the $^{86}Sr/^{87}Sr$ isotope ratio (Almeida and Vasconcelos, 2001; Barbaste et al., 2002) and Pb isotope ratios (Augagneur et al., 1997; Dean et al., 1990) could be used to identify regional variations. The $^{86}Sr/^{87}Sr$ isotope ratio is an important parameter for rock dating and does not change during biological processes, thus reflecting its environment. Pb's isotopic distribution is composed of four stable isotopes, three of which have radio-genic origin; their respective abundances, originating from rock genesis and ore deposits, vary with geological age and therefore with geographical location. Pb isotope ratios can then be a way to identify the source of lead in a sample. $^{208}Pb/^{207}Pb$, $^{206}Pb/^{207}Pb$ and $^{208}Pb/^{206}Pb$ ratios are found to be more efficient in dis-criminating samples from different countries. A major drawback of isotope ratio analysis is that the necessary resolution, i.e. the ability to discriminate between two atomic species differing by a small fraction of mass, is only provided by highly expensive techniques, such as thermal ionization mass spectrometry (TIMS) or double-focusing sector field ICP-MS (ICP-SMS).

Sources of metals in wine

As previously stated, various factors determine metal content in wines. First of all, there is the original amount absorbed from soil and found in grapes; then there are several augmentative and decreasing factors connected with vinification pro-cesses which affect the final concentrations in wine. As a general rule, it is possible to identify two main sources: natural or *primary*, and artificial or *secondary*.

Among the decreasing factors that apply to all metals, the most important is alcoholic fermentation (Eschnauer et al., 1989; Salati, 1999), as can be seen in Table 9.7. From must to wine, most metals have their concentrations decreased to 5–10% of the original amount, due to decreased solubility and precipitation as sulfides. Another decreasing factor is the so-called *blue-fining* practice, in which potassium ferrocyanide is used to precipitate copper, iron and other metals that cause troublesome hazes and catalyze oxidation. The overall decontamination

Table 9.7 Lowering of metal content in wine after fermentation and blue-fining

Element	Fermentation (%)	Blue-fining (%)
Aluminum	20–30	0
Cadmium	29–41	~80
Cobalt	17–24	77–100
Chromium	24–30	0
Copper	88–90	~100
Iron	0–19	63–80
Manganese	0–6	46–73
Lead	32–40	0–12
Vanadium	0–20	50–80
Zinc	0–31	78–89

effects of these two processes on metal content were summarized by Bauer *et al.* (1994). Further decrease is caused by other materials used for treating wine, such as clarifying agents.

While decrease of metal content is not a problem, increase of metal ions should be carefully checked because of two aspects: sanitary (toxic metals) and enological (alterations in organoleptic features). The main increasing factors are fining treatments and storage. Fifty years ago, most winemaking equipment was made of iron or brass. Wine acids are strong enough to dissolve small amounts of Fe and Cu, and in the past, hazes were common problems throughout the wine industry. In recent years, the prevalent use of stainless steel and plastic materials has virtually eliminated metal haze problems, though steel might release small amounts of Fe, Ni, Cr, Mo, and Ti.

We shall now describe separately the main sources for every metal. Additional information will be given on:

- effects on vine growth
- role (if any) and effects in wine
- chemical form in wine.

Alkaline metals

Lithium

It is a natural mineral constituent of wines, though minor; its physiological role in plants and humans is not fully understood. It comes mainly from plant root uptake, and to a lesser extent from storage in glass bottles. Its concentration ranges between 1 and 50 µg/L, and it is used in Italy as a denaturating agent to mark wines not allowed for consumption (Zerbinati *et al.*, 2000). An excess of Li could therefore be seen as a sign of adulteration. Higher levels of Li are reported for aged wines as a consequence of extraction from glass (Ough and Amerine, 1988).

Li in wine is present as a free ion.

Potassium

K is one of the three major elements required by vines for healthy growth (the other two are N and P). It constitutes about 3% of the vine's dry weight, and is an important component of grape juice, as it is the principal counter-ion of carboxylic acids and proteins. Its decrease after alcoholic fermentation is due to precipitation as hydrogen tartrate. Among metals, K has the highest concentration in wine, which is why it is widely regarded as the most important element directly affecting wine quality. In fact, elevated K levels in grape juice cause high pH, which adversely affects wine quality, but low K levels seem to produce a certain insipidity; within proper concentration ranges, K seems to reinforce a pleasant acid sapidity.

Grapes contain high levels of K, with concentration in the skin four to five times higher than in the pulp. Its content in must depends on several variables, which include grape varieties, soil conditions, and time of harvest. Besides natural sources, K content is also determined by the addition of several chemical compounds during vinification. The following are some examples:

- K sorbate, added as wine stabilizer to prevent refermentation in bottle
- K hydrogensulfite or metahydrogensulfite for sterilization
- K caseinate for clarification
- K tartrate or hydrogencarbonate for deacidification
- K tartrate for precipitating excess calcium
- K ferrocyanide for blue-fining.

K is present partly as free ion in wine, and is partly bound to organic compounds as pigments or complexed with hydrogen tartrate and sulfate (Bertrand *et al.*, 1978).

Sodium

It is not a required nutrient for vine growth; indeed, Na chloride is a major hazard for vine-growers, particularly in hot, irrigated areas where ground waters are saline, or where salty irrigation water is applied to the leaves. Similar effects can occasionally be found in coastal vineyards affected by wind-borne salt.

Grape juice, and hence wine, can contain elevated Na and chloride levels. As previously stated, primary sources can be sprinkler irrigation with saline water, uptake from soil in wines from vineyards with saline soils, and marine spray in wines from coastal vineyards. Secondary sources can be the following:

- Na metabisulfite for sterilization
- Na chloride, an illicit addition in salting treatments to increase sapidity of immature wines
- Na benzoate as wine stabilizer to prevent refermentation
- release from bentonite and gelatines
- common impurity in other salts used in vinification processes.

Though it is not a toxic element, Na needs to be kept under control because its content is important for people on low Na diets. For this reason, several countries have issued legal limits, generally indicating a maximum value for Na, in excess of the chloride already present in wines. For example, for Na, a limit of 60 mg/L was proposed by the Office International de la Vigne et du Vin which stoichiometrically exceeds chloride concentration (Organisation International de la Vigne et du Vin, 1990).

Na in wine is present mainly as a free ion.

Rubidium

Rb is considered essential as a trace element due to its ability to act as a nutritional substitute for potassium.

Caesium

As with Rb, Cs has a physiological role due to its close physicochemical relationship to potassium.

Alkali-earth metals

Calcium

Ca is a natural constituent of musts and a major element required for vine growth, and it is hardly ever deficient in vineyards. Ca is very important to many aspects of the vine's metabolism; it acts mainly as a catalyst in enzymatic reactions and as a basic constituent of cell walls, as it is a counter-ion of pectin compounds.

The passage from must to wine causes a decrease of Ca because of precipitation reactions: its compounds, in fact, are generally less soluble than Mg compounds, whose concentration is generally lower in must, but can be similar or higher in wine. Precipitation as tartrate is both spontaneous, due to alcoholic fermentation, and induced, due to intentional addition of tartaric acid to lower Ca concentration further and to avoid precipitations in bottle. It is indeed known that Ca has a role in favoring precipitation of colloids in the iron-phosphate *haze*, and of pectin salts. Ca concentration in wine is determined by:

- natural content of grapes
- residues of use of Ca, Cu oxychloride as fungicidal
- addition of Ca carbonate and sulfate as disacidificants
- addition of Ca tartrate as a technological adjuvant to assist the precipitation of tartar and the tartaric stabilization of the wine by reducing the final K hydrogen tartrate and Ca tartrate concentrations
- addition of Ca phytate as a sequestering agent
- release from cement containers
- clarification treatments with bentonite
- ion-exchange treatments.

Ca is present as free ion or complexed in wine, and possible complexing agents can be dicarboxylic acids or polyuronic acids.

Magnesium

Like Ca, it is a natural constituent of musts and a mineral element essential for healthy vine growth, due to its role in the formation of chlorophyll molecule and of some enzymes; moreover, it is involved in the composition of cell walls as a counter-ion of pectin compounds. Unlike Ca, Mg concentration does not decrease significantly from must to wine due to the higher solubility of its compounds; a small amount is consumed by yeasts feeding. According to Ough and Amerine (1988), Mg may be important in tartrate stability and to the acid taste of wine.

Clarification treatments with bentonites or deodorizing carbon, ion-exchange treatments or storage in concrete containers, are all factors that can cause an increase of Mg in wine. Apart from this, Mg content is generally uniform.

Its chemical form in wine is similar to that of Ca.

Strontium

Sr's biological behavior resembles that of Ca (which Sr can substitute in some enzyme systems) and this supports the hypothesis of its essentiality, although it has not yet been fully verified.

Sr content in wines is affected mainly by the type of soil from which vines get their nourishment; it therefore has a natural source. Secondary sources are possibly as impurities in phosphate-based fertilizers.

It could be present in wine as Sr^{2+} ion complexed by rhamnogalacturonan II, according to Pellerin and O'Neill (1998) and Tahiri *et al.* (2001).

Barium

There is no conclusive evidence that Ba performs any essential function in living organisms; in any case, as for strontium, its close resemblance to calcium makes it possible to think of Ba as a micronutrient. It is present in very small quantities and its concentration in wines is regulated by soil composition.

As with Sr, in wine it could be present as Ba^{2+} ion complexed by rhamnogalacturonan II (Pellerin and O'Neill, 1998; Tahiri, 2001).

Transition metals

Titanium

It is a non-essential, non-toxic element to humans and plants.

Vanadium

V is probably essential for plants, though its role is still unknown. It is present in wines at very low concentrations, most probably due to the interaction of musts and wines with metallic containers rather than from natural sources.

Teissedre *et al.* (1998a) determined V levels in French and Californian wines, and found that wine storage conditions may increase V content.

Chromium

It is a naturally occurring element in soil that can be absorbed by vines. Its role in plant physiology is strictly dependent on the chemical species: Cr(VI) compounds can reduce plant growth, while the role of Cr(III) is not fully understood.

Extended maceration of husks tends to extract Cr, causing red wines to have a higher content than white wines. As for V, dissolution of Cr^{3+} from stainless steel used in metallic containers constitutes a major source in wine (for this reason Cr content in wine has increased in recent years), a minor source being the use of metallic oxides in bottle pigmentation. As a consequence of these contamination sources, Cabrera-Vique *et al.* (1997) reported that Cr tends to increase with the age of the wine. Pertoldi-Marletta *et al.* (1989) demonstrated the influence of pollution carried by vehicular traffic on Cr concentration in wines: the contamination effect on vines was detectable up to a distance of 50 m from the road.

Cr levels can increase by a factor of two to ten in relation to Cr concentrations in musts.

In wine it is mainly present as a non-toxic Cr^{3+} ion.

Manganese

It is a soil nutrient essential for vine growth in very low quantities. Mn's principal function is to catalyze enzymatic reactions. Its content in wine is generally constant.

Considering redox potentials, Mn should be present as an Mn^{2+} ion.

Iron

It is a mineral element essential for healthy vine growth in trace amounts, mainly for chlorophyll synthesis. Fe can be intentionally added to soils suffering from iron deficiency (when vine is grown on wet, alkaline soils where Fe is present in a chemical form, which makes it unavailable to the vine roots). In those cases, fertilizers containing Fe in a protected form could be added, such as a chelate, a form in which Fe is bound in an organic complex preventing it from oxidation.

Much of Fe present in must is lost during fermentation by absorption and adsorption by yeasts. Various sources are possible:

- primary sources: absorbed from soil by vines or coming from soil particles residues
- secondary sources: vinification equipment, containers, use of fossil meals and bentonites.

Due to human physiological needs, an excess of Fe in wine does not constitute a sanitary problem. However, the same is not true from an enological point of view: beyond 10–15 mg/l, ferric haze can occur due to oxidation of Fe^{2+} to Fe^{3+} and its interaction with phosphates (*white haze*) or tannins (*blue haze*); a color change is another undesired effect of a large excess of Fe.

Fe is present as Fe^{2+} and Fe^{3+} aquoions with prevalence of the reduced form in wine, due to the presence in wine of many reducing substances. Wines kept out of contact with air have 80–95% of Fe in the ferrous state (Ough and Amerine, 1988). For the problems cited above, it is important to discriminate between oxidation states of Fe, as a major concentration of Fe^{3+} is a potential hazard in wine preservation. Other forms are negatively charged soluble complexes with organic acids such as tartaric, malic, and citric (Weber, 1991) that can become insoluble in the presence of an excess of Fe, by causing haze formation, as previously stated. Speciation studies carried out with adsorptive stripping voltammetry (Wang and Mannino, 1989) and ion exchange chromatography–flame atomic absorption spectrometry (Ajlec and Štuar, 1989) allowed quantitative discrimination between total Fe, Fe^{2+} and Fe^{3+} species. Interaction with the tannin component of red wines has also been reported (McKinnon and Scollary, 1997).

Cobalt

The role of Co in plant physiology is yet unknown. The only known function is its participation in metabolism as a component of vitamin B_{12}.

Co is present in wines at very low concentrations, coming more probably from the interaction of musts and wines with metallic containers than from natural sources.

Nickel

Ni is a trace mineral nutrient, essential to all higher plants that require it for seeds to germinate. Its role is to aid in liberating nitrogen from soil and absorb iron. As with many trace minerals, minute amounts may be essential nutrients, but a high-level exposure is hazardous.

It is present in wines at very low concentrations, coming more probably from the interaction of musts and wines with metallic containers than from natural sources. Together with Cr, Ni content in wine has gone up in recent years, as a consequence of the increased use of stainless steel equipment. In a study by Pertoldi Marletta *et al.* (1989), vehicular traffic was found to generate an Ni contamination effect on vines located up to a distance of 50 m from the road. A study by Teissedre *et al.* (1998b) determined Ni concentration in French wines and grapes and traced possible sources of contamination: for a given vineyard and winery, Ni content increased with the period of storage, suggesting contamination from stainless steel storage tanks and Ni-containing pigments in bottles during the wine storage.

A speciation study by means of filtration and liquid–liquid extraction (Weber and Schwedt, 1982) showed that a high fraction of Ni is present as bound to organic compounds.

Copper

It is a trace element required in very small concentrations for healthy vine growth; due to the widespread use of fungicides containing copper, deficiencies of this element in vineyards are uncommon. Its physiological functions are different, being a key factor in the constitution of a high content of polyphenoloxydase and in some non-enzymatic oxidations.

The natural content of Cu in grape is generally low. During fermentation, Cu is fixed by yeasts (though at high levels it can poison them) or is precipitated as sulfide or tartrate; its natural content in wine should therefore be at μg/L levels.

The principal secondary source of Cu is, of course, use of cupric fungicides. Examples are Cu(I) oxide, Cu(I) hydroxide, Cu(II) oxychloride and, most of all, Cu(II) sulfate pentahydrate mixed with lime to form the famous *Bordeaux mixture*. Other artificial sources can be the release of Cu by contact with vinification equipment (tank taps, pumps), though the use of stainless steel could limit this, and the addition of copper sulfate to eliminate taste defects or smell in the wine. It should be pointed out that wines maintaining a high Cu content (8–10 mg/L) reveal a bitter, metallic taste that is unsuitable for drinking. Moreover, a concentration of 0.5–0.8 mg/L is high enough to generate Cu haze that can sometimes occur in white and rosé wines, with precipitation of copper sulfide; even ferric haze is influenced by Cu that acts as catalyst. Finally, it is known that Cu, like Fe, has a role in wine oxidation, i.e. a wine rich in Cu and Fe ions tends to age more quickly.

Cu in wine is present as Cu^+ and Cu^{2+} ion, with Cu^+ stabilized by the presence of some component of wine (Cl^-); free ions should be a minor fraction, the greater part being complexed by oxyacids, phenolic compounds (catechin, caffeic acid), peptides and macromolecules present in wine. Lability of Cu ions seems to increase in older wines, where organic matter is more oxidized (Arcos et al., 1993). In a study by Wiese and Schwedt (1997), Cu speciation was studied with electrochemical techniques: free Cu^{2+} ions, labile bound and tightly bound Cu fractions could be determined in white wine samples.

Rather than the total concentration of Cu in wine, the knowledge of its chemical forms in wine should be taken into consideration, as this is a better indicator of potential spoilage, and thus demonstrates the importance of speciation studies.

Zinc

It is an element essential for healthy vine growth, as it is a constituent of carbonic anydrase enzyme, and it becomes phytotoxic at high concentrations in soil. Moreover, high content in wine may cause acute or chronic toxication. Zn concentration in wine seems to be related to astringency (Finoli et al., 1986).

Zn comes naturally from soil; secondary sources can be fungicidal treatments (Bordeaux mixture, zinc dithiocarbamates) or vinification equipment.

In wine it is mainly present as a free or highly labile Zn^{2+} ion (Arcos et al., 1993).

Molybdenum

It is an element essential for healthy vine growth for its role as a constituent of several metalloenzymes.

Heavy metals

Cadmium

Cd is not an essential element in plant nutrition and is indeed a highly toxic element with no known biological function. It can be easily transferred from soil to the plant, which absorbs and accumulates it. In any case, its content in wines is generally quite low and well below the maximum allowable levels; moreover, it has been demonstrated that today's wines have considerably lower Cd concentrations than older wines (Eschnauer *et al.*, 1996; Teissedre *et al.*, 1994a).

Cd content in must is strongly decreased after fermentation because yeasts tend to accumulate it. Blue-fining treatment is another effective means to reduce Cd concentration in contaminated wines. Teissedre *et al.* (1994a) studied variation of Cd levels during vinification processes in Côtes du Rhône wines: they found that during alcoholic fermentation Cd elimination is almost complete, with losses between 87 and 100%.

Sources of Cd in wine were reviewed by Eschnauer *et al.* (1996). Secondary sources can be residues of agrochemical products, such as insecticides and fungicides, contact of wine with apparatus used in production or in packaging processes, environmental contamination from industrial activities close to vineyards; higher values of Cd can be found in wines produced from vines grown near Pb and Cd pigment factories.

Most Cd present in wine is complexed by carboxylic acids (Spiess *et al.*, 1984) or by inorganic ligands present in wine.

Lead

Pb is the most checked metal in wine. It is a widely dispersed heavy metal which occurs naturally in trace amounts in all plants, therefore in grapes, and consequently in wines, usually only in µg/L quantities. In minimal part, it naturally comes from soil; it mostly derives from anthropogenic activities. It has no known biological function in vines; high concentrations in soil can promote inhibition of plant growth, especially in the case of organolead compounds. Due to its toxicological relevance, we will deal with Pb in wine more broadly.

Pb has been associated with wine since the time of Ancient Rome. Poisoning could result from the willful addition of lead to wine. The Romans used to heat grape juice in lead vessels to produce *sapa*, a sweet concentrate used as a wine additive and in cooking; even in the nineteenth century wine bottles were still cleaned with lead shots, thereby contaminating the wine.

Most of the traces of lead from grapes are precipitated out during winemaking: a major fraction is lost during fermentation and blue-fining treatment, so that only 42–62% is found in wine (Ough and Amerine, 1988).

The primary and secondary sources of Pb were elucidated by Eschnauer and Sachgebiet (1986), Eschnauer and Scollary (1996), and Augagneur (1996), among others. There are four principal secondary sources.

- Pb-rich car exhaust particles settling on both grapes and soil: this is a problem for roadside vineyards in particular, in which an asymptotic decrease of Pb content is generally observed within 100 m; this source is declining as the use of unleaded fuels increases.
- Prior use of the now-banned chemical insecticide Pb arsenate, which has contaminated many vineyard soils, especially where soil acidity is high.
- Impurities in copper-based fungicide or in alloys-based materials (brass, bronze).
- Pb capsules used to protect corks: seepage of wine around the cork can corrode the foil and, if the lip of the bottle is not thoroughly cleaned before pouring, the wine may be contaminated by some of the Pb salt. Research by Dean *et al.* (1990) revealed that Pb can be released during pouring by Pb-containing capsules used in wine storage. However, the use of Pb capsules or foils is now declining or prohibited in many regions.

The equipment used in modern wineries should not result in any Pb contamination. Besides sources connected with vinification or with environmental pollution, another source was identified in crystal decanters: release of Pb was demonstrated to occur from Pb silicate crystal wine glasses (Hight, 1996). Lengthy storage of wines in Pb crystal decanters provides time for the wine acids to leach some Pb from the glass, but the usual period of few hours is too short to produce dangerous amounts of contamination. In any case, modern bottles are made of Pb-free glass.

Because of the public health aspects involved, Pb has been and continues to be the subject of active research regarding its content in wines and grapes. Several reviews have been published in the past 30 years, reporting average values in samples and providing hypotheses on possible contamination sources. Teissedre *et al.* (1993) investigated possible sources of Pb contamination in wines from Côtes du Rhône and Vallee du Rhône, determining Pb content at the various steps of winemaking. Kaufmann (1998) reported values from analyses of 7000 wines, showing that contamination from atmospheric pollution (leaded gasoline) was not responsible for elevated Pb concentrations in wine; brass tubes and faucets were instead found to be the main contamination source. It was also shown that the presence or absence of Sn–Pb capsules, as well as their corrosion, had only a very minor influence on Pb concentration in wine. A positive correlation between wine age and Pb concentration was found; however, vintage and wine color, rather than age, were the most significant contributing factors. Medina *et al.* (2000) determined Pb content in samples of French wines from the end of the eighteenth century, finding a strong decrease from ~1 mg/L to ~0.25 mg/L around the 1950s to less than 0.1 mg/L nowadays, or even lower. Utilizing ICP-MS, they estimated the isotopic signatures of the pollutant that could be determined as atmospheric fallout, industrial and gasoline origin.

The chemical forms of Pb in wine have been the subject of several studies in recent years. Up to the mid-1990s there was concern that wine could be considered as a major source of Pb intake (Elinder et al., 1988; Pedersen et al., 1994); the recent development of speciation techniques, though, contributed greatly to the knowledge that the risk of heavy metals intake associated with wine assumption was highly dependent on these elements' chemical forms in wine. Some studies concerning Pb speciation concentrated on the identification of organolead compounds, which are liposoluble (unlike Pb^{2+}), and are therefore more easily adsorbed by humans. Łobinski et al. (1993) and Teissedre et al. (1994b) found that organolead compounds were relevant in wines made from grapes grown close to large industrialized centers or highways. $(CH_3)_3Pb^+$, $(C_2H_5)_3Pb^+$ and $(C_2H_5)_2Pb^{2+}$ were the analytes detected. The source of contamination was considered to be of atmospheric origin; this hypothesis was supported by much larger concentrations of organolead compounds found in older vintages than in the present ones, a fact attributed to the decreasing use of leaded gasoline.

Organolead fraction accounts for only 0.1–1% of total Pb in wine: from a toxicological point of view, this makes it irrelevant. Most of the interest was then devoted to the quantification of the *bioavailable* fraction, considered to be the most intrinsically toxic. Since this could be related to the *electrochemically labile* fraction, some authors studied the distribution of Pb species by applying electrochemical techniques: there was general agreement on the fact that a very minor percentage of free Pb^{2+} ion was present in wine (Baldo et al., 1997; Fournier et al., 1998; Scollary, 1997; Vasconcelos et al., 2000). Complexing agents present in wine, and particularly in red wine, were thought to be responsible for keeping the labile fraction of Pb minimal. These results are consistent with further researches: McKinnon and Scollary (1997), using the ultrafiltration technique to examine size fractionation, found a markedly different distribution for Pb than those observed in other metals studied. Potential binding agents for Pb in white wines were thought to be proteins and procyanidins, while in red wines a polymeric species, probably tannin, could be the binding agent; French researchers (Pellerin et al., 1997; Szpunar et al., 1998), using size-exclusion chromatography, found evidence that a pectic polysaccharide called rhamnogalacturonan II (RG-II) was a predominant anionic molecule, existing in wine as a dimer (dRG-II) and responsible for complexing Pb for a major fraction of the total Pb content. This polymeric species is not degraded during vinification and could act as a detoxification agent for Pb, though the stability of the Pb–RG–II complex in the gastrointestinal system is yet to be investigated. The properties of rhamnogalacturonan II were further investigated by Vidal et al. (1999): it was found to be stable in red wines for up to 10 years, with a content of 50–150 mg/L that was enough to complex a Pb content 10 times the average content. Tahiri et al. (2001) found a decrease of Pb intestinal absorption and tissue retention in rats provoked by rhamnogalacturonan II. Finally, Azenha and Vasconcelos (2000) studied wines subjected to *in vitro* gastrointestinal digestion, finding that Pb was less bioavailable in red wines than in white wines.

Mercury

It is a highly toxic element whose toxicity depends strongly on the chemical species, with effects increasing in the series inorganic ions < mercury vapor < organic ions and compounds. Hg is not very phytotoxic in normally occurring concentrations, perhaps due to some protection mechanism.

Hg in must, independent of the initial level, is nearly completely eliminated during the fermentation and the subsequent processing steps of wine production. For these reasons, the primary Hg content in wine is very low, on average 0.02 µg/L or lower (Enkelmann *et al.*, 1984).

Platinum-group metals

The elements termed platinum group elements (PGEs) have become of interest in the environmental field since the introduction in 1975 of catalytic cleaning of exhaust gases from cars. Little is known about their biological effects, though only in exceptional cases is their toxicity significant.

Investigations of Pt content in wines produced before and after the introduction of catalysts in the early 1980s yielded no significant difference (Alt *et al.*, 1997); otherwise, Pt content was found to be lower in vineyards located in traffic-free areas than in vineyards located near high-traffic roads. It therefore seems that vehicular traffic could be the main secondary source of Pt in wine. Other sources can be bentonite and active charcoal.

As for most metals, depletion of Pt by fermentation is close to 100%; Pt in wine is therefore an ultra-trace element. In any case, its determination may be useful in understanding the impact of catalysts in the future.

Silver

It is not an essential element for plants, but at present it does not seem to cause health risks.

The enological importance of Ag was discussed by Alt *et al.* (2000). The natural Ag content in wine is below 0.1 µg/L; secondary sources were found to be the use of Ag-containing materials (silver plated devices) and agents for wine treatment, e.g. Ag chloride used as a deodorizer.

Thallium

Tl seems to have no nutritional importance. Its presence can lead to health problems for plants and humans, with an acute toxicity comparable to that of

Pb and Hg; however, contamination is highly improbable due to its low occurrence in the environment.

Tl is found in very low quantities in wine. Average content is about 0.1 μg/L in white wines and about twice as much in red wines, probably due to the different winemaking treatments. Higher levels are found in wines produced in areas next to cement plants or on abandoned mines (Eschnauer *et al.*, 1984).

Other metals or metalloids

Aluminum

There is no conclusive evidence that Al has any essential function in plants. It has recently been the object of major attention due to its possible relationship with Alzheimer's disease and other physiological dysfunctions (World Health Organization, 1989).

Sources of Al were elucidated by Eschnauer and Scollary (1995). The use of bentonite for clarification is a major secondary source of Al contamination, with possible increases of 100% after bentonite treatment. Other sources are kaolin (another clarification agent), damaged aluminum casks, illicit use of alum or other Al salts for fining, and of Al-containing preservatives.

Elevated contents of Al have negative effects on wine quality: as little as 10 mg/L is sufficient to spoil wine; concentrations of 10–20 mg/L cause it to become cloudy because of haze formation (perhaps because of its interaction with Fe ions) and give wine a characteristic harsh metallic taste.

Al in wine is bound to small compounds such as tartaric, malic, gallic or other carboxylic acids (Eschnauer and Scollary, 1995; McKinnon and Scollary, 1997).

Antimony

Sb is a non-essential element in plants. Its toxicity depends on chemical species, with Sb(III) being more active than Sb(V).

Sb can be released in wine by contact with old rubber hoses.

It can be present in wine in both III and V oxidation states, as suggested by Wifladt *et al.* (1997), who found an increase in the signal of Sb(III) upon addition of thiourea to the samples by determining Sb with hydride generation–atomic absorption spectrometry. Moreover, the ease of generation of Sb hydride indicated that this element in wine is not strongly bound to organic compounds, but is present in a more available species.

Arsenic

As is a toxic element that can impair growth of plants; its toxicity is strongly dependent on chemical form, with As(III) species more phytotoxic than As(V) ones, and inorganic compounds more toxic than most organic ones.

It can be present in wines in ultra-trace concentrations, but wines produced with grapes treated with arsenical compounds can have higher values. It is mostly present in wine as As(III). A speciation study by Wangkarn and Pergantis (2000), performed with HPLC–ICP–MS, revealed that the only As species present in wine was arsenite, except for one sample that contained dimethylarsinic acid. A more recent study by Herce-Pagliai *et al.* (2002) analyzed wine samples from the south of Spain, finding that, besides As(III) and As(V) inorganic species, organic compounds such as monomethylarsonic acid and dimethylarsinic acid were the predominant species.

Boron

It is a mineral element required in small quantities for healthy vine growth, as it is required for the movement of sugars and the synthesis of auxins in the plant. B toxicity is also possible, sometimes due to over-application of fertilizers, from irrigation water or from fraudulent addition of boric acid as anti-fermentative agent.

Wines from vineyards close to volcanoes have high B levels, due to the high B content in volcanic soils (Eschnauer, 1982).

In wine B should be present as boric acid or its esters.

Phosphorus

It is one of the most important mineral elements required for vine growth, yet the amounts required are so small that for most vineyards, the supply from the soil is sufficient. P in vines is an essential component of compounds involved in photosynthesis and sugar–starch transformations as well as the transfer of energy.

It is present naturally as both organic and inorganic phosphates, but can be added to musts as calcium or ammonium salts to encourage the growth of yeasts. The phosphate content is remarkable in the formation of ferric-phosphate casse.

Rare earths elements

Rare earths elements (REEs) or lanthanides constitute a group of fifteen elements with similar physicochemical properties; they are not known to be nutritionally essential.

The concentration distribution of REE can be altered by bentonite treatment that increases their natural content upon contact with wine (Jakubowski *et al.*, 1999).

They could be present in wine as trivalent cations complexed by rhamno-galacturonan II (Pellerin and O'Neill, 1998; Tahiri *et al.*, 2001).

Selenium

It is an essential element for humans due to its antioxidant properties, but it is not clear whether it is also essential for plants. It has a narrow range of intake consistent with good health, outside of which deficiency diseases and toxicity occur; its effects depend on the chemical species.

Red wines contain more Se, as the skins and pulps of these grapes contain higher concentrations. During fermentation, 30–60% of the contents in must are precipitated (Eschnauer *et al.*, 1989a).

Silicon

It is an essential element for good health in small quantities. As it is a major component of soil, musts generally have high concentrations of it which tend to decrease in wine due to alcoholic fermentation.

Sources of Si were described by Bauer *et al.* (1995). Secondary sources can be:

- cement containers
- bentonite, kaolin, silicon dioxide as a gel or colloidal solution for clarification
- fossil meal.

High Si content is a potential contamination risk: concentrations higher than 20 mg/L can cause haze.

Si can be present in wine as orthosilicic acid (in monomer or oligomer forms).

Tin

Sn is considered non-toxic and essential as a trace element, but its compounds have biological effects that are strictly determined by their chemical species, with organo-Sn compounds being mostly toxic.

Secondary sources of Sn can be tinplate containers or storage in untreated PVC bottles.

It can be present in wine in different forms; those of toxicological relevance are organo-Sn compounds such as monobutyl-, dibutyl- and tributyl-Sn, monooctyl- and dioctyl-Sn (Forsyth *et al.*, 1994).

Analytical techniques for metal determination in wine

The contribution of analytical chemistry to understanding metal behavior in wines is strong and improving, essentially due to the increasing interest in the production of quality wines, which in this context can be defined as wines with a very low content of undesired metals and the right content of essential or useful metals. We will now describe the most used techniques for metal determination in wine.

Atomic spectrometric techniques

These are without a doubt the most used techniques for metal determination in wines, as witnessed by more than 200 papers published in the literature in the past 20 years. They generally require small volumes of sample (from a few microliters to a few milliliters), and little or no sample pretreatment. A review of the conditions needed for optimal determination of metals with the different techniques was recently published (Aceto *et al.*, 2002).

Flame atomic absorption spectrometry

This technique is frequently used in enological laboratories, due to the low cost of instruments and ease of use. Alkaline, alkali-earths and most concentrated transition metals (Mn, Fe, Cu, and Zn) can easily be determined. It is noteworthy that EU official methods of analysis for determination of Ag, Ca, Fe, K, Mg, Na, and Zn in wines (European Union, 1990) explicitly require use of Flame-AAS.

Electrothermal atomic absorption spectrometry

Electrothermal or graphite furnace-atomic absorption spectrometry (GF-AAS) is widely used for metal determination in wines, though its instruments are more expensive than Flame-AAS instruments. Indeed, its high sensitivity allows determination of As, Cd, and Pb. Moreover, GF-AAS is the method of choice indicated by EU regulation for the determination of Cd and Pb in wines (European Union, 1990).

Inductively-coupled plasma–atomic emission spectrometry

This technique has been increasingly applied to wine analysis in the past 15 years, and it is now well established for the determination of a wide range of elements (Eschnauer *et al.*, 1989b; Thiel and Danzer, 1997). Wide linear dynamic range (five–six orders of concentrations), excellent robustness and good sensitivity make its use suitable for routine wine analyses, though its instruments' costs are still inaccessible to most enological laboratories.

Inductively-coupled plasma–mass spectrometry

The application of this technique to wine analysis has greatly improved in the past 10 years (Perez-Jordan *et al.*, 1999; Stroh *et al.*, 1994) and, apart from its high price, it could be the ideal technique for metal determination in wine. Its combination of ultra-high sensitivity and wide linear dynamic range (up to eight orders of concentrations) allows sequential determination of nearly all metals of interest in wine, either toxicological (Cu, Pb, and Zn but also Cd, Hg, and Tl, among others) or geochemical (lanthanides). Pretreatment procedures have been proposed for its routine use in wine analysis, ranging from simple dilution of samples to microwave or UV irradiation. The suitability of ICP–MS semi-quantitative procedures in wine analysis has recently been demonstrated (Almeida and Vasconcelos, 2002; Castiñeira *et al.*, 2001). This mode of operation allows rapid determination of many elements with good accuracy.

Electrochemical techniques

Stripping voltammetry, polarography and potentiometry have been proposed for determination of metals in wine as ions. As the detection limits of these techniques are very low, it is possible to determine some toxic metal ions occurring in wine at trace concentration levels, such as Cd^{2+} and Pb^{2+}, together with the principal transition metal ions, such as Mn^{2+}, Fe^{2+}, Fe^{3+}, Cu^{2+}, and Zn^{2+}.

Voltammetric techniques

Anodic stripping voltammetry (ASV) is a well-established technique for metal determination and has frequently been applied to wine analysis (Baldo et al., 1997; Buldini et al., 1999). Pretreatment of sample is the major challenge, due to the need to destroy the organic matrix of wine that can interfere with the electrochemical processes through adsorption on electrodes or can cause alteration of peak currents and of potentials (Arcos et al., 1993). Moreover, the presence of several complexing agents in wine can cause a shift of potentials towards more positive values. An acidification or an acid digestion step is required in order to release metal ions (unless speciation is the scope). Baldo et al., (1997) found that UV irradiation in presence of hydrogen peroxide was the most efficient method in releasing metal ions, probably because of the complete degradation of organic matrix to simpler molecules. Results of ASV determination of Cd^{2+} and Pb^{2+} are comparable to GF-AAS for accuracy and precision. Ultra-trace metals can also be determined (Ostapczuk et al., 2000).

Potentiometric techniques

The other class of electrochemical techniques commonly applied to wine analysis is potentiometry. Ion-selective electrodes are used to determine free ions with minimal sample perturbation, a major advantage over voltammetric techniques (Wiese and Schwedt, 1997). Recently, potentiometric stripping analysis (PSA) has been applied to wine analysis, with some advantages over the ASV technique: the instrumentation is simpler, mercury films for the electrodes are easier to prepare, and no sample pretreatment is required (Töben and Ostapczuk, 1995; Ostapczuk et al., 1997).

Speciation studies

An interesting feature of the electrochemical techniques is the possibility of speciation studies of metals in wine that can be performed with or without minimal sample pretreatment. The significance of speciation has been highlighted above. Stripping potentiometry, differential pulse anodic stripping voltammetry and ion-selective electrodes potentiometry have been used in wine speciation studies of Cu (Green et al., 1997: 711; Scollary, 1997; Wiese and Schwedt, 1997), Pb (Green et al., 1997; Scollary, 1997), and Ca (Scollary, 1997).

Chromatographic techniques

Among chromatographic techniques, ion chromatography (IC) is the most suitable for metal determination in wine (Buldini *et al.*, 1997). Keeping in mind the concentration levels reported in Table 9.2, this technique, when coupled with conductimetric detection, allows the sequential determination of nearly all alkaline and alkali-earth metal ions (Li^+, Na^+, K^+, Rb^+, Ca^{2+}, Mg^{2+}, Sr^{2+}, and Ba^{2+}), and, when coupled with UV-visible spectrophotometric detection or with amperometric detection, of the principal transition and heavy metal ions (Cu^{2+}, Fe^{3+}, Mn^{2+}, Ni^{2+}, Pb^{2+}, and Zn^{2+}). Samples of wine analyzed with IC should be diluted with water (at least 1:20) and filtered on reverse-phase adsorbents before injection, to remove organic compounds that can saturate the separation column. An interesting alternative to dilution is oxidative UV photolysis (Buldini *et al.*, 1999), in which wine samples are treated with hydrogen peroxide (to supply free OH radicals) and subjected to UV irradiation: this causes the rapid decomposition of organic compounds present in wine, while metal ions are quantitatively recovered. Samples can then be injected after regulating pH to the proper value.

Speciation studies

Chromatographic techniques are frequently used in speciation studies and some studies report the application of separation systems to wine analysis. In most cases speciation is obtained by interfacing a separation system, either liquid (Ajlec and Štuar, 1989; Szpunar *et al.*, 1998; Wangkarn and Pergantis, 2000) or gas (Forsyth *et al.*, 1994; Łobinski *et al.*, 1993) with an atomic spectroscopic detector in the so-called *hyphenated* systems.

Other techniques

Capillary electrophoresis (CE) has recently been applied to the determination of some cations in wine (Arellano *et al.*, 1997; Nuñez *et al.*, 2000). Li^+, Na^+, K^+, Ca^{2+}, Mg^{2+}, and Mn^{2+} can be determined in red wines with separation on a fused silica capillary column, using α-hydroxyisobutyric acid (creatinine) and 18-crown-6-ether as eluent buffered at pH 4.5 (4.1) and indirect UV detection at 214 nm (230 nm). The only sample pretreatment required is 1:10 (1:50) dilution with ultrapure water. The main advantages of CE when applied to wine analysis are its low cost (capillary fibers can perform 600–1000 analyses), low consumption of solvents, and buffers, and high automation facility.

References

Aceto, M., Abollino, O., Bruzzoniti, M.C., Mentasti, E., Sarzanini, C., and Malandrino, M. (2002) Determination of metals in wine with atomic spectroscopy (Flame-AAS, GF-AAS and ICP-AES); a review, *Food Additives and Contaminants*, **19**: 126–133.

Ajlec, R. and Štuar, J. (1989) Determination of iron species in wine by ion-exchange chromatography–flame atomic absorption spectrometry, *The Analyst*, **114**: 137–142.

Almeida, C.M.R. and Vasconcelos, M.T.S.D. (2001) ICP-MS determination of strontium isotope ratio in wine in order to be used as a fingerprint of its regional origin, *Journal of Analytical Atomic Spectrometry*, **16**: 607–611.

Almeida, C.M.R. and Vasconcelos, M.T.S.D. (2002) Advantages and limitations of the semi-quantitative operation mode of an inductively coupled plasma-mass spectrometer for multi-element analysis of wines, *Analytica Chimica Acta*, **463**: 165–175.

Alt, F., Eschnauer, H.R., Mergler, B., Messerschmidt, J., and Tölg, G. (1997) A contribution to the ecology and enology of platinum, *Fresenius' Journal of Analytical Chemistry*, **357**: 1013–1019.

Alt, F., Messerschmidt, J., Görtges, S., Eichler, P., and Eschnauer, H.R. (2000) Enological and ecological importance of silver, *Viticultural and Enological Sciences*, **55**: 102–105.

Arcos, M.T., Ancin, M.C., Echeverria, J.C., Gonzalez, A., and Garrido, J.J. (1993) Study of lability of heavy metals in wines with different degrees of aging through differential pulse anodic stripping voltammetry, *Journal of Agricultural and Food Chemistry*, **41**: 2333–2339.

Arellano, M., Siméon, N., Puig, P., and Couderc, F. (1997) Diverses applications de l'électrophorèse capillaire à l'analyse des vins. Dosage des acides organiques et inorganiques, de cations minéraux, des acides aminés et amines biogènes, *Journal International des Sciences de la Vigne et du Vin*, **31**: 213–218.

Augagneur, S. (1996) *Étude de la composition isotopique du plomb dans une serie séculaire de vins: mise en évidence de la pollution d'origine anthropique*, thesis, University of Bordeaux I.

Augagneur, S., Medina, B., and Grousset, F. (1997) Measurement of lead isotope ratios in wine by ICP-MS and its applications to the determination of lead concentration by isotope dilution, *Fresenius' Journal of Analytical Chemistry*, **357**: 1149–1152.

Azenha, M.A. and Vasconcelos, M.T. (2000) Pb and Cu speciation and bioavailability in Port wine, *Journal of Agricultural and Food Chemistry*, **48**: 5740–5749.

Baldo, M.A., Bragato, C., and Daniele, S. (1997) Determination of lead and copper in wine by ASV with mercury microelectrodes: assessment of the influence of sample pre-treatment procedures, *The Analyst*, **122**: 1–5.

Barbaste, M., Robinson, K., Guilfoyle, S., Medina, B., and Łobinski, R. (2002) Precise determination of the strontium isotope ratios in wine by inductively coupled plasma sector field multicollector mass spectrometry (ICP-SF-MC-MS), *Journal of Analytical Atomic Spectrometry*, **17**: 135–137.

Bauer, K.H., Hinkel, S., Neeb, R., Eichler, P., and Eschnauer, H.R. (1994) Gehalte von Fe, Cu, Zn, Mn and Al in deutschen Weinen – Simultan-Bestimmung mit ICP-OES, *Viticultural and Enological Sciences*, **49**: 209–214.

Bauer, K.H., Hinkel, S., Neeb, R., Eichler, P., and Eschnauer, H.R. (1995) Silicium in Wein. Ein Spurenelement – Vinogram, *Viticultural and Enological Sciences*, **50**: 118–122.

Baxter, M.J., Crews, H.M., Dennis, M.J., Goodall, I., and Anderson, D. (1997) The determination of the authenticity of wine from its trace element composition, *Food Chemistry*, **60**: 443–450.

Bertrand, G.L., Carroll, W.R., and Miller Foltyn, E. (1978) Tartrate stability of wines. I. Potassium complexes with pigments, sulphate and tartrate ions, *American Journal of Enology and Viticulture*, **29**: 25–29.

Buldini, P.L., Cavalli, S., and Trifirò, A. (1997) State-of-the-art ion chromatographic determination of inorganic ions in food, *Journal of Chromatography*, **789**: 529–548.

Buldini, P.L., Cavalli, S., and Sharma, J.L. (1999) Determination of transition metals in wine by IC, DPASV-DPCSV and ZGFAAS coupled with UV photolysis, *Journal of Agricultural and Food Chemistry*, **47**: 1993–1998.

Cabrera-Vique, C., Teissedre, P.L., Cabanis, M.T., and Cabanis, J.C. (1997) Determination and levels of chromium in French wine and grapes by graphite furnace atomic absorption spectrometry, *Journal of Agricultural and Food Chemistry*, **45**: 1808–1811.

Castiñeira, M.M., Brandt, R., Von Bohlen, A., and Jakubowski, N. (2001) Development of a procedure for the multi-element determination of trace elements in wine by ICP-MS, *Fresenius' Journal of Analytical Chemistry*, **370**: 553–558.

Darret, G., Couzy, F., Antoine, J., Magliola, C., and Mareschi, J. (1986) Estimation of minerals and trace elements provided by beverages for the adult in France, *Annals of Nutrition and Metabolism*, **30**: 335–344.

Dean, J.R., Ebdon, L., and Massey, R.C. (1990) Isotope ratio and isotope dilution analysis of lead in wine by inductively coupled plasma-mass spectrometry, *Food Additives and Contaminants*, **7**: 109–116.

De la Torre, M.C. (1997) Les contaminants du vin, aspects toxicologiques et de la securité alimentaire, *Analusis*, **25**: M21–M26.

Elinder, C.G., Lind, B., Nilsson, B., and Oskarsson, A. (1988) Wine – an important source of lead exposure, *Food Additives and Contaminants*, **5**: 641–644.

Enkelmann, R., Eschnauer, H.R., May, K., and Stoeppler, M. (1984) Quecksilberspuren in Most und Wein, *Fresenius' Zeitschrift für Analitische Chemie*, **317**: 478–480.

Eschnauer, H.R. (1974) *Spurenelemente in Wein und anderen Getränken*. Weinheim: Verlag Chemie.

Eschnauer, H.R. (1982) Trace elements in must and wine: primary and secondary contents, *American Journal of Enology and Viticulture*, **33**: 226–230.

Eschnauer, H.R. (1986) Spurenelemente und Ultra-spurenelemente in Wein, *Naturwissenschaften*, **73**: 281–290.

Eschnauer, H.R., Alt, F., Messerschmidt, J., and Tölg, G. (1989a) Ein Beitrag zur Oenologie und Oekologie von Selen. Spurenelement-Vinogramm, *Fresenius' Zeitschrift für Analitische Chemie*, **332**: 874–879.

Eschnauer, H.R., Gemmer-Colos, V., and Neeb, R. (1984) Thallium in Wein – Spurenelement-Vinogramm des Thalliums, *Zeitschrift für Lebensmitteluntersuchung und Forschung*, **178**: 453–460.

Eschnauer, H.R., Jakob, L., Meierer, H., and Neeb, R. (1989b) Use and limitations of ICP-OES in wine analysis, *Mikrochimica Acta*, **III**: 291–298.

Eschnauer, H.R., Ostapczuk, P., and Scollary, G.R. (1996) Cadmium in Wein – Ein Ultra-Spurenelement-Vinogramm, *Viticultural and Enological Sciences*, **51**: 63–69.

Eschnauer, H. and Sachgebiet, L. (1986) Lead in wine from tin-leaf capsules, *American Journal of Enology and Viticulture*, **37**: 158–162.

Eschnauer, H.R. and Scollary, G.R. (1995) Aluminium in Wein, *Viticultural and Enological Sciences*, **50**: 24–30.

Eschnauer, H. and Scollary, G.R. (1996) Zur Oenologie und Oekologie von Blei, *Viticultural and Enological Sciences*, **51**: 6–12.

European Union (1990) Commission Regulation no. 2676/90 of 17-09-1990, *Official Journal*, **L272**: 1.

Finoli, C., Galkina Benelli, T., and Vecchio, A. (1986) Microelementi del vino, *Tecnologie alimentari-Imbottigliamento*, **11**: 39–42.

Food and Nutrition Information Center (2002) *Dietary Reference Intakes (DRI) and Recommended Dietary Allowances (RDA).* Beltsville, MD: Food and Nutrition Information Center. http://www.nal.usda.gov/fnic/etext/000105.html (accessed 4 June 2002).

Forsyth, D.S., Sun, W.F., and Dalglish, K. (1994) Survey of organotin compounds in blended wines, *Food Additives and Contaminants,* 11: 343–350.

Fournier, J.B., El Hourch, M., and Martin, G.J. (1998) Analyse du Zinc, du Cuivre et du Plomb dans le vin. Rapport entre les concentrations totales analysees par spectrometrie d'absorption atomique et les concentrations des ions libres determinees par polarographie, *Journal International des Sciences de la Vigne et du Vin,* 32: 45–50.

Friberg, L., Nordberg, G.F., and Vouk, V.B. (1986) *Handbook on the Toxicology of Metals,* 2nd edn, vol. II. Amsterdam: Elsevier.

Green, A.M., Clark A.C., and Scollary, G.R. (1997) Determination of free and total copper and lead in wine by stripping potentiometry, *Fresenius' Journal of Analytical Chemistry,* 358: 711–717.

Greenough, J.D., Longerich, H.P., and Jackson, S.E. (1996) Trace element concentrations in wines by ICP-MS: evidence for the role of solubility in determining uptake by plants, *Canadian Journal of Applied Spectroscopy,* 41: 76–80.

Greenough, J.D., Longerich, H.P., and Jackson, S.E. (1997) Element fingerprinting of Okanagan Valley wines using ICP-MS: relationships between wine composition, vineyard and wine colour, *Australian Journal of Grape and Wine Research,* 3: 75–83.

Gulson, B.L., Stockley, C.S., Lee, T.H., Gray, B., Mizon K.J., and Patison, N. (1998) Contribution of lead in wine to the total dietary intake of lead in humans with and without a meal: a pilot study, *Journal of Wine Research,* 9: 5–14.

Heard, M.J., Chamberlain, A.C., and Sherlock, J.C. (1983) Uptake of lead by humans and effects of minerals and food, *Science of the Total Environment,* 30: 245–253.

Herce-Pagliai, C., Moreno, I., González, G., Repetto, M., and Cameán, A.M. (2002) Determination of total arsenic, inorganic and organic arsenic species in wine, *Food Additives and Contaminants,* 19: 542–546.

Hight, S.C. (1996) Lead migration from lead crystal wine glasses, *Food Additives and Contaminants,* 13: 744–765.

Jakubowski, N., Brandt, R., Stuewer, D., Eschnauer, H.R., and Görtges, S. (1999) Analysis of wines by ICP-MS: is the pattern of the rare earth elements a reliable fingerprint for the provenance?, *Fresenius' Journal of Analytical Chemistry,* 364: 424–428.

Kaufmann, A. (1998) Lead in wine, *Food Additives and Contaminants,* 15: 437–445.

Kieffer, F. (1991) Metals as essential trace elements for plants, animals and humans. In *Metals and their Compounds in the environment* (ed. E. Merian), pp. 481–489. Weinheim, Germany: VCH.

Kwan, W.O., Kowalski, B.R., and Skogerboe, R.K. (1979) Pattern recognition analysis of elemental data. Wines of *Vitis vinifera* cv. Pinot Noir from France and the USA, *Journal of Agricultural and Food Chemistry,* 27: 1321–1326.

Łobinski, R., Szpunar-Łobinska, J., Adams, F.C., Teissedre, P.L., and Cabanis, J.C. (1993) Speciation analysis of organolead compounds in wine by capillary gas chromatography/microwave-induced-plasma atomic emission spectrometry, *Journal of AOAC International,* 76: 1262–1267.

Lopez, F.F., Cabrera, C., Lorenzo, M.L., and Lopez, M.C. (1998) Aluminium levels in wine, beer and other alcoholic beverages consumed in Spain, *Science of the Total Environment,* 220: 1–9.

McCurdy, E., Potter, D., and Medina, B. (1992) Trace elements in wine, *Laboratory News,* September: 10–11.

McKinnon, A.J. and Scollary, G.R. (1997) Size filtration of metals in wine using ultrafiltration, *Talanta*, **44**: 1649–1658.

Martin, G.J., Mazure, M., Jouitteau, C., Martin, Y.L., Aguile, L., and Allain, P. (1999) Characterization of the geographic origin of Bordeaux wines by a combined use of isotopic and trace element measurements, *American Journal of Enology and Viticulture*, **50**: 409–417.

Medina, B., Augagneur, S., Barbaste, M., Grouset, F.E., and Buat-Meard, P. (2000) Influence of atmospheric pollution on the lead content of wines, *Food Additives and Contaminants*, **17**: 435–445.

Mena, C., Cabrera, C., Lorenzo, M.L., and Lopez, M.C. (1996) Cadmium levels in wine, beer and other alcoholic beverages: possible sources of contamination, *Science of the Total Environment*, **181**: 201–208.

Mertz, W. and Cornatzer, W.E. (1971) *Newer Trace Elements in Nutrition.* New York: Marcel Dekker.

Nuñez, M., Peña, R.M., Herrero, C., and Garcia-Martin, S. (2000) Analysis of some metals in wine by means of capillary electrophoresis. Application to the differentiation of Ribeira Sacra Spanish red wines, *Analusis*, **28**: 432–437.

Organisation International de la Vigne et du Vin (1990) *Recueil des Methods Internationales d'Analyses des Vins et des Moûts.* Paris: OIV.

Ostapczuk, P., Eschnauer, H.R., and Scollary, G.R. (1997) Determination of cadmium, lead and copper in wine by potentiometric stripping analysis, *Fresenius' Journal of Analytical Chemistry*, **358**: 723–727.

Ostapczuk, P., Alt, F., Bauer, K.H., Eschnauer, H.R., Neeb, R., and Scollary, G.R. (2000) Electrochemical traces (Pb, Cd, Cu) and ultratraces (Tl, Bi, Pt) determination in wine, *Viticultural and Enological Sciences*, **55**: 106–109.

Ough, C. and Amerine, M. (1988) *Methods for Analysis of Musts and Wine*, 2nd edn. New York: Wiley.

Pedersen, G.A., Mortensen, G.K., and Larsen, E.H. (1994) Beverages as a source of toxic trace element intake, *Food Additives and Contaminants*, **11**: 351–363.

Pellerin, P. and O'Neill, M.A. (1998) The interaction of the pectic polysaccharide Rhamnogalacturonan II with heavy metals and lanthanides in wines and fruit juices, *Analusis*, **26**: M32–M36.

Pellerin, P., O'Neill, M.A., Pierre, C., Cabanis, M.T., Darvill, A.G., Albersheim, P., and Moutounet, M. (1997) Complexation du plomb dans les vins par les dimères de rhamnogalacturonane II, un polysaccharide pectique du raisin, *Journal International des Sciences de la Vigne et du Vin*, **31**: 33–41.

Pereira, C.F. (1988) The importance of metallic elements in wine, *Zeitschrift für Lebensmitteluntersuchung und Forschung*, **186**: 295–300.

Perez-Jordan, M.Y., Soldevilla, J., Salvador, A., Pastor, A., and De la Guardia, M. (1999) Inductively coupled plasma mass spectrometry analysis of wines, *Journal of Analytical Atomic Spectrometry*, **14**: 33–39.

Pertoldi-Marletta, G., Gabrielli-Favretto, L., and Favretto, L. (1989) Chromium and nickel in roadside grapes, *Food Additives and Contaminants*, **6**: 219–225.

Rebolo, S., Peña, R.M., Latorre, M.J., García, S., Botana, A.M., and Herrero, C. (2000) Characterisation of Galician (NW Spain) Ribeira Sacra wines using pattern recognition analysis, *Analytica Chimica Acta*, **417**: 211–220.

Salati, V. (1999) *Atomi, Molecole e Vino.* Occimiano: Gimar Tecno.

Scollary, G.R. (1997) Metals in wine: contamination, spoilage and toxicity, *Analusis*, **25**: M26–M30.

Siegmund, H. and Bachmann, K. (1978) The application of numerical taxonomy for the classification of wines, Zeitschrift für Lebensmitteluntersuchung und Forschung, 166: 298–303.

Smart, G.A., Pickford, C.J., and Sherlock, J.C. (1990) Lead in alcoholic beverages: a second survey, Food Additives and Contaminants, 7: 93–99.

Spiess, B., Harraka, E., Wencker, D., and Laugel, P. (1984) Theoretical approach of the iron(III), lead and cadmium repartition in wine and precipitation by the hexacyanoferrate(II), Analusis, 12: 290–297.

Stockley, C. and Lloyd-Davies, S. (2001) Analytical Specifications for the Export of Australian Wine. Glen Osmond, South Australia: The Australian Wine Research Institute.

Stroh, A., Brückner, P., and Völlkopf, U. (1994) Multielement analysis of wine samples using ICP-MS, Atomic Spectroscopy, 15: 100–106.

Szpunar, J., Pellerin, P., Makarov, A., Doco, T., Williams, P., Medina, B., and Łobinski, R. (1998) Speciation analysis for biomolecular complexes of lead in wine by size-exclusion high-performance liquid chromatography–inductively coupled plasma mass spectrometry, Journal of Analytical Atomic Spectrometry, 13: 749–754.

Tahiri, M., Doco, T., Tressol, J.C., Pellerin, P., Pépin, D., Rayssiguier, Y., and Coudray, C. (2001) Rhamnogalacturonan II, a pectic polysaccharide, decreases intestinal absorption and tissue retention of lead in rats, Bulletin de l'Office de la Vigne et de Vin, 74(841–842): 228–235.

Tahvonen, R. (1998) Lead and cadmium in beverages consumed in Finland, Food Additives and Contaminants, 15: 446–450.

Teissedre, P.L., Cabanis, M.T., Daumas, F., and Cabanis, J.C. (1993) Evolution de la teneur en plomb au cours de l'elaboration des vins des Côtes du Rhône et de la Vallee du Rhône, Revue Française d'Œnologie, 33: 6–18.

Teissedre, P.L., Cabanis, M.T., Daumas, F., and Cabanis, J.C. (1994a) Evolution des teneurs en cadmium au cours de l'elaboration des vins des côtes du Rhône et de la vallée du Rhône, Sciences des Aliments, 14: 741–749.

Teissedre, P.L., Łobinski, R., Cabanis, M.T., Szpunar-Łobinska, J., Cabanis, J.C., and Adams, F.C. (1994b) On the origin of organolead compounds in wine, Science of the Total Environment, 153: 247–252.

Teissedre, P.L., Krosniak, M., Portet, K., Gasc, F., Waterhouse, A.L., Serrano, J.J., Cabanis, J.C., and Cros, G. (1998a) Vanadium levels in French and Californian wines: influence on vanadium dietary intake, Food Additives and Contaminants, 15: 585–591.

Teissedre, P.L., Vique, C.C., Cabanis, M.T., and Cabanis, J.C. (1998b) Determination of nickel in French wines and grapes, American Journal of Enology and Viticulture, 49: 205–210.

Thiel, G. and Danzer, K. (1997) Direct analysis of mineral components in wine by inductively coupled plasma optical emission spectrometry (ICP-AES), Fresenius' Journal of Analytical Chemistry, 357: 553–557.

Töben, L. and Ostapczuk, P. (1995) Bestimmung von Kupfer, Cadmium und Blei im Wein mit Hilfe der potentiometrischen Stripping Analyse (PSA), Viticultural and Enological Sciences, 50: 123–126.

Vasconcelos, M.T.S.D., Azenha, M., and de Freitas, V. (2000) Electrochemical studies of complexation of Pb in red wines, The Analyst, 125: 743–748.

Vidal, S., Doco, T., Moutounet, M., and Pellerin, P. (1999) Rhamnogalacturonane II, a complex polysaccharide of wine with remarkable properties, Revue Française d'Œnologie, 178: 12–17.

Wang, J. and Mannino, S. (1989) Application of adsorptive stripping voltammetry to the speciation and determination of iron(III) and total iron in wines, *The Analyst*, **114**: 643–645.

Wangkarn, S. and Pergantis, S.A. (2000) High-speed separation of arsenic compounds using narrow-bore high-performance liquid chromatography on-line with inductively coupled plasma mass spectrometry, *Journal of Analytical Atomic Spectrometry*, **15**: 627–633.

Weber, G. (1991) Speciation of iron using HPLC with electrochemical and flame-AAS detection, *Fresenius' Journal of Analytical Chemistry*, **340**: 161–165.

Weber, G. and Schwedt, G. (1982) Zur analytik chemischer Aindungsformen von Nickelspuren in Kaffee, Tee und Rotwein mit chromatographischen und spektroskopischen Methoden, *Analytica Chimica Acta*, **134**: 81–92.

Wennig, R. and Kirsch, N. (1988) Vanadium. In *Handbook on the Toxicity of Inorganic Compounds* (eds Seiler, H.G., Sigel, H., and Sigel, A.), pp. 749–765. New York: Marcel Dekker.

Wiese, C. and Schwedt, G. (1997) Strategy for copper speciation in white wine by differential pulse anodic stripping voltammetry, potentiometry with an ion-selective electrode and kinetic photometric determination, *Fresenius Journal of Analytical Chemistry*, **358**: 718–722.

Wifladt, A.M., Wibetoe, G., and Lund, W. (1997) Determination of antimony in wine by hydride generation graphite furnace atomic absorption spectrometry, *Fresenius' Journal of Analytical Chemistry*, **357**: 92–96.

World Health Organization (1989) *Toxicological Evaluation of Certain Food Additives and Contaminants*, WHO Food Additives Series 24. Cambridge: Cambridge University Press.

Zerbinati, O., Balduzzi, F., and Dell'Oro, V. (2000) Determination of lithium in wines by ion chromatography, *Journal of Chromatography*, **881**: 645–650.

10 Toxic considerations related to ingestion of carrageenan

Joanne K. Tobacman

Summary

Carrageenan has been widely used as a food additive in the Western diet for several decades. Its unique ability to solubilize milk proteins has led to its use in many processed foods, including both low-fat and high-fat and low-calorie and high-calorie foods. Hence, individuals who follow dietary recommendations with regard to cholesterol and calories may still have significant exposure to carrageenan. In experimental animal models, ingestion of carrageenan has been associated consistently with development of gastrointestinal ulcerations and neoplasms. It has been used as a model of human ulcerative colitis, an inflammatory bowel disorder that is pre-neoplastic. In addition, it has been used to induce inflammation in animal models of arthritis and pleuritis and to study effectiveness of anti-inflammatory therapies. Observation of cells exposed to carrageenan from inflammatory models and from tissue culture has demonstrated development of intracellular inclusions, consistent with incomplete metabolism of carrageenan within endosomes and lysosomes of the exposed cells, including macrophages, intestinal epithelial cells, and mammary cells in tissue culture. Subsequent vacuolation and disruption of the lysosomes appear to lead to cellular destruction due to release of the lysosomal contents. These changes may be associated with subsequent development of ulcerations and neoplasms.

Characteristics of carrageenan

Carrageenan has been used as a food additive for centuries. During the twentieth century, its incorporation into a wide variety of food products in the Western diet increased markedly, and coincident with marked increases in diseases often associated with the Western lifestyle, including atherosclerotic cardiovascular disease and malignancies of the colon, lung, breast, and prostate. In 1997, annual consumption of carrageenan in Western Europe and the United States was estimated to be 15 200 tonnes, and is projected to be over 18 000 tonnes in these regions in 2002 (Will *et al.*, 1999).

Carrageenan is a naturally occurring gum, derived from red seaweed. For several centuries in Ireland and other parts of Europe, red seaweed extracts have been incorporated into foods and medications due to their gelling and thickening properties. Carrageenan has been used in the United States since at least 1835, when it was brought by Irish immigrants. The process for its extraction and purification from Irish moss was patented in the US in 1871, and it became commercially available in the US in 1937. Carrageenan's uses increased when supplies of other gums were reduced during the Second World War (IARC, 1983; Moirano, 1977).

Unlike the other naturally occurring gums, carrageenan has an unusual ability to solubilize milk proteins. This property has led to its wide use as a thickener and stabilizer in a variety of milk-based products, including ice cream, yogurt, whipped cream, infant formula, soymilk, and dietetic beverages. Increasingly, other applications have emerged for carrageenan, including in processed meats, candy, toothpaste, laxatives, room deodorizers, and cosmetics.

Carrageenans are predominantly in one of three forms: kappa (κ), lambda (λ), or iota (ι). These are composed of disaccharides of two D-galactose residues (λ) or D-galactose and 3,6-anhydrose D-galactose residues (κ and ι) that may be sulfated at 0–3 residues. Alpha-1,4 and beta-1,3 linkages of the sugar residues form the backbone. The lambda form is the most highly sulfated, with sulfate groups on up to two carbons and three sulfates per disaccharide. The general characteristics of these carrageenans are indicated in Table 10.1. Kappa carrageenan forms gels with potassium ions, and iota carrageenan with calcium ions, unlike lambda carrageenan which does not form gels. The kappa and iota carrageenans form double right-handed helices; kinks can occur in this structure, leading to complex three-dimensional structures. Lambda carrageenan has the distinct property of being soluble in either cold or hot solutions, whereas the kappa and iota forms are soluble only in heated conditions. Small quantities of mu, nu, and theta carrageenans are found in nature as well. Carrageenan's attractiveness to food manufacturers involves its ability to form gels by the association of helical chains. The helix structure is promoted by stabilization of the C1 chair conformation of the residues, related to the 3,6 anhydro-bridge formations (Daniel, 1994; Marrs, 1998; Moirano, 1977).

In the following text, the toxic effects of carrageenan will be considered, including:

1   the harmful gastrointestinal effects associated with ingestion in animal experiments
2   the effects on cells in tissue culture, including mammary myoepithelial cells
3   the inflammatory effects associated with carrageenan and its use to model inflammation in animal experiments
4   extra-intestinal manifestations of toxicity, including renal, hepatic, immunologic, and anticoagulant effects
5   data about teratogenicity
6   potential toxicity related to human consumption and the extent of human exposure.

Table 10.1 Characteristics of carrageenan and specific characteristics of κ-, λ-, and ι-carrageenans

	κ-carrageenan	λ-carrageenan	ι-carrageenan
Chemical composition	3,6-anhydro-D-galactose and D-galactose-4 sulfate residues as disaccharide unit with β-1,4 link	D-galactose-2,6 sulfate and D-galactose-2 sulfate residues as disaccharide unit with β-1,4 link	3,6-anhdyro-D-galactose-2 sulfate and D-galactose-4 sulfate residues as disaccharide unit with β-1,4 link
	α-1,3 glycosidic linkage of disaccharide to other disaccharide units; hydrocolloid with ammonium, calcium, magnesium, potassium, or sodium salts		
Structure	Forms right-handed double helices; may have complex tertiary structure due to branching	No helices	Forms right-handed double helices; may have complex tertiary structure due to branching
Gelling	Forms gels with potassium ions	Does not form gels	Forms weak gels with calcium ions
Viscosity	Ranges from 5 to 800 cps for 1.5% solution; near logarithmic increase in viscosity with increasing concentration	5% solution at 75°C; food-grade carrageenan defined as not less than 5 cps at 75°C for 1.5% solution	
Solubility	Only in hot aqueous solutions	In hot or cold aqueous solutions	Only in hot aqueous solutions
Sulfate content	25–30%	32–39%	28–35%
Sources	Red seaweeds, including Chondrus, Gigartina, Eucheuma species; from North America, Philippines, Denmark, Japan		
Metabolism	Acid hydrolysis of glycosidic linkages that is accelerated by heat, carrageenases, sulfatases		
Other	More susceptible to acid hydrolysis than iota; has marked synergism with locust bean gum; gel network forms with casein		More resistant to hydrolysis in gelled state

Harmful gastrointestinal effects of carrageenan

Evidence about the harmful effects associated with carrageenan consumption has been acquired from many studies in animals performed over the past half-century. At least 45 published studies document the results of feeding carrageenan of different molecular weights and types to animals, including rats, mice, guinea pigs, monkeys, and rabbits. Review of these studies indicates that harmful effects were reported in 43/45 studies. The results of exposure were erosions, ulcerations, and neoplasms. These were often associated with macrophage infiltration, crypt abscesses, and macrophage vacuolation. Effects were seen with both degraded (<40 000 MW) and undegraded carrageenan, and undegraded carrageenan was found to be a tumor promoter in several experiments (Tobacman, 2001).

Gastrointestinal ulceration

The pattern of changes seen in the colon in the majority of these investigations suggests a consistent underlying mechanism that produces marked inflammation, epithelial cell death, erosions, and ulcerations with macrophage participation in the inflammatory process. Intestinal lesions were often seen proximally, but could be obtained more distally if carrageenan were introduced directly more distally in the intestinal tract. In guinea pigs and rabbits, the lesions occurred initially in the cecum; however, when carrageenan was introduced directly into the colon after ileotransversostomy, the lesions occurred more distally in the colon (Olsen *et al.*, 1983). Ulcerations occurred initially in distal colon and rectum in rats (Marcus, 1981).

Watt and Marcus (1969) observed ulcerations following carrageenan ingestion over three decades ago. 100% of guinea pigs fed 2% degraded carrageenan as liquid for 20–30 days developed colonic ulcerations; 75% of the animals had over 200 ulcerations. With 1% undegraded carrageenan as liquid for 20–30 days, 80% of the exposed guinea pigs developed colonic ulcerations. Lesions developed routinely with concentrations of 0.2%–1%, similar content to that of some food products that humans commonly consume.

Development of the ulcerations following carrageenan exposure appeared to be dose- and duration-dependent. Small epithelial ulcerations were found in guinea pigs that had carrageenan in their drinking fluid for two days (Kitsukawa *et al.*, 1992). Cecal lesions were identified after 24 h, and confluent ulcerations after seven days in pigs that drank a 5% solution (Olsen and Poulsen, 1980). In rats, superficial erosions at the anorectal junction arose at 24 h after 10% dietary carrageenan; over time, these extended more proximally (Oohashi *et al.*, 1979). Jensen *et al.* (1984) observed as many as 111 ulcerations/cm^2 over the mucosal surface of the cecum after five days of feeding a 5% carrageenan solution.

When concentrations of carrageenan between 0.5%–2% in drinking fluid were given to rhesus monkeys for 7–14 weeks, a dose effect was evident (Benitz *et al.*, 1973). Watt and Marcus (1970a) observed that 60% of rabbits exposed to 0.1% degraded carrageenan developed ulcerations, whereas 100% of those given 1% carrageenan had lesions with exposures of 6–12 weeks.

Macrophage infiltration appears as a common feature of carrageenan exposure. Infiltrating macrophages were observed to have metachromatic staining, and the macrophage lysosomes took up fibrillar material, associated with lysosomal distortion and vacuolation. Release of lysosomal contents and associated macrophage lysis appeared to provoke epithelial ulceration. Alterations in the macrophages were observed with exposure to undegraded carrageenan with molecular weight of 800 000 as a 1% solution (Mankes and Abraham, 1975). Marcus et al. (1992) evaluated pre-ulcerative lesions in guinea pigs, after exposure to degraded carrageenan for only two to three days, with an average daily consumption of 5.8 g/kg. Early focal lesions appeared macroscopically in the cecum in one of the animals tested, and all test animals had a diffuse cellular infiltrate with macrophages and polymorphonuclear leukocytes that was apparent microscopically. The inflammatory changes in cecum and ascending colon were present in all animals and in the distal colon and rectum of three of four animals. Metachromatic staining material was found in the lamina propria of the colon and surface epithelium from cecum to rectum and in colonic macrophages. Controls were unaffected. The early lesions observed differed from more advanced lesions because the surface epithelial cells and the macrophages contained vacuoles filled with the metachromatic material; this was not seen previously in more advanced lesions. Ulceration, hence, was associated with the breakdown of the mucosa by a direct toxic effect on the epithelial cells (Marcus et al., 1992).

Carrageenan model of human ulcerative colitis

The experimental findings presented above provided the basis for many investigators to use a carrageenan model for study of the inflammatory bowel disease (IBD) ulcerative colitis (UC) and for assessment of response to various treatments. The ulcerative lesions and associated inflammatory changes in the animal experiments resemble the histopathological changes seen in the human disease ulcerative colitis. Clinical features associated with the carrageenan model in animals have included weight loss, anemia, diarrhea, mucus in stools, and occult or visible blood in stools. Small intestinal lesions and spontaneous remission are not features of the carrageenan model, nor of ulcerative colitis. Additional histopathologic features of the animal models included loss of haustral folds, mucosal granularity, crypt abscesses, lymphocytic infiltration, capillary congestion, pseudopolyps and strictures. Transition from colitis to squamous metaplasia to neoplasms occurred in the colorectum. Findings of atypical epithelial hyperplasia associated with carrageenan-induced ulcerations resemble changes associated with human ulcerative colitis and provide a link with mechanisms of intestinal neoplasia (Ishioka et al., 1987; Kim and Berstad, 1992; Mottet, 1971; Onderdonk, 1985; Ottet, 1972; Sharratt et al., 1971; Watt and Marcus, 1973).

Frequently, medications used to treat ulcerative colitis have been tested in the carrageenan model. For example, testing of mesalazine microgranules was done in rabbits with carrageenan-induced colitis. The impact of mesalazine was determined in relation to its effect on colonic mucosal damage, leukotriene B5 concentrations, and concentrations of mesalazine derivatives. The benefits in this model were anticipated to correspond to therapeutic benefits to patients with ulcerative colitis and Crohn's disease (Kitano *et al.*, 1996).

Anti-inflammatory effects of 5-aminosalicylic acid (ASA) conjugates with chenodeoxycholic acid and ursodeoxycholic acid were studied in the carrageenan model of intestinal ulceration in guinea pigs. The number of ulcers in the cecum and colon, body weights and bleeding scores of occult blood in feces were measured. The ASA conjugates were begun on the 15th day after carrageenan was started and continued for four weeks, looking for improvement, in order to address the question of dose for treatment of ulcerative colitis (Goto *et al.*, 2001).

Although inflammatory bowel disease has been explored by many investigators, no causative agent in man has been established. Epidemiological data indicate that inflammatory bowel disease is predominantly a disorder of the West, associated with the Western lifestyle and diet (Whelan, 1990).

Gastrointestinal neoplasia

Similarly, the increased incidence of colon carcinoma in the West may have a relation to the consumption of carrageenan. IBD has been identified as pre-neoplastic, frequent colonoscopies are recommended in order to screen for malignancies in patients with ulcerative colitis, and colectomy is often performed prophylactically. The basis for the development of the malignancies appears to be related to the inflammation and the associated mucosal changes. Although study of the relationship between carrageenan-induced lesions and other pathways associated with development of colonic polyps, including genetic factors such as adenomatous polyposis coli (APC) and p53, have not yet been reported, further characterization of any genetic changes associated with exposure to carrageenan may be informative. Polypoid lesions in the intestinal mucosa have been identified in relation to the inflammation induced by carrageenan exposure, suggesting that there may be a continuum related to erosions, ulcerations, polyps, adenomas, adenocarcinomas, in which the stimulus for development of the neoplasms may arise in relation to the changes introduced by inflammation with its associated release of intracellular contents. In addition, the ulcerative lesions introduced in the intestine may provide a mechanism of entry for carrageenan, both in relation to the macrophage uptake of carrageenan in the inflammatory lesions and by loss of the normal epithelial barrier (Fabian *et al.*, 1973; Oohashi *et al.*, 1979, 1981; Watt and Marcus, 1970b).

Investigation of the carcinogenicity of degraded carrageenan has demonstrated that colonic tumors developed in 32% of rats fed 10% degraded carrageenan in the diet for less than 24 months. The lesions observed included adenocarcinomas, adenomas, and squamous cell carcinomas. With exposure to 5% degraded carrageenan in the drinking water, 20% incidence of colonic metaplasia occurred after 15 months. In this experiment, metastatic squamous cell carcinoma was observed in retroperitoneal lymph nodes. Macrophages with metachromatic staining consistent with carrageenan uptake were observed in liver and spleen (Wakabayashi et al., 1978).

Polypoid lesions and marked irreversible squamous metaplasia of the rectal mucosa have occurred, the extent of which appear related to duration and concentration of carrageenan exposures. Oohashi et al. (1981) observed 100% incidence of colorectal metaplasia that progressed even after discontinuing exposure to degraded carrageenan in rats fed 10% degraded carrageenan for two, six or nine months and sacrificed at 18 months. Adenomatous and hyperplastic polyps and metaplasia of the anorectal region and the distal colon were seen after 5% carrageenan as drinking fluid. Hyperplastic mucosal changes and polypoidal lesions were observed in rabbits given carrageenan as a drink for 6–12 weeks at a concentration of 0.1–5% (Watt and Marcus, 1970b). Focal and severe dysplasia of the mucosal epithelium was observed in rabbits after 28 months of 1% degraded carrageenan in drinking fluid (Kitano et al., 1986).

Promotion of neoplasia

Undegraded or degraded carrageenan ingestion in association with exposure to a known carcinogen has led to increased occurrence of neoplasia. In rats treated with azoxymethane (AOM) and nitrosomethylurea (NMU), the addition of carrageenan to the diet increased markedly the incidence of colonic tumors. Groups included controls, controls with 15% carrageenan, 15% carrageenan plus 10 injections of AOM given weekly, carrageenan plus NMU, NMU alone and AOM alone. Undegraded carrageenan with either AOM or NMU was associated with 100% incidence of tumors, versus 57% with AOM alone and 69 with NMU alone. Controls had 0% and undegraded carrageenan alone had 7%. When undegraded carrageenan was combined with AOM, a 10-fold increase in the number of tumors per rat was seen (Wakabayashi et al., 1978).

Other work has also demonstrated promotion of neoplasms. Using degraded carrageenan as a solid gel at 2.5% concentration for 100 days, promotion of aberrant crypt foci increased by 15% following exposure to azoxymethane (Corpet et al., 1997). Tumors increased from 40% to 75%, and larger and more proximal tumors occurred following exposure of rats to 6% undegraded carrageenan in the diet for 24 weeks with 1,2-dimethylhydrazine (DMH) injections weekly (Arawaka et al., 1986).

Experiments with degraded carrageenan in the diet of rats at a 10% concentration, in combination with 1,2-DMH weekly for 15 weeks, led to an increase in small intestinal tumors from 20% to 50% and in colonic tumors from 45% to 60% (Kawaura et al., 1982). Degraded carrageenan in the drinking water for less than 30 weeks, in association with 1,2-DMH weekly injections, was associated with increases in poorly differentiated adenocarcinomas and in tumors of the ascending and transverse colon, as well as increased proliferation of cells in the deep glandular areas (Iatropoulos et al., 1975).

A five-fold increase in thymidine kinase activity was observed in colon cells with exposure to 5% undegraded or degraded carrageenan. There was an associated 35-fold increase in proliferating cells in the upper third of crypts with degraded carrageenan and an eight-fold increase with undegraded carrageenan (Wilcox *et al.*, 1992). Five percent undegraded lambda carrageenan fed to rats for four weeks led to a four-fold increase in thymidine kinase activity in the distal 12 cm of the colon (Calvert and Reicks, 1988). There was a two-fold increase in colonic epithelial cells proliferating in both proximal and distal colon and extensive increase in proliferation in the proximal colon to the upper third of the intestinal crypt after exposure of mice to 10% degraded carrageenan for 10 days in drinking water (Fath *et al.*, 1984).

Effects of intestinal bacteria

The composition of the intestinal microflora may have a significant role in the development of intestinal lesions. Investigators have examined the impact of antibiotics and alteration of the resident microbial flora on the activity of carrageenan. Carrageenan, as well as other sulfated polysaccharides, has been shown to stimulate H_2S production from fecal slurries (Gibson *et al.*, 1990). Sulfide has been implicated in the development of ulcerative colitis, perhaps by interference with butyrate oxidation by colonic epithelial cells (Richardson *et al.*, 2000; Roediger *et al.*, 1993).

The mechanism of the carrageenan-associated colonic changes may be related to the production of toxic sulfur-containing gases, such as hydrogen sulfide, methanethiol, and dimethyl sulfide, following carrageenan feeding in a rat model of ulcerative colitis. Hydrogen sulfide production increased five-fold following carrageenan exposure, based on measurement of cecal accumulation in rats. Between the cecum and rectum, over 90% of the sulfur-containing gases were absorbed or metabolized (Suarez *et al.*, 1998).

Extra-colonic effects of carrageenan in animal experiments

In addition to localized lesions in the intestine, circulation to the spleen and liver of macrophages that had taken up metachromatic particles, consistent with carrageenan, has been determined in animal experiments. Degraded carrageenan was taken up and stored in lysosomes of intestinal macrophages of guinea pigs, rats, and monkeys (Abraham *et al.*, 1974) and in macrophages and reticuloendo-thelial cells of rhesus monkey (Abraham *et al.*, 1972; Mankes and Abraham, 1975). This uptake was noted not only with exposures to low molecular weight, but also with higher molecular weight carrageenan. Uptake by intestinal macrophages with migration of the macrophages to lymph nodes, spleen, and liver can provide a mechanism for extra-intestinal actions of carrageenan (Benitz *et al.*, 1973; Fabian *et al.*, 1973; Grasso *et al.*, 1975; Nicklin and Miller, 1989; Oohashi *et al.*, 1981; Pittman *et al.*, 1976). In addition, carrageenan-induced intestinal ulcerations have been associated with an increase in permeability to large molecules (polyethylene glycol-900), suggesting another mechanism for uptake and extraintestinal effects (Delahunty *et al.*, 1987).

Table 10.2 Carrageenan effects in experimental animal models

Gastrointestinal	Destruction of intestinal epithelial cells, intestinal ulcerations, intestinal neoplasms, promotion of intestinal neoplasia
Immunologic	Uptake by macrophages and destruction of macrophages; depression of cell-mediated immunity and prolongation of graft survival
Tissue culture	Destruction of mammary myoepithelial cells in tissue culture; destruction of small intestinal epithelial cells in tissue culture; destruction of other cells in tissue culture, including LNCaP, endothelial cell line, rat mammary adenocarcinoma cell line; reduced cellular adhesion; inhibit gap junctional communication
Neoplastic	Potentiation of tumor growth; induction of sarcomas, breast, and testicular malignancies
Systemic	Death at high concentrations, anticoagulant effect, hepatotoxicity, nephrotoxicity, anaphylaxis
Infectious	Reduced infectivity of viruses; diminished delayed hypersensitivity; macrophage vacuolation and lysis
Inflammatory	Induction of inflammation in models of inflammation including hindpaw, pleural space, peritoneum; increased TNF-alpha; increased IL-1 beta, increased PGE2, increased iNOS activity
Reproductive	Mouse fetal toxicity with increased fetal deaths, decreased pup weight; abnormalities in skeletal maturation

Many experiments have been performed in the past several decades to study effects of carrageenan on different organs and cellular processes. These have included studies of lethal effects, nephrotoxicity, hepatotoxicity, anaphylaxis, direct effects with regard to tumors, alteration of immune function, virucidal properties, effects on coagulation, and teratogenic effects. A summary of effects related to experimental carrageenan exposure is presented in Table 10.2.

Intravenous undegraded (native) carrageenan at 15 mg/kg body weight caused death in two of three dogs within 24 h (Houck *et al.*, 1957). In rabbits, 1–5 mg/ kg bw lambda carrageenan or 3–15 mg/kg bw kappa carrageenan intravenously caused death within 24 h (Anderson and Duncan, 1965).

Undegraded kappa carrageenan was found to be nephrotoxic based on increased serum creatinine and urea and hepatotoxic based on increased serum aspartate aminotransferase activity and reduced albumin, whereas undegraded lambda and iota did not affect these functions (Thomson and Whiting, 1981).

Anaphylaxis has been observed following exposure to barium contrast medium in which carrageenan was used as a suspending agent. Positive skin puncture testing and specific IgE antibodies to carrageenan were found in serum (Tarlo *et al.*, 1995).

Carrageenan by subcutaneous injection (5 ml of a 1% solution) in rats produced local sarcomas at 19.6 times the expected level at 650 days and 16.2 times the expected level at 825 days. Mammary and testicular tumors have also been observed (Cater, 1961; Hopkins, 1981; Informatics, 1972; Rustia *et al.*, 1980).

Prolongation of graft survival, depression of cell-mediated immunity, and potentiation of tumor growth have been attributed to the selective cytopathic effect of carrageenan on macrophages (Thomson and Fowler, 1981). Local injection of carrageenan into a tissue site containing tumor cells in mice produced an accelerated growth of tumor, with reduced percentage of apoptotic cells and increased proportion of cells at the S and G2/M phases of the cell cycle. The effects were dose-dependent and aborted by indomethacin, suggesting prostaglandin mediation (Raz et al., 2000).

In addition to depression of cell-mediated immunity in association with carrageenan exposure, impairment of complement activity and of humoral responses was reported. Carrageenan via the intraperitoneal route was associated with reduced primary antibody responses against T-cell dependent antigens. Oral administration of food-grade carrageenan was associated with depressed systemic humoral immunity against a heterologous T-cell dependent antigen (Nicklin and Miller, 1989). These alterations may have been the result of modified antigen processing by macrophages. The carrageenan treated macrophages *in vitro* could release stimulatory and/or inhibitory factors. Exposure to undegraded carrageenan has been found to inhibit binding of basic fibroblast growth factor, transforming growth factor beta-1 and platelet derived growth factor, but not insulin-like growth factor-1 or transforming growth factor-alpha (Hoffman, 1993).

Carrageenan has been associated with reduced infectivity of viruses, such as HIV-1 and herpesvirus, and been introduced experimentally into contraceptives to attempt to reduce infectivity associated with HIV. Carrageenan's activity inhibitory to HIV appears due to its polyanionic characteristics, molecular weight, and sulfate content, with the lambda carrageenan most active (Yamada et al., 1997). Iota carrageenan, at concentrations of 1–2 µg/ml, is able to block infection of epithelial cell lines by HIV-1, and is a more effective blocker of adhesion of monocytes to epithelial cells than other sulfated polysaccharides studied (Pearce-Pratt and Phillips, 1996). Antiviral effects of carrageenan on herpes simplex virus (HSV) types 1 and 2 have been demonstrated, with the predominant antiviral action upon virus adsorption, rather than internalization or protein synthesis. However, lambda carrageenan had greater virucidal properties than kappa or iota, remaining active after adsorption, and not interfering only with interaction between the HSV particles and the cell (Carlucci et al., 1999).

Teratogenicity and fetal loss effects

Fetal toxicity has been observed in studies with rats and mice. In studies evaluating fetal status in female mice, an increase in the number of fetal deaths and a decrease in the number of live pups and pup weight was noted following exposure to doses of 470–900 mg/kg per day. Abnormalities in skeletal maturation were observed in fetuses from mice, rats, and hamsters, suggesting a teratogenic effect (Informatics, 1972).

These data were referred to in the 1979 report in the Federal Register that indicated the planned reconsideration of the status of carrageenan (Federal

Register, 1979). Effects on reproduction, fetal development, and prenatal toxicity in rats and hamsters were limited to reduced birth weight and weight at weaning in rats (Collins *et al.*, 1977a, 1977b, 1979).

Carrageenan was non-mutagenic in *Salmonella* mutagenicity testing and non-genotoxic by DNA repair tests (Ishioka *et al.*, 1987; Mori *et al.*, 1984).

Effects on coagulation

Both carrageenan and heparin are highly sulfated polysaccharide molecules with anticoagulant properties. Unlike heparin and heparanases, carrageenan is not spontaneously made by cells and naturally occurring carrageenases do not exist in human cells. In general, the anticoagulant properties of the sulfated polysaccharides appear related to the percentage sulfate, and the carrageenans can be sulfated by as much as 40% by weight (Carlucci *et al.*, 1997; Dace *et al.*, 1997).

Effects in tissue culture

In tissue culture, carrageenan has been associated with the disruption and destruction of mammary myoepithelial cells (Tobacman, 1997), small intestine epithelial cell monolayers (Ling *et al.*, 1988), androgen-dependent malignant prostate cells (Hoffman *et al.*, 1995), bFGF-dependent endothelial cell line (Hoffman *et al.*, 1995), and rat mammary adenocarcinoma 13762 MAT cells (Coombe *et al.*, 1987). Carrageenan inhibited the proliferation of normal breast epithelial cells and breast cancer epithelial cell lines (MCF-7 and MDA-MB-231). In addition, carrageenan inhibited FGF-2 binding in normal, MCF-7, and MDA-MB-231 cells and inhibited urokinase plasminogen activation in the MDA-MB-231 cells (Lambrecht *et al.*, 1998).

Ability of MCF-7 and MDA-MB231 adenocarcinoma breast cells to adhere to different substrata was investigated using different sulfated polysaccharides. The most effective in inhibiting cell adhesion was iota carrageenan, attributable to the charge density related to the sulfate groups, molecular weight, and carbohydrate structure. These properties may impair the usual interaction between the glycosaminoglycan portion of proteoglycans and the extracellular matrix proteins, blocking adhesion (Liu *et al.*, 2000).

When rat liver epithelial cells were exposed to carrageenan, inhibition of gap-junctional intercellular communication occurred, similar to that associated with phorbol ester, although phosphorylation and localization of connexin 43 were not altered (Suzuki *et al.*, 2000).

Effects on mammary myoepithelial cells

In primary cultures of human mammary myoepithelial cells derived from reduction mammoplasty, we have determined that carrageenan has a profound detrimental effect on the mammary myoepithelial cells. Exposure to concentrations as low as 10^{-5}g% led to rapid and irreversible loss. This was observed with lambda, kappa, and iota carrageenans, although the solubility of lambda in either warm or cold solutions and its lack of gel formation make it easier to use in the laboratory. Exposure to lower molecular weight derivatives of kappa, lambda, and iota appears also to be associated with destruction of the mammary myoepithelial cells in tissue culture (unpublished data).

The appearance of endosomal and lysosomal inclusions in the mammary myoepithelial cells resembles to some extent the lysosomal inclusions observed in the mucopolysaccharidoses or lysosomal storage diseases (LSDs) and in macrophages and intestinal epithelial cells following exposure to carrageenan (Abraham *et al.*, 1972, 1974; Marcus *et al.*, 1992; Tobacman and Walters, 2001b). As in the LSD, there appears to be accumulation of partially metabolized molecules that, due to deficiency of the required enzyme, cannot be further broken down, similar to the accumulation of sulfated mucopolysaccharides that accumulate in deficiency of arylsulfatase A (metachromatic leukodystrophy), arylsulfatase B (Maroteaux-Lamy Syndrome), or multiple sulfatase deficiency. The lamellated inclusions resemble to some extent the thylakoid membrane of algae, which contains sulfated galactose residues among other components. The intracellular trafficking of the carrageenan involves membrane uptake and incorporation into vesicles that fuse into endosomal or lysosomal compartments, apparently by a process of membrane folding. Subsequent appearance of vacuolations within the endosomal–lysosomal organelles suggests that mechanical distortion and increased oxidative processes have led to lysosomal disruption. These changes are associated with other intracellular changes, including disruption of the myofilaments with diminished staining of alpha-smooth muscle specific actin and gelsolin. The cellular destruction appears attributable to direct cytopathic effects, rather than overexpression of pro-apoptotic oncogenes or mutations (Tobacman, 1997; Tobacman and Walters, 2001).

The mammary myoepithelial cells are known to have very high levels of steroid sulfatase activity (Tobacman *et al.*, 2002a). Downregulation of steroid sulfatase mRNA occurs following exposure to carrageenan, suggesting that increased sulfate in the cells from the carrageenan exposure may impact on sulfatase expression (Tobacman *et al.*, 2002b). In turn, this may lead to less active estrogenic hormone available to the adjacent epithelial cells, and to imbalance between the normal estrogen/progesterone processes within the cell. Hence, it is possible that carrageenan effects may interfere with some of the basic metabolic processes related to steroid and sulfatase metabolism within the cell.

Extra-intestinal models of inflammation associated with carrageenan exposure

In addition to the effectiveness of carrageenan ingestion as a model of inflammatory bowel disease, carrageenan has been used to study inflammation at other sites and for other purposes. Models have been developed to induce inflammation to study mediators and mechanisms of inflammation and pain, as well as pharmacologic interventions to reduce inflammation. Over 30 years ago, carrageenan was observed to induce acute inflammatory responses in rats, forming the basis for its use as a model system to study inflammation and anti-inflammatory drugs (Di Rosa, 1972). Subcutaneous injection of carrageenan into guinea pigs was observed to lead to granulomas, and acute inflammation has been produced experimentally by injection of carrageenan directly into confined spaces, such as the plantar surface of rat's hind paw, pleural space, peritoneal cavity, joint space, subacromial bursa, or subcutaneous air bleb. In general, the inflammatory response to carrageenan is characterized by edema, migration of inflammatory cells, including polymorphonuclear leukocytes, macrophages and lymphocytes, and increased release of cytokines.

The acute inflammatory response evoked by carrageenan injection into the pleural cavity of rats was associated with fluid accumulation and infiltration of polymorphonuclear leukocytes into lung tissues, lipid peroxidation and increased production of prostaglandin E2, tumor necrosis factor (TNF)-alpha and inter-leukin (IL)-1 beta. In addition, there was upregulation of the adhesion molecules ICAM-1 and P-selectin, as well as nitrotyrosine, and poly ADP-ribose synthetase (PARS) (Cuzzocrea *et al.*, 2002).

TNF-alpha and IL-1 beta have critical roles in cell migration and exudation following injection of carrageenan into the mouse pleural cavity. Intrapleural injection of TNF-alpha or IL-1 beta shortly prior to carrageenan caused graded increase in the early and late exudation phases of the inflammatory response. When antibodies against TNF-alpha and IL-1 beta were injected 30 min prior to intrapleural injection of carrageenan, exudation and cell migration charac-teristic of the early phase response (4 h) were reduced, but there was potentiation or no effect on the 48 h response. An IL-1 receptor antagonist (RA) reduced exudation by about 50% and abolished early and late cell migration (Frode *et al.*, 2001). It is interesting to note that TNF-alpha has been found to convert CD44 from its inactive form to its active form by inducing the sulfation of CD44, thereby enabling CD44-mediated leukocyte adhesion at inflammatory sites (Maiti *et al.*, 1998). Since carrageenan is so highly sulfated, the association between carrageenan exposure and subsequent sulfation of inflammatory med-iators may help understanding of the inflammatory process associated with carrageenan.

In IL-6 knockout mice injected with carrageenan into the pleural space, the degree of lung injury was reduced, and the intensity and degree of staining for cyclo-oxygenase-2 and iNOS were markedly reduced, compared to normal mice. The resistance of the IL-6 KO mice to the carrageenan-induced inflammation suggests a role for IL-6 in mediating the inflammatory response to carrageenan (Cuzzocrea *et al.*, 1999b). Carrageenan-induced local inflammation can also be inhibited by soluble murine IL-15 receptor alpha that contains a Sushi domain with four cysteines forming two disulfide bonds, but not by a mutant IL-15 receptor alpha with an amino acid substitution for the first or fourth cysteine (Wei *et al.*, 2001).

In carrageenan-induced pleurisy in rats, oophorectomy enhanced the degree of pleural exudation and polymorphonuclear leukocyte migration, as well as myeloeperoxidase activity and lipid peroxidation. iNOS was increased and correlated with increased production of TNF-alpha and IL-1 beta, as well as increased immunohistochemical staining for P-selectin, ICAM-1, nitrotyrosine, and PARS. Intraperitoneal injection of 17-beta estradiol reversed these effects (Cuzzocrea *et al.*, 2001b).

Oxidative stress may be a major factor in carrageenan-associated inflammation, and in carrageenan-induced pleurisy, all parameters of inflammation were attenuated by treatment with N-acetylcysteine (NAC), a free radical scavenger. This treatment was associated with a partial restoration of the cellular level of NAD$^+$ in *ex vivo* macrophages harvested from the pleural cavity. Altered morphology of red blood cells was also observed 24 h after carrageenan administration and diminished by the NAC treatment (Cuzzocrea *et al.*, 2001a). In the rat model of carrageenan-induced pleurisy, depletion of endogenous glutathione pools enhanced the carrageenan-induced degree of exudate and polymorphonuclear leukocyte migration, as well as myeloperoxidase activity and lipid peroxidation. iNOS was not altered, nitrotyrosine staining was increased, and the cellular level of NAD$^+$ in harvested *ex vivo* macrophages from the pleural cavity was reduced. Administration of glutathione led to anti-inflammatory effects (Cuzzocrea *et al.*, 1999a).

In rat carrageenan pleurisy induced by injection of 0.2 ml of 1% lambda carrageenan into the pleural cavity, the nitric oxide synthase (NOS) inhibitor, NG-nitro-L-arginine methyl ester (L-NAME), reduced the amounts of NOx (NO$_2^-$ and NO$_3^-$) and PGE2 in a dose-dependent manner, and L-arginine increased these substances. In the carrageenan-induced pleural exudate, the amount of NOx correlated with the amount of PGE2 (Sautebin *et al.*, 1998).

When wild type mice and knockout mice lacking inducible NOS were compared following carrageenan exposure, reduced pleural exudation and polymorphonuclear cell migration were seen in the knockout mice. Lung myeloperoxidase activity and lipid peroxidation were significantly reduced in the knockout mice, and intensity and degree of staining for nitrotyrosine and poly-ADP-ribose synthetase in alveolar macrophages and in airway epithelial cells were reduced in tissue sections from the carrageenan-exposed iNOS-KO mice. (Cuzzocrea *et al.*, 2000). Hence, the carrageenan associated pleurisy was less damaging in the iNOS-KO mice or in rats given NOS inhibitor, suggesting a role for iNOS in carrageenan-induced inflammation.

In the rat hindpaw model of inflammation, carrageenan appeared to induce peripheral release of nitric oxide, the production of which was mediated by different nitric oxide synthase isoforms. The early production was mediated by (neuronal) nNOS, and in the late phase by both nNOS and (inducible) iNOS (Omote *et al.*, 2001).

In rat paw inflammation induced by carrageenan, there was a time-dependent increase in edema, neutrophil infiltration and increased levels of NO$_2^-$ and NO$_3^-$ and PGE2. Nonselective nitric oxide synthase inhibitors given intravenously before or after carrageenan inhibited paw edema at all time points, in contrast to selective inducible NOS inhibitors that suppressed paw edema at later time points (5–10 h). Inhibition of paw edema by use of the NOS inhibitors was associated with reduction of NO_2^- and NO_3^- and PGE2 levels in the exudate (Salvemini *et al.*, 1996).

Intra-articular injection of carrageenan into the rat knee joint was used to study early and late phase inflammation, the roles of cyclo-oxygenase (COX)-1 and -2, and the impact of indomethacin, a nonselective COX inhibitor. Prostaglandin production by COX-2 appeared to mediate the development of the acute inflammatory hyperemia induced by carrageenan, with increased urinary prostaglandins by 6 h, but back to baseline by 24 h. Urinary NOx levels increased progressively over the 24 h time period studied, associated with induction of iNOS in 3 and 24 h samples, suggesting that the acute inflammatory effects associated with carrageenan were mediated by prostaglandins (Egan *et al.*, 2002).

In summary, the inflammatory potential of carrageenan in these models appears related predominantly to its ability to stimulate TNF-alpha, PGE2, IL-1 beta, and possibly other interleukins, its induction of NOS, and its impact on oxidative stress. The effect of carrageenan on the viscosity of joint or compartmental fluid or on ionic characteristics of these fluids has not been elaborated.

Human exposure to carrageenan

Carrageenans are widely used in foods due to their ability to improve the consistency of food products. World production of carrageenan in 1971 was about 4500 tons; 2300 tons was produced in the US, with most of the rest from Denmark and France, and some from Japan, Spain, and the UK (Towle, 1973). This has increased to 17 000 tons in worldwide production in 1997 (Will *et al.*, 1999).

Increasing uses for carrageenan have expanded the extent and type of exposures of humans to carrageenan. Carrageenan has been used in bath oil tablets; make-up preparations; toothpaste; deodorants; cleansing creams; face, body and hand preparations; moisturizing creams; air fresheners; wrinkle smoothing preparations; etc., as well as food products and pharmaceuticals. It has been used as an emulsifier in laxatives, in liquid petrolatum, in cod liver oil and in some antibiotics. It is used as a thickening agent in pesticides. It may be used as an oil well drilling fluid component. Increased use in meat products has occurred, with carrageenans contributing to gel formation and water retention. This is particularly important in low-fat meat products, since lack of fat leads to tough texture and reduced juiciness (Trius and Sebranek, 1996). Human exposure to carrageenan can occur by ingestion in food, but also by other routes, including inhalation and topical application. The food uses include both low- and high-fat and low- and high-calorie foods; hence, attention to low-fat or low-calorie diet does not preclude significant dietary exposure to carrageenan.

The increase in consumption corresponds to an increase in breast cancer incidence from 74.6 cases per 100 000 population (1947) to 110.7 cases per 100 000 in 1996. Correlation data have demonstrated that with incorporation of lag times of 25 and 30 years before occurrence of malignancy, significant positive correlations (Pearson correlation coefficients = 0.8812 and 0.9576) are obtained between carrageenan consumption and breast cancer incidence. The Spearman correlation coefficient for 30-year lag is 1.000 with $p = 0.0001$ (Tobacman *et al.*, 2001).

Carrageenan intake levels

Previous estimates of carrageenan use in the US include Food and Drug Administration (FDA) data collected when application was made for processed *Eucheuma* seaweed (PES) from the Philippines in the 1990s. The PES is composed of carrageenan and more undigestible fiber than previous products. In FDA documents from this time, the average processed Eucheuma seaweed (PES) consumption was estimated as 3.837 g/day for eaters for all age groups, male and female. This involved the assumption that the amount of PES in these foods was the same as the use levels of carrageenan, indicating that carrageenan intake among eaters was over 3.8 g/day. The 90th percentile consumption was 7.487 g/day (FDA unpublished data). These intake values for carrageenan-eaters far exceed the estimate of 100 mg/day made by the National Academy of Sciences (NAS) panel in the 1970s (Food and Nutrition Board, 1976), probably reflecting a marked increase in consumption of carrageenan in recent decades. When Informatics prepared a summary for the FDA of carrageenan intake in the 1970s, they determined that the mean consumption for the average user and eater was 334.98 mg/day of carrageenan. Very high intake rose to 1623.97 mg/day (Informatics, 1972).

Degraded and undegraded carrageenan exposures

Regulatory issues pertaining to the incorporation of carrageenan in foods have largely been confined to considerations related to degraded carrageenan. This appears to be due to the many studies that have been conducted in animals that clearly demonstrated the toxic effects of exposure to lower molecular weight carrageenan. By lower molecular weight, investigators have generally considered carrageenan of under 30 000–40 000 molecular weight, although others consider low molecular weight carrageenan to have molecular weight less than 100 000 (Marrs, 1998).

The available evidence suggests that ingestion of food-grade carrageenan invariably is associated with exposure to low molecular weight forms. The reasons for this include:

1   food products that contain food-grade carrageenan contain degraded carrageenan (Ekstrom, 1985; Ekstrom *et al.*, 1983; Marrs, 1998)
2   acid digestion such as occurs in the stomach is sufficient to break down higher MW forms of carrageenan to lower MW (Ekstrom, 1985; Ekstrom *et al.*, 1983; Yu *et al.*, 2002)

3   bacterial action is able to break down carrageenan (Sarwar *et al.*, 1987; Weigl and Yaphe, 1986)

4   heat exposure, such as can occur with consumption of warmed beverages or preparation of food products, leads to degradation of carrageenan (Marrs, 1998).

These four processes lead to the availability of low molecular weight carrageenan from the higher molecular weight forms.

Gastrointestinal metabolism of carrageenan to form smaller molecular weight components has been observed by several investigators, who reported that carrageenan of high molecular weight changed during intestinal passage, compatible with a process of hydrolysis yielding lower molecular weight components (Ekstrom, 1985; Ekstrom *et al.*, 1983; Engster and Abraham, 1976; Pittman *et al.*, 1976; Taché *et al.*, 2000).

Under conditions such as might occur in the process of digestion, 17% of food-grade carrageenan degraded to MW less than 20 000 in 1 h at pH 1.2 at 37°C. At pH 1.9 for 2 h at 37°C, 10% of the carrageenan had MW less than 20 000 (Ekstrom *et al.*, 1983). These and other data (Yu *et al.*, 2002) reveal that substantial fractions of lower molecular weight carrageenan are likely to arise during the normal process of digestion.

Data describing contamination of food-grade carrageenan by degraded carrageenan indicate that 25% of total carrageenans in eight food-grade carrageenans were found to have molecular weight less than 100 000, and 9% had molecular weight less than 50 000 (Ekstrom *et al.*, 1983). Native carrageenans have been shown to contain a broad distribution of molecular weights, extending to 20 kD; and in commercial products, carrageenans with molecular weight less than 20 kD composed up to 3% (Marrs, 1998).

Experiments with heating to 75°C and varying the pH have been performed to determine the degradation of food-grade carrageenan. Reasonable stability to heating down to pH 4 was found, but the rate of depolymerization increased significantly from pH 4 to pH 3. When the pH fell to 3.6 from 4.1, there was a marked increase in the degradation of kappa carrageenan. The proportion of material with molecular weight less than 100 000 increased to 30%–40% at pH 3.6–3.7 in water jellies made with commercial carrageenan products. With brief processing at high temperatures (specifically, 15 s at 115°C), 18% of the carrageenan had molecular weight <100 000. At 140°C for 10 s, the fraction with molecular weight less than 100 000 increased to 35%. Kappa carrageenan is more susceptible to acid hydrolysis than the iota form (Marrs, 1998).

Several bacteria have been identified that are able to hydrolyze carrageenan into smaller products, including tetracarrabiose. These bacteria, including *Cytophaga* species and *Pseudomonas carrageenovora*, are of marine origin; it is unknown if the human microbial flora can perform similar hydrolysis reactions. Some human bacteria are known to have sulfatases that can generate H_2S and other products from the metabolism of sulfates (Johnston and McCandless, 1973; McLean and Williamson, 1979; Potin *et al.*, 1991; Sarwar *et al.*, 1987; Weigl and Yaphe, 1986).

Extent of human exposure

Analysis suggests that the percentage of degraded carrageenan that may be expected to be derived either by gastric acid digestion or by consumption of a carrageenan-containing food product that is contaminated by degraded carrageenan is of the order of 10%. If about 9 mg of carrageenan with MW < 50 000 is likely to contaminate 100 mg of food-grade carrageenan and at least 8 mg with MW < 20 000 is likely to arise in the process of normal digestion of 100 mg food-grade carrageenan (simulated by exposure to pH 1.9 with pepsin for 1 h at 37°C), it is likely that at least 10 mg of degraded carrageenan will be derived from every 100 mg consumed. This suggests an average intake of degraded carrageenan of 380 mg/day for eaters in the United States, based on the FDA estimate of 3.8 g consumed/day. The reported TD_{50} (tumorigenic dose 50% = the dose-rate, in mg/kg body weight per day, which will halve the probability of remaining tumorless over the lifespan of the exposed animal) by the Carcinogenic Potency Database for degraded carrageenan is 2310, based on rodent experiments (*Handbook of Carcinogenic Potency*, 1997). This extrapolates to 138.6 g for a 60 kg individual. An important issue is whether 380 mg/day (or even 10 mg/day) of degraded carrageenan is safe to ingest. By the Delaney clause, no carcinogen should be permitted in food. The Food Quality Protection Act (FQPA) established a usage level for "negligible risk" associated with pesticide residue in food at one part per million (Food Quality Protection Act, 1996; Food Additives Amendment, 1958). Applying this standard to carrageenan, an anticipated average intake of 10 mg/day of degraded carrageenan (using the consumption data compiled by the Food and Nutrition Board of the Committee on GRAS for the NAS in the 1970s) is 70-fold greater than this standard (138.6 g/10^6 per day = 0.14 mg), 35 mg/day (using the data compiled by Informatics in the 1970s) is 245-fold greater, and an intake of 380 mg/day as indicated by the FDA data is nearly 2700-fold greater. These calculations do not take into consideration possible exposure to furcellaran (MW 20 000–80 000), or the wide range of possible intakes of carrageenan among consumers, up to almost 7.5 g/day by the FDA data.

When compared to saccharin, for example, it is noteworthy that the TD_{50} for saccharin is comparable at 2140 mg/kg per day (*Handbook of Carcinogenic Potency*, 1997); however, the expected daily intake of saccharin in the adult US population was estimated to be 120 µg/kg per day in average users (7.2 mg for a 60 kg person) (National Research Council, 1996). Inadvertent exposure to saccharin is much less likely to occur than for degraded carrageenan, since the use of artificial sweeteners is clearly marked and is by choice, whereas the carrageenan content may not be clearly distinguished if it is a component of another ingredient, such as condensed milk.

With these findings in mind, it is not expected that human exposure to low molecular weight carrageenans could be eliminated by introduction of a minimum molecular weight requirement.

Commercial food products differ in the extent of their incorporation of carrageenan. Exact descriptions of carrageenan content are difficult to obtain,

Table 10.3 Estimates of carrageenan content of some common food products*

Food	Percentage carrageenan (g/100g food)
Bakery products	0.01–0.1
Beer	0.03–0.05
Chocolate milk	0.01–0.2
Cottage cheese	0.02–0.50
Fish gels	0.5–1.0
Frosting base mix	3–4
Ice cream, frozen custard, sherbets, etc.	0.01–0.05
Infant formula	0.02–0.3
Jams and jellies	0.5–1.5
Liquid coffee whitener	0.1–0.3
Pie filling	0.1–1.0
Processed cheese (includes cream cheese)	0.011–1.00
Processed meat or fish	0.2–1.0
Pudding (non-dairy)	0.1–0.5
Ready-to-eat canned pudding	0.10–0.20
Relishes, pizza, barbecue sauces	0.2–0.5
Salad dressing	0.2–0.6
Sour cream	0.50
Syrups	0.1–0.3
Whipped cream	0.05–0.20
Yogurt	0.20–0.50

*Since manufacturing processes vary and there can be substitutions of one hydrocolloid for another, the content of carrageenan for any individual product may differ from these estimates.

due to variation in formulations, use of combinations of gums, and proprietary considerations. In general, carrageenan content of various food products has been established to vary between 0.05% and 0.2% by weight. Some of these estimates are presented in Table 10.3. Over time, specific brands may vary the carrageenan content, and variation among different brands is likely. Hence, accurate calculation of individual or population-based intake values is not possible at this time.

Issues for further investigation

Several areas remain for further investigation and further substantiation of already acquired evidence. These include:

1   identification of a biochemical marker associated with exposure to carrageenan
2   identification and characterization of carrageenan in blood and in cells
3   determination of the unique components of carrageenan that determine the extent of metabolism or lack of metabolism of carrageenan
4   analysis of the impact *in vivo* of accumulation of carrageenan or its byproducts in lysosomes of mammary myoepithelial cells, prostate basal cells, and other cells, especially those absent in invasive malignancies, and the relationship

between accumulation in these cells, their destruction, and human pathology, including invasive malignancies

5 specification of the intracellular and extracellular biochemical reactions affected by carrageenan exposure, with particular attention to sulfatases, sulfotransferases and galactosidases

6 specific consideration of the effects of carrageenan on steroid sulfatase expression and activity and the impact on the hormonal milieu of mammary tissue

7 determination of the genetic effects, either related to activation of protooncogenes or reduction of normal tumor suppressor gene activity, associated with carrageenan exposure

8 possible formulation of a designer carrageenan that would retain the useful properties of carrageenan, but not the harmful ones.

References

Abraham, R., Fabian, R.J., Golberg, M.B., and Coulston, F. (1974) Role of lysosomes in carrageenan-induced cecal ulceration, *Gastroenterology*, **67**: 1169–1181.

Abraham, R., Golberg, L., and Coulston, F. (1972) Uptake and storage of degraded carrageenan in lysosomes of reticuloendothelial cells of the rhesus monkey, *Experimental Molecular Pathology*, **17**: 77–93.

Anderson, W. and Duncan, J.G.C. (1965) The anticoagulant activity of carrageenan, *Journal of Pharmacy and Pharmacology*, **17**: 647–654.

Arakawa, S., Okumua, M., Yamada, S., Ito, M., and Tejima, S. (1986) Enhancing effect of carrageenan on the induction of rat colonic tumors by 1,2-dimethylhydrazine and its relation to β-glucuronidase activities in feces and other tissues, *Journal of Nutrition Science and Vitaminology*, **32**: 481–485.

Benitz, K.-F., Golberg, L., and Coulston, F. (1973) Intestinal effects of carrageenans in the rhesus monkey, *Food and Cosmetic Toxicology*, **11**: 565–575.

Calvert, R.J. and Reicks, M. (1988) Alterations in colonic thymidine kinase enzyme activity induced by consumption of various dietary fibers, *Proceedings of the Society for Experimental Biology and Medicine*, **189**: 45–51.

Carlucci, M.J., Pujol, C.A., Ciancia, M., Noseda, M.D., Matulewicz, M.C., Damonte, E.B., and Cerezo, A.S. (1997) Antiherpetic and anticoagulant properties of carrageenans from the red seaweed *Gigartina skottsbergii* and their cyclized derivatives: correlation between structure and biological activity, *International Journal of Biological Macromolecules*, **20**: 97–105.

Carlucci, M.J., Ciancia, M., Matulewicz, M.C., Cerezo, A.S., and Damonte, E.B. (1999) Antiherpetic activity and mode of action of natural carrageenans of diverse structural types, *Antiviral Research*, **43**: 93–102.

Cater, D.B. (1961) The carcinogenic action of carrageenin in rats, *British Journal of Cancer*, **15**: 607–614.

Collins, T.F.X., Black, T.N., and Prew, J.H. (1977a) Long-term effects of calcium carrageenan in rats – I. Effects on reproduction, *Food and Cosmetic Toxicology*, **15**: 533–538.

Collins, T.F.S., Black, T.N., and Prew, J.H. (1977b) Long-term effects of calcium carrageenan in rats – II. Effects on foetal development, *Food and Cosmetic Toxicology*, **15**: 539–545.

Collins, T.F.X., Black, T.N., and Prew, J.H. (1979) Effects of calcium and sodium carrageenan and iota-carrageenan on hamster foetal development, *Food and Cosmetic Toxicology*, **17**: 443–449.

Coombe, D.R., Parish, C.R., Ramshaw, I.A., and Snowden, J.M. (1987) Analysis of the inhibition of tumour metastasis by sulphated polysaccharides, *International Journal of Cancer*, **39**: 82–88.

Corpet, D.E., Taché, S., and Préclaire, M. (1997) Carrageenan given as a jelly, does not initiate, but promotes the growth of aberrant crypt foci in the rat colon, *Cancer Letters*, **114**: 53–55.

Cuzzocrea, S., Costantino, G., Zingarelli, B., Mazzon, E., Micali, A., and Caputi, A.P. (1999a) The protective role of endogenous glutathione in carrageenan-induced pleurisy in the rat, *European Journal of Pharmacology*, **372**: 187–197.

Cuzzocrea, S., Mazzon, E., Calabro, G., Dugo, L., De Sarro, A., van De Loo, F.A., and Caputi, A.P. (2000) Inducible nitric oxide synthase-knockout mice exhibit resistance to pleurisy and lung injury caused by carrageenan, *American Journal of Respiratory and Critical Care Medicine*, **162**: 1859–1866.

Cuzzocrea, S., Mazzon, E., Dugo, L., Serraino, I., Ciccolo, A., Centorrino, T., De Sarra, A., Caputi, A.P. (2001a) Protective effects of n-acetylcysteine on lung injury and red blood cell modification induced by carrageenan in the rat, *FASEB Journal*, **15**: 1187–1200.

Cuzzocrea, S., Mazzon, E., Sautebin, L., Dugo, L., Serraino, I., De Sarro, A., and Caputi, A.P. (2002) Protective effects of Celecoxib on lung injury and red blood cells modification induced by carrageenan in the rat, *Biochemical Pharmacology*, **63**: 785–795.

Cuzzocrea, S., Mazzon, E., Sautebin, L., Serraino, I., Dugo, L., Calabro, G., Caputi, A.P., and Maggi, A. (2001b) The protective role of endogenous estrogens in carrageenan-induced lung injury in the rat, *Molecular Medicine*, **7**: 478–487.

Cuzzocrea, S., Sautebin, L., De Sarro, G., Costantino, G., Rombola, L., Mazzon, E., Ialenti, A., De Sarro, A., Ciliberto, G., Di Rosa, M., Caputi, A.P., and Thiemermann, C. (1999b) Role of IL-6 in the pleurisy and lung injury caused by carrageenan, *Journal of Immunology*, **163**: 5094–5104.

Dace, R., McBride, E., Brooks, K., Gander, J., Buszko, M., and Doctor, V.M. (1997) Comparison of the anticoagulant action of sulfated and phosphorylated polysaccharides, *Thrombosis Research*, **87**: 113–121.

Daniel, J.R., Voragen, A.C.J., and Pilnik, W. (1994) Starch and other polysaccharides. In *Ullmann's Encyclopedia of Industrial Chemistry* (eds Elvers, B., Hawkins, S., and Russey, W.). New York: VCH Verlagsgesellschaft, Vol. A25, pp. 21–62.

Delahunty, T., Recher, L., and Hollander, D. (1987) Intestinal permeability changes in rodents: a possible mechanism for degraded carrageenan-induced colitis, *Food Chemistry and Toxicology*, **25**: 113–118.

Di Rosa, M. (1972) Review: biological properties of carrageenan, *Journal of Pharmacy and Pharmacology*, **24**: 89–102.

Egan, C.G., Lockhart, J.C., Ferrell, W.R., Day, S.M., and McLean, J.S. (2002) Pathophysiological basis of acute inflammatory hyperaemia in the rat knee: roles of cyclo-oxygenase-1 and -2. *Journal of Physiology*, **539** (Pt 2): 579–587.

Ekstrom, L.-G. (1985) Molecular weight distribution and the behavior of kappa-carrageenan on hydrolysis, *Carbohydrate Research*, **135**: 283–289.

Ekstrom, L.-G., Kuivinen, J., and Johansson, G. (1983) Molecular weight distribution and hydrolysis behavior of carrageenans, *Carbohydrate Research*, **116**: 89–94.

Engster, M. and Abraham, R. (1976) Cecal response to different molecular weights and types of carrageenin in the guinea pig, *Toxicology and Applied Pharmacology*, **38**: 265–212.

Fabian, R.J., Abraham, R., Coulston, F., and Golberg, L. (1973) Carrageenan-induced squamous metaplasia of the rectal mucosa in the rat, *Gastroenterology*, **65**: 265–276.

Fath, R.B., Deschner, E.E., Winawer, S.J., and Dworkin, B.M. (1984) Degraded carrageenan-induced colitis in CF_1 mice, *Digestion*, **29**: 197–203.

Federal Register (1979) 44 Fed. Reg. 40343–40345 (10 July 1979).

Food Additives Amendment of 1958. Pub. L. 85-929, 72 Stat. 1784.

Food and Nutrition Board, National Research Council (1976) Committee on GRAS List Survey – Phase III. Estimating Distribution of daily intakes of *Chondrus* extract (carrageenan). Appendix C, pp. 1–7. Washington, DC: National Academy of Sciences.

Food Quality Protection Act of 1996 (FQPA) Pub. L. 104-170, 110 Stat. 1489.

Frode, T.S., Souza, G.E., and Calixto, J.B. (2001) The modulatory role played by TNF-alpha and IL-1 beta in the inflammatory responses induced by carrageenan in the mouse model of pleurisy, *Cytokine*, **13**: 162–168.

Gibson, G.R., Macfarlane, S., and Cummings, J.H. (1990) The fermentability of polysaccharides by mixed human faecal bacteria in relation to their suitability as bulk-forming laxatives, *Letters in Applied Microbiology*, **11**: 251–254.

Goto, M., Okamoto, Y., Yamamoto, M., and Aki, H. (2001) Anti-inflammatory effects of 5-aminosalicylic acid conjugates with chenodeoxycholic acid and ursodeoxycholic acid on carrageenan-induced colitis in guinea-pigs, *Journal of Pharmacy and Pharmacology*, **53**: 1711–1720.

Grasso, P., Gangolli, S.D., Butterworth, K.R., and Wright, M.G. (1975) Studies on degraded carrageenan in rats and guinea-pigs, *Food and Cosmetic Toxicology*, **13**: 195–201.

Handbook of Carcinogenic Potency and Genotoxicity Databases (1997) (eds Gold, L.S. and Zeiger, E.), pp. 116–117, 629. New York: CRC Press.

Hoffman, R. (1993) Carrageenans inhibit growth-factor binding, *Biochemical Journal*, **289**: 331–334.

Hoffman, R., Burns, W.W., and Paper, D.H. (1995) Selective inhibition of cell proliferation and DNA synthesis by the polysulphated carbohydrate ι-carrageenan, *Cancer Chemotherapy and Pharmacology*, **36**: 325–334.

Hopkins, J. (1981) Carcinogenicity of carrageenan, *Food and Cosmetic Toxicology*, **19**: 779–788.

Houck, J.C., Morris, R.K., and Lazaro, E.J. (1957) Anticoagulant, lipemia clearing and other effects of anionic polysaccharides extracted from seaweed, *Proceedings of the Society for Experimental Biology and Medicine*, **96**: 528–530.

IARC Working Group on the Evaluation of the Carcinogenic Risk of Chemicals to Humans (1983) Carrageenan. In *IARC Monographs on the Evaluation of the Carcinogenic Risk of Chemicals to Humans*, Vol. 31, pp. 79–94. Lyon: IARC.

Iatropoulos, M.J., Golberg, L., and Coulston, L. (1975) Intestinal carcinogenesis in rats using 1,2-dimethylhydrazine with or without degraded carrageenan, *Experimental Molecular Pathology*, **23**: 386–401.

Informatics, Inc. (1972) *Carrageenan*, pp. 1–68. Arlington, VA: National Technical and Information Service.

Ishioka, T., Kuwabara, N., Oohashi, Y., and Wakabayashi, K. (1987) Induction of colorectal tumors in rats by sulfated polysaccharides, *CRC Critical Reviews in Toxicology*, **17**: 215–244.

Jensen, B.H., Andersen, J.O., Poulsen, S.S., Olsen, P.S., Rasmussen, S.N., Hansen, S.H., and Hvidberg, D.F. (1984) The prophylactic effect of 5-aminosalicylic acid and salazosulphapyridine on degraded-carrageenan-induced colitis in guinea pigs, *Scandinavian Journal of Gastroenterology*, **19**: 299–303.

Johnston, K.H. and McCandless, E.L. (1973) Enzymic hydrolysis of the potassium chloride soluble fraction of carrageenan: properties of "lambda carrageenases" from *Pseudomonas carrageenovora*, *Canadian Journal of Microbiology*, **19**: 779–788.

Kawaura, A., Shibata, M., Togei, K., and Otsuka, H. (1982) Effect of dietary degraded carrageenan on intestinal carcinogenesis in rats treated with 1,2-dimethylhydrazine dihydrochloride, *Tokushima Journal of Experimental Medicine*, **29**: 125–129.

Kim, H.-S. and Berstad, A. (1992) Experimental colitis in animal models, *Scandinavian Journal of Gastroenterology*, **27**: 529–537.

Kitano, A., Matsumoto, T., Hiki, M., Hashimura, H., Yoshiyasu, K., Okawa, K., Kuwajima, S., and Kobayashi, K. (1986) Epithelial dysplasia of the rabbit colon induced by degraded carrageenan, *Cancer Research*, **46**: 1374–1376.

Kitano, A., Matsumoto, T., Oshitani, N., Nakagawa, M., Yasuda, K., Wanatabe, Y., Tomobuchi, M., Obayashi, M., Tabata, A., Fukushima, R., Okabe, H., Nakamura, S., Obata, A., Okawa, K., and Kobayashi, K. (1996) Distribution and anti-inflammatory effect of mesalazine on carrageenan-induced colitis in the rabbit, *Clinical and Experimental Pharmacology and Physiology*, **23**: 305–309.

Kitsukawa, Y., Saito, H., Suzuki, Y., Kasanuki, J., Tamura, Y., and Yoshida, S. (1992) Effect of ingestion of eicosapentaenoic acid ethyl ester on carrageenan-induced colitis in guinea pigs, *Gastroenterology*, **102**: 1859–1866.

Lambrecht, V., Boilly, B., and Le Bourhis, X. (1998) Regulation of cell proliferation and urokinase plasminogen activation of human breast epithelial cells by carrageenans, *International Journal of Oncology*, **12**: 1397–1401.

Ling, K.-Y., Bhalla, D., and Hollander, D. (1988) Mechanisms of carrageenan injury of IEC18 small intestinal epithelial cell monolayers, *Gastroenterology*, **95**: 1487–1495.

Liu, J.M., Haroun-Bouhedja, F., and Boisson-Vidal, C. (2000) Analysis of the *in vitro* inhibition of mammary adenocarcinoma cell adhesion by sulphated polysaccharides, *Anticancer Research*, **20**: 3265–3271.

McLean, M.W. and Williamson, F.B. (1979) κ-Carrageenase from *Pseudomonas carrageenovora*, *European Journal of Biochemistry*, **93**: 553–558.

Maiti, A., Maki, G., and Johnson, P. (1998) TNF-alpha induction of CD44-mediated leukocyte adhesion by sulfation, *Science*, **282**: 941–943.

Mankes, R. and Abraham, R. (1975) Lysosomal dysfunction in colonic submucosal macrophages of rhesus monkeys caused by degraded iota carrageenan, *Proceedings of the Society for Experimental Biology and Medicine*, **150**: 166–170.

Marcus, R. (1981) Harmful effects of carrageenan fed to animals, *Cancer Detection and Prevention*, **4**: 129–134.

Marcus, S.N., Marcus, A.J., Marcus, R., Ewen, S.W.B., and Watt, J. (1992) The pre-ulcerative phase of carrageenan-induced colonic ulceration in the guinea pig, *International Journal of Experimental Pathology*, **73**: 515–526.

Marcus, R. and Watt, J. (1969) Seaweeds and ulcerative colitis in laboratory animals, *Lancet*, **2**: 489–490.

Marcus, R. and Watt, J. (1980) Potential hazards of carrageenan, *Lancet*, **1**: 602–603.

Marrs, W.M. (1998) The stability of carrageenan to processing. In *Gums and Stabilisers for the Food Industry* (eds Williams, P.A. and Phillips, G.O.), pp. 345–357. Cambridge: The Royal Society of Chemistry.

Moirano, A.L. (1977) Sulfated seaweed polysaccharides. In *Food Colloids* (ed. Graham, H.D.), pp. 347–381. Westport, CT: Avi Publishing Co.

Mori, H., Ohbayashi, F., Hirono, I., Shimada, T., and Williams, G.M. (1984) Absence of genotoxicity of the carcinogenic sulfated polysaccharide carrageenan and dextran sulfate in mammalian DNA repair and bacterial mutagenicity assays, *Nutrition and Cancer*, **6**: 92–97.

Mottet, N.K. (1971) On animal models for inflammatory bowel disease, *Gastroenterology*, **62**: 1269–1271.

National Research Council (1996) *Carcinogens and Anti-carcinogens in the Human Diet*, p. 398. Washington, DC: National Academy Press.

Nicklin, S. and Miller, K. (1989) Intestinal uptake and immunological effects of carrageenan – current concepts, *Food Additives and Contaminants*, **6**: 425–436.

Olsen, P.S., Kirkegaard, P., and Poulsen, S.S. (1983) The effect of ileotransversostomy on carrageenan-induced colitis in guinea pig, *Scandinavian Journal of Gastroenterology*, **18**: 407–410.

Olsen, P.S. and Poulsen, S.S. (1980) Stereomicroscopic and histologic changes in the colon of guinea pigs fed degraded carrageenan, *Acta Path Microbiol Scand Sect*, **88**: 135–141.

Omote, K., Hazama, K., Kawamata, T., Kawamata, M., Nakayaka, Y., Toriyabe, M., and Namiki, A. (2001) Peripheral nitric oxide in carrageenan-induced inflammation, *Brain Research*, **912**: 171–175.

Onderdonk, A.B. (1985) The carrageenan model for experimental ulcerative colitis, *Progress in Clinical and Biological Research*, **186**: 237–245.

Oohashi, Y., Ishioka, T.T., Wakabayashi, K., and Kuwabara, N. (1981) A study of carcinogenesis induced by degraded carrageenan arising from squamous metaplasia of the rat colorectum, *Cancer Letters*, **14**: 267–272.

Oohashi, Y., Kitamura, S., Wakabayashi, K., Kuwabara, N., and Fukuda, Y. (1979) Irreversibility of degraded carrageenan-induced colorectal squamous metaplasia in rats, *Gann*, **70**: 391–392.

Ottet, N.K. (1972) On animal models for inflammatory bowel disease, *Gastroenterology*, **62**: 1269–1272.

Pearce-Pratt, R. and Phillips, D.M. (1996) Sulfated polysaccharides inhibit lymphocyte-to-epithelial transmission of human immunodeficiency virus-1, *Biology of Reproduction*, **54**: 173–182.

Pittman, K.A., Golberg, L., and Coulston, F. (1976) Carrageenan: the effect of molecular weight and polymer type on its uptake, excretion and degradation in animals, *Food and Cosmetic Toxicology*, **14**: 85–93.

Potin, P., Sanseau, A., LeGall, Y., Rochas, C., and Bloareg, B. (1991) Purification and characterization of a new κ-carrageenase from a marine *cytophaga*-like bacterium, *European Journal of Biochemistry*, **201**: 241–247.

Raz, A., Levine, G., and Khomiak, Y. (2000) Acute local inflammation potentiates tumor growth in mice, *Cancer Letters*, **148**: 115–120.

Richardson, C.J., Magee, E.A.M., and Cummings, J.H. (2000) A new method for the determination of sulphide in gastrointestinal contents and whole blood by microdistillation and ion chromatography, *Clinica Chimica Acta*, **293**: 115–125.

Roediger, W.E.W., Duncan, A., Kapaniris, O., and Millard, S. (1993) Reducing sulfur compounds of the colon impair colonocytes nutrition: implications for ulcerative colitis, *Gastroenterology*, **104**: 802–809.

Rustia, M., Shubik, P., and Patil, K. (1980) Lifespan carcinogenicity tests with native carrageenan in rats and hamsters, *Cancer Letters*, **11**: 1–10.

Salvemini, D., Wang, Z.Q., Wyatt, P.S., Bourdon, D.M., Marino, M.H., Manning, P.T., and Currie, M.G. (1996) Nitric oxide: a key mediator in the early and late phase of carrageenan-induced rat paw inflammation, *British Journal of Pharmacology*, **118**: 829–838.

Sarwar, G., Matoyoshi, S., and Oda, H. (1987) Purification of a κ-carrageenase from marine *Cytophaga* species, *Microbiology and Immunology*, **31**: 869–877.

Sautebin, L., Ialenti, A., Ianara, A., and Di Rosa, M. (1998) Relationship between nitric oxide and prostaglandins in carrageenin pleurisy, *Biochemical Pharmacology*, **55**: 1113–1117.

Sharratt, M., Grasso, P., Carpanini, F., and Gangolli, S.D. (1971) Carrageenan ulceration as a model for human ulcerative colitis, *Lancet*, **1**: 192–193.

Suarez, F., Furne, J., Springfield, J., and Levitt, M. (1998) Production and elimination of sulfur-containing gases in the rat colon, *American Journal of Physiology*, **274**(4, Pt 1): G727–G733.

Suzuki, J., Na, H.K., Upham, B.L., Chang, C.C., and Trosko, J.E. (2000) Lambda-carrageenan-induced inhibition of gap-junctional intercellular communication in rat liver epithelial cells, *Nutrition and Cancer*, **36**: 122–128.

Taché, S., Peiffer, G., Millet, A.-S., and Corpet, D.E. (2000) Carrageenan gel and aberrant crypt foci in the colon of conventional and human flora-associated rats, *Nutrition and Cancer*, **37**: 193–198.

Tarlo, S.M., Dolovich, J., and Lostgarten, C. (1995) Anaphylaxis to carrageenan: a pseudo-latex allergy, *Journal of Allergy and Clinical Immunology*, **95**: 933–936.

Thomson, A.W. and Fowler, E.F. (1981) Carrageenan: a review of its effect on the immune system, *Agents and Actions*, **1**: 265–273.

Thomson, A.W. and Whiting, P.H. (1981) A comparative study of renal and hepatic function in Sprague-Dawley rats following systemic injection of purified carrageenans (kappa, lambda, and iota), *British Journal of Experimental Pathology*, **62**: 207–213.

Tobacman, J.K. (1997) Filament disassembly and loss of mammary myoepithelial cells after exposure to lambda-carrageenan, *Cancer Research*, **57**: 2823–2826.

Tobacman, J.K. (2001) Review of harmful gastrointestinal effects of carrageenan in animal experiments, *Environmental Health Perspectives*, **109**: 983–994.

Tobacman, J.K., Hinkhouse, M., and Khalkhali-Ellis, Z. (2002a) Steroid sulfatase activity and expression in mammary myoepithelial cells, *Journal of Steroid Biochemistry and Molecular Biology*, **81**: 65–68.

Tobacman, J.K., Khalkhali-Ellis, Z., and Walters, K. (2002b) Reduced expression of steroid sulfatase in mammary myoepithelial cells following exposure to λ-carrageenan, *Proceedings of the American Association for Cancer Research*, **43**: 1079.

Tobacman, J.K., Wallace, R.B., and Zimmerman, B. (2001) Consumption of carrageenan and other water-soluble polymers used as food additives and incidence of mammary carcinoma, *Medical Hypotheses*, **56**: 589–598.

Tobacman, J.K. and Walters, K. (2001) Carrageenan-induced inclusions in mammary myoepithelial cells, *Cancer Detection and Prevention*, **25**: 520–526.

Towle, G.A. (1973) Carrageenan. In *Industrial Gums: Polysaccharides and their Derivatives* (ed. Whistler, R.L.), pp. 84–109. New York: Academic Press.

Trius, A. and Sebranek, J.G. (1996) Carrageenans and their use in meat products, *Critical Reviews in Food Science and Nutrition*, **35**: 69–85.

Wakabayashi, K., Inagaki, T., Fujimoto, Y., and Fukuda, Y. (1978) Induction by degraded carrageenan of colorectal tumors in rats, *Cancer Letters*, **4**: 171–176.

Watanabe, K., Reddy, B.S., Wong, C.Q., and Weisburger, J.H. (1978) Effect of dietary undegraded carrageenan on colon carcinogenesis in F344 rats treated with azoxymethane or methylnitrosourea, *Cancer Research*, **38**: 4427–4430.

Watt, J. and Marcus, R. (1969) Ulcerative colitis in the guinea-pig caused by seaweed extract, *Journal of Pharmacy and Pharmacology*, **21**: 187S–188S.

Watt, J. and Marcus, R. (1970a) Ulcerative colitis in rabbits fed degraded carrageenan, *Journal of Pharmacy and Pharmacology*, **22**: 130–131.

Watt, J. and Marcus, R. (1970b) Hyperplastic mucosal changes in the rabbit colon produced by degraded carrageenin, *Gastroenterology*, **59**: 760–768.

Watt, J. and Marcus, R. (1973) Progress report: experimental ulcerative disease of the colon in animals, *Gut*, **14**: 506–510.

Wei, Xq, Orchardson, M., Gracie, J.A., Lelung, B.O., Gao, B.M., Guan, H., Niedbala, W., Paterson, G.K., McInnes, I.B., and Liew, F.Y. (2001) The Sushi domain of soluble IL-15 receptor alpha is essential for binding IL-15 and inhibiting inflammatory and allogenic responses *in vitro* and *in vivo*, *Journal of Immunology*, **167**: 277–282.

Weigl, J. and Yaphe, W. (1986) The enzymic hydrolysis of carrageenan by *Pseudomonas carrageenovora*: purification of a κ-carrageenase, *Canadian Journal of Microbiology*, **12**: 939–947.

Whelan, G. (1990) Epidemiology of inflammatory bowel disease, *Medical Clinics of North America*, **74**: 1–12.

Wilcox, D.K., Higgins, J., and Bertram, T.A. (1992) Colonic epithelial cell proliferation in a rat model of nongenotoxin-induced colonic neoplasia, *Laboratory Investigations*, **67**: 405–411.

Will, R., Zuanich, J., De Boo, A., and Ishikawa, Y. (1999) Water-soluble polymers (582.0). In *Chemical Economics Handbook*. Menlo Park, CA: SRI International.

Yamada, T., Ogano, A., Saito, T., Watanabe, J., Uchiyama, H., and Nakagawa, Y. (1997) Preparation and anti-HIV activity of low-molecular-weight carrageenans and their sulfated derivatives, *Carbohydrate Polymers*, **32**: 51–55.

Yu, G., Guan, H., Ioanoviciu, A.S., Sikkander, S.A., Thanawiroon, C., Tobacman, J.K., Toida, T., and Linhardt, R.J. (2002) Structural studies on kappa carrageenan derived oligosaccharides, *Carbohydrate Research*, **337**: 433–440.

11 Interpreting and communicating health and risk information on chemicals in breast milk

DDT as a case study

Judy S. LaKind

Introduction

Humans carry body burdens of a wide array of environmental chemicals, including persistent organic chemicals. These chemicals may be found in different compartments of the body, including blood, adipose tissue, organs such as the liver, and for women, in breast milk. Despite the fact that the presence of these chemicals in breast milk was first reported about 50 years ago, and hundreds of papers on this issue have appeared in the scientific literature, with a few exceptions it is only relatively recently that the popular press and others have focused on this issue. Past qualms about discussing the issue of environmental chemicals in breast milk were due, in part, to a reluctance to contribute unnecessarily to a decline in breastfeeding rates. With the increased visibility of this issue, some have raised new questions regarding the safety of breast milk as a nutrition source for infants. While the American Academy of Pediatrics (AAP) and others strongly support breast milk as the preferred nutrition for infants, their statements on breastfeeding only indirectly address questions regarding safety/ risk for specific chemical contaminants (AAP, 1997, 2001). The AAP statements address the issue indirectly because its conclusions are based on examinations of infants breastfed milk that likely contained a mixture of environmental chemicals. Despite this, benefits to the breastfed infant were numerous.

Other organizations, such as the World Health Organization, have addressed the issue more directly by using a risk assessment approach (i.e. comparing the infant's exposure to an acceptable dose) (WHO, 1998). Their conclusions on breastfeeding safety and risk were based on analyses using "safe" levels that may not be entirely appropriate for the nursing infant; this shortcoming is partly due to the lack of toxicological information developed specifically for the neonate. Examinations of breastfeeding risks and benefits due to chemical contaminants have been undertaken for specific endpoints such as cancer (Hoover, 1999; Rogan et al., 1991) and noncancer endpoints (Hoover, 1999). The risk assessments for cancer are especially useful, since the relative rarity and long latency make cancer epidemiology studies infeasible (Rogan *et al.*, 1991). To evaluate cancer risk to breastfed infants from exposure to contaminants in breast milk, standard risk assessment methodologies were utilized, which include inherent uncertainties associated with cancer risk assessments (e.g. use of lifetime studies with laboratory animals to estimate risks from short-term human exposures). Cancer risk was compared to excess risk of postneonatal mortality associated with not breastfeeding. Rogan *et al.* (1991, p. 235) concluded that "on the basis of lifetime cancer risk alone, there is not sufficient evidence to advise against breast feeding on the basis of the commonly observed range of contaminant concentrations". A similar conclusion was reached by Hoover (1999) in a cancer risk assessment for Canadian breast milk. The methods included state-of-the-science approaches to understanding health risks as compared to benefits of breastfeeding. Hoover (1999, p. 541) also assessed noncancer health risks to infants, using a quantitative risk assessment approach as well as a qualitative approach, and concluded that "most chemicals in Canadian breast milk are not present at high enough levels to cause concern".

Fundamental questions remain. How can a pediatrician or other healthcare provider interpret the information in the scientific literature on the meaning of current levels of environmental chemicals in human milk? How can they respond to questions that arise from information gleaned from the media and advocacy organizations? How should healthcare providers respond when asked by new mothers whether they should test their breast milk for the presence of environmental contaminants?

In this chapter, an interpretation and pictorial presentation of risks from environmental chemicals in breast milk is provided by synopsizing the scientific literature in a manner that is accessible to the medical and lay audience. It is emphasized that any assessment of risks and benefits of breastfeeding must consider that infants must be fed, and that the alternative to breastfeeding (use of infant formulas) is not without its own risks (LaKind *et al.*, 2002).

This chapter will not describe in detail the world of environmental chemicals found in human milk, or the literature on the health benefits of breastfeeding. Excellent reviews may be found in Jensen and Slorach (1991), Lawrence and Lawrence (1999), Schanler (2001), and Sonawane (1995). In addition, for health-care providers concerned about specific occupational or residential exposures to the mother, Schreiber (2001) provides example questions which can be asked of the mother in order to better ascertain the potential for risks from breastfeeding.

The methodology used here is to compare current concentrations of a specific group of chemicals in breast milk with health outcomes from studies of mother/infant pairs. The focus of this chapter is dichlorodiphenyltrichloroethane (DDT) and related compounds. The information on concentrations of DDT compounds and health outcomes is synthesized into a visual presentation. It can be argued that by presenting the information on a chemical-by-chemical basis, the concept of mixtures is ignored; that is, breast milk contains more than one environmental chemical, along with a diverse group of proteins, fats and other substances, which may exert an effect on the nursing infant. However, studies which explore associations between one chemical (or a small group of chemicals) and a health outcome inadvertently consider mixtures, simply by the fact that other chemicals, not specifically analyzed for, are in any event likely present in the milk of the mother at the time of the study.

Most of the research on environmental chemicals in human milk and potential adverse health effects to the nursing infant has focused on a relatively small number of environmental chemicals. The chemicals for which the preponderance of data exist are DDT and related chemicals and polychlorinated biphenyls (PCBs). This chapter focuses on DDT and related chemicals; a similar assessment and pictorial presentation for PCBs in breast milk is in preparation and will appear elsewhere. A large mother/infant cohort, followed for several years, forms the basis for this review. Reported clinical or subclinical effects that may be associated with prenatal exposures are not included in this assessment, because the focus here is on the safety of human milk. Potential effects on the mother's ability to lactate are also discussed.

What are DDT compounds?

DDT was one of the most heavily utilized pesticides in the US before its ban in 1972. Its use continues in several countries for control of malaria, principally by application to the inside of homes (WHO, 1998). While an effective pesticide, certain other characteristics of DDT resulted in public concern, including its toxicity, its persistence in the environment, and its lipophilicity, that is, its ability to accumulate in the fatty tissues of animals. Because of the persistence and extensive use of DDT (1.35 billion pounds used in the US before its uses were cancelled) (USEPA, 1975), its presence (or the presence of its metabolites) in fatty tissues in humans is essentially ubiquitous.

DDT, its major metabolite DDE (dichlorodiphenyl dichloroethylene), and a further metabolite, DDD (dichlorodiphenyl dichloroethane) are referred to collectively as DDT compounds (see Figure 11.1). The presence of DDT in breast milk suggests recent exposures. DDE is more commonly detected in breast milk in countries which banned the use of DDT as early as the 1970s. For these

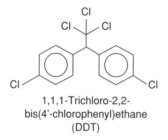

1,1,1-Trichloro-2,2-
bis(4'-chlorophenyl)ethane
(DDT)

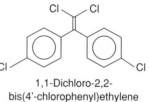

1,1-Dichloro-2,2-
bis(4'-chlorophenyl)ethylene
(DDE)

Figure 11.1 Structures of DDT and metabolite DDE. Reproduced by permission of The University of Minnesota Biocatalysis/Biodegradation Database. http://umbbd.ahc.umn.du/ddt/ddt_map.html.

countries (including the US and Canada), levels of DDT compounds in breast milk have declined considerably (Smith, 1999).

DDT compounds in human milk – studies with mothers and infants

The most comprehensive examination of potential adverse health effects from exposure to DDE in human milk began in 1978 with the recruitment of the first infant in the North Carolina Breast Milk and Formula Project (North Carolina Project), with recruitment ending in 1982 with the 856th infant (Rogan and Gladen, 1985). Maternal blood, cord blood, and placenta were collected from each mother, as was a sample of the infant's nutrition source (colostrum, early milk, or formula). Newborns were examined, and then re-examined at six weeks, three months, six months, one year, 18 months, and two years, and then yearly up to five years. Follow-up of children at puberty was also performed (Gladen *et al.*, 2000). Levels of DDT compounds in human milk and infant/lactation effects are summarized here.

Effects of DDT compounds in breast milk on infants

Medical histories for each child in the North Carolina Project were reviewed at every visit (Rogan *et al.*, 1987). Illnesses such as upper respiratory illness (e.g., cold, flu, sore throat), otitis media, gastroenteritis, eczema, asthma, allergies and lower respiratory infections were not related to levels of DDE in breast milk. Children were assessed at six and 12 months of age using Bayley Scales of Infant Development (Mental Development Index, or MDI, and Psychomotor Development Index, or PDI) (Gladen *et al.*, 1988); no adverse effects on scores for these tests were associated with breastfeeding. Children were further evaluated at 18 months and two years of age with Bayley Scales of Infant Development (MDI and PDI) (Rogan and Gladen, 1991). Again, no adverse effects on test scores from exposure to DDE in breast milk were reported. A follow-up examination of the children at the age of puberty (from 10 to 15 years of age) was also performed (Gladen *et al.*, 2000). DDE in breast milk did not affect height, weight, or stage of pubertal development. In this study, the median concentration (lipid basis) of DDE in milk at time of birth was 2.43 ppm, the maximum was 25.4 ppm, and the 95th percentile was 6.72 ppm (Rogan *et al.*, 1986).

Effects of DDT compounds on lactation

Rogan and Gladen (1985) have postulated that DDE exerts an estrogenic effect on the mother, resulting in reduced lactation duration or lactational failure. Healthcare providers should note that the operational definition of lactation failure was quite broad (Rogan *et al.*, 1987, p. 1296): "at most one month mostly breast-fed and two months until final weaning", where the causes included insufficient milk, poor weight gain, the baby was allergic to milk, the baby had

Table 11.1 Concentrations of DDT compounds in breast milk from women in the North Carolina Project (1978–1982) and percentage of women with lactational failure (as defined in the text) (Rogan *et al.*, 1987)

DDE concentration (parts per million)	Duration of lactation (median number of weeks)	% with lactation failure	Standard deviation for % lactation failure
0.31–0.99	26	5	3.0
1.0–1.99	26	6	1.6
2.0–2.99	23	6	1.6
3.0–3.99	24	8	2.3
4.0–4.99	18	15	5.2
5.0–5.99	9	24	8.2
6.00–23.80	10	10	4.3

difficulty breastfeeding, or the baby became ill. Percent lactational failure is shown in Table 11.1. It would not be possible to establish a control group for this type of study in order to determine "background" levels of lactational failure; however, there appears to be a natural cut-off below 4.0 ppm DDE in human milk. That is, at levels above 3.99 ppm, percent lactational failure almost doubles, while below that level, percent failures do not change substantially and are quite low. For example, in the 0.31 to 0.99 ppm group, of 54 women, approximately three fit the description of lactational failure. This number is fewer than the number of potential reasons given for lactational failure; with no additional information, it is difficult to know whether, for example, the infants of these women were unable to breastfeed due to illness. In addition, at levels below 4.0 ppm, the duration of lactation was fairly constant at 23–26 weeks. The relatively small numbers of women in each concentration range contribute to the considerable statistical uncertainty as to the magnitude of the difference in lactational failure rates among women with different DDE concentrations in their milk. This uncertainty can be shown with standard deviations (see Table 11.1, where standard deviations are based on the binomial distribution). In order to quantify the degree of statistical uncertainty associated with the observation differences in a simple way, concentration categories in Table 11.1 were combined; lactation failure rates were compared for women with low DDE exposure (below 4 ppm) and high exposure (at or above 4 ppm). While the lactation failure rate for women with DDE concentrations below 4 ppm is 6.4% with a standard deviation of 1.0%, the rate for women with concentration above 4 ppm is 14.8% with a standard deviation of 3.2%. Thus, for the purposes of this discussion, a guidance value of 4 ppm DDT compounds in breast milk is used. In other words, below this level, it is not anticipated that a healthcare provider would observe any influence of DDT compounds on lactation. Until studies can control for some of the many influences on breastfeeding duration, and until a generally agreed-upon definition for lactation failure is available, a connection between concentrations of environmental chemicals and weaning will be very difficult.[1]

Levels of DDT compounds in human milk

Breast milk from countries in which DDT has been banned for several years will exhibit a different profile for concentrations of DDT compounds than that from countries which either only recently prohibited its use or continue to permit its use. In order to compare any health effects discerned from the North Carolina Project (described above) with levels of DDT compounds in breast milk, two types of descriptors are necessary. First, since the North Carolina cohort was composed of women who were lactating approximately 20 years ago, it is important to describe current DDT compound levels as compared to those at the time of the study. This is because over 20 years have passed since the ban on DDT in the US, and current levels of DDT compounds in breast milk are likely to be substantially lower than those seen in the North Carolina Project. Second, since some countries still permit the limited use of DDT for malarial control, levels of DDT compounds in the milk of women from these countries must be described separately. An overall description of worldwide trends of DDT compounds in breast milk was provided by Smith (1999).

In Figure 11.2, levels of DDT compounds from studies of women in the US and Canada (spanning the time of the North Carolina cohort to 1991) and

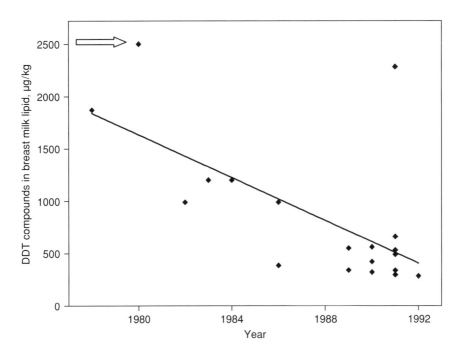

Figure 11.2 Declines in levels of DDT compounds in human milk in the US, Canada, and Western Europe. The North Carolina cohort breast milk level, from samples taken from 1978 to 1982, is indicated by the arrow. Data from summary table in Smith (1999).

Western Europe (from 1990 to 1992) are shown (data from summary table in Smith, 1999). Limitations inherent in interstudy comparison have been described previously (LaKind and Berlin, 2002; LaKind et al., 2001; Sim and McNeil, 1992; Smith, 1999), and include:

1   variations in protocols for collecting human milk samples (for example, collection of pooled versus individual samples)
2   incomplete reporting of information (such as methods used for collection of human milk samples or characteristics of the mother)
3   non-representative sampling when considering sample population size and geography
4   timing of sampling of the milk (breast milk concentrations of persistent chemicals decline over the course of lactation).

Despite these limitations, it is clear that mean levels of DDT compounds in human milk in the US, Canada and Western Europe have declined considerably since the time of the North Carolina cohort study.

Figure 11.3 shows recent data on levels of DDT compounds in breast milk from women residing in countries where DDT is still in use or was only recently phased out. It is clear that for these countries, DDT compounds in human milk may be found at comparatively high levels. The information in Figure 11.3 is not meant to be all-encompassing, but rather to alert healthcare providers in countries where DDT has only relatively recently been prohibited, or is currently used to control malaria, that mothers' levels of DDT compounds may be in the range where reports of adverse effects on lactation have been reported.

Comparison of current levels of DDT compounds in breast milk with effect levels

Potential adverse effects on infant health and mother's lactation were evaluated by the North Carolina Project. The results are compared to current levels of DDT compounds in breast milk.

Infant health

To date, no adverse effects on infant health associated with DDT compounds in breast milk have been reported. Figure 11.4 contains this straightforward message. This figure includes information for healthcare providers on (i) levels of DDT compounds in the milk of women from countries such as the US where DDT use has been prohibited for decades; and (ii) levels of DDT compounds in the milk of women from countries where DDT is still in use for malaria control or has been prohibited relatively recently.

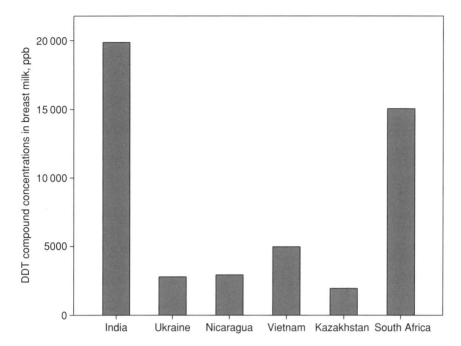

Figure 11.3 Levels of DDT compounds in human milk in countries with relatively recent DDT restrictions or current DDT use. Samples were collected in the 1990s. Values provided as DDT in whole milk were converted to lipid basis assuming 2.5% lipid. Data from the following: India, Siddiqui *et al.*, 2002; Ukraine, Gladen *et al.*, 1999; Nicaragua, Romero *et al.*, 2000; Vietnam, Nakamura *et al.*, 1994; Kazakhstan, Lutter *et al.*, 1998; South Africa, Bouwman *et al.*, 1992.

Lactation

Figure 11.5 compares current levels of DDT compounds in breast milk with levels at which decreases in duration of lactation have been reported. Current levels of DDT compounds in breast milk from the US and Canada appear to be well below levels that would result in observable effects on lactation.

Conclusions

Questions by expecting and new mothers regarding the potential health implications of environmental chemicals in human milk will continue to arise. Healthcare providers need a method for conveying information to those in their care regarding the preferred source of infant nutrition. In this chapter, the available information on DDT compounds as they relate to health outcomes to the infant and effects on lactation was summarized. Graphical presentation of

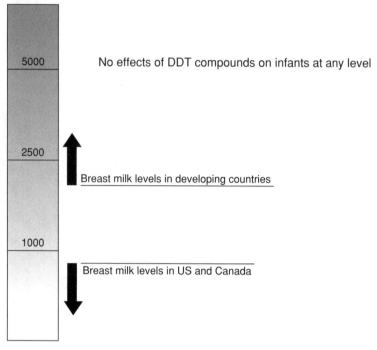

DDT compounds, ppb

Figure 11.4 DDT compounds in breast milk: effects on the breastfed infant. With some
exceptions, levels of DDT compounds in breast milk in countries with current use of DDT compounds, or with recent restrictions, tend to be above
1000 ppb. In the US and Canada, levels tend to be below 1000 ppb.

the information should assist in placing current levels of these chemicals in the
milk of women in the US and other developed countries, as well as in developing countries, in perspective. Clearly, data gaps still exist in terms of health
endpoints which could be examined, and a better picture of current levels of
these and other chemicals is needed (LaKind *et al.*, 2001). In the meantime,
these graphs support the American Academy of Pediatrics' (AAP) recommen-
dation of "breast milk as the preferred source of feeding for almost all babies for
at least the first year of life" because "breastfeeding provides health, nutritional,
immunologic, developmental, psychological, social, economic and environmental advantages unmatched by other feeding options" and because "epidemiologic
research shows that human milk and breastfeeding provide advantages with
regard to general health, growth, and development, while significantly decreasing risk for a large number of acute and chronic diseases" (AAP, 1997). Despite
the fact that this conclusion did not explicitly address environmental chemicals
in breast milk, it is important to note that, given the ubiquitous nature of these
chemicals, the breastfed infants in the clinical research which formed the basis

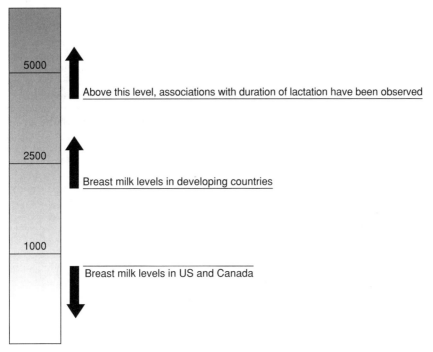

DDT compounds, ppb

Figure 11.5 DDT compounds in breast milk: effects on the mother. With some exceptions, levels of DDT compounds in breast milk in countries with current use
of DDT compounds, or with recent restrictions, tend to be above 1000 ppb.
In the US and Canada, levels tend to be below 1000 ppb.

for the AAP's conclusions were likely exposed to DDT compounds and other
lipophilic environmental chemicals in breast milk.

Acknowledgments

The contributions of Dr Cheston M. Berlin and Dr Daniel Q. Naiman to this
chapter are greatly appreciated. I would also like to thank Dr Jan Koppelman,
Ms Amina Wilkins, and Ms Ann Mason for their insightful comments. Permission to reproduce the structures of the DDT compounds was kindly given by the
University of Minnesota Biocatalysis/Biodegradation Database.

Note

1 The issue of lactation failure is complex (Berlin, 2002). There is lack of agreement on
terms to describe breastfeeding: exclusive, partial, mixed. The term "lactation failure" as
used in studies of environmental chemicals and breastfeeding must be first separated
from the failure to initiate lactation (lactogenesis). The latter is caused by a variety of

maternal and infant factors. Maternal causes are: anatomic problems with the breasts (tubular or hypoplastic breasts) (Neifert et al., 1985), maternal illness, previous breastfeeding failure, flat or inverted nipples, and breast surgery (Neifert, 1996). Infant factors include illness, prematurity, poor latch, and sucking problems (Lawrence and Lawrence, 1999). It is unlikely for lactation failure to occur outside the immediate postnatal period in a nursing mother and her child for whom lactation has been well established. It is possible in rare instances that the infant's demand after one or two months may exceed the capacity of the small-breasted mother. Any significant illness in the mother including depression may decrease milk supply. Perhaps the most important reason for stopping breastfeeding within the first three to four months of the infant's age is that the mother's breasts are not completely emptying often enough. It is quite clear that for maximum milk production the breasts need to be emptied with each feeding and frequently throughout the day (Daly and Hartmann, 1995; Lawrence and Lawrence, 1999, Chapter 3; Powers and Slusser, 1997). Recent work has identified a number of reasons for the decrease in the incidence of breastfeeding during the first six months of life. Many of these are social (e.g., need to return to work, inadequate pumping facilities at work, lack of support both at home and at work), but there are other risk factors that need to be considered as confounding variables in any study that attempts to assign an external reason for stopping nursing. Hoddinott et al. (2000) found the following factors in mothers least likely to be breastfeeding at three months: smoking during pregnancy, younger mothers who had left school before 16, and less social support. In mothers from a lower socio-economic group, breastfeeding beyond one month was associated with the mother having herself been breastfed, and also having successfully breastfed a previous infant (Meyerink and Marquis, 2002). Other positive associations were with older mothers and mothers with relatives who breastfed. Use of pacifiers and supplements may significantly influence breastfeeding duration. Victora et al. (1997) showed that for breastfeeding babies, the introduction of teas or water decreased the rate of breastfeeding at three months from 78.5% to 70.9%; at six months the rate was decreased from 51.3% to 37.7%. Use of the feeding bottle decreased the rate from 93.1% to 65.9% at three months and from 64% to 37.3% at six months. Most significant was the decrease with the use of cow milk or formula: the rate decreased from 84.6% to 34.0% at three months and from 52.2% to 8.3% at six months. The use of pacifiers has been shown to decrease the incidence of breastfeeding (Howard et al., 1999). The presence of formula advertising material during prenatal visits influences the rate of breastfeeding (Howard et al., 2000). It may be very difficult to tease out the precise reason for women ceasing breastfeeding before the infant is six months old. Many women may be reluctant to give the reason for weaning, especially for social/ work reasons. Recall of what other foods may have been offered during breastfeeding, thus influencing the duration of nursing, may be imprecise (Aarts et al., 2000).

References

Aarts, C., Kylberg, E., Hörnell, A., Hofvander, Y., Gebre-Medhin, M., and Greiner, T. (2000) How exclusive is exclusive breastfeeding? A comparison of data since birth with current status data, International Journal of Epidemiology, 29: 1041–1046.

American Academy of Pediatrics (AAP) (1997) Breastfeeding and the use of human milk (RE9729). Policy Statement. Pediatrics, 100: 1035–1039.

American Academy of Pediatrics (AAP) (2001) The transfer of drugs and other chemicals into human milk. AAP Committee on Drugs, Pediatrics, 108: 776–789.

Berlin, C.M. (2002) The discussion on lactation failure was provided by Cheston M. Berlin, Jr, MD, Department of Pediatrics, Children's Hospital, Milton S. Hershey Medical Center, Pennsylvania State University College of Medicine.

Bouwman, H., Becker, P.J., Cooppan, R.M., and Reinecke, A.J. (1992) Transfer of DDT used in malarial control to infants via breast milk, *Bulletin of WHO*, **70**: 241–250.

Daly, S.E.J. and Hartmann, P.E. (1995) Infant demand and milk supply. Part 1: infant demand and milk production in lactating women, *Journal of Human Lactation*, **11**: 21–23.

Gladen, B.C., Rogan, W.J., Hardy, P., Thullen, J. Tingelstad, J., and Tully, M. (1988) Development after exposure to polychlorinated biphenyls and dichlorodiphenyl dichloroethene transplacentally and through human milk, *Journal of Pediatrics*, **113**: 991–995.

Gladen, B.C., Monaghan, S.C., Lukyanova, E.M., Hulchiy, O.P., Shkyryak-Nyzhnyl, Z.A., Sericano, J.L., and Little, R.E. (1999) Organochlorines in breast milk from two cities in Ukraine, *Environmental Health Perspectives*, **107**: 459–462.

Gladen, B.C., Ragan, N.B., and Rogan, W.J. (2000) Pubertal growth and development and prenatal and lactational exposure to polychlorinated biphenyls and dichlorodiphenyl dichloroethene, *Journal of Pediatrics*, **136**: 490–496.

Hoddinott, P., Pill, R., and Hood, K. (2000) Identifying which women will stop breastfeeding before three months in primary care: a pragmatic study, *British Journal of General Practice*, **50**: 888–891.

Hoover, S.M. (1999) Exposure to persistent organochlorines in Canadian breast milk: a probabilistic assessment, *Risk Analysis*, **19**: 527–545.

Howard, C.R., Howard, F.M., Lanphear, B., deBlieck, E.A., Eberly, S. and Lawrence, R.A. (1999) The effects of early pacifier use on breastfeeding duration, *Pediatrics*, **103**: e33.

Howard, C.R., Howard, F.M., Lawrence, R.A., Andersen, E., DeBlieck, E., and Weitzman, M. (2000) Office prenatal formula advertising and its effect on breast-feeding patterns, *Obstetrics and Gynecology*, **95**: 296–303.

Jensen, A.A. and Slorach, S.A. (eds) (1991) *Chemical Contaminants in Human Milk*. Boca Raton, FL: CRC Press.

LaKind, J.S. and Berlin, C.M. (2002) Technical Workshop on Human Milk Surveillance and Research on Environmental Chemicals in the United States: an overview, *Journal of Toxicology and Environmental Health*, **65**: 1829–1838.

LaKind, J.S., Berlin, C., and Naiman, D.Q. (2001) Infant exposure to chemicals in breast milk in the United States: what we need to learn from a breast milk monitoring program, *Environmental Health Perspectives*, **109**: 75–88.

LaKind, J.S., Birnbach, N., Borgert, C.J., Sonawane, B.R., Tully, M.R., and Friedman, L. (2002) Human milk surveillance and research of environmental chemicals: concepts for consideration in interpreting and presenting study results, *Journal of Toxicology and Environmental Health*, **65**: 1909–1928.

Lawrence, R.A. and Lawrence, R.M. (1999) *Breastfeeding: a Guide for the Medical Profession*, 5th edn. St Louis, MO: Mosby.

Lutter, C., Iyengar, V., Barnes, R., Chuvakova, T., Kazbekova, G., and Sharmanov, T. (1998) Breastmilk contamination in Kazakhstan: Implications for infant feeding, *Chemosphere*, **17**: 1761–1772.

Meyerink, R.R. and Marquis, G.S. (2002) Breastfeeding initiation and duration among low-income women in Alabama: the importance of personal and familial experiences in making infant-feeding choices, *Journal of Human Lactation*, **18**: 38–45.

Nakamura, H., Matsuda, M., Quynh, H.T., Cau, H.D., Chi, H.T.K., and Wakimoto, T. (1994) Levels of polychlorinated dibenzo-p-dioxins, dibenzofurans, PCBs, DDTs and HCHs in human adipose tissue and breast milk from the south of Vietnam, *Organohalogen Compounds*, **21**: 71–76.

Neifert, M. (1996) Early assessment of the breastfeeding infant, *Contemporary Pediatrics*, **13**: 142–166.

Neifert, M.R., Seacat, J.M., and Jobe, W.E. (1985) Lactation failure due to insufficient glandular development of the breast, *Pediatrics*, **76**: 823–828.

Powers, N.G. and Slusser, W. (1997) Breastfeeding update 2: clinical lactation management, *Pediatrics in Review*, **18**: 147–161.

Rogan, W.J., Blanton, P.J., Portier, C.J., and Stallard, E. (1991) Should the presence of carcinogens discourage breast feeding?, *Regulatory Toxicology and Pharmacology*, **13**: 228–240.

Rogan, W.J. and Gladen, B.C. (1985) Study of human lactation for effects of environmental contaminants: the North Carolina Breast Milk and Formula Project and some other ideas, *Environmental Health Perspectives*, **60**: 215–221.

Rogan, W.J. and Gladen, B.C. (1991) PCBs, DDE, and child development at 18 and 24 months, *Annals of Epidemiology*, **1**: 407–413.

Rogan, W.J., Gladen, B.C., McKinney, J.D., Carreras, N., Hardy, P., Thullen, J., Tingelstad, J., and Tully, M. (1986) Polychlorinated biphenyls (PCBs) and dichlorodiphenyl dichloroethene (DDE) in human milk: effects of maternal factors and previous lactation, *American Journal of Public Health*, **76**: 172–177.

Rogan, W.J., Gladen, B.C., McKinney, J.D., Carreras, N., Hardy, P., Thullen, J., Tingelstad, J., and Tully, M. (1987) Polychlorinated biphenyls (PCBs) and dichlorodiphenyl dichloroethene (DDE) in human milk: effects on growth morbidity and duration of lactation, *American Journal of Public Health*, **77**: 1294–1297.

Romero, M.L., Dorea, J.G., and Granja, A.C. (2000) Concentrations of organochlorine pesticides in milk of Nicaraguan mothers, *Archives of Environmental Health*, **55**: 274–278.

Schanler, R.J. (ed.) (2001) Breastfeeding 2001, Part I: The evidence for breastfeeding, *Pediatric Clinics of North America*, **48**: 1.

Schreiber, J.S. (2001) Parents worried about breast milk contamination. What is best for baby?, *Pediatric Clinics of North America*, **48**: 1113–1127.

Siddiqui, M.K.J., Nigam, U., Srivastava, S., Tejeshwar, D.S., and Chandrawati, (2002) Association of maternal blood pressure and hemoglobin level with organochlorines in human milk, *Human and Experimental Toxicology*, **21**: 1–6.

Sim, M.R. and McNeil, J.J. (1992) Monitoring chemical exposure using breast milk: a methodological review, *American Journal of Epidemiology*, **136**: 1–11.

Smith, D. (1999) Worldwide trends in DDT levels in human breast milk, *International Journal of Epidemiology*, **28**: 179–188.

Sonawane, B.R. (1995) Chemical contaminants in human milk: an overview, *Environmental Health Perspectives*, **103**(S6): 197–205.

USEPA (US Environmental Protection Agency) (1975) *DDT regulatory history: a brief survey (to 1975)*. www.epa.gov/history/topics/ddt/02.htm

Victora, C.G., Behague D.P., Barros, F.C., Olinto, M.T.A., and Weiderpass, E. (1997) Pacifier use and short breastfeeding duration: cause, consequence or coincidence?, *Pediatrics*, **99**: 445–453.

World Health Organization (WHO) (1998) *GEMS/Food International Survey: Infant exposure to certain organochlorine contaminants from breast milk – a risk assessment.* D. Schutz, G.G. Moy and F.K. Käferstein. WHO Food Safety Unit, Programme of Food Safety and Food Aid. WHO/FSF/FOS/98.4.

12 Parenteral nutrition as a source of toxicity

Roland N. Dickerson

Summary

The critically ill hospitalized patient as well as the long-term home nutrition support patient can experience various toxic effects associated with the parenteral nutrition support. The intent of this review is to provide an overview of the most common toxicities associated with parenteral nutrition. The adverse effects of dextrose, lipids, amino acids, water, electrolytes, vitamins, trace minerals, and contaminants as well as issues concerning parenteral nutrition-associated liver and bone disease have been reviewed. Practitioners should continue to anticipate and potentially avoid these adverse effects whenever possible.

Introduction

There have been numerous advances regarding the safe and efficacious provision of parenteral nutrition since its inception in the late 1960s; however, parenteral nutrition has its own inherent complications. The toxicity of parenteral nutrition is not only related to provision of excesses of its ingredients, but also omission of essential nutrients that lead to deficiencies. The intent of this overview is to focus on the former: the toxicity of parenteral nutrition as related to its provision of nutrients or byproducts of other additives leading to various adverse effects and complications in adult patients. The toxicities of parenteral nutrition in the critically ill patient were reviewed about a decade ago (Phelps *et al.*, 1991); however, numerous new findings warrant this update.

Dextrose

Dextrose is the major non-protein calorie source in a parenteral nutrition regimen. The body requires about 100 to 125 g/day for glucose-requiring tissues such as the central nervous system, bone marrow, leukocytes, erythrocytes and the renal medulla (Dickerson *et al.*, 1986). This obligatory glucose requirement must be met or increased protein breakdown will occur for the generation of carbon chains for the hepatic synthesis of glucose. For the critically ill patient, these obligatory glucose requirements may be greater, particularly if the patient has a thermal injury or other type of wound. Glucose consumption across a burned limb may account for an additional 80 to 150 g/day of glucose depending on the burn wound size (Wilmore et al., 1977). Despite the obvious beneficial effects of glucose, there are numerous toxicities associated with dextrose/glucose.

Examination of glucose oxidation rates in critically ill patients indicates that the percentage of carbon dioxide production coming from the direct oxidation of glucose plateaus at about 5 mg/kg per min (25 kcal/kg per day) (Burke et al., 1979). In unstressed patients, the mean oxidation rate may be only about 4 mg/kg per min (Wolfe et al., 1979). Further increases in dextrose infusion beyond these rates result in significant increases in the respiratory quotient to greater than 1.0 which reflects net fat synthesis (Burke et al., 1979). In addition to increased net fat synthesis, hyperglycemia (serum glucose >200 mg/dl) has been shown to occur in about half of all parenterally fed patients receiving greater than 5 mg/kg per min of dextrose (Rosmarin et al., 1996). Accentuated gluconeogenesis and glycogenolysis that is less suppressible with glucose infusion than in normal controls and a post-receptor insulin resistance (Black et al., 1982; McCowen et al., 2001) has been demonstrated in seriously ill patients. Therefore, critically ill non-diabetic patients requiring parenteral nutrition are often predisposed to developing hyperglycemia upon feeding with parenteral nutrition.

Hyperglycemia can lead to glycosuria, dehydration, and possibly even hyperglycemic hyperosmolar non-ketotic dehydration, coma and death in some individuals. There are data to indicate that hyperglycemia may also impair immune function (McCowen et al., 2000; Pomposelli et al., 1998; Pomposelli and Bistrian, 1994) and increase endogenous body protein catabolism (Gore et al., 2002). Recent data from van den Berghe and colleagues clearly illustrate the detrimental effect of hyperglycemia in 1548 critically ill patients (van den Berghe et al., 2001). In this large prospective, randomized, multi-center trial, critically ill, intensive care unit patients received intensive insulin therapy to maintain a blood glucose level between 80 and 110 mg/dl or were assigned to the conventional treatment group. Conventional treatment was whereby insulin therapy was not initiated until the blood glucose exceeded 215 mg/dl and the blood glucose was maintained between 180 and 200 mg/dl. The intensive insulin therapy group had a mortality rate of half that of the conventional group (4.6% versus 8%, respectively). The benefit of intensive insulin therapy appeared more remarkable in those sicker patients who remained in the intensive care unit for greater than five days (10.6% versus 20.2%, respectively). The greatest reduction in mortality involved deaths due to multiple organ failure with a proven infectious source.

Another potential toxicity of dextrose, when given in abundance, is excess production of carbon dioxide. This may be pertinent in the carbon dioxide-retaining, ventilator-dependent patient who is being weaned from the ventilator. When feeding patients at 1.35 to 2.25 times the mean resting energy expenditure as dextrose, Askanazi et al. (1980) have shown that carbon dioxide production increases by 56% in seriously ill patients. In a subsequent study, these investigators showed that when 50% of the non-protein calories were given as lipid, carbon dioxide production was reduced by 24% compared to the same patients given all their non-protein calories as dextrose (Askanazi *et al.*, 1981). All patients were fed at 1.5 times the measured resting energy expenditure in that study (Askanazi *et al.*, 1981). These intakes relative to measured energy expenditure are particularly important, as Talpers *et al.* (1992) have shown that the proportion of glucose to lipid calories is not as important as the total caloric intake with regard to carbon dioxide production in mechanically ventilated patients. Patients fed a 60% glucose/20% fat/20% amino acids parenteral nutrition regimen at 1, 1.5, and 2 times the Harris-Benedict equations for estimated energy expenditure had marked differences in CO_2 production. However, when patients were fed three different isocaloric (at 1.3 times the Harris-Benedict equations for estimated energy expenditure) regimens with 40% dextrose/40% fat, 60% dextrose/20% fat, and 75% dextrose/5% fat, no significant difference was noted among groups in carbon dioxide production rates. Combined, these data would indicate that when overfeeding, proportion of lipid calories can alter carbon dioxide production; however, a more conservative caloric intake is more important for reducing carbon dioxide production than the individual contributions of dextrose and lipid for a given parenteral nutrition regimen. Also of particular note is whether the infusion is given continuously or by cyclic infusion. Cyclic hypercapnia has been demonstrated for those patients receiving intermittent parenteral nutrition with inability to wean from the ventilator (Jannace *et al.*, 1988). Continuous infusion of parenteral nutrition may be preferable in these patients.

Parenteral nutrition-associated liver disease may be another complication of excessive dextrose intake. This complication is of particular concern as it may not always be reversible (Bowyer *et al.*, 1985). However, parenteral nutrition-associated liver disease is a complex, multifactorial process usually from continuous, excessive intakes of glucose, lipid, or excessive total calories in the absence of oral intake (Allardyce, 1982; Chan *et al.*, 1999; Dickerson and Karwoski, 2002; Lowry and Brennan, 1979; Sheldon *et al.*, 1978). A listing of proposed etiologies for parenteral nutrition-associated liver disease is given in Table 12.1.

Table 12.1 Proposed etiologies for parenteral nutrition-associated liver disease in adults

Excess total caloric intake
Excess glucose intake
Excess lipid intake
Continuous glucose infusion
Tryptophan breakdown products
Lack of enteral nutrition
Intestinal toxins due to bacterial overgrowth (e.g. blind loop)
Manganese intoxication
Essential fatty acid deficiency
Choline deficiency
Carnitine deficiency
Aluminum accumulation?

Parenteral nutrition-associated liver disease also appears to be accentuated by the presence of inflammation and infection (Chan et al., 1999; Dickerson and Karwoski, 2002; Lowry and Brennan, 1979; Sheldon et al., 1978) which may be a chronic complication of the patients' primary disease process. Parenteral nutrition-associated liver dysfunction in adults classically presents as a fatty infiltration of the liver or a non-specific triaditis usually resulting in cholestatic jaundice (Allardyce, 1982; Bowyer et al., 1985; Chan et al., 1999; Dickerson and Karwoski, 2002; Lowry and Brennan, 1979; Sheldon et al., 1978). Biochemical evidence for parenteral nutrition-associated liver disease often occurs within the first seven to ten days of parenteral nutrition. It is classically associated with a significant rise in serum alkaline phosphatase or gamma glutamyl transferase followed by a rise in serum total bilirubin a couple weeks later (Sheldon et al., 1978). When presented with a patient with potential parenteral nutrition-associated liver disease, the clinician should assess whether the patient is able to eat or initiate enteral nutrition support. If this is not possible, the amount of dextrose administered to the patient should be scrutinized and efforts undertaken to insure that the glucose intake has not exceeded 4 to 5 mg/kg per min (Tulikoura and Huikuri, 1982). Meguid et al. (1984) found that substitution of 30% of the glucose calories with intravenous lipid calories resulted in fewer liver chemistry abnormalities; however, others found no effect of altering the proportion of non-protein calories (Wagner et al., 1983). In some cases, the continuous infusion of glucose can be changed to a cyclic regimen whereby the patient is free of any dextrose-containing solutions for a portion of the day (Maini et al., 1976). All of these techniques to address parenteral nutrition-associated liver disease have had some limited success. Probably the most important intervention from the nutrition support perspective is to not overfeed in general, particularly in critically ill patients (Guenst and Nelson, 1994).

As a result of these data, some clinician-researchers have opted for a more conservative caloric and glucose intake when feeding hospitalized patients with specialized nutrition support (McCowen et al., 2000; Patino et al., 1999). A more rigorous use of insulin and conservative dosing of dextrose in an effort to gain more precise control of serum glucose concentrations are also recommended. Parenteral nutrition regimens are often composed of both dextrose and lipid emulsions as the non-protein caloric sources. Hypocaloric feeding as a means to achieve better glucose control may be particularly useful in obese patients with predisposition to or with existing diabetes mellitus (Dickerson et al., 1986, 2002). Others have adopted this conservative hypocaloric feeding approach to all patients requiring parenteral nutrition (McCowen et al., 2000; Patino et al., 1999). However, this generic approach to caloric requirements for most hospitalized patients requiring parenteral nutrition may be considered controversial.

Lipid emulsion

Since the availability of lipid emulsions in the mid-1970s, the use of mixed fuel systems (glucose, lipids, and amino acids) is prevalent in practice. Lipid has been shown to be anabolically equivalent to dextrose in terms of nitrogen balance when given up to 50% of the non-protein caloric intake (Nordenstrom *et al.*, 1983). However, there have been numerous reported toxicities associated with intravenous lipid emulsion and many of these reports have become the subject of considerable controversy among nutritional support practitioners and researchers.

It is important to differentiate between the composition and metabolism of intravenous lipid emulsion and enterally absorbed chylomicrons. Chylomicrons contain a central core of triglycerides plus small amounts of cholesterol that is surrounded by a layer of phospholipids and apoproteins acquired during gastrointestinal absorption. Intravenous fat emulsion consists of droplets of triglycerides emulsified with egg phospholipids and suspended in glycerol and water. The intravenous fat emulsion contains virtually no cholesterol except for the minimal amounts contained within the egg phospholipids. After hydrolysis of the triglyceride, the intravenous fat particle is now composed of an unstable layer of phospholipid and lacks the cholesterol core. Some of these phospholipids are cleared whereas others extract preexisting cholesterol from body tissue pools for the stabilization of the phospholipids. This cholesterol–phospholipid particles are often referred to as lipoprotein-X and may accumulate if the dose of intravenous lipid exceeds clearance (Griffin *et al.*, 1979). Disruption of the plasma lipid profiles appears to be directly related to the dose of infused phospholipids. These remnants accumulate in the reticuloendothelial system (RES) and are phagocytized by the Kupffer cells of the liver. Accumulation of fat emulsion remnants and impaired clearance of the triglyceride derived from an omega-6 long chain triglyceride, with aggressive dosing has been suggested to cause fat overload syndrome, cholestatic liver disease, respiratory dysfunction, immune dysfunction, pancreatitis, and acalculous cholecystitis.

Fat overload syndrome is the culmination of multiple organ dysfunction syndrome in the presence of aggressive intravenous lipid dosing for patients with impaired clearance of fat emulsion. Taylor and Buckner (1982) describe a case where a critically ill bone marrow transplant patient was given 1 L daily of 10% lipid emulsion while experiencing liver dysfunction, ascites, and large volumes of bloody diarrhea. The patient was given Amphotericin B for candidemia and his renal function declined. After 71 days of parenteral nutrition his serum was noted to be lipemic. The lipid emulsion was discontinued and two days later his serum triglyceride was 483 mg/dl. On day 72, he became short of breath and it was felt that he had developed iatrogenic fat overload syndrome leading to respiratory insufficiency, hemolytic anemia, liver and renal failure. He died 27 days later of disseminated aspergillosis and graft-versus-host disease.

Excessive lipid intake has also been shown to cause cholestatic liver disease (Table 12.1). Allardyce (1982) assigned 35 patients to receive intravenous fat emulsion at a dose of either 1 or 3 g/kg per day provided as 10% fat emulsion. Biochemical evidence for cholestasis was noted in 10 out of 18 patients who received lipid emulsion at 3 g/kg per day as opposed to one in 17 patients who received 1 g/kg per day after greater than 20 days of therapy. In addition, significant increases were noted in serum cholesterol in the high dose group, implying increased lipoprotein-X appearance.

It has also been suggested that intravenous fat emulsion may cause adverse pulmonary effects. Investigators have shown in animals and humans that rapid administration of large doses of intravenous lipid results in ventilation and perfusion defects resulting in less oxygen delivery to arterial blood. The etiology for this phenomenon is unclear; however, it may be related to a flux in eicosanoid precursors from the lipid emulsion that may alter pulmonary hemodynamics and oxygen transfer. Indomethacin appears to block the intravenous fat emulsion-induced pO_2 decrease, supporting a prostaglandin-mediated etiology (Hageman et al., 1983). There also have been numerous cases of intrapulmonary (vascular and/or alveolar) fat deposition at autopsy in immature infants receiving intravenous fat emulsion (Levene et al., 1984). However, these cases of pulmonary fat emboli have been questioned as a postmortem artifact. The lungs of 22 immature infants were fixated in situ immediately after death with glutaraldehyde, which was instilled through an endotracheal tube (Schroder et al., 1984). Nine of the 22 newborns had been fed formula and given supplemental amounts of amino acids and glucose intravenously, but not intravenous fat emulsion. The remaining neonates received an average of 2 g/kg per day (range, 0.5 to 3.6 g/kg per day) of intravenous fat emulsion for a mean of 20 days (range, 3 h to 75 days). Neither the intravenous lipid emulsion group nor the non-lipid parenteral nutrition controls exhibited pulmonary intravascular fat accumulation. The data suggest that the previously described fat globules found in the lungs of premature infants receiving intravenous lipid emulsion were likely postmortem artifacts (Hageman et al., 1983). These data, combined with the other data previously discussed in this chapter regarding the effects of glucose and lipid on carbon dioxide production, suggest that intravenous lipid emulsion, if given at a conventional rate and dose and without inducing hypertriglyceridemia, will likely not have significant adverse pulmonary effects.

Infection is a major cause of morbidity and mortality in the intensive care unit setting and therapy that might be toxic to the normal immune response would be considered detrimental. Malnutrition is associated with immune dysfunction and efforts to avoid malnutrition often include the use of specialized nutrition support. When giving parenteral nutrition, this would also include the use of intravenous lipid emulsion. Some of the earlier work in animals suggested that lipid emulsion impaired immune function; however, many of these early studies offered conflicting results. In addition, many of these early studies were performed with very high, clinically irrelevant doses, that led to extremes in serum triglyceride concentrations and impaired clearance (Fischer et al., 1980).

There are various plausible explanations of the observed effect of intravenous fat emulsions on the immune system, particularly the reticuloendothelial system (RES). Soybean and safflower oil contain large amounts of the linoleic acid, which serves as precursor for arachidonic acid, prostaglandins, and leukotrienes (Pomposelli and Bistrian, 1994). Several of the prostaglandins have shown to inhibit cytokine release, thus influencing immune function. A second mechanism includes a slowing in the rate of clearance of bacteria from the recticuloen-dothelial system due to various chylomicron remnants causing a mechanical blockage. However, the rate of appearance of these chylomicron remnants and eicosanoids from the administration of intravenous lipid emulsion appears to be dose- and rate-dependent (Pomposelli and Bistrian, 1994). Clinical studies that address dosage and rate may provide further insight as to the significance of this potential toxicity of lipid emulsion.

To assess the effect of fat emulsion on neutrophil chemiluminescence, 18 chronically ill patients receiving glucose-based parenteral nutrition were studied before and after a 4 to 6 h infusion of 500 ml of 10% lipid emulsion (Robin *et al.*, 1989). A significant suppression in neutrophil oxidant release (reflective of bactericidal activity) was observed post-infusion. Pre-incubation of activated neutrophils with lipid emulsion resulted in no difference in activity. These data suggested that this depression was not due to a direct effect of the lipid *per se* but rather due to inhibitory substances released in response to lipid emulsion infusion. Nordenstrom *et al.* (1979) examined the effect of a 20% lipid emulsion on leukocyte migration in 12 normal subjects. The adults received 50, 100, or 200 ml/h of lipid emulsion over a 2 h infusion period. All patients were hypertriglyceridemic during the infusion with slow return back to normal baseline values by 24 h. Only the 200 ml/h group demonstrated significant differences in leukocyte chemotaxis at 1 and 2 h with a return to baseline by 24 h. These data indicate a transient adverse effect of lipid emulsion at the highest infusion rate. Ota *et al.* (1985) examined neutrophil function (chemotaxis, phagocytosis, bactericidal index) and lymphocytic blastogenic response to mitogens in 40 malnourished patients who were randomized to receive either a dextrose-based or total nutrient admixture system with 3.3% lipid concentration. Measurements were taken prior to starting parenteral nutrition and at the end of therapy (average duration of parenteral nutrition therapy was 10.3 and 9.0 days for each group, respectively). No significant differences were noted for any of the markers in immune function between groups. Collectively, these three studies demonstrate that the inhibitory cellular effects of lipid emulsion are dose- and rate-related and are transient. When the lipid is infused continuously at a moderate dose, no significant detrimental effects on cellular immune function are observed.

To examine the effect of a 10 h infusion of intravenous lipid emulsion (comprising 43% of the non-protein calories) on the RES, the serum clearance of ^{99m}Tc-sulfur colloid was studied before the lipid infusion was initiated and on the first day after lipid therapy in 10 patients and on the third day of lipid infusion in eight patients (Seidner *et al.*, 1989). Their data showed no significant reduction in sulfur colloid clearance after one day (0.27 ± 0.1/min to 0.26 ± 0.1/min, respectively). However, a significant decrease was observed after three days of lipid infusion (0.46 ± 0.08/min to 0.27 ± 0.03/min). Of concern with these data were the marked differences in baseline clearance between the two control periods for each study; these differences confound the interpretation of their data. In a follow-up study by the same group, sulfur colloid clearance was assessed in eight patients given a continuous intravenous infusion of soybean lipid (1.3 g/kg per day) via a total nutrient admixture system (Jensen et al., 1990). Measurements were conducted at baseline and after three days of therapy. Clearance of the sulfur colloid was unchanged with continuous lipid therapy (0.38 ± 0.09/min and 0.41 ± 08/min, respectively). These data regarding lipid emulsion and RES function are analogous to the cellular immune function findings. There appears to be some impairment in RES clearance of sulfur colloid when lipid is given intermittently at a higher infusion rate, but no adverse effects on RES clearance when given continuously at a more moderate rate/dosage.

Another issue in regard to conventional lipid emulsions commercially available in the United States is whether the basis of using oils that are predominantly ω-6 based is optimal for critically ill patients. The long chain triglycerides of the ω-6 series are substrates for the production of arachidonic acid which are substrates for the production of pro-inflammatory prostaglandins such as prostaglandin E2 and leukotrienes of the B4 series. These substances are mediators of the inflammatory response that may be an issue for patients with systemic inflammatory response syndrome or adult respiratory distress syndrome. Further clinical research is necessary to elucidate any beneficial effects to reducing ω-6 and increasing ω-3 fatty acids for parenteral nutrition.

Peroxidation reactions from lipid emulsion administration have also been suggested to be a detrimental complication. Lipid peroxidation may lead to tissue damage, increased inflammatory response, and impairment of the immune response. The latter two areas have been previously addressed. Although the exact tissues damaged were not identified, increased breath pentane (reflective of increased lipid peroxidation) was noted in nine home parenteral nutrition patients compared to 10 normal controls (Lemoyne et al., 1988). Further research is necessary to elucidate the clinical ramifications of these findings.

There are some case reports suggesting that intravenous lipid emulsions can induce acute pancreatitis in selected patients (Buckspan et al., 1984; Lashner et al., 1986). Most of the published case reports are somewhat anecdotal as details are lacking with regard to triglyceride concentrations before and after the infusion, lipid emulsion concentration and administration details including duration of infusion, and lack of a rechallenge after recovery. Lashner et al. (1986) reported a young patient with Crohn's disease with a surgically-confirmed edematous and inflamed pancreas after six weeks of parenteral nutrition therapy that included lipid emulsion. The patient was rechallenged with 500 ml of 20% fat emulsion after complete resolution of the pancreatitis (Lashner et al., 1986). Thirty-six hours after the rechallenge, mild epigastric pain had developed; serum amylase and triglycerides were increased. The serum triglyceride concentration was 492 mg/dl and the serum appeared lipemic. The event quickly resolved after discontinuation of the lipid emulsion. Differentiation between hyperlipidemia associated with pancreatitis and hyperlipidemia-induced pancreatitis can be difficult (Cameron et al., 1973). Other clinician investigators have reported the safe and efficacious use of intravenous lipid emulsion as part of the parenteral nutrition regimen in patients with pancreatitis for numerous patients (Robin *et al.*, 1990; Silberman *et al.*, 1982; Sitzmann *et al.*, 1989). However, some patients with acute pancreatitis may be hyperlipidemic and have impaired clearance of lipid emulsion (Guzman *et al.*, 1985; Rollan *et al.*, 1990). As a result, it has been our approach to ascertain if the patient with pancreatitis is hypertriglyceridemic prior to implementation of lipid emulsion and then obtain subsequent triglyceride concentrations to insure the patient has adequate clearance of the emulsion.

Acalculous cholecystitis has also been suggested as a toxicity or complication of using intravenous lipid emulsions for patients requiring parenteral nutrition. Lipid emulsion has been suggested to increase bile lithogenicity in animals (Gimmon *et al.*, 1982). However, gallbladder disease in patients receiving long-term parenteral nutrition is more likely due to the lack of enteral nutrition resulting in gallbladder stasis and not the parenteral nutrition solution or lipid component of the parenteral nutrition solution (Doty *et al.*, 1985; Roslyn *et al.*, 1983).

Other uncommon adverse effects of lipid emulsion reported in the literature include eosinophilia, urticaria and pruritis, nausea, bradycardia, fever, wheezing, tachycardia, thrombocytopenia, tachypnea, and diarrhea.

Because of these complications, clinicians will often use 20% or 30% fat emulsion products instead of 10%, as the same concentration of phospholipid emulsifiers is contained in each product despite increasing amounts of triglyceride. Twice or three times the amount of triglycerides can be provided to the patient with the same dose of phospholipids. In addition, the amount of lipid emulsion may be limited depending on body clearance. Critically ill patients should be monitored closely to insure adequate clearance of the lipid emulsion. One may argue that it may be preferential to administer the fat emulsion empirically over a 12 to 24 h period to minimize adverse effects and to optimize lipid oxidation (Abbott *et al.*, 1984). This would be particularly pertinent in the patient with suspected impaired clearance of intravenous lipid emulsion (e.g. immature, small for gestational age newborns, patients with hyperlipidemia, pancreatitis, renal failure, advanced liver disease, HIV disease, or end-stage sepsis) (Dickerson, 1986). Patients with suspected alterations in lipid emulsion clearance should have a baseline serum triglyceride concentration performed with a repeat level soon after initiation of lipid emulsion therapy. This procedure may need to be repeated once to twice weekly thereafter.

Amino acids

Nutritional support of the critically ill patient often requires an aggressive protein intake as they are often highly catabolic. Unstressed malnourished patients will also benefit by sufficient protein intake to facilitate replenishment of body cell mass. However, protein when provided as crystalline amino acids, as in parenteral nutrition solutions, may cause adverse effects in certain patients.

Optimal protein intake for patients with acute or chronic renal failure continues to generate controversy. Nevertheless, if patients are given too much protein (which is dependent on the patient's severity of uremia and renal dysfunction), it is likely to be detrimental. Protein intake, in such patients, is often titrated to type and frequency of dialysis, appearance of uremic symptomatology, and serum urea nitrogen concentration. Commercially available products for patients with renal failure have been suggested to promote anabolism, yet be less ureagenic in an effort to reduce the toxic effect of amino acids in renal failure. These products contained only essential amino acids or a higher proportion of essential amino acids relative to non-essential amino acids when compared to conventional formulations. The premise for use of these formulations was the suggestion that there would be increased efficiency for use of urea and other nitrogenous waste substances for tissue synthesis when a predominantly essential amino acid enriched product was used. Mirtallo et al. (1982) randomized 45 patients with compromised renal function to receive either an essential amino acid or conventional amino acid product. Both groups were given isocaloric, isonitrogenous parenteral nutrition support. Urea nitrogen appearance, mortality, and electrolyte imbalances were not significantly different between groups. The authors concluded that there was no demonstrable advantage to the use of an essential amino acid solution as opposed to a conventional amino acid formulation for parenterally-fed patients with renal impairment.

Protein intake can also be potentially harmful for patients with hepatic encephalopathy. It has been contended that 50% to 60% of patients with chronic liver failure will tolerate 60 to 80 g/day of a standard amino acid mixture as part of the parenteral nutrition regimen. Additional protein intake may result in worsening of the encephalopathy. However, more protein than 60 to 80 g/day is required in many hospitalized patients. A commercially available parenteral amino acid solution, composed of a higher amount of branched chain amino acids (e.g. 36% of the amino acids) and lower sulfur-containing and aromatic amino acids than conventional formulations, has been developed for patients with hepatic encephalopathy. The theoretical basis for this amino acid modification was based on some studies that suggest patients with cirrhosis and hepatic encephalopathy have a low serum essential amino acid to elevated aromatic amino acid acid ratio when compared to normals. Correction of this abnormal amino acid profile has led to resolution of encephalopathy in some patients. In a controlled study of 70 patients with acute hepatic encephalopathy, use of conventional amino acids versus a branched chain enriched product was evaluated (Michel et al., 1985). Patients in both groups received isocaloric, isonitrogenous parenteral nutrition regimens. Of the 34 patients who received conventional amino acids, 10 patients' encephalopathy improved, 14 were unchanged, 10 deteriorated and seven died. In the modified amino acid group of 36 patients, 12 improved, 14 were unchanged, 10 deteriorated and seven died. The authors concluded that branched chain enriched/low sulfur, aromatic amino acid solutions were ineffective in the treatment of acute hepatic encephalopathy in cirrhotic patient. However, a meta-analysis of the literature suggested an improvement in mental status recovery with use of the specialized formulation (Naylor et al., 1989). Further research is warranted.

Table 12.2 Proposed contributing factors to the
development of parenteral nutrition-associated bone
disease in adults

Calcium deficiency
Magnesium deficiency
Vitamin D toxicity
Vitamin D deficiency
Aluminum toxicity
Chronic acidemia
Excessive protein intake
Cyclic parenteral nutrition therapy
Vitamin K deficiency
Medications (corticosteroids, heparin)
Copper deficiency
Immobility
Menopause
Phosphorus excess
Phosphorus deficiency

Photodegradation products of tryptophan have been suggested to be
hepatotoxic and a potential etiology in the pathogenesis of parenteral-nutrition
associated liver disease (Grant *et al.*, 1977). However, given current methods
for storage and protection of parenteral solutions from long-term exposure to
light, this pathogenic effect is likely minimized.

Amino acids may contribute a detrimental role in the pathogenesis of parenteral nutrition associated bone disease. Parenteral nutrition-associated metabolic
bone disease is complex and its etiology is multifactorial (Table 12.2). It has
been suggested that 40% to 100% of patients on long-term parenteral nutrition
may have decreased bone density or evidence of metabolic bone disease. Bone
pain and spontaneous fractures are hallmarks of this disorder, which may occur
as early as three months or as late as several years after starting long-term parenteral nutrition. Part of the difficulty in defining the most appropriate treatment
for patients with suspected metabolic bone disease is due to the heterogeneity of
bone histology associated with this disorder (Table 12.3). Hypercalciuria is a
common finding for patients with parenteral nutrition associated bone disease
(Klein *et al.*, 1980; Lipkin *et al.*, 1988; Shike *et al.*, 1980, 1986; Wood *et al.*,
1985). Amino acids induce hypercalciuria in patients receiving total parenteral
nutrition. Bengoa *et al.* (1983) demonstrated these effects by examining calcium
excretion in five long-term parenterally fed patients by giving the patients
either 1 or 2 g/kg per day of protein in a randomized, crossover fashion. The
parenteral calcium intake was kept constant at 12 mEq/day. Three of the five
patients were in positive calcium balance at a protein intake of 1 g/kg per day.
All five were in negative balance at 2 g/kg per day. The administration of
protein has been known to increase glomerular filtration rate markedly, which
may partially explain the increase in calciuria. However, the investigators normalized the calcium clearance to creatinine clearance and still found that this

Table 12.3 A summary of case series for parenteral nutrition-associated bone disease

Author/Year	N	Bone disease	Proposed etiology
Klein et al., 1980	11	Osteopenia	Unknown
Shike et al., 1980	16	Osteomalacia	Vitamin D toxicity
Ott et al., 1983	16	Osteopenia/low turnover	Aluminum toxicity/ hypoparathyroidism
de Vernejoul, 1985	7	Osteopenia/reduced bone formation	Aluminum/high protein intake
Shike et al., 1986	13	Osteopenia/low bone formation	Unknown, multifactorial
Lipkin et al., 1987	26	Heterogenity of bone histology findings	Aluminum and unknown
Foldes, 1990	10	Osteoporosis	Multifactorial
Pironi, 2000	16	Hyperkinetic bone (early, <4 months) Osteopenia/low bone formation (>12 months)	Unknown, multifactorial

ratio was significantly increased. The data indicate that other metabolic effects account for this increased calcium excretion beyond protein-induced increases in glomerular filtration rate. Other data suggest that the sulfur amino acids may be partially responsible for this increase in calciuria (Cole and Zlotkin, 1983). However, it is possible that the increased calciuria may be due to the increased acid load associated with an increase in amino acids given to the patient that the bone may be required to buffer (with subsequent release of calcium). Some of the earlier reports regarding parenteral nutrition associated liver disease involved patients who received casein hydrolysates as the protein source instead of crystalline amino acids (Klein *et al.*, 1980). Casein hydrolysates were heavily contaminated with aluminum and have also been implicated in the potential etiology of parenteral nutrition associated bone disease (Table 12.2) (Klein *et al.*, 1980; Ott *et al.*, 1983).

The administration of amino acids has been shown to alter ventilatory drive in nutritionally depleted patients who required parenteral nutrition. In a crossover design, eight nutritionally depleted patients were randomized to receive either a high nitrogen intake (15 mg nitrogen per kcal of measured energy expenditure) or low nitrogen intake (7.5 mg nitrogen per kcal of measured energy expenditure) for seven days with each regimen (Askanazi *et al.*, 1984). Total energy intake was given at 1.3 times the measured energy expenditure. Half of the non-protein calories were administered as glucose and the other half as lipid. Breathing patterns were assessed at rest and during inhalations of 2% and 4% carbon dioxide. With the increased nitrogen intake regimen, the patients demonstrated an increased ventilatory sensitivity to CO_2 as evidenced by a marked shift in the relationship between minute ventilation and $PaCO_2$. Some clinicians would regard that increased ventilatory sensitivity to $PaCO_2$ as beneficial, whereas others have hypothesized that this effect may result in earlier fatigue in some patients who are trying to be weaned from the ventilator and that this effect could be potentially detrimental. Further research is warranted to differentiate these theoretical from clinically relevant considerations.

Water

A substantial amount of fluid must often be provided to the patient in an effort to meet parenteral nutrition needs. However, some hospitalized patients have diseases such as congestive heart failure, renal failure with oliguria/anuria, cirrhotic ascites, or syndromes of inappropriate anti-diuretic hormone which can result in impaired urinary water excretion and could potentially lead to water intoxication. Another clinical scenario whereby excess fluid may be toxic is in the patient with adult respiratory distress syndrome (ARDS) (Simmons *et al.*, 1987). The investigators demonstrated improved survival for patients whose fluids were restricted and had a low cumulative fluid balance over a 14 day observation period (Simmons *et al.*, 1987). Patients should be closely monitored for fluid balance and hemodynamic monitoring should be utilized if possible to optimize fluid therapy, avoid fluid overload, and avoid pulmonary congestion. To maximize fluid restriction, the parenteral nutrition solution should be compounded using the most concentrated macronutrient components commercially available: 70% dextrose, 15% amino acids, and 30% lipid emulsion.

Electrolytes

Any of the electrolytes, when given in excess of requirements, can lead to toxicity. This can be further complicated by administration of certain medications that may alter urinary excretion of minerals resulting in a change in requirements (Brown and Dickerson, 1999). For example, the presence of therapeutic doses of heparin, trimethoprim, octreotide, potassium-sparing diuretics such as triamterene or spironolactone, or angiotensin-converting enzyme inhibitors (e.g. captopril, enalapril, lisinopril) may predispose the patient to develop a clinically significant hyperkalemia. Despite conventional dosing of potassium (0.5 to 1.2 mEq/kg per day for patients with normal renal function), patients receiving these drugs often necessitate a readjustment in potassium intake to prevent toxicity. Weinsier *et al.* (1982) observed a 5% incidence of severe hyperkalemia (as defined by a serum potassium >6.5 mEq/L) in 42 surgical patients receiving parenteral nutrition with a potassium intake of ≥60 mEq/day. None of the patients had hypermagnesemia, hypercalcemia, or hyperphosphatemia; however, the incidence of these electrolyte imbalances is dependent upon the institution's population. In our Level 1 Trauma Center and Burn Center at the Regional Medical Center at Memphis, we observe a greater variety of electrolyte abnormalities due to the patients' acuity of illness, alterations in acid–base homeostasis, and varying levels of renal impairment than in the population described by Weinsier *et al.* (1982).

Veech (1986) has theoretically questioned the use of conventional fluid and electrolyte therapy given to hospitalized patients. His argument stems from the presumption that the prescribing of parenteral fluids (and electrolytes) has become so routine that most clinicians have become oblivious to the toxic impact of current practices on the cellular metabolism of patients. The theoretical basis of his discussion relates to the understanding of the metabolic and ionic organization of the cells to control the inherent metabolic energy of the cells. He has classified the errors in fluid/electrolyte therapy of hospitalized patients into four major classes of toxicity:

1   hyperchloremic acidosis from the use of normal saline or other fluids with an $[Na^+]$ to $[Cl^-]$ ratio above the physiologically normal ratio of 1.38
2   lactic acidosis and the inappropriate use of lactated Ringer's solution
3   pathological accumulation of normal metabolites that occurs during routine dialysis with high acetate containing fluids
4   ineffectual treatment of hemorrhage and the replacement of blood with artificial plasma expanders which lack charge.

The first error is probably most germane to this review on the toxicity of parenteral nutrition. Hyperchloremic metabolic acidosis has been classically reported as an adverse effect with parenteral nutrition solutions. Parenteral nutrition is often included in the differential diagnosis for assessing a patient with a normal anion gap metabolic acidosis. Parenteral nutrition solutions tend to be acidotic in nature due to the titratable acidity of the amino acids and low pH of the dextrose solutions. The manufacturers of amino acid solutions reformulated their solutions a couple of decades ago to include more acetate salts than chloride salts to compensate partially for this acid load. However, the astute clinician must balance the chloride and acetate salts of the parenteral nutrition solution in relation to the patient's current acid–base status and to the patient's overall clinical progress to prevent this or other acid–base abnormalities from occurring.

Vitamins

Vitamin D

Hypervitaminosis D is unlikely in hospitalized or long-term parenteral nutrition patients receiving conventional multivitamin supplementation. However, hypervitaminosis D has been questioned as a potential etiology for parenteral nutrition-associated metabolic bone disease (Table 12.2). The Toronto group withdrew vitamin D for six months from 11 patients with histologic evidence of osteomalacia/parenteral nutrition-associated metabolic bone disease (Shike et al., 1981). Prior to withdrawal of vitamin D, serum levels of 1,25 dihydroxy vitamin-D and parathyroid hormone were low whereas 25-hydroxy vitamin D levels were normal despite provision of 500 IU of vitamin D_2 per day. Current multivitamin formulations for parenteral nutrition in adults provide 200 IU of vitamin D_2 per day. Intermittent hypercalcemia with calciuria and phosphaturia were also observed. Withdrawal of the vitamin D from the parenteral nutrition solution resulted in an improvement in histologic findings, including an increase in the mineralization/tetracycline uptake and a decrease in osteoid bone tissue. In the three patients with symptoms, bone pain subsided, fractures healed, and the urinary loss of phosphate and calcium decreased. Conversely, the UCLA group discontinued vitamin D_2 for six months in two patients. Neither patient had any change in their symptoms or hypercalciuria (Klein *et al.*, 1981). The University of Pennsylvania group found their population to exhibit hyperkinetic bone with osteoclast activity that was greater than osteoblast activity; patients responded well to supplemental vitamin D and calcium beyond what was contained in the parenteral nutrition solutions (unpublished observations). In a follow-up study by the lead author for the vitamin D toxicity paper (relocated to New York City from Toronto), 13 long-term parenterally fed patients exhibited osteopenia without a mineralization defect and had a normal 1,25 dihydroxy vitamin D level (Shike *et al.*, 1986). It is this widespread heterogeneity of metabolic bone abnormalities associated with the use of parenteral nutrition (Table 12.3) that continues to baffle clinicians and prevents definition of the most appropriate therapy for this complication. These data indicate that vitamin D toxicity may not necessarily be universal among all parenterally fed patients with symptomatic metabolic bone disease.

Vitamin A

Chronic vitamin A intoxication, rare in the general population, classically presents with skin dryness, fissures, pruritis, hair loss, generalized fatigue, bone tenderness, anorexia, headache, diplopia, and hepatomegaly (Muenter *et al.*, 1971). Hypervitaminosis A is rare for patients receiving conventional doses of vitamin A during long-term parenteral nutrition. However, a case report of a four-year-old boy with intestinal pseudo-obstruction and normal renal function developed classical signs of vitamin A toxicity while on long-term parenteral nutrition (Seibert *et al.*, 1981). He received 6000 IU/day, which was about two and a half times the suggested maintenance requirements for children on long-term parenteral nutrition. The symptoms resolved upon discontinuation of the vitamin A supplementation. Patients with renal failure requiring dialysis who receive long-term parenteral nutrition are more likely to be at risk of developing hypervitaminosis A. Failure of the kidney to metabolize retinol to retinoic acid may cause diminished excretion via the bile and urine, leading to elevated serum and hepatic vitamin A concentrations. Gleghorn *et al.* (1986) reported a case series of three patients (seven, 13, and 26 years of age) with renal failure who received long-term parenteral nutrition with 5000 IU/day of vitamin A (retinol). The current recommended daily parenteral intake for retinol in adults is 3300 IU/day. All patients had elevated serum vitamin A levels in the range normally reported for patients with renal failure; however, all three patients also exhibited the hallmark signs and symptoms of hypervitaminosis A. Clinical improvement followed discontinuation of the retinol in the parenteral nutrition solution. These cases also illustrate a point regarding interpretation of vitamin A levels for patients with renal disease. Their vitamin A levels were similar to other renal failure patients reported in the literature, yet these other patients were asymptomatic. Retinol-binding protein is excreted in the urine and its concentration is elevated for patients with renal failure. Examination of serum total vitamin A levels in dialysis-treated patients with end-stage renal disease has demonstrated that total vitamin A concentrations and retinol-binding protein concentrations to be elevated. However, free retinol concentrations were within normal limits (Cundy *et al.*, 1983). Therefore, long-term parenterally fed patients who may be at risk for hypervitaminosis A should have further laboratory evaluation beyond a total vitamin A serum concentration. This evaluation should include a free retinol concentration or, alternatively, the vitamin A to retinol binding protein ratio if free concentrations are not available, to ascertain if the patient is at risk for vitamin A toxicity.

Trace minerals

It is common practice among clinicians to withhold or reduce the amount of copper and manganese supplementation in the parenteral nutrition solution of patients who have advanced liver disease since these minerals are excreted predominantly by the hepatobiliary system. Conversely, selenium is withheld from the parenteral nutrition solutions of patients who have renal failure. Data regarding copper and selenium toxicity in long-term, parenterally fed patients are lacking. However, there is abundant literature regarding manganese intoxication in long-term parenterally fed patients and some limited toxicity information concerning zinc.

Manganese

Hypermanganesemia and its associated complications have become an issue in the patient receiving long-term parenteral nutrition (Dickerson, 2001). Table 12.4 provides a summary of some of the larger case series in parenterally fed adult patients that have been reported in the literature. Since intestinal absorption has a significant role in manganese homeostasis, receiving manganese by the parenteral route bypasses this important regulatory feedback mechanism and may make the patient susceptible to the complications of hypermanganesemia. Manganese poisoning presents clinically as parkinsonian-like symptoms whereby the subjects have muscular weakness, stiffness, tremors, ataxia, abnormal gait, asthenia, and difficulty with speech. Psychological changes including mental irritability, headaches, nervousness, compulsive actions, and hallucinations can also occur. Manganese accumulation occurs in the basal ganglia as evidenced by symmetric increased signal intensity on T-1 weighted magnetic resonance images for patients receiving parenteral nutrition with manganese.

The literature suggests that the presence of hypermanganesemia and the clinical symptoms from manganese toxicity are dependent upon the dose of parenteral

Table 12.4 Selected case series of manganese intoxication in parenterally-fed adult patients (adapted from Dickerson, 2001)

Investigator	N	Age	Disease condition	Mn intake	Duration of intake	Laboratory findings
Alves et al., 1997	1	Adult	SBS	1–2 mg/day	19 months	Increased serum and urine Mn; abnormal MRI
Bertinet et al., 2000	4	Adults	SBS	1 mg/day	18 months (16 months–7 years)	Serum Mn normal; increased MRI signals
	15	54 years (32–74)	SBS (n = 12), chronic intestinal obstruction (n = 3)	0.17–0.8 mg/day	3.8 years (1.7–10 years) d/c Mn × 1 year	10/15 increased MRI signals decreased MRI signals, decreased blood Mn levels
Fitzgerald et al., 1999	36	Adults	Numerous	500 µg/day	<48 h of PN	RBC Mn: low to normal
	30	Adults	Numerous	500 µg/day	2–28 days	Increased RBC Mn in 2 patients
	21	Adults (14–87)	(18 home PN patients)	500	36–5075 days	Increased RBC Mn in 15/21 patients 3 selected cases of abnormal MRI
Forbes and Jawhari, 1996	29	Adults	Home PN patients (11 patients with biochemical evidence of cholestasis)	3–17 µg/kg per day	4 years (3 months– 14 years)	25/29 had increased whole blood Mn levels; no relationship to levels with cholestasis
Mirowitz et al., 1991	9	58.9 years (51–74)	Crohn's disease, scleroderma, intestinal infarction, esophageal stricture	0.3–0.4 mg/day	5.3 years (5 months–11 years)	Increased T1 weighted MRI signals in all 9 patients; intensity not correlated with PN duration
Reimund et al., 2000	21	55 ± 14 years	IBD (n = 6), radiation enteritis (n = 7), ischemic bowel (n = 5), pseudo-obstruction (n = 3)	1 mg/day	30 ± 37 months (3–132 months)	Increased plasma Mn compared to controls
	10	Matched	Healthy controls			11/11 increased T1 MRI signals in basal ganglia
Wardle et al., 1999	20	43 years (24–66)	Crohn's disease (n = 15), SBS (n = 13), intestinal failure (n = 2)	1 mg/day	43 months (3–168 months)	Increased whole blood Mn in 26/30 patients; MRI normal (n = 2)

d/c, discontinued; IBD, inflammatory bowel disease; MRI, magnetic resonance imaging; PN, parenteral nutrition; RBC, red blood cell; SBS, short bowel syndrome.

manganese, duration of use, and the presence of significant liver disease (Table 12.4). Others have suggested age as a risk factor for development of toxicity, with infants/children and older adults being more susceptible to manganese toxicity. However, it is difficult to be certain that age is an important determinant for risk of toxicity, as published case reports and series are limited. Manganese, like copper, is eliminated predominantly via the hepatobiliary system. Patients with significant hepatobiliary disease may have impaired excretion of these minerals and, intuitively, may be particularly predisposed to manganese toxicity. Some of the first cases of clinical symptoms from hypermanganesemia associated with parenteral nutrition therapy were described in patients with cholestatic liver disease (Mehta and Reilly, 1990; Taylor and Manara, 1994). Close inspection of the onset and resolution of signs and symptoms of manganese toxicity suggest that patients with liver disease receiving parenteral manganese tend to develop signs and symptoms of intoxication more rapidly than the long-term parenteral nutrition patient without cholestatic liver disease. Conversely, the symptoms tend to resolve sooner over a period of several days to few weeks, whereas the long-term patient may take months and may exhibit some residual symptomatology (Dickerson, 2001).

Dosage of parenteral manganese is also an important determinant of risk factor for toxicity. Many of the case reports of manganese intoxication are in those adults who received ≥ 1 mg/day of parenteral manganese or >40 µg/kg per day in pediatric patients. However, elevated manganese levels, abnormal MRI signals, or symptoms of hypermanganesemia have occurred at more "conventional doses" (the AMA NAG recommendations (American Medical Association, 1979)) from 0.15 to 0.8 mg/day in patients without liver disease when taken over a prolonged period of time (>3 months to several years). Although safe and sufficient quantities of parenteral manganese intake are generally unknown, supplementation of 0.1 to 0.3 mg/day (lower dosage range of the AMA NAG recommendations) may be sufficient in many long-term adult parenteral nutrition patients without liver disease (Dickerson, 2001).

Zinc

Zinc is an essential trace element, is involved in numerous enzymatic functions in humans and is essential for normal protein synthesis, and in the elaboration of the immune response to critical illness. Zinc losses are exaggerated during critical illness and in patients with gastrointestinal fluid losses (Wolman et al., 1979). However, parenteral zinc, when given in excess, exhibits toxicities. One of the first reports of the toxicity of parenteral zinc in parenteral nutrition solutions was given by Faintuch and Faintuch et al. (1978). Seven patients receiving parenteral nutrition were inadvertently given 100 mg/day of zinc sulfate (instead of 10 mg/day) for 26 to 60 days. Six of the seven patients exhibited hyperamylasemia during most of the period of excessive zinc administration and in one patient, hyperamylasemia persisted for several weeks after discontinuation of zinc administration. Peak hyperamylasemia occurred approximately at 12 to 60 days of excessive zinc supplementation. None of the patients had clinical signs of pancreatitis; however, pancreatic damage has been noted in animals given large doses of zinc over a prolonged time period (Scott and Fisher, 1938). Mortality was very high in this population, with five out of the seven patients dying from septic complications. The authors suggested that the septic deaths and zinc therapy were not related, as the infectious complications occurred before the appearance of the hyperamylasemia.

However, Faintuck *et al.*'s conclusions may be potentially erroneous as more recent data suggest that zinc intoxication may have some detrimental effects on the patient's metabolic response to infection. Parenteral zinc supplementation at 30 mg/day of zinc chloride may increase the febrile response in parenterally-fed infected patients (Braunschweig *et al.*, 1997). Aggressive oral zinc supplementation has been shown to impair polymorphonuclear leukocyte function in healthy subjects (Chandra, 1984) and monocyte function during nutritional rehabilitation in marasmic infants (Schlesinger *et al.*, 1993). It is pertinent to view these data in light of Wolman *et al.*'s (1979) estimation of zinc losses in gastrointestinal fluids. Their data suggest that between 12 and 17 mg of zinc is lost for every liter of gastrointestinal fluid lost – depending on the site of the gastrointestinal fluids. However, the authors state that a positive zinc balance was readily achieved with 12 mg/day. Therefore, erroneous conclusions could be easily drawn from their data if their estimates were applied to a patient with massive gastrointestinal fluid losses (e.g. secretory diarrhea). Theoretically, evidence of zinc toxicity may occur at these high doses. Further research is necessary before conclusions can be drawn between zinc supplementation, immune function, and infectious events in hospitalized patients.

Iron

The American Medical Association National Advisory Group did not provide any guidelines for parenteral iron needs of parenterally-fed adult patients. It has been estimated that men may require 0.5 to 1 mg/day of elemental iron and menstruating women may require up to 2.8 mg/day. However, these estimates may be higher than actual needs as there is a reduced loss of iron from decreased turnover of intestinal cells in the parenterally-fed patient. Parenteral iron is not as efficiently used for hematopoiesis as orally absorbed iron. Only about 40% of the parenterally delivered iron is incorporated into new erythrocytes of anemic subjects, compared to 80% to 90% of enterally absorbed iron. Parenteral iron (dextran) has a propensity to be taken up by the recticuloendothelial system. Excessive iron is stored in the body as ferritin or hemosiderin which a non-toxic forms of iron. Hemosiderosis and hepatomegaly have occurred in patients given excessive iron dextran (Pitts and Barbour, 1978). Another classic presentation of significant hemosiderosis with parenteral iron excess is the bronzing/sun tan color of the skin in caucasians caused by hemosiderin deposition in the skin. Although hemochromatosis (inflammation and fibrosis) from parenteral iron therapy has been demonstrated in animal models, a literature search by the author did not reveal any cases of hemochromatosis from parenteral iron therapy in patients without genetic predisposition to thalassemia.

Aluminum

Aluminum has been a known contaminant of parenteral nutrition solutions for over two decades (Klein *et al.*, 1982). As discussed in the amino acids section, a major source of aluminum contamination came from the now defunct casein hydrolysates protein source. Metabolic bone disease appeared to improve in some long-term patients after withdrawal from the casein hydrolysates and then provided crystalline amino acids (Klein *et al.*, 1982; Ott *et al.*, 1983; Vargas *et al.*, 1988). Aluminum exerts toxic effects on tissues other than bone, notably the central nervous system and the liver. Although aluminum-induced encephalopathy has been noted in chronic dialysis patients, this toxicity has not been reported in long-term parenterally fed adult patients (Klein, 1995). Additionally, aluminum accumulates in the liver of parenterally fed patients and has caused cholestasis in animals. However, it is not clear whether aluminum may cause hepatotoxicity in parenterally-fed humans (Klein, 1995). Unfortunately, aluminum contamination is abundant in many parenteral nutrition solution additives such as calcium gluconate, calcium gluceptate, sodium phosphate, potassium phosphate, and albumin (Klein, 1995; Koo *et al.*, 1986). The variability of aluminum contamination is even different in the same product by the same manufacturer from lot to lot (Klein, 1995). In an effort to regulate the amount of contaminants that may pose a toxic threat, the FDA has proposed an upper limit of 25 µg/L in large-volume parenteral drug products. For small-volume parenteral products, the proposed labeling on the immediate container is the quantity of aluminum in the product at the time the product was released. Pharmacists could then estimate the total aluminum load of the compounded parenteral nutrition solution. The FDA developed some suggested guidelines to define the "safe", "unsafe", and "toxic" amounts of aluminum in a parenteral nutrition solution (Klein, 1995). These guidelines are provided in Table 12.5.

Table 12.5 Guidelines for the definition of safe, unsafe, and toxic amounts of aluminum in parenteral nutrition solutions (adapted from Klein, 1995)

	Safe	*Unsafe*	*Toxic*
Definition	Results in neither tissue loading nor dysfunction	Results in tissue loading without clear evidence of tissue dysfunction	Results in both tissue loading and dysfunction
Dose	~2 µg/kg/per day (0.074 µmol/kg per day)	15–30 µg/kg per day (0.56–1.11 µmol/kg per day)	~60 µg/kg per day (2.24 µmol/kg per day)

Other miscellaneous toxic substances

Di (2-ethylhexyl) phthalate

Di (2-ethylhexyl) phthalate (DEHP) is a plasticizer incorporated into polyvinyl chloride (PVC) to make intravenous containers and tubing more pliable. Some medical devices, such as PVC tubing, contain up to 40% DEHP by weight (Dickerson, 1997a, 1997b) Contamination of intravenous solutions can occur in solutions containing lipid emulsion which are not administered in DEHP-free containers and tubing. Substances that contain large amounts of phthalates may be harmful if significant leaching from the tubing and container occurs. It has been suggested that phthalate exposure can lead to increased potential for carcinogenicity, hepatic peroxisome proliferation, gonadal toxicity, and hepatic toxicity in animals (Dickerson, 1997a). Because of DEHP leaching into lipid containing solutions, manufacturers are designing containers and tubing that do not use DEHP as a plasticizer. Although the toxicity of DEHP in humans remains an enigma, the potential for long-term exposure would be greatest in the home or long-term parenteral nutrition patient. These patients should receive DEHP-free containers and tubing for provision of their parenteral nutrition solutions. Neonates and infants may be another population for which DEHP-free plastics should be used, as the dwell time for the parenteral nutrition solution in the tubing is prolonged. This would result in increased contact time and increased potential for leaching of the DEHP. Given the controversy over adverse effects in humans, the avoidance of potential adverse effects is likely worth the additional cost of a DEHP-free delivery system.

Anti-oxidants and preservatives

A few case reports of hypersensitivity reactions to parenteral nutrition have appeared in the literature (Dalton-Bunnow, 1985; Nagata, 1993; Udall and Richardson, 1986). Most of these reports have attributed these effects to either lipid emulsion or iron dextran. Some of these patients may have been allergic to soybean protein (the oil source) or to eggs (the source of phospholipid). Those lipid-free parenteral nutrition solutions that have caused mild adverse hyper-sensitivity reactions could be managed with antihistamine pharmacotherapy if the parenteral nutrition solution could not be discontinued. It has been suggested that the multivitamin preparations and specific allergic reactions to thiamine or other vitamins in the preparation may be the culprit with regard to these lipid-free parenteral nutrition solutions (Nagata, 1993); however, it is possible that other preservative/additives may be responsible for these reactions. Although these adverse events are generally mild, they should be considered seriously lest we forget the fatal "gasping syndrome" reactions to the preservative, benzyl alcohol, that occurred in premature infants (Gershanik *et al.*, 1982). To determine which parenteral nutrition component is responsible for the adverse effect, elimination of suspected allergens from the solutions followed by conservative rechallenge is required. If the adverse effect was severe, some clinicians have employed skin testing to determine the potential causative allergen.

Effect of parenteral nutrition on the efficacy of drug therapy

The effect of parenteral nutrition on drug disposition (absorption, distribution, metabolism, and elimination) has not been adequately studied; however, significant potential exists in its ability to alter the pharmacokinetics of drugs. During total parenteral nutrition, various morphologic and physiologic changes occur in the gastrointestinal tract that may potentially alter enteral absorption of medications. Additionally, various components of the parenteral nutrition solution can directly alter drug metabolism and elimination. Fat emulsion has been shown to alter the binding characteristics of drugs to serum proteins as the increase in free fatty acids concentrations following lipid administration has been reported to displace highly protein bound drugs such as morphine, valproic acid, and phenytoin (Phelps et al., 1991). The suppressive effects of parenteral nutrition on hepatic cytochrome P450 concentration and various isozyme activities have been established in animal models (Dickerson and Charland, 2002). A "high index of suspicion" for a potential alteration in drug pharmacokinetics, efficacy, or toxicity should be considered for patients who receive a medication with a narrow therapeutic range when the patient's nutritional regimen is changed to either the parenteral or enteral route.

Conclusion

Patients receiving parenteral nutrition support should be closely evaluated to assess the efficacy and potential toxicities of their therapy. The critically ill hospitalized patient as well as the long-term home nutrition support patient can experience various adverse effects. Practitioners should continue to anticipate and potentially avoid these adverse effects whenever possible. Knowledge of the effects, along with appropriate clinical assessment of a patient's course of disease and therapy, can help facilitate optimal nutrition support for the patient.

References

Abbott, W.C., Grakauskas, A.M., Bistrian, B.R., et al. (1984) Metabolic and respiratory effects of continuous and discontinuous lipid infusions. Occurrence in excess of resting energy expenditure, *Archives of Surgery*, **119**: 1367–1371.

Allardyce, D.B. (1982) Cholestasis caused by lipid emulsions, *Surgical Gynecology and Obstetrics*, **154**: 641–647.

Alves, G., Thiebot, J., Tracqui, A., et al. (1997) Neurologic disorders due to brain manganese deposition in a jaundiced patient receiving long-term parenteral nutrition, *Journal of Parenteral and Enteral Nutrition*, **21**: 41–45.

American Medical Association (1979) Guidelines for essential trace element preparations for parenteral use: a statement by the Nutrition Advisory Group, *Journal of the American Medical Association*, **241**: 2051–2054.

Askanazi, J., Carpentier, Y.A., Elwyn, D.H., *et al.* (1980) Influence of total parenteral nutrition on fuel utilization in injury and sepsis, *Annals of Surgery*, **191**: 40–46.

Askanazi, J., Nordenstrom, J., Rosenbaum, S.H., *et al.* (1981) Nutrition for the patient with respiratory failure: glucose vs. fat, *Anesthesiology*, **54**: 373–377.

Askanazi, J., Weissman, C., LaSala, P.A., *et al.* (1984) Effect of protein intake on ventilatory drive, *Anesthesiology*, **60**: 106–110.

Bengoa, J.M., Sitrin, M.D., Wood, R.J., *et al.* (1983) Amino acid-induced hypercalciuria in patients on total parenteral nutrition, *American Journal of Clinical Nutrition*, **38**: 264–269.

Bertinet, D.B., Tinivella, M., Balzola, F.A., *et al.* (2000) Brain manganese deposition and blood levels in patients undergoing home parenteral nutrition, *Journal of Parenteral and Enteral Nutrition*, **24**: 223–227.

Black, P.R., Brooks, D.C., Bessey, P.Q., *et al.* (1982) Mechanisms of insulin resistance following injury, *Annals of Surgery*, **196**: 420–435.

Bowyer, B.A., Fleming, C.R., Ludwig, J., *et al.* (1985) Does long-term home parenteral nutrition in adult patients cause chronic liver disease?, *Journal of Parenteral and Enteral Nutrition*, **9**: 11–17.

Braunschweig, C.L., Sowers, M., Kovacevich, D.S., *et al.* (1997) Parenteral zinc supplementation in adult humans during the acute phase response increases the febrile response, *Journal of Nutrition*, **127**: 70–74.

Brown, R.O. and Dickerson, R.N. (1999) Drug–nutrient interactions, *American Journal of Managed Care*, **5**: 345–352; quiz 353–355.

Buckspan, R., Woltering, E., and Waterhouse, G. (1984) Pancreatitis induced by intravenous infusion of a fat emulsion in an alcoholic patient, *South Medical Journal*, **77**: 251–252.

Burke, J.F., Wolfe, R.R., Mullany, C.J., *et al.* (1979) Glucose requirements following burn injury. Parameters of optimal glucose infusion and possible hepatic and respiratory abnormalities following excessive glucose intake, *Annals of Surgery*, **190**: 274–285.

Cameron, J.L., Capuzzi, D.M., Zuidema, G.D., *et al.* (1973) Acute pancreatitis with hyperlipemia: the incidence of lipid abnormalities in acute pancreatitis, *Annals of Surgery*, **177**: 483–489.

Chan, S., McCowen, K.C., Bistrian, B.R., *et al.* (1999) Incidence, prognosis, and etiology of end-stage liver disease in patients receiving home total parenteral nutrition, *Surgery*, **126**: 28–34.

Chandra, R.K. (1984) Excessive intake of zinc impairs immune responses, *Journal of the American Medical Association*, **252**: 1443–1446.

Cole, D.E. and Zlotkin, S.H. (1983) Increased sulfate as an etiological factor in the hypercalciuria associated with total parenteral nutrition, *American Journal of Clinical Nutrition*, **37**: 108–113.

Cundy, T., Earnshaw, M., Heynen, G., *et al.* (1983) Vitamin A and hyperparathyroid bone disease in uremia, *American Journal of Clinical Nutrition*, **38**: 914–920.

Dalton-Bunnow, M.F. (1985) Review of sulfite sensitivity, *American Journal of Hospital Pharmacy*, **42**: 2220–2226.

Dickerson, R.N. (1986) Intravenous lipid emulsion in pulmonary disease: beneficial or detrimental? *Hospital Pharmacy*, **21**: 348–352.

Dickerson, R.N. (1997a) Di(2-ethylhexyl)phthalate as a plasticizer for intravenous bags and tubing: a toxicological quandary, *Nutrition*, **13**: 1010–1012.

Dickerson, R.N. (1997b) Leaching of di (2-ethylhexyl) phthalate from plastic bags and tubing, *Hospital Pharmacology*, **32**: 737–738.

Dickerson, R.N. (2001) Manganese intoxication and parenteral nutrition, *Nutrition*, **17**: 689–693.

Dickerson, R.N., Boschert, K.J., Kudsk, K.A., *et al.* (2002) Hypocaloric enteral tube feeding in critically ill obese patients, *Nutrition*, **18**: 241–246.

Dickerson, R.N. and Charland, S.L. (2002) The effect of sepsis during parenteral nutrition on hepatic microsomal function in rats, *Pharmacotherapy*, **22**: 1084–1090.

Dickerson, R.N. and Karwoski, C.B. (2002) Endotoxin-mediated hepatic lipid accumulation during parenteral nutrition in rats, *Journal of the American College of Nutrition*, **21**: 351–356.

Dickerson, R.N., Rosato, E.F., and Mullen, J.L. (1986) Net protein anabolism with hypocaloric parenteral nutrition in obese stressed patients, *American Journal of Clinical Nutrition*, **44**: 747–755.

Doty, J.E., Pitt, H.A., Porter-Fink, V., *et al.* (1985) Cholecystokinin prophylaxis of parenteral nutrition-induced gallbladder disease, *Annals of Surgery*, **201**: 76–80.

Faintuch, J., Faintuch, J.J., Toledo, M., *et al.* (1978) Hyperamylasemia associated with zinc overdose during parenteral nutrition, *Journal of Parenteral and Enteral Nutrition*, **2**: 640–645.

Fischer, G.W., Hunter, K.W., Wilson, S.R., *et al.* (1980) Diminished bacterial defenses with Intralipid, *Lancet*, **2**: 819–820.

Fitzgerald, K., Mikalunas, V., Rubin, H., *et al.* (1999) Hypermanganesemia in patients receiving total parenteral nutrition, *Journal of Parenteral and Enteral Nutrition*, **23**: 333–336.

Foldes, J., Rimon, B., Muggia-Sullam, M., *et al.* (1990) Progressive bone loss during long-term home total parenteral nutrition, *Journal of Parenteral and Enteral Nutrition*, **14**: 139–142.

Forbes, A. and Jawhari, A. (1996) Manganese toxicity and parenteral nutrition, *Lancet*, **347**: 1774.

Gershanik, J., Boecler, B., Ensley, H., *et al.* (1982) The gasping syndrome and benzyl alcohol poisoning, *New England Journal of Medicine*, **307**: 1384–1388.

Gimmon, Z., Kelley, R.E., Simko, V., *et al.* (1982) Total parenteral nutrition solution increases bile lithogenicity in rat, *Journal of Surgical Research*, **32**: 256–263.

Gleghorn, E.E., Eisenberg, L.D., Hack, S., *et al.* (1986) Observations of vitamin A toxicity in three patients with renal failure receiving parenteral alimentation, *American Journal of Clinical Nutrition*, **44**: 107–112.

Gore, D.C., Wolf, S.E., Herndon, D.N., *et al.* (2002) Relative influence of glucose and insulin on peripheral amino acid metabolism in severely burned patients, *Journal of Parenteral and Enteral Nutrition*, **26**: 271–277.

Grant, J.P., Cox, C.E., Kleinman, L.M., *et al.* (1977) Serum hepatic enzyme and bilirubin elevations during parenteral nutrition, *Surgical Gynecology and Obstetrics*, **145**: 573–580.

Griffin, E., Breckenridge, W.C., Kuksis, A., *et al.* (1979) Appearance and characterization of lipoprotein X during continuous Intralipid infusions in the neonate, *Journal of Clinical Investigation*, **64**: 1703–1712.

Guenst, J.M. and Nelson, L.D. (1994) Predictors of total parenteral nutrition-induced lipogenesis, *Chest*, **105**: 553–559.

Guzman, S., Nervi, F., Llanos, O., *et al.* (1985) Impaired lipid clearance in patients with previous acute pancreatitis, *Gut*, **26**: 888–891.

Hageman, J.R., McCulloch, K., Gora, P., *et al.* (1983) Intralipid alterations in pulmonary prostaglandin metabolism and gas exchange, *Critical Care Medicine*, **11**: 794–798.

Jannace, P.W., Lerman, R.H., Dennis, R.C., *et al.* (1988) Total parenteral nutrition-induced cyclic hypercapnia, *Critical Care Medicine*, **16**: 727–728.

Jensen, G.L., Mascioli, E.A., Seidner, D.L., *et al.* (1990) Parenteral infusion of long- and medium-chain triglycerides and reticuloendothelial system function in man, *Journal of Parenteral and Enteral Nutrition*, **14**: 467–471.

Klein, G.L. (1995) Aluminum in parenteral solutions revisited – again, *American Journal of Clinical Nutrition*, **61**: 449–456.

Klein, G.L., Alfrey, A.C., Miller, N.L., *et al.* (1982) Aluminum loading during total parenteral nutrition, *American Journal of Clinical Nutrition*, **35**: 1425–1429.

Klein, G.L., Ament, M.E., and Coburn, J.W. (1981) Metabolic bone disease in total parenteral nutrition, *Lancet*, **1**: 835.

Klein, G.L., Targoff, C.M., Ament, M.E., *et al.* (1980) Bone disease associated with total parenteral nutrition, *Lancet*, **2**: 1041–1044.

Koo, W.W., Kaplan, L.A., Horn, J., *et al.* (1986) Aluminum in parenteral nutrition solution – sources and possible alternatives, *Journal of Parenteral and Enteral Nutrition*, **10**: 591–595.

Lashner, B.A., Kirsner, J.B., and Hanauer, S.B. (1986) Acute pancreatitis associated with high-concentration lipid emulsion during total parenteral nutrition therapy for Crohn's disease, *Gastroenterology*, **90**: 1039–1041.

Lemoyne, M., Van Gossum, A., Kurian, R., *et al.* (1988) Plasma vitamin E and selenium and breath pentane in home parenteral nutrition patients, *American Journal of Clinical Nutrition*, **48**: 1310–1315.

Levene, M.I., Batisti, O., Wigglesworth, J.S., *et al.* (1984) A prospective study of intrapulmonary fat accumulation in the newborn lung following Intralipid infusion, *Acta Paediatrica Scandinavia*, **73**: 454–460.

Lipkin, E.W., Ott, S.M., and Klein, G.L. (1987) Heterogeneity of bone histology in parenteral nutrition patients, *American Journal of Clinical Nutrition*, **46**: 673–680.

Lipkin, E.W., Ott, S.M., Chesnut, C.H., 3rd, *et al.* (1988) Mineral loss in the parenteral nutrition patient, *American Journal of Clinical Nutrition*, **47**: 515–523.

Lowry, S.F. and Brennan, M.F. (1979) Abnormal liver function during parenteral nutrition: relation to infusion excess, *Journal of Surgical Research*, **26**: 300–307.

Maini, B., Blackburn, G.L., Bistrian, B.R., *et al.* (1976) Cyclic hyperalimentation: an optimal technique for preservation of visceral protein, *Journal of Surgical Research*, **20**: 515–525.

McCowen, K.C., Friel, C., Sternberg, J., *et al.* (2000) Hypocaloric total parenteral nutrition: effectiveness in prevention of hyperglycemia and infectious complications – a randomized clinical trial, *Critical Care Medicine*, **28**: 3606–3611.

McCowen, K.C., Malhotra, A., and Bistrian, B.R. (2001) Stress-induced hyperglycemia, *Critical Care Clinics*, **17**: 107–124.

Meguid, M.M., Akahoshi, M.P., Jeffers, S., *et al.* (1984) Amelioration of metabolic complications of conventional total parenteral nutrition. A prospective randomized study, *Archives of Surgery*, **119**: 1294–1298.

Mehta, R. and Reilly, J.J. (1990) Manganese levels in a jaundiced long-term total parenteral nutrition patient: potentiation of haloperidol toxicity? Case report and literature review, *Journal of Parenteral and Enteral Nutrition*, **14**: 428–430.

Michel, H., Bories, P., Aubin, J.P., *et al.* (1985) Treatment of acute hepatic encephalopathy in cirrhotics with a branched-chain amino acids enriched versus a conventional amino acids mixture. A controlled study of 70 patients, *Liver*, **5**: 282–289.

Mirowitz, S.A., Westrich, T.J., and Hirsch, J.D. (1991) Hyperintense basal ganglia on T1-weighted MR images in patients receiving parenteral nutrition, *Radiology*, **181**: 117–120.

Mirtallo, J.M., Schneider, P.J., Mavko, K., *et al.* (1982) A comparison of essential and general amino acid infusions in the nutritional support of patients with compromised renal function, *Journal of Parenteral and Enteral Nutrition*, **6**: 109–113.

Muenter, M.D., Perry, H.O., and Ludwig, J. (1971) Chronic vitamin A intoxication in adults. Hepatic, neurologic and dermatologic complications, *American Journal of Medicine*, **50**: 129–136.

Nagata, M.J. (1993) Hypersensitivity reactions associated with parenteral nutrition: case report and review of the literature, *Annals of Pharmacotherapy*, **27**: 174–177.

Naylor, C.D., O'Rourke, K., Detsky, A.S., *et al.* (1989) Parenteral nutrition with branched-chain amino acids in hepatic encephalopathy. A meta-analysis, *Gastroenterology*, **97**: 1033–1042.

Nordenstrom, J., Askanazi, J., Elwyn, D.H., *et al.* (1983) Nitrogen balance during total parenteral nutrition: glucose vs. fat, *Annals of Surgery*, **197**: 27–33.

Nordenstrom, J., Jarstrand, C., and Wiernik, A. (1979) Decreased chemotactic and random migration of leukocytes during Intralipid infusion, *American Journal of Clinical Nutrition*, **32**: 2416–2422.

Ota, D.M., Jessup, J.M., Babcock, G.F., *et al.* (1985) Immune function during intravenous administration of a soybean oil emulsion, *Journal of Parenteral and Enteral Nutrition*, **9**: 23–27.

Ott, S.M., Maloney, N.A., Klein, G.L., *et al.* (1983) Aluminum is associated with low bone formation in patients receiving chronic parenteral nutrition, *Annals of Internal Medicine*, **98**: 910–914.

Patino, J.F., de Pimiento, S.E., Vergara, A., *et al.* (1999) Hypocaloric support in the critically ill, *World Journal of Surgery*, **23**: 553–559.

Phelps, S.J., Brown, R.O., Helms, R.A., *et al.* (1991) Toxicities of parenteral nutrition in the critically ill patient, *Critical Care Clinics*, **7**: 725–753.

Pironi, L., Zolezzi, C., Ruggeri, E., *et al.* (2000) Bone turnover in short-term and long-term home parenteral nutrition for benign disease, *Nutrition*, **16**: 272–277.

Pitts, T.O. and Barbour, G.L. (1978) Hemosiderosis secondary to chronic parenteral iron therapy in maintenance hemodialysis patients, *Nephron*, **22**: 316–321.

Pomposelli, J.J., Baxter, J.K., 3rd, Babineau, T.J., *et al.* (1998) Early postoperative glucose control predicts nosocomial infection rate in diabetic patients, *Journal of Parenteral and Enteral Nutrition*, **22**: 77–81.

Pomposelli, J.J. and Bistrian, B.R. (1994) Is total parenteral nutrition immunosuppressive?, *New Horizons*, **2**: 224–229.

Reimund, J.M., Dietemann, J.L., Warter, J.M., *et al.* (2000) Factors associated to hypermanganesemia in patients receiving home parenteral nutrition, *Clinical Nutrition*, **19**: 343–348.

Robin, A.P., Arain, I., Phuangsab, A., *et al.* (1989) Intravenous fat emulsion acutely suppresses neutrophil chemiluminescence, *Journal of Parenteral and Enteral Nutrition*, **13**: 608–613.

Robin, A.P., Campbell, R., Palani, C.K., *et al.* (1990) Total parenteral nutrition during acute pancreatitis: clinical experience with 156 patients, *World Journal of Surgery*, **14**: 572–579.

Rollan, A., Guzman, S., Pimentel, F., *et al.* (1990) Catabolism of chylomicron remnants in patients with previous acute pancreatitis, *Gastroenterology*, **98**: 1649–1654.

Roslyn, J.J., Pitt, H.A., Mann, L.L., *et al.* (1983) Gallbladder disease in patients on long-term parenteral nutrition, *Gastroenterology*, **84**: 148–154.

Rosmarin, D.K., Warlaw, G.M., and Mirtallo, J. (1996) Hyperglycemia associated with high, continuous infusion rates of total parenteral nutrition dextrose, *Nutrition in Clinical Practice*, **11**: 151–156.

Schlesinger, L., Arevalo, M., Arredondo, S., *et al.* (1993) Zinc supplementation impairs monocyte function, *Acta Paediatrica*, **82**: 734–738.

Schroder, H., Paust, H., and Schmidt, R. (1984) Pulmonary fat embolism after intralipid therapy – a post-mortem artefact? Light and electron microscopic investigations in low-birth-weight infants, *Acta Paediatrica Scandinavia*, **73**: 461–464.

Scott, D.A. and Fisher, A.M. (1938) Studies on the pancreas and liver of normal and zinc-fed cats, *American Journal of Physiology*, **121**: 253–260.

Seibert, J.J., Byrne, W.J., and Golladay, E.S. (1981) Development of hypervitaminosis A in a patient on long-term parenteral hyperalimentation, *Pediatric Radiology*, **10**: 173–174.

Seidner, D.L., Mascioli, E.A., Istfan, N.W., *et al.* (1989) Effects of long-chain triglyceride emulsions on reticuloendothelial system function in humans, *Journal of Parenteral and Enteral Nutrition*, **13**: 614–619.

Sheldon, G.F., Peterson, S.R., and Sanders, R. (1978) Hepatic dysfunction during hyperalimentation, *Archives of Surgery*, **113**: 504–508.

Shike, M., Harrison, J.E., Sturtridge, W.C., *et al.* (1980) Metabolic bone disease in patients receiving long-term total parenteral nutrition, *Annals of Internal Medicine*, **92**: 343–350.

Shike, M., Shils, M.E., Heller, A., *et al.* (1986) Bone disease in prolonged parenteral nutrition: osteopenia without mineralization defect, *American Journals of Clinical Nutrition*, **44**: 89–98.

Shike, M., Sturtridge, W.C., Tam, C.S., *et al.* (1981) A possible role of vitamin D in the genesis of parenteral-nutrition-induced metabolic bone disease, *Annals of Internal Medicine*, **95**: 560–568.

Silberman, H., Dixon, N.P., and Eisenberg, D. (1982) The safety and efficacy of a lipid-based system of parenteral nutrition in acute pancreatitis, *American Journal of Gastroenterology*, **77**: 494–497.

Simmons, R.S., Berdine, G.G., Seidenfeld, J.J., *et al.* (1987) Fluid balance and the adult respiratory distress syndrome, *American Review of Respiratory Diseases*, **135**: 924–929.

Sitzmann, J.V., Steinborn, P.A., Zinner, M.J., *et al.* (1989) Total parenteral nutrition and alternate energy substrates in treatment of severe acute pancreatitis, *Surgical Gynecology and Obstetrics*, **168**: 311–317.

Talpers, S.S., Romberger, D.J., Bunce, S.B., *et al.* (1992) Nutritionally associated increased carbon dioxide production. Excess total calories vs high proportion of carbohydrate calories, *Chest*, **102**: 551–555.

Taylor, R.F. and Buckner, C.D. (1982) Fat overload from 10 percent soybean oil emulsion in a marrow transplant recipient, *West Journal of Medicine*, **136**: 345–349.

Taylor, S. and Manara, A.R. (1994) Manganese toxicity in a patient with cholestasis receiving total parenteral nutrition [letter] [see comments], *Anaesthesia*, **49**: 1013.

Tulikoura, I. and Huikuri, K. (1982) Morphological fatty changes and function of the liver, serum free fatty acids, and triglycerides during parenteral nutrition, *Scandinavian Journal of Gastroenterology*, **17**: 177–185.

Udall, J.N. and Richardson, D.S. (1986) Allergic reactions to parenteral nutrition solutions, *Nutritional Support Services*, **6**: 20–22.

Van den Berghe, G., Wouters, P., Weekers, F., et al. (2001) Intensive insulin therapy in the critically ill patients, New England Journal of Medicine, 345: 1359–1367.

Vargas, J.H., Klein, G.L., Ament, M.E., et al. (1988) Metabolic bone disease of total parenteral nutrition: course after changing from casein to amino acids in parenteral solutions with reduced aluminum content, American Journal of Clinical Nutrition, 48: 1070–1078.

Veech, R.L. (1986) The toxic impact of parenteral solutions on the metabolism of cells: a hypothesis for physiological parenteral therapy, American Journal of Clinical Nutrition, 44: 519–551.

de Vernejoul, M.C., Messing, B., Modrowski, D., et al. (1985) Multifactorial low remodeling bone disease during cyclic total parenteral nutrition, Journal of Clinical Endocrinol Metabolism, 60: 109–113.

Wagner, W.H., Lowry, A.C., and Silberman, H. (1983) Similar liver function abnormalities occur in patients receiving glucose-based and lipid-based parenteral nutrition, American Journal of Gastroenterology, 78: 199–202.

Wardle, C.A., Forbes, A., Roberts, N.B., et al. (1999) Hypermanganesemia in long-term intravenous nutrition and chronic liver disease, Journal of Parenteral and Enteral Nutrition, 23: 350–355.

Weinsier, R.L., Bacon, J., and Butterworth, C.E., Jr (1982) Central venous alimentation: a prospective study of the frequency of metabolic abnormalities among medical and surgical patients, Journal of Parenteral and Enteral Nutrition, 6: 421–425.

Wilmore, D.W., Aulick, L.H., Mason, A.D., et al. (1977) Influence of the burn wound on local and systemic responses to injury, Annals of Surgery, 186: 444–458.

Wolfe, R.R., Allsop, J.R., and Burke, J.F. (1979) Glucose metabolism in man: responses to intravenous glucose infusion, Metabolism, 28: 210–220.

Wolman, S.L., Anderson, G.H., Marliss, E.B., et al. (1979) Zinc in total parenteral nutrition: requirements and metabolic effects, Gastroenterology, 76: 458–467.

Wood, R.J., Bengoa, J.M., Sitrin, M.D., et al. (1985) Calciuretic effect of cyclic versus continuous total parenteral nutrition, American Journal of Clinical Nutrition, 41: 614–619.

13 Safety of probiotic bacteria

Seppo Salminen, Erika Isolauri, and
Atte von Wright

Background

Probiotics

Probiotic bacteria, by definition, are living microbial food components or inactivated microbes or parts of microbes that have a beneficial effect on human health (Isolauri *et al.*, 2002; Salminen *et al.*, 1998). The probiotic definition requires that the efficacy and safety of probiotics be verified, and thus the assessment of probiotic safety is an important part of their characterization for human use.

Generally the microbes used in food fermentations have a long history of safe use. There are a few published case reports of rare infections involving lactobacilli and bifidobacteria, species among which the most common probiotics have been selected. Therefore, the safety of probiotics needs to be assessed especially when new, more adhesive or more effective strains are selected and characterized. Evidence-based data on safety and efficacy for human use should be required for all future probiotics.

Safety: how should it be defined?

Safety is defined as the state of being protected from the risk of experiencing or causing injury or disease. The safety of lactic acid bacteria in foods and food fermentations has never been in question; rather, the use of lactic acid bacteria in food fermentations has resulted in food products with longer shelf life and enhanced safety profile. However, the more recent use of intestinal isolates of various bacteria as probiotics to be delivered in high numbers to consumers with potentially suppressed immune function or chronic diseases has raised the question of safety. Thus, by the recent probiotic definition, safety assessment should address both viable and inactivated or nonviable probiotics.

At present probiotics consist mostly of *Lactobacillus* and *Bifidobacterium* species and thus the safety discussion is focused on them. However, new genera and species, such as clostridia, *Bacillus* and others, are suggested as potential probiotics. The emergence of new probiotics challenges the safety assessment procedures in the future. The assurance of safety and the future safety assessment procedures are important factors guiding probiotic development and the confidence of consumers on probiotic use.

History of safe use of food microbes

The safety of lactobacilli and bifidobacteria has been discussed in both probiotic use and food fermentation or starter culture use (Adams and Marteau, 1995; Salminen and Arvilommi, 2002; Salminen *et al.*, 1998a, 1998b; Sipsas *et al.*, 2002). In general, the pathogenic potential of lactobacilli and bifidobacteria appears quite low. The conclusion is based on the extensive presence of these microbes in many fermented foods, as commensal colonizers of the mucous surfaces of the human body and as part of the normal healthy human intestinal microbiota, and the concomitant low level of infection attributed to them. However, reports of association of lactobacilli and bifidobacteria with human infection (commonly endocarditis) in patients with compromised health has been considered to suggest that some of these microbes may have opportunistic detrimental properties. A report from the Lactic Acid Bacteria Industrial Platform (LABIP) concluded that the overall risk of infection from lactic acid bacteria (excluding enterococci) is very low, but that *Lactobacillus rhamnosus* deserved particular surveillance due to the greater proportion of infections attributed to this species compared to other lactobacilli (Adams and Marteau, 1995). One commercial strain, *Lactobacillus rhamnosus* GG (ATCC 53013), has been used safely and extensively in clinical trials and human studies, including one involving enteral feeding of premature infants with no indication of pathogenic potential. These conclusions have been also supported by the ILSI Europe working group on functional food science and intestinal health (Salminen *et al.*, 1998a) and the European probiotic research consortium PROBDEMO (Salminen *et al.*, 1998b) as well as several international working groups and reports (Holzapfel *et al.*, 2001; Ishibashi and Yamazaki, 2001; Marteau and Adams, 1997; O'Brien *et al.*, 1999; Saarela *et al.*, 2000; Salminen and Arvilommi, 2002; Salminen *et al.*, 1998a, 2001; von Wright and Salminen, 1999).

Regarding the safety of enterococci, the picture is less clear-cut. Foods containing enterococci have been traditionally consumed in different parts of the world. However, safety reports seem to agree that the enterococci pose a greater threat than other lactic acid bacteria. Enterococci have been isolated from clinical infections as well as bloodstream and endocarditis infections much more frequently than lactic acid bacteria or bifidobacteria. *Enterococcus*-mediated infections of the biliary tract, urogenital tract, the abdomen, burn wounds, surgical wounds, and many others have been reported. Often, enterococci are isolated as pure cultures from these infections, showing their primary pathogenic nature. In the USA, vancomycin-resistant enterococci are the number one cause of hospital-acquired infections. Enterococci have been reported to transfer antibiotic resistance properties to other microbes within the intestinal milieu. These observations and contradictory characteristics of enterococci justify the scrutiny of these microorganisms as probiotic agents.

Epidemiological studies and history of safe use of probiotics

Epidemiological surveillance of probiotic related infections forms a basis for safety assessment of current probiotic strains. Such surveillance studies have been reported for lactic acid bacteria and bifidobacteria indicating that extremely rare bacteremia cases exist with these bacteria identified in blood samples, Reported cases have not been associated with probiotic use (Saxelin *et al.*, 1996a, 1996b). Moreover, such bacteremia cases are often preceded by serious other underlying diseases and often previous bacteremia episodes treated with antibiotics. Other studies have collected epidemiological information and indicated that infections caused by lactic acid bacteria are very rare (Aquirre and Collins, 1993). It has been proposed that immunocompromised patients would be more prone to infection and especially opportunistic infections. At present, no information is available on potentially increased risk when assessing epidemiology studies on bacteremia (Apostolou *et al.*, 2001; Saxelin *et al.*, 1996a, 1996b). At least two studies on probiotic use by immunocompromised subjects and the epidemiology studies together attest to the safety of currently used probiotics (Cunningham-Rundles *et al.*, 2000; Saxelin *et al.*, 1996a, 1996b; Wolf *et al.*, 1998). The recent study from Finland summarizes a decade of rapidly increasing probiotic consumption with increases in bacteremia cases associated with lactic acid bacteria. Some changes in case numbers are indicated and they suggest the need for further epidemiological surveillance studies, especially in subjects with severe underlying diseases (Salminen *et al.*, 2002).

Safety criteria for microbes

Taxonomy as a determinant

Identification of a probiotic strain and deposition in an international culture collection for future reference are important factors related to safety. Species identification alone may not be sufficient and probiotics and starter cultures should always be characterized to strain level. Proper identification may also be associated with safety and the occurrence of the species or strain in intestinal environments. Most current probiotics belong to a limited number of species of mainly the genera *Bifidobacterium* and *Lactobacillus*, other genera are increasingly introduced and used as probiotics.

Most species in the genera *Bifidobacterium* and *Lactobacillus* are considered safe (Adams and Marteau, 1995; Salminen *et al.*, 1998a). There is some concern that *L. rhamnosus* may be more often associated with bacteremia than other *Lactobacillus* species (Adams and Marteau, 1995; Berufsgenossenschaft de chemischen Industrie, 1998). However, since *L. rhamnosus* is among the most common *Lactobacillus* species in the human intestine (Adawi *et al.*, 2001;

Apostolou *et al.*, 2001) this may be secondary to the extensive presence in the intestine. Among bifidobacteria, only *B. dentium*, *B. denticolens* and *B. inopinatum* are of potential concern as they have been found to be associated with human caries.

Potential risk factors

Virulence factors have always been described for pathogens, but defining virulence factors or even risk factors for non-pathogenic lactic acid bacteria and bifidobacteria has been unsuccessful. Several possible risk factors have been proposed for the assessment of the safety of probiotics. Such factors include strong adherence to intestinal mucosa and other mucosal surfaces suggested to relate to translocation potential, production of harmful metabolites, direct acute toxicity, and factors such as platelet aggregation possibly predisposing to endocarditis (Salminen *et al.*, 1998b; Salminen and von Wright, 1998). However, none of the suggested factors have been proved to be risk factors for lactic acid bacteria.

Traditional toxicity studies

One of the most direct ways to assess the safety of a probiotic is to determine the LD_{50}. This gives general information on the potential toxicity, or absence of it. Acute and chronic toxicity tests have been performed for a number of probiotic strains. The LD_{50} for mice was found to be high for all tested strains, for some even more than 50 g/kg body weight (Donohue *et al.*, 1993). Despite the high exposure, no translocation outside the intestine was observed and the toxicity measured by this test system can be considered extremely low (Zhou *et al.*, 2000).

Microbial metabolism

Many of the suggested risk factors have been related to the metabolism of the microbe. Hyaluronidase and gelatinase activity may damage the extracellular matrix proteins, thereby causing direct tissue damage. Not much is known about this enzymatic activity in lactobacilli and bifidobacteria, but it is a relatively common property of enterococci (Franz *et al.*, 1999).

Degradation of intestinal mucus is a normal phenomenon in the cecum and colon whereby several microorganisms are involved. However, excessive degradation may cause damage to the intestinal mucosal barrier function. The ability of probiotics to degrade intestinal mucus has been investigated for several strains *in vitro*. So far no degradation has been observed for any of the tested strains (Ruseler-van Embden *et al.*, 1995; Zhou *et al.*, 2000). In human studies, no change in excretion of mucus was observed upon consumption of probiotics (Ouwehand *et al.*, 2002) suggesting that probotics do not take part in the degradation of intestinal mucus.

Intrinsic microbial properties

Some suggested virulence factors are related to specific intrinsic properties of lactobacilli and bifidobacteria: the ability to produce a capsule or the ability to transfer genetic material. With the exception of enterococci, the ability to transfer genetic material is low in lactic acid bacteria. The presence of antibiotic resistance plasmids and transposable genetic elements has been reported to be rare among lactobacilli and bifidobacteria (von Wright and Sibakov, 1998), but it may occur and plasmids carrying resistance for erythromycin and related macrolides have been observed (Teuber et al., 1999). Thus, although the spread of antibiotic resistance through lactobacilli is far less likely than with enterococci, it should be considered as one of the first steps of safety assessment.

Mucosal adhesion

Adhesion and differences in adhesion properties to the intestinal mucosa have been among the main selection criteria for probiotics. These are thought to be important for local effects, prolonged transient colonization of the intestinal mucosal surfaces and contents, modulation of the host immune system and competitive exclusion of pathogens (Ouwehand et al., 2001a). However, adhesion to the intestinal mucosa is also the first step in pathogenesis. Strong adhesion has been suggested to act as a risk factor for platelet aggregation with harmful health properties (Harty et al., 1993, 1994). However, in comparative studies with bacteremia *Lactobacillus* isolates, no correlation between harmful properties and adherence properties could be observed. On the contrary, the strains causing platelet aggregation exhibited a low level of adhesion, indicating that adhesion is not associated with platelet aggregation (Kirjavainen et al., 1999).

Enterococci as a special safety concern

Enterococci (previously group D streptococci) are ubiquitously present as harmless commensals in the intestinal tract of humans and animals. They can also be found in various other habitats such as in plant material or in various foods, either as contaminants and spoilage organisms or as deliberately used starters (Giraffa, 2002; Giraffa et al., 1997). Some strains are also used as probiotics (Fris-Møller and Hey, 1983). However, in recent years enterocci have emerged as important pathogens in hospital environment (Moellering, 1992).

The factors that contribute to the virulence of enterococcal strains are not well understood, but adhesins, haemolysin, hyaluronidase, aggregation substances, and gelatinase have been implicated in the pathogenicity (Franz et al., 1999). Recently the occurrence of several supposed virulence factors has been screened among food and clinical enterococcal isolates (Franz et al., 2001). Although clinical isolates tended to have virulence factors more frequently than food isolates or starter strains, there was no clearcut difference between strains of clinical and food origin. In one of the studies two *Enterococcus faecium* strains used as probiotics were included and were found not to contain any of the virulence factors tested (Franz *et al.*, 2001). Interestingly, no comparable screens of intestinal strains appear to have been published.

An additional safety aspect with enterococci is that many strains are multi-resistant to antibiotics (Landman and Quale, 1997). Enterococcal transferable vancomycin resistance has been a cause of special concern, since vancomycin is one of the few reserve antibiotics effective against multiresistant staphylococci, and vancomycin resistant enterococcal strains have been frequently isolated from fecal, clinical, and food sources (Jordens *et al.*, 1994; Wegener *et al.*, 1997). Of the main genetic mechanisms behind the enterococcal transferable vancomycin resistance (*VanA*, *VanB*, *VanC*, *VanD*, and *VanE*; Fines *et al.*, 1999; Perichón *et al.*, 1997) at least *VanA* and *VanB* are usually associated with specific transposons (Arthur *et al.*, 1996). The fact that enterococci apparently can very effectively transfer antibiotic resistance elements by conjugation (Clewell, 1999), and the fact that conjugative transfer of certain putative virulence factors have been experimentally observed make the spread of both antibiotic resistance and virulence among enterococcal populations a possibility that has to be taken into account in safety evaluation.

Antibiotic resistance and probiotics

The relevance of antibiotic resistance for safety is highlighted above in the special case of enterococci. In general, if a bacterium is a pathogen or an opportunistic pathogen, its range of antibiotic resistance and sensitivity is of crucial clinical concern. In those cases the distinction between an intrinsic resistance – resulting from natural physiological or structural properties of the organism or from a mutational event – and acquired resistance based on transmissible genetic elements is of secondary importance, with the exception in the latter case of the risk of resistance being transferred to even previously susceptible strains.

Because lactobacilli and bifidobacteria, which represent the most important groups of human probiotics so far, have, in contrast to enterococci, had only a limited role as opportunistic pathogens, relatively little attention has been paid to the antibiotic resistance among these organisms. Plasmids conveying resistance to antibiotics such as erythromycin and other macrolides, tetracycline and chloramphenicol have been occasionally detected in various lactobacillar isolates from mainly fecal sources (Axelsson *et al.*, 1988; Morelli *et al.*, 1983) but also from food (Ahn *et al.*, 1992). These findings have not, so far, triggered any systematic antibiotic resistance screening among the strains used as starters or probiotics.

The increased safety concerns linked with the use of antibiotics as animal growth promoters have, however, focused attention also on the antibiotic resistance factors in the specific case of animal probiotics. Because subtherapeutic concentrations of antibiotics used in animal feeds could select for resistance factors in intestinal bacteria and cause the spreading of resistance to clinically important pathogens, the use of antibiotics as growth promoters is being phased out in the EU.[1] Since the aim has been to eliminate transferable antibiotic resistance determinants from the food chain, it has also been considered necessary to ensure that they do not enter there via strains used as animal probiotics and potentially harboring these genes. Therefore the EU Scientific Committee on Animal Nutrition has published an opinion[2] recommending that the transferability and genetic basis (intrinsic versus acquired) of any observed resistance against a range of representative antibiotics should be elucidated before a strain could be accepted as an animal probiotic. This policy is currently being pursued in the EU evaluation procedure for animal feed additives. (So far, no measures to expand this practice to human probiotics have been suggested.) In practice, the lack of data on the intrinsic levels of resistance in various genera and species of lactic acid bacteria often makes differentiation between the intrinsic and acquired resistance difficult. An illustrative example of the importance of this distinction is the case of intrinsic vancomycin resistance typical to many lactobacilli, pediococci, and leuconostocs (Billot-Klein *et al.*, 1994; Evers *et al.*, 1996) and different from the enterococcal transmissible type.

Summary of enterococci and antibiotic resistance

The potential of pathogenic potential of enterococci together with their tendency to exchange genetic material and acquire antibiotic resitance determinants make their food or probiotic use problematic. It is to be hoped that a better understanding of factors affecting their virulence will emerge in the near future (a special ongoing EU project, FAIR-CT97-3078, "Enterococci in Food Fermentations: Functional and Safety Aspects", is devoted to this end) and allow for a rational selection of safe strains.

There is obviously a need for further studies on the spectra of antibiotic resistance among the probiotic species and strains used. Avoiding transmissible antibiotic resistance determinants is a sensitive precautionary measure. However, as long as the intrinsic background levels of resistance among food and intestinal strains are poorly known, there is little scientific basis for regulatory measures, at least in the case of human probiotics.

New aspects of safety

The history of safe use has been always used as a criterion for safety assessment, but the history of safe use has never been properly defined. Recently, an attempt has been made and work is in progress to further define dairy cultures with a safe history of use in Europe. This listing with its literature referenced information on the safe use of dairy starters and probiotics can provide a basis for future developments and regulatory definition of "safe" (Mogensen *et al.*, 2002a; Mogensen *et al.*, 2002b). Such an assessment needs to be updated coninuously and checked in different parts of the world.

Intestinal microbiota and probiotic safety

The establishment of the gut microbiota, commencing immediately after birth, is a gradual and well-regulated process (Kirjavainen *et al.*, 2002; McCracken and Lorenz, 2001). The predominant fecal organisms by the end of the first week of life have been reported to comprise bifidobacteria, bacteroides, clostridia, enterobacteria, and streptococci. Breastfed infants harbor a natural predominance of bifidobacteria with specific strains present, while the formula-fed have a profile more complex and similar to the adult microbiota, with enterobacteria, lactobacilli, bacteroides, clostridia, bifidobacteria, and streptococci. Thus the normal microbiota appears to be determined by both the maturational state of the host as well as the environment (Isolauri *et al.*, 2002).

The "normality" of normal balanced gut microbiota may be also seen from the angle of tolerance, as oral tolerance mechanisms have been shown to apply to the resident microbiota as well. Healthy individuals are tolerant to their own gut microbiota, and such tolerance is abrogated in patients with inflammatory disease (Duchmann *et al.*, 1995). Altered gut microbiota is reported in patients with inflammatory bowel disease, rheumatoid arthritis (Linskens *et al.*, 2001) and allergic disease (Kalliomäki *et al.*, 2001; Kirjavainen *et al.*, 2001, 2002), implying that the gut normal microbiota constitutes an ecosystem responding to inflammation in the gut and elsewhere in the human body. Consequently, normalization of the properties of the indigenous microbiota by specific strains of the healthy gut microbiota forms the basis of probiotic therapy, one mechanism being the control of the balance between pro- and anti-inflammatory cytokine generation.

An important new question arises for the safety of probiotic use at an early age: what are the long-term effects on the overall composition of the gut microbiota and gut immunity during the maturation phase? Clearly, once a probiotic strain is adopted by the normal microbiota, as has been documented during infancy, the potential to stimulate an immune response may be abolished and so consequently the probiotic potential. Moreover, not all *Lactobacillus* and *Bifidobacterium* strains are health-promoting. For example, recent data indicate that allergic infants have different species of bifidobacteria compared to healthy infants (He *et al.*, 2001), carrying a different immunoregulatory potential (Christensen *et al.*, 2002; He *et al.*, 2002). Therefore, the strain-specific probiotic properties need to be characterized by, firstly, *in vitro* pilot testing of the immunomodulatory effects, followed by the assessment of the immunological effects in human studies in the development of prophylactic and therapeutic interventions. The documentation is required in the target population, as the "normal" gut microbiota and the responsiveness to probiotic intervention varies according to the age and the clinical status of the host. Assessment of the long-term health effects will form an important part of the probiotic selection and characterization studies. For specific targets different probiotics may have to be identified and characterized to assure the development of a health-promoting intestinal microbiota.

Conclusions

The history of safe use of food microorganisms has been reviewed recently, specifically for dairy foods through the International Dairy Federation. As a result a list of cultures with safe history of use has been produced (Seifert and Mogensen *et al.*, 2002b). Such assessments are required in other food industry areas and they may provide the future reservoir for the use of lactic acid bacteria and bifidobacteria in foods and the basis for genera, species and strains to be characterized as probiotic organisms.

Probiotic safety assessment programs should be risk-based to ensure the consumers are protected from health risks. Decisions on safety should be science-based and involve risk analyses. Risk assessment may be useful both in understanding the potential problems and to assist in determining appropriate safety assessment studies and risk management response when new probiotics are taken into use.

Notes

1 Opinion of the Scientific Steering Committee on Antimicrobial Resistance of 28 May 1999, and the second SSC Opinion on antimicrobial resistance of 10–11 May 2001; White Paper on Food Safety of 12 January 2000.
2 Opinion of the Scientific Committee on Animal Nutrition on the criteria for assessing the safety of microorganisms resistant to antibiotics of human clinical and veterinary importance (adopted on 3 July 2001, revised on 18 April 2002).

Bibliography

Adams, M.R. (1999) Safety of industrial lactic acid bacteria, *Journal of Biotechnology*, **68**: 171–178.

Adams, M.R. and Marteau, P. (1995) On the safety of lactic acid bacteria from food, *International Journal of Food Microbiology*, **27**: 263–264.

Adawi, D., Ahrne, S., and Molin, G. (2001) Effects of different probiotic strains of *Lactobacillus* and *Bifidobacterium* on bacterial translocation and liver injury in an acute liver injury model, *International Journal of Food Microbiology*, **8**: 213–220.

Ahn, C., Collins-Thompson, D., Duncan, C., and Stiles, M.E. (1992) Mobilization and location of the genetic determinant of chloramphenicol resistance from *Lactobacillus plantarum* caTC2R, *Plasmid*, **27**: 169–176.

Aquirre, M. and Collins, M.D. (1993) Lactic acid bacteria and human clinical infections, *Journal of Applied Bacteriology*, **75**: 95–107.

Apostolou, E., Kirjavainen, P.V., Saxelin, M., Rautelin, H., Valtonen, V., Salminen, S.J., and Ouwehand, A.C. (2001) Good adhesion properties of probiotics: a potential risk for bacteremia? *FEMS Immunology Medical Microbiology*, **31**: 35–9.

Apostolou, E., Pelto, L., Kirjavainen, P., Isolauri, E., Gibson, G., and Salminen, S. (2001) Differences in the bacterial flora of healthy and milk hypersensitive adults measured by fluorescent in situ hybridisation, *FEMS Immunology Medical Microbiology*, **30**: 217–221.

Arthur, M., Reynold, P., and Courvalin, P. (1996) Glycopeptide resistance in enterococci, *Trends in Microbiology*, **4**: 401–407.

Arvola, T., Laiho, K., Torkkeli, S., Mykkanen, H., Salminen, S., Maunula, L., and Isolauri, E. (1999) Prophylactic Lactobacillus GG reduces antibiotic-associated diarrhea in children with respiratory infections: a randomized study, Pediatrics, 104: e64.

Axelsson, L.T., Ahrne, S.I.S., Andersson, M.C., and Stahl, S.R. (1988) Identification and cloning of a plasmid encoded erythromycin resistance from Lactobacillus reuteri, Plasmid, 20: 171–174.

Bernardeau, M., Vernoux, J.P., and Gueguen, M. (2002) Safety and efficacy of probiotic lactobacilli in promoting growth in post-weaning Swiss mice, International Journal of Food Microbiology, 77: 19–27.

Berufsgenossenschaft der Chemischen Industrie (1998) Sichere Biotechnologie: Eingruppierung biologischer Agenzien: Baterien, Merkblatt B 006.

Billot-Klein, D., Gutman, L., Sablé, S., Guittet, E., and van Heijenoort, J. (1994) Modification of peptidoglycan precursors is a common feature of the low-level vancomycin-resistant VanB-type Enterococcus D366 and of the naturally glycopeptide-resistant species Lactobacillus casei, Pediococcus pentosaceus, Leuconostoc mesenteroides and Enterococcus gallinarum, Journal of Bacteriology, 176: 2398–2405.

Christensen, H., Fokier, H., and Petska, J. (2002) Lactobacilli differentially modulate expression of cytokines and maturation surface markers in murine dendritic cells, Journal of Immunology, 168: 171–178.

Clewell, B.D. (1999) Movable genetic elements and antibiotic resistance in enterococci, European Journal of Microbiological Infectious Diseases, 9: 90–102.

Cunningham-Rundles, S., Ahrne, S., Bengmark, S., Johann-Liang, R., Marshall, F., Metakis, L., Califano, C., Dunn, A., Grassey, C., Hinds, G., and Cervia, J. (2000) Probiotics and immune response, American Journal of Gastroenterology, 95 (1 Suppl.): S22–S25.

Dong, M., Chang, T., and Gorbach, S.L. (1987) Effects of feeding Lactobacillus GG on lethal irradiation in mice, Diagnostic Microbiology Infectious Diseases, 7: 1–7.

Donohue, D., Deighton, M., Salminen, S., and Ahokas, J. (1993) Toxicity of lactic acid bacteria. In Lactic Acid Bacteria (eds Salminen, S. and von Wright, A.), pp. 136–148. New York: Marcel Dekker.

Duchmann, R., Kaiser, I., Hermann, E., Mayet, W., Ewe, K., and Meyer zum Buschenfelde, K.H. (1995) Tolerance exists towards resident intestinal flora but is broken in active inflammatory bowel disease (IBD), Clinical and Experimental Immunology, 102: 448–455.

Evers, S., Casadewall, B., Charles, M., Dutka-Malen, S., Galimand, M., and Courvalin, P. (1996) Evolution of structure and substrate specificity in D.alanine:D-alanine ligases and related enzymes, Journal of Molecular Evolution, 42: 706–712.

Fines, M., Perichon, B., Reynolds, P., Sahm, D., and Courvalin, P. (1999) VanE, a new type of acquired glycopeptide resistance in Enterococcus faecalis BM4405, Antimicrobial Agents and Chemotherapy, 43: 2161–2164.

Franz, C.M., Holzapfel, W.H., and Stiles, M.E. (1999) Enterococci at the crossroads of food safety, International Journal of Food Microbiology, 47: 1–24.

Franz, C.M., Muscholl-Silberhorn, A.B., Yousif, N.M.K., Vancanneyt, M., Swings, J., and Holzapfel, W.H. (2001) Incidence of virulence factors and antibiotic resistance among enterococci isolated from food, Applied and Environmental Microbiology, 67: 4385–4389.

Fris-Møller, A. and Hey, H. (1983) Colonization of the intestinal canal with a Streptococcus faecium preparation (Paraghurt), Current Therapeutic Research, 33: 807–815.

Gasser, F. (1994) Safety of lactic acid bacteria and their occurrence in human clinical infections, Bulletin Institut Pasteur, 92: 45–67.

Giraffa, G. (2002) Enterococci from foods, FEMS Microbiology Reviews, 26: 163–171.

Giraffa, G., Carminati, D., and Neviani, E. (1997) Enterococci isolated from dairy products: a review of risks and potential technological use, *Journal of Food Protection*, **60**: 732–738.

Harty, D.W.S., Oakey, H.J., Patrikakis, M., Hume, E.B.H., and Knox, K.W. (1994) Pathogenic potential of lactobacilli, *International Journal of Food Microbiology*, **24**: 179–189.

Harty, D.W.S., Patriakis, M., and Knox, K.W. (1993) Identification of *Lactobacillus* strains isolated from patients with infective endocarditis and comparison of their surface-associated properties with those of other strains of the same species, *Microbial Ecology in Health and Disease*, **6**: 191–201.

He, F., Ouwehand, A., Isolauri, E., Hashimoto, H., Benno, Y., and Salminen, S. (2001) Comparison of mucosal adhesion and species identification of bifidobacteria isolated from healthy and allergic infants, *FEMS Immunology and Medical Microbiology*, **1285**: 43–47.

He, F., Morita, H., Hashimoto, H., Hosoda, M., Kurisaki, J., Ouwehand, A.C., Isolauri, E., Benno, Y., and Salminen, S. (2002) Intestinal *Bifidobacterium* species induce varying cytokine production, *Journal of Allergy Clinical Immunology*, **109**: 1035–1036.

Holzapfel, W.H., Haberer, P., Geisen, R., Bjorkroth, J., and Schillinger, U. (2001) Taxonomy and important features of probiotic microorganisms in food and nutrition, *American Journal of Clinical Nutrition*, **73** (Suppl. 2): 365S–373S.

Ishibashi, N. and Yamazaki, S. (2001) Probiotics and safety, *American Journal of Clinical Nutrition*, **73** (Suppl. 2): 465S–470S.

Isolauri, E., Rautava, S., Kalliomaki, M., Kirjavainen, P., and Salminen, S. (2002) Role of probiotics in food hypersensitivity, *Current Opinion in Allergy Clinical Immunology*, **2**: 263–271.

Jordens, J.Z., Bates, J., and Griffiths, D.T. (1994) Faecal carriage and nosocomial spread of vancomycin-resistant *Enterococcus faecium*, *Journal of Antimicrobial Chemotherapy*, **44** (Suppl.), 25–30.

Kalliomäki, M., Kirjavainen, P., Eerola, E., Kero, P., Salminen, S., and Isolauri, E. (2001) Distinct patterns of neonatal gut microflora in infants developing or not developing atopy, *Journal of Allergy and Clinical Immunology*, **107**: 129–134.

Kaur, I.P., Chopra, K., and Saini, A. (2002) Probiotics: potential pharmaceutical applications, *European Journal of Pharmaceutical Science*, **15**: 1–9.

Kirjavainen, P.V., Apostolou, E., Arvola, T., Salminen, S., Gibson, G., and Isolauri, E. (2001) Characterizing the composition of intestinal microflora as a prospective treatment target in infant allergic disease, *FEMS Immunology and Medical Microbiology*, **32**: 1–7.

Kirjavainen, P.V., Tuomola, E.M., Crittenden, R.G., Ouwehand, A.C., Harty, D.W.S., Morris, L.F., Rautelin, H., Playne, M.J., Donohue, D.C., and Salminen, S.J. (1999) In vitro adhesion and platelet aggregation properties of bacteremia-associated lactobacilli, *Infection and Immunity*, **67**: 2653–2655.

Kirjavainen, P., Arvola, T., Salminen, S., and Isolauri, E. (2002) Aberrant composition of gut microbiota of allergic infants: a target of bifidobacterial therapy at weaning? *Gut*, **51**: 51–55.

Klein, G., Hallmann, C., Casas, I.A., Abad, J., Louwers, J., and Reuter, G. (2000) Exclusion of vanA, vanB and vanC type glycopeptide resistance in strains of *Lactobacillus reuteri* and *Lactobacillus rhamnosus* used as probiotics by polymerase chain reaction and hybridization methods, *Journal of Applied Microbiology*, **89**: 815–824.

Landman, D. and Quale, J.M. (1997) Management of infections due to resistant enterococci: a review of therapeutic options, *Journal of Antimicrobial Chemotherapy*, **40**: 161–170.

Lemay, M.J., Rodrigue, N., Gariepy, C., and Saucier, L. (2000) Adaptation of *Lactobacillus alimentarius* to environmental stresses, *International Journal of Food Microbiology*, **55**: 249–253.

Linskens, R.K., Huijsdens, X.W., Savelkoul, P.H., Vandenbroucke-Grauls, C.M., and Meuwissen, S.G. (2001) The bacterial flora in inflammatory bowel disease: current insights in pathogenesis and the influence of antibiotics and probiotics, *Scandinavian Journal of Gastroenterology*, **234**: 29–40.

McCracken, V. and Lorenz, R. (2001) The gastrointestinal ecosystem: a precarious alliance among epithelium, immunity and microbiota, *Cellular Microbiology*, **3**: 1–11.

Millar, M.R., Bacon, C., Smith, S.L., Walker, V., and Hall, M.A. (1993) Enteral feeding of premature infants with *Lactobacillus* GG, *Archives of Diseases in Children*, **69**: 483–487.

Moellering, R.C. (1992) Emergence of *Enterococcus* as a significant pathogen, *Clinical Infectious Diseases*, **14**: 1173–1176.

Mogensen, G., Salminen, S., O'Brien, J., Ouwehand, A., Holtzapfel, W., Shortt, C., Fondén, R., Miller, G., Donohue, D., Playne, M., Crittenden, R., and Bianchi Salvadori, B. (2002a) Food microorganisms – health benefits, safety evaluation and strains with documented history of use in foods, *IDF Bulletin*, **377**: 4–9.

Mogensen, G., Salminen, S., O'Brien, J., Ouwehand, A., Holtzapfel, W., Shortt, C., Fondén, R., Miller, G., Donohue, D., Playne, M., Crittenden, R., and Bianchi Salvadori, B. (2002b) Inventory of microorganisms with a documented history of use in food, *Bulletin of the IDF*, **377**: 10–19.

Morelli, L., Vescovo, M., and Bottazzi, V. (1983) Identification of chloramphenicol resistance plasmids in *Lactobacillus reuteri* and *Lactobacillus acidophilus*, *International Journal of Microbiology*, **1**: 1–5.

Nanji, A., Khettry, U., and Sadrzaedh, M. (1994) *Lactobacillus* feeding reduces endotoxemia and severity of experimental alcoholic liver (disease), *Proceedings of the Society for Experimental Biology and Medicine*, **205**: 243–247.

O'Brien, J., Crittenden, R., Ouwehand, A., and Salminen, S. (1999) Demonstrating the safety of probiotics, *Trends in Food Science Technology*, **10**: 418–424.

Ouwehand, A.C., Tuomola, E.M., Lee, Y.K., and Salminen, S. (2001a) Microbial interactions to intentinal mucosal models, *Methods Enzymology*, **337**: 200–212.

Ouwehand, A.C., Isolauri, E., He, F., Hashimoto, H., Benno, Y., and Salminen, S. (2001b) Differences in *Bifidobacterium* flora composition in allergic and healthy infants, *Journal of Allergy Clinical Immunology*, **108**: 144–145.

Ouwehand, A.C., Lagstrom, H., Suomalainen, T., and Salminen, S. (2002) Effect of probiotics on constipation, fecal azoreductase activity and fecal mucin content in the elderly. *Annals of Nutrition and Metabolism*, **46**: 159–162.

Perichon, B., Reynolds, P., and Courvalin, P. (1997) VanD-type glycopeptide-resistant *Enterococcus faecium* BM4339, *Antimicrobial Agents and Chemotherapy*, **41**: 2016–2018.

Pidcock, K., Heard, G.M., and Henriksson, A. (2002) Application of nontraditional meat starter cultures in production of Hungarian salami, *International Journal of Food Microbiology*, **76**: 75–81.

Reid, G. (2002) Safety of *Lactobacillus* strains as probiotic agents, *Clinical Infectious Diseases*, **35**: 349–350.

Ruseler-van Embden, J.G., van Lieshout, L.M., Gosselink, M.J., and Marteau, P. (1995) Inability of *Lactobacillus casei* Strain GG, *L. acidophilus*, and *Bifidobacterium bifidum* to degrade intestinal mucus glycoproteins, *Scandinavian Journal of Gastroenterology*, **30**: 675–680.

Saarela, M., Mogensen, G., Fonden, R., Matto, J., and Mattila-Sandholm, T. (2000) Probiotic bacteria: safety, functional and technological properties, *Journal of Biotechnology*, **84**: 197–215.

Salminen, S. and Arvilommi, H. (2002) Safety of *Lactobacillus* strains: discussion, *Clinical Infectious Diseases*, **34**: 1284–1285.

Salminen, S. and Von Wright, A. (1998) Current human probiotics – safety assured? *Microbial Ecology in Health and Disease*, **10**: 68–77.

Salminen, S., Bouley, M.C., Boutron-Rualt, M.C., Cummings, J., Franck, A., Gibson, G., Isolauri, E., Moreau, M-C., Roberfroid, M., and Rowland, I. (1998a) Functional food science and gastrointestinal physiology and function. *British Journal of Nutrition*, **Suppl. 1**: 147–171.

Salminen, S., Von Wright, A., Morelli, L., Marteau, P., Brassard, D., de Vos, W., Fondén, R., Saxelin, M., Collins, K., Mogensen, G., Birkeland, S.-E., and Mattila-Sandholm, T. (1998b) Demonstration of safety of probiotics – a review, *International Journal of Food Microbiology*, **44**: 93–106.

Sanders, M.E. and Klaenhammer, T.R. (2001) Invited review: the scientific basis of *Lactobacillus acidophilus* NCFM functionality as a probiotic, *Journal of Dairy Science*, **84**: 319–331.

Saxelin, M., Chuang, N.H., Chassy, B., Rautelin, H., Mäkelä, P.H., Salminen, S., and Gorbach, S.L. (1996a) Lactobacilli and bacteremia in Southern Finland. 1989–1992, *Clinical Infectious Diseases*, **22**: 564–566.

Saxelin, M., Rautelin, H., Salminen, S., and Mäkelä, P. (1996b) The safety of commercial products with viable *Lactobacillus* strains, *Infectious Diseases in Clinical Practice*, **5**: 331–335.

Sipsas, N.V., Zonios, D.I., and Kordossis, T. (2002) Safety of *Lactobacillus* strains used as probiotic agents, *Clinical Infectious Diseases*, **34**: 1283–1284.

Soboleva, T.K., Pleasants, A.B., and le Roux, G. (2000) Predictive microbiology and food safety, *International Journal of Food Microbiology*, **57**: 183–192.

Teuber, M., Meile, L., and Schwarz, F. (1999) Acquired antibiotic resistance in lactic acid bacteria from food, *Antonie Van Leeuwenhoek*, **76**: 115–137.

Tuomola, E., Crittenden, R., Playne, M., Isolauri, E., and Salminen, S. (2001) Quality assurance criteria for probiotic bacteria, *American Journal of Clinical Nutrition*, **73** (Suppl. 2): 393S–398S.

Ventura, M., Reniero, R., and Zink, R. (2001) Specific identification and targeted characterization of *Bifidobacterium lactis* from different environmental isolates by a combined multiplex–PCR approach, *Applied and Environmental Microbiology*, **67**(6): 2760–2765.

Von Wright, A. and Salminen, S. (1999) Probiotics: established effects and open questions, *European Journal of Gastroenterology and Hepatology*, **11**: 1195–1198.

Von Wright, A. and Sibakov, M. (1998) Genetic modification of lactic acid bacteria, in S. Salminen and A. Von Wright (eds.) *Lactic Acid Bacteria; Microbiology and Functional Aspects*, New York: Marcel Dekker Inc.

Wegener, H.C., Madsen, M., Nielsen, N., and Aarestrup, F.M. (1997) Isolation of vancomycin resistant *Enterococcus faecium* from food, *International Journal of Food Microbiology*, **35**: 57–66.

Wolf, B.W., Wheeler, K.B., Ataya, D.G., and Garleb, K.A. (1998) Safety and tolerance of *Lactobacillus reuteri* supplementation to a population infected with the human immunodeficiency virus. *Food Chemistry Toxiciology*, **36**: 1085–1094.

WHO/FAO (2001) *Health and Nutritional Properties of Probiotics in Food including Powder Milk with Live Lactic Acid Bacteria*, Report of a Joint FAO/WHO Expert Consultation on Evaluation of Health and Nutritional Properties of Probiotics in Food Including Powder Milk with Live Lactic Acid Bacteria, Córdoba, Argentina, 1–4 October 2001. http://www.fao.org/es/ESN/probio/probio.htm

Zhou, J.S., Shu, Q., Rutherfurd, K.J., Prasad, J., Birtles, M.J., Gopal, P.K., and Gill, H.S. (2000) Safety assessment of potential probiotic lactic acid bacterial strains *Lactobacillus rhamnosus* HN001, *Lb. acidophilus* HN017, and *Bifidobacterium lactis* HN019 in BALB/c mice, *International Journal of Food Microbiology*, **56**: 87–96.

14 Dietary alcohol and xenobiotics

Danièle Lucas

Summary

Alcohol and xenobiotics share the same metabolic microsomal pathway, which is mainly located in the endoplasmic reticulum of hepatocytes. This pathway involves enzymes that belong to the super family of cytochrome P450, and elucidates many pharmacokinetic or toxic interactions between alcohol and xenobiotics. Cytochrome P450 2E1 (CYP2E1) is the key enzyme of the microsomal pathway of ethanol oxidation. It is inducible by chronic ethanol consumption and its activity is increased three- to five-fold in liver from alcoholic subjects. This induction is also accompanied by enhanced activity of other enzymes resulting in accelerated metabolism of other drugs. Furthermore, CYP2E1 has a high capacity to activate numerous xenobiotics into toxic or carcinogenic compounds, often free radicals. These include common drugs such as paracetamol, anesthetics (enflurane, halothane), industrial solvents (benzene or its derivatives), halogenated solvents (carbon tetrachloride, trichlorethylene, chlorofluorocarbons), and N-nitrosamines which are present in food or tobacco smoke. Therefore, heavy consumption of alcohol, which results in CYP2E1 induction, increases individual susceptibility to the toxic or carcinogenic effects of these xenobiotics.

Introduction

In humans, more than 90% of the ingested ethanol is degraded in the liver by oxidative and non-oxidative pathways. The major enzymes involved are alcohol dehydrogenase (ADH), aldehyde dehydrogenase (ALDH) and cytochrome P450 2E1 (CYP2E1). Catalase and free radicals, generated throughout metabolism of ethanol, are also considered to be involved in ethanol degradation (Figure 14.1). All these enzymes are located in different compartments of the cell: ADH is cytosolic and contributes to 70–90% of ethanol oxidation whereas CYP2E1 is microsomal, i.e. located in the endoplasmic reticulum, and contributes to only 10% (Lieber, 1999). The microsomal ethanol metabolic pathway, called MEOS (microsomal ethanol-oxidizing system) by Lieber, is increased after chronic ethanol intoxication. Although CYP2E1 is the key-enzyme of the

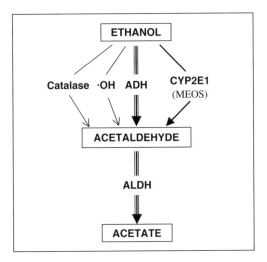

Figure 14.1 Main pathways for ethanol metabolism. Ethanol is metabolized into
acetaldehyde by various pathways: the major enzymes involved are alcohol
dehydrogenase (ADH) and cytochrome P450 2E1 (CYP2E1), which is the
key enzyme of the microsomal ethanol oxidizing system (MEOS). Catalase
and free radicals (•OH), generated during the metabolism of ethanol, are of
limited quantitative importance. Acetaldehyde is mainly metabolized into
acetate by aldehyde dehydrogenase (ALDH).

MEOS, other cytochromes P450 (CYPs) such as CYP1A2 or CYP3A4 can also
contribute to ethanol metabolism.

However, several xenobiotics such as drugs or industrial solvents are also
metabolized by CYPs. Most xenobiotics are hydrophobic and need biotransformation to facilitate their excretion from the body. These processes may be
classically broken down into three phases (Figure 14.2). Phase I metabolic transformations are catalyzed by the CYP system: they consist of reduction, oxidation,
and hydrolysis in order to reveal or introduce functional or reactive groups in
the molecules. Phase II transformations are generally conjugation reactions of
the parent xenobiotics or of phase I metabolites with inorganic sulfate, acetate,
glucuronic acid, or glutathione. Conjugation reactions facilitate transport and
enhance elimination via the renal and biliary routes. Phase III enzymes are
involved in the transport out of the cell of the products derived from phase II
conjugation reactions (Vermeulen, 1996). The liver is quantitatively the most
important organ in the process of biotransformation, though other organs and
tissues are also relevant. Thus, CYPs favor xenobiotics' elimination and constitute
the first line of defense against their toxic effects.

Since alcohol and xenobiotics share the same metabolic pathway, which is in
addition inducible, pharmacokinetic and/or toxic interactions can be expected.
In the presence of high ethanol concentrations, xenobiotics metabolism is

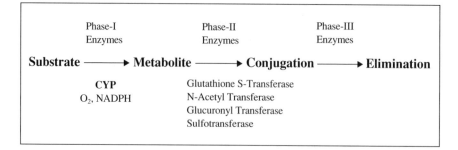

Figure 14.2 Biotransformation of xenobiotics. Most xenobiotics are hydrophobic and need biotransformation to facilitate their excretion. Phase I metabolic transformations involve the CYP system in order to introduce functional or reactive groups in the molecules. Phase II transformations are generally conjugation reactions of the parent xenobiotics or of phase I metabolites with inorganic sulfate, acetate, glucuronic acid, or glutathione. Phase III enzymes are involved in the transport of the products derived from phase II conjugation reactions outside the cell.

inhibited because of a competition for a common oxidation pathway. Conversely, when ethanol is lacking, ethanol-mediated microsomal induction will account for drug tolerance; this has been often noticed in alcoholics (Lieber, 1991). If the metabolites are still biologically active or have toxicological concern, chronic alcohol intake increases the risk of adverse events (organ toxicity or carcinogenicity). This may explain the enhanced susceptibility of alcoholics to the adverse effects of some industrial solvents. For example, high ethanol consumption has been reported to potentiate the toxicity of carbon tetrachloride in humans (Manno *et al.*, 1996).

After recalling the main properties of CYPs, this review will more particularly focus on CYP2E1 because of its inducibility by chronic ethanol consumption together with its role in the bioactivation of numerous xenobiotics, including therapeutic agents, environmental contaminants, and industrial solvents.

The superfamily of cytochromes P450

Cytochromes P450 are ubiquitous hemeproteins. The entire set of genes coding for these proteins belongs to the cytochrome P450 superfamily. Over 100 genes have been identified and classified on the basis of their structural relationships. Their complementary DNA sequences with at least 40% identity have been grouped into families (given the numbers 1, 2, 3 . . .). Sequences within families that are at least 60% identical are called subfamilies (A, B, C . . .). Individual enzymes are then given specific numbers. Thus, for example, a particular enzyme can be referred to as cytochrome P450 2E1. Cytochrome P450 proteins are named CYPs, and the corresponding genes *cyp* in the mouse and

CYP in other species. In humans, 49 CYP genes have been identified and distributed in 16 families (Nelson *et al.*, 1996). A specialized CYP database has been constructed recently and is available online (http://drnelson.utmem.edu/cytochromeP450.html).

Cytochromes P450 play two main roles in living organisms. Some CYPs catalyze oxidation steps in the biosynthesis or biodegradation of endogenous compounds such as steroids, fatty acids, or prostaglandins. However, the largest number of CYPs (families 1 to 3) are involved in the metabolism of foreign chemicals such as drugs, pollutants, and food additives ingested from environment. They facilitate their elimination from living organisms. The CYP enzymes are predominantly found in the endoplasmic reticulum of most cells, the greatest abundance being in the liver (Ioannides, 1996). The first activity of these enzymes is the so-called monooxygenase activity which catalyzes the transfer of one atom of oxygen from O_2 to various substrates. It works in conjunction with other microsomal enzymes such as NADPH-cytochrome P450 reductase and cytochromes b5. However, CYPs can also function as oxidases, peroxidases, and reductases and catalyze a great diversity of reactions (Mansuy, 1998). The oxidase activity involves direct electron transfer from reduced cytochrome P450 to molecular oxygen with the concomitant formation of superoxide anion radicals and hydrogen peroxide. This phenomenon is particularly important when CYPs are involved in the metabolism of xenobiotics that are not perfectly positioned in their active site to receive the oxygen atom. It occurs during the microsomal oxidation of ethanol (Nordmann *et al.*, 1992). CYP2E1 effectively reduces dioxygen and is capable of undergoing futile cycling to produce active oxygen species. The reductase activity involves direct electron transfer to reducible substrates such as halogenated alkanes to produce free radical intermediates. The reductive reactions proceed more readily under cellular conditions of low oxygen tension, in the presence of NADPH (Vermeulen, 1996). The substrates of CYP-catalyzed reactions are usually hydrophobic compounds, although some CYPs such as CYP2E1 can oxidize hydrophilic substrates too. The internal pocket of cytochrome P450 molecule is surrounded by hydrophobic aminoacid residues and can accommodate various bulky hydrophobic molecules, which bind to the substrate-binding site. Different apoprotein structures of the numerous CYP isoforms are responsible for the broad and overlapping substrate specificity.

Families 1 to 3 of cytochrome P450 exhibit the phenomenon of enzyme induction, i.e. the increased synthesis of a specific enzyme protein in response to exposure to substrates of that particular cytochrome. The mechanisms of induction involve increased transcription, increased stabilization of mRNA, or increased stabilization of the protein by controlling the rate of its degradation (Ioannides, 1996).

Many of the parent chemicals are not toxic by themselves but can be activated through metabolic transformations into toxic reactive intermediates (Guengerich *et al.*, 1991). In most cases, toxic intermediates are detoxified or bioinactivated at their site of formation. However, in the case of inefficient

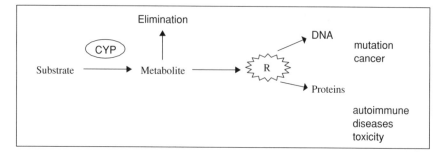

Figure 14.3 Metabolism of exogenous compounds. Xenobiotics can be activated through metabolic transformations into toxic reactive intermediates. In most cases, toxic intermediates will be detoxified or bioinactivated at their site of formation, but in the case of inefficient detoxification they can covalently bind to proteins or DNA, causing cytotoxicity or genotoxicity.

detoxification, they can covalently bind to proteins or DNA and then cause cytotoxicity and genotoxicity (Parke *et al.*, 1991) (Figure 14.3). The occurrence of a toxic effect due to toxic parent chemicals or to reactive intermediates generally depends on the balance between toxification and detoxification processes (Vermeulen, 1996).

Metabolism of ethanol and xenobiotics by CYP2E1

Microsomal ethanol oxidation mainly involves CYP2E1 and requires phospholipids and NADPH-cytochrome P450 reductase (Lieber, 1999). CYP2E1 oxidizes ethanol to acetaldehyde mainly through a typical monooxygenase reaction. In addition to this mechanism, CYP2E1 displays an oxidase activity which involves direct electron transfer from reduced cytochrome P450 to molecular oxygen, and give rise to free radicals (Cederbaum, 1987). Formation of superoxide anion and hydrogen peroxide produce through a Fenton-type reaction very reactive hydroxyl radicals ($^{\bullet}$OH) that oxidize ethanol into hydroxyethyl radicals, an intermediate between ethanol and acetaldehyde (Albano *et al.*, 1991). This likely explains the reported activity of ethanol as a hydroxyl radical scavenger (Cederbaum, 1987). In another way, hydroxyethyl radicals may be directly formed by cytochrome P450 (Albano *et al.*, 1991; Reinke *et al.*, 1997). However, the $^{\bullet}$OH-dependent pathway for microsomal ethanol oxidation represents only a minor contribution (about 10%) under normal conditions (Poupon *et al.*, 2002; Stoyanovski and Cederbaum 1998).

CYP2E1 plays a significant role in ethanol metabolism at concentrations higher than 10 mM ethanol, in contrast with ADH, which is active for concentrations less than 0.5 mM. CYP2E1 Km of ethanol is about 10 mM (Lieber, 1997). Therefore, CYP2E1 involvement in ethanol oxidation increases as blood ethanol concentration increases. Among the CYPs, CYP2E1 has the highest activity for oxidizing ethanol to acetaldehyde but CYP1A2 and CYP3A4 can also participate (Salmela *et al.*, 1998). CYP3A is quantitatively the most important CYP in the liver (approximately 30%, compared to CYP1A2 or CY2E1, 10% each (Vermeulen, 1996)) and is involved in the metabolism of 50% of the drugs.

Besides ethanol, CYP2E1 can oxidize many other compounds of low molecular weight (Table 14.1) including endogenous substrates (fatty acids, acetone, acetaldehyde, etc.), drugs (chlorzoxazone, paracetamol, salicylate, anesthetics) or industrial solvents (benzene, trichlorethylene, etc.) (for a review, see Lieber, 1997). Most of these substrates are oxidized through a mono-oxygenase pathway, but

Table 14.1 Main CYP2E1 substrates, inducers, and inhibitors

Substrates	Inducers	Inhibitors
Endogenous substrates	*Pathophysiological states*	*Dietary inhibitors*
Acetaldehyde	Diabetes	Diallylsulfide
Acetone	Obesity	Dihydrocapsaicin
Fatty acids	Fasting	Phenethylisothiocyanate
Ethanol		
Glycerol		
Drugs	*Drugs*	*Drugs*
Acetaminophen (paracetamol)	Isoniazid	Chlormethiazole
Caffeine	Pyrazole	Disulfiram
Chlorzoxazone		Malotilate
Dapsone		
Enflurane, sevoflurane, methoxyflurane		
Halothane		
Salicylic acid		
Trimethadione		
Organic solvents/chemicals	*Organic solvents*	*Chemicals*
Acrylonitrile	Ethanol	3-Amino-1,2,4-triazole
Alcohols, acetone, ether, alkanes	Acetone	Diethyldithiocarbamate
Aniline	Benzene, xylene	4-Methylpyrazole
Benzene and derivatives	Isopropanol	
Butadiene	Diethyl ether	
Carbontetrachloride	Dimethylsulfoxide	
Halogenated hydrocarbons	Pyridine	
Chloroform	Pyrazole	
Trichloroethylene		
Nitrosamines (N-nitrosodimethylamine)		
Pyrazole		
Pyridine		
Styrene		
Urethan (ethyl carbamate)		
Vinyl bromide, carbamate, chloride		

some of them, such as halogenated solvents, can undergo a reduction and lead to reactive free radicals (Raucy *et al.*, 1993). CYP2E1 has the unusual capacity to activate many xenobiotics to their toxic metabolites (Guengerich *et al.*, 1991).

The typical range of catalytic activity of CYP2E1 varies from six to 20 times in human liver microsomes (Guengerich and Turvy, 1991; Lucas *et al.*, 1993, 1999); any variation in enzyme concentration and hence in activity may increase the risk of toxicity and carcinogenicity. Therefore, the knowledge of the factors involved in CYP2E1 regulation along with the way to determine the enzyme activity in humans are of the highest interest in order to assess the risks in relation with exposure to xenobiotics.

Regulation of CYP2E1

The regulation of CYP2E1 expression is complex and involves transcriptional, post-transcriptional, translational and post-translational mechanisms (for reviews, see Koop and Tierney, 1990; Novak and Woodcroft, 2000; Ronis *et al.*, 1996).

Induction by chronic ethanol consumption

CYP2E1 is easily inducible by chronic ethanol consumption, as demonstrated in several species: rat, rabbit, hamster, and humans. Due to the worldwide consumption of ethanol, this compound is the most relevant CYP2E1 inducer in humans. Recently drinking alcoholics display three- to five-fold increased amount or activity of CYP2E1 in the liver (Lucas *et al.*, 1995b; Perrot *et al.*, 1989; Takahashi *et al.*, 1993). In rats, ethanol chronic treatment *per os* or by inhalation for four weeks increases the CYP2E1 level three- to ten-fold (Zerilli *et al.*, 1995). Consumption of 40 g ethanol per day for one to four weeks is enough to induce CYP2E1 in humans (Oneta *et al.*, 2002). In fact, a single dose is able to induce CYP2E1 content or activity in mice (Petersen *et al.*, 1982) as in humans (Plee-Gautier *et al.*, 2001). This observation can be related to the regulation of CYP2E1 by ethanol, which involves two mechanisms.

The first mechanism is protein stabilization by its substrate through reduced degradation and protection of the enzyme against proteolysis by the proteasome complex (French *et al.*, 2001; Roberts *et al.*, 1995b); it is worth noting that this mechanism is not fully understood, but seems to occur at low blood alcohol levels. The second mechanism involves transcriptional activation of the *CYP2E1* gene under high ethanol concentrations (Badger *et al.*, 1993; Ronis *et al.*, 1993) or long-term consumption (Takahashi *et al.*, 1993). This likely explains why CYP2E1 protein content or activity and mRNA levels are correlated (Takahashi *et al.*, 1993) or not (Powell *et al.*, 1998). CYP2E1 induction during ethanol treatment is enhanced when it is associated with a diet rich in polyunsaturated fatty acids (Takahashi *et al.*, 1992). In fact, potentiation is observed only when the fat-to-carbohydrate ratio is high (Korourian *et al.*, 1999).

CYP2E1 levels correlate with blood ethanol levels in animals (Badger *et al.*, 1993; Raucy *et al.*, 1995), but this correlation is rather low in humans (Dupont *et al.*, 2000), probably because of environmental factors (diet, hormonal status, pollutants, etc.) and short half-life of proteins (Roberts *et al.*, 1995a). When ethanol consumption is stopped, CYP2E1 protein returns to basal level in 24 h in rats whereas it takes five days in humans (Lucas *et al.*, 1995b; Oneta *et al.*, 2002).

Induction by xenobiotics or environmental factors

Many CYPs are induced by their substrates. This helps to remove the xenobiotics from the body. Most xenobiotics, e.g. acetone, pyridine, pyrazole, and isoniazid (Table 14.1) are able to increase CYP2E1 protein levels but without a concomitant increase of mRNA levels (Ronis *et al.*, 1996). Thus, xenobiotic-mediated CYP2E1 induction occurs via post-transcriptional mechanisms such as increased translational efficiency or protein stabilization. In contrast, certain physiopathological states, e.g. starvation, obesity, and diabetes, enhance CYP2E1 expression at both mRNA and protein levels both in experimental animals and in humans. CYP2E1 is also negatively and positively regulated by some hormones, e.g. insulin, glucagon, growth hormone, leptin, and growth factors; such observations provide evidence that CYP2E1 expression is under tight homeostatic control (Novak and Woodcroft, 2000).

In addition, diet can also modulate CYP2E1 expression (Ioannides, 1999). Generally, fat levels affect CYP levels; indeed, diets rich in polyunsaturated fatty acids are more effective than those rich in saturated fatty acids. The lipid-to-carbohydrate ratio seems to be an important parameter (Korourian *et al.*, 1999; Yoo *et al.*, 1991). Fasting is known to induce CYP2E1 in animals (Hong *et al.*, 1987) but not in humans (O'Shea *et al.*, 1994) and sugar or lipid restriction in obese individuals decreases CYP2E1 activity in humans (Leclercq *et al.*, 1999).

Enzyme expression after induction takes place in the centrilobular region of the liver (Ingelman-Sundberg *et al.*, 1988). The regioselective hepatic CYP2E1 expression is of interest because ethanol, acetaminophen, N-nitrosamines, solvents, and other CYP2E1 substrates that are metabolized into toxic reactive intermediates mainly destroy the centrilobular liver region. CYP2E1 induction also takes place at the peripheral level, in extrahepatic tissues where CYP2E1 is expressed, i.e. nasal mucosa, lung, kidney, small intestine, colon, brain, lymphocytes, and mononuclear cells (Ronis *et al.*, 1996).

Inhibition

Because of the toxicological implication of CYP2E1, research on inhibitors has been developed: the rationale is to prevent CYP2E1-mediated production of reactive metabolites. Among the inhibitors known so far, one should cite malotilate, a hepatoprotectant (Kim *et al.*, 1994), chlormethiazole, a drug used for its sedative effects during ethanol withdrawal (Gebhardt *et al.*, 1997), and disulfiram, an inhibitor of aldehyde dehydrogenase, used in the past in alcohol detoxification programs. This last compound is metabolized by CYP2E1 into diethyldithiocarbamate, an irreversible inhibitor of CYP2E1, effective both *in vitro* (Guengerich *et al.*, 1991) and *in vivo* (Frye and Branch, 2002; Kharash *et al.*, 1999). Polyenylphosphatidylcholine, an innocuous inhibitor of CYP2E1 induction by chronic ethanol, has been tested in humans (Lieber, 1999) in order to counteract the deleterious effects of ethanol. Diet may also provide inhibitors and substrates (competitive inhibitors) for CYP2E1. Vegetables such as the Cruciferae or garlic contain phenethylisothiocyanate and diallylsulfide which decrease CYP2E1 activity in humans (Ioannides, 1999; Leclercq *et al.*, 1998; Le Marchand *et al.*, 1999). Dihydrocapsaicin, a constituent of red pepper, is an irreversible inhibitor of CYP2E1 (Gannett *et al.*, 1990).

Genetic polymorphism

In addition to the multiple regulation described above, several *CYP2E1* genetic polymorphisms have been described and suspected to lead to different protein expressions. All these polymorphisms have been found in the promoter region as well as in introns. However, the coding regions of *CYP2E1* appeared to be well conserved among different ethnic groups and species (Ronis *et al.*, 1996). The most studied restriction fragment length polymorphisms are: the *PstI/RsaI* polymorphism in the 5′-flanking region of the gene (Hayashi *et al.*, 1991); the *DraI* polymorphism in intron 6 (Hirvonen *et al.*, 1993); and a repeat polymorphism in the promoter region of the gene (McCarver *et al.*, 1998), giving rise to different alleles. A new nomenclature for CYP alleles has recently been recommended (http://www.imm.ki.se/CYPalleles). Significant interethnic differences exist in *CYP2E1* polymorphisms (Garte *et al.*, 2001), but there is still no clear evidence that any of them are related to altered function of the enzyme *in vivo* (Lucas *et al.*, 1995a; Plee-Gautier *et al.*, 2001) or alcohol-related diseases or cancers (Wong *et al.*, 2000). Therefore, environmental factors such as physiological or hormonal status and diet may be additional determinants for the interindividual differences observed in CYP2E1 activity in humans.

Determination of CYP2E1 levels in humans

CYP2E1 levels can be assessed using *in vitro* or *in vivo* methods (Lucas *et al.*, 1996). *In vitro* methods refer to direct determination of enzyme activity in liver microsomes using chlorzoxazone (Peter *et al.*, 1990), p-nitrophenol (Tassaneeyakul *et al.*, 1993) or N-nitrosodimethylamine (Yoo *et al.*, 1988) as the most selective substrates in humans. However, alternative and non-invasive approaches have been developed. Chlorzoxazone, a centrally acting muscle relaxant, can be used *in vivo* as a safe probe in humans. It is mainly metabolized into 6-hydroxychlorzoxazone by CYP2E1. Various chlorzoxazone pharmacokinetic measures have been proposed to assess CYP2E1 activity after administration of 250, 500 or 750 mg chlorzoxazone (Streetman *et al.*, 2000). The best choice appears to be 500 mg when considering the Km of CYP2E1 for chlorzoxazone (40–70 μM) and the possible involvement of other CYPs for lower or higher substrate concentrations (Lucas *et al.*, 1999). Fully pharmacokinetic studies revealed a good correlation with the blood metabolite/drug concentration ratio, determined 2 h after drug intake. This metabolic ratio has been validated in recent years by several groups of researchers (Streetman *et al.*, 2000) and can be used for determination of CYP2E1 activity in large numbers of individuals. Its selectivity has been recently reassessed in humans (Lucas *et al.*, 1999). Other *in vivo* probes such as salicylate (Dupont *et al.*, 1999) or trimethadione (Kurata *et al.*, 1998) have been tested but are less specific since other CYPs intervene in their metabolism.

As CYP2E1 is expressed in lymphocytes at the protein and mRNA levels (Raucy *et al.*, 1999), the use of a surrogate tissue to liver such as blood has been suggested to screen CYP2E1 activity in large populations. Indeed, a correlation was observed in alcoholic subjects between CYP2E1 content in lymphocytes, chlorzoxazone clearance rates and mRNA expression in lymphocytes (Raucy *et al.*, 1999). Recent studies using quantitative RT-PCR techniques are now arising (Haufroid *et al.*, 2001; Rodriguez-Antona *et al.*, 2001). CYP2E1 mRNA levels in lymphocytes are increased in actively drinking chronic alcoholics; they rapidly decrease after ethanol withdrawal (Yano *et al.*, 2001). However, CYP2E1 expressions are not always correlated between liver and lymphocytes (Finnstrom *et al.*, 2001).

Increased xenobiotic toxicity and carcinogenicity

CYP2E1 catalyzes the metabolism of more than 100 low molecular weight compounds, many of which are industrial solvents, chemical additives of toxicological and carcinogenic significance, or therapeutic agents. However, as already indicated, CYP2E1 has the unusual capacity to activate these xenobiotics to hepatotoxic or carcinogenic products. For example, ethanol, acetaminophen (paracetamol), a commonly prescribed drug, or carbon tertrachloride, an industrial solvent, lead to hepatotoxic metabolites whereas N-nitrosodimethylamine, an environmental carcinogen, is activated into a methyl carbonium ion suspected to initiate carcinogenesis. In contrast, some substrates and metabolites are innocuous and may eventually be used as markers of heavy drinking: this is the case for chlorzoxazone. Increased vulnerability of chronic alcoholics to drugs, industrial solvents, or chemical carcinogens can be attributed to microsomal induction since induced CYP2E1 increases xenobiotic metabolism and activates most of them to their toxic metabolites. This susceptibility occurs particularly after ethanol withdrawal, when microsomal induction persists, but alcohol no longer has an inhibitory effect. In fact, toxicity depends on the balance between production of the toxic metabolites by CYPs and their elimination by phase-II enzymes.

Interactions of ethanol with xenobiotics metabolism

Alcohol–xenobiotics interactions are highly important in medical prescription and in occupational medicine because of concomitant exposure to alcohol and drugs or environmental pollutants. But these interactions radically differ between chronic and acute alcohol abuse. Chronic ethanol can induce both CYP2E1 and related microsomal detoxifying enzymes, as suggested by observation of accelerated hepatic metabolism of various compounds that act as microsomal substrates but without being specifically metabolized by CYP2E1. In fact, metabolism by CYP2E1 concerns only a few drugs, e.g. chlorzoxazone, acetaminophen, and volatile anesthetics such as halothane, enflurane, methoxyflurane, and sevoflurane. Thus, an increase in the clearance of acetaminophen (Girre et al., 1993), chlorzoxazone (Lucas et al., 1995b) but also of meprobamate, pentobarbital, warfarin, phenytoin, tolbutamide, propranolol, rifampin, and methadone has been linked to long-term ethanol consumption, as reviewed elsewhere (Lieber, 1991). This "metabolic tolerance" is more obvious during the withdrawal of ethanol, especially in the early phase of abstinence where the half-life of each of these drugs is 50% shorter. In contrast, since the microsomal enzymes metabolize both ethanol and xenobiotics, high ethanol concentration causes inhibitory effects partly due to competition for a common oxidation pathway. Accordingly, simultaneous administration of drugs and ethanol slows down drug metabolism and increases drug concentration leading to overdose: this has been shown for some benzodiazepines (diazepam, chlordiazepoxide), phenothiazines, tricyclic antidepressants, barbiturates, morphine, and methadone (Lieber, 1991). Pharmacodynamic effects can be added to metabolic effects, especially for drugs having sedative effects such as barbiturates, neuroleptics, and analgesics (Lieber, 1991). As with drugs, ethanol interacts with industrial solvents. For example, ethanol decreases the metabolic clearance of xylene by about one half (Riihimaki et al., 1982). Acute interactions of this type have also been described for other industrial solvents.

Activation of xenobiotics into reactive compounds

Much evidence suggests that the toxicity associated with CYP2E1 involves the production of free radicals. CYP2E1 displays the capacity to generate reactive oxygen intermediates, such as superoxide anions, hydroxyl radicals, and hydrogen peroxide (Nordmann et al., 1992) and to activate many xenobiotics to toxic metabolites, which are generally free radicals. This has been demonstrated for ethanol, which leads to hydroxyethyl radicals (Albano et al., 1991; Dupont et al., 1998), but also for carbon tetrachloride (McCay et al., 1984), halogenated hydrocarbons such as trichlorethylene (Halmes et al., 1997), fluorinated anesthetics such as halothane (Gut et al., 1993), or hydrochlorofluorocarbons used as substitutes for the ozone-depleting chlorofluorocarbons (Ferrara et al., 1997) that are metabolized via reductive pathways to free radicals. Toxicity of halogenated hydrocarbons may arise at either cytotoxicity or carcinogenesis and generally occurs in the liver or the kidneys (Raucy *et al.*, 1993). Free radical intermediates have also been observed after metabolism of alkylhydrazines by CYP2E1 (Albano *et al.*, 1995). Pyridine, a constituent of tobacco, has been shown to undergo sequential oxidation, resulting in the generation of reactive oxygen species and damages in DNA (Novak and Woodcroft, 2000). Many quinones also exert their toxic action through radical formation. Other reactive intermediates such as electrophilic epoxides can also be produced: CYP2E1 is the major catalyst of acrylonitrile epoxidation to the mutagen 2-cyanoethylene oxide (Kedderis *et al.*, 1993) or of epoxidation of ethylcarbamate (urethane), present in alcoholic beverages (Guengerich *et al.*, 1991). Most free radicals are generally detoxicated by glutathione but stores of glutathione in alcoholics are depleted, which favors accumulation of toxic compounds.

Growing bodies of evidence, mainly gained through animal studies, have shown that induction of a CYP by one chemical can result in enhanced toxicity of another compound. Therefore, prior exposure to ethanol or to CYP2E1 inducers can elicit cytotoxic and/or carcinogenic effects of xenobiotics metabolized by this CYP. Conversely, prior or concomitant exposure to CYP inhibitors can reduce or abolish the production of the reactive metabolite and hence the toxicity.

Enhanced susceptibility to hepatotoxicity

CYP2E1 plays a key role in the pathogenesis of liver injury. Ethanol-mediated microsomal induction promotes toxicity through increased formation of radical oxygen species and enhanced lipid peroxidation (Lieber, 1997). It is involved in the enhanced toxicity of therapeutic agents, e.g. acetaminophen (paracetamol), fluorinated anesthetics, and industrial solvents such as carbon tetrachloride or benzene.

Acetaminophen is a generally safe analgesic and antipyretic drug. However, therapeutic amounts of 2.5 to 6 g/day have been incriminated as the cause of hepatic injury in alcoholic patients (Seeff *et al.*, 1986). Acetaminophen is converted in N-acetyl-p-benzoquinone imine (NAPQI), a highly reactive free radical, by CYP2E1, CYP1A2 and CYP3A4 (Holtzman, 1995). NAPQI, normally detoxicated by glutathione, can bind covalently to proteins and hence cause severe hepatoxicity or nephrotoxicity. Detoxification of the toxic metabolite NAPQI may be impaired in chronic alcoholics by the depletion of reduced glutathione or alternatively by defective regulation of hepatic glutathione homeostasis after ethanol consumption (Lieber, 1991). Contribution of CYP1A2 and CYP3A4 to NAPQI formation has recently been shown to be negligible *in vivo* in humans (Manyike *et al.*, 2000). Pretreatment of volunteers by disulfiram, a CYP2E1 inhibitor, decreases the formation of NAPQI by 74% (Manyike *et al.*, 2000). In addition, it has recently been shown that CYP2E1 inhibitors used in human therapy, namely disulfiram and diethyldithiocarbamate, are also potent inhibitors of NAPQI formation in human liver microsomes (Hazai *et al.*, 2002). Enhanced metabolism (Girre *et al.*, 1993) and toxicity (Johnston and

Pelletier, 1997) of this drug have been observed after chronic ethanol consumption and have been related to CYP2E1 induction. In animals chronically fed with ethanol, the potentiation of acetaminophen hepatotoxicity occurred after ethanol withdrawal (Sato *et al.*, 1981). In fact, ethanol prevents acute acetaminophen-induced toxicity because of the inhibition of acetaminophen biotransformation into reactive metabolites.

Fluorinated anesthetics have also been shown to be activated by CYP2E1 into hepatotoxic compounds. CYP2E1 is the major catalyst in the formation of trifluoroacetylated proteins from halothane (Eliasson and Kenna, 1996), which have been implicated as target antigens responsible for stimulation of an immune reaction leading to severe hepatic necrosis (halothane hepatitis). Inhibition of CYP2E1 by disulfiram greatly reduces the production of the halothane metabolite responsible for the neoantigen formation (Kharash *et al.*, 1996).

Enhanced susceptibility to carcinogenicity

Alcohol abuse is associated with an increased incidence of upper alimentary and respiratory tract cancers. Enhancement of cytochrome P450-dependent carcinogen activation has been shown using microsomes from different tissues including the liver, principal site of xenobiotics metabolism, the lungs and intestines, entry for tobacco smoke and dietary or occupational carcinogens, and the esophagus, where ethanol consumption is a major risk in cancer development (Lieber, 1997).

Ethanol markedly increases the microsomal metabolism of benzene, a carcinogenic compound in humans, and aggravates its hematopoietic toxicity. Metabolism of benzene in human microsomes is associated with individual variations in CYP2E1 expression (Nedelcheva *et al.*, 1999). Toxicity of benzene has been related to the formation of benzene oxide by CYP2E1 in the liver; this oxide can form DNA-adducts (Soucek *et al.*, 1994). Benzene oxide spontaneously forms phenol which is further metabolized by CYP2E1 in hydroquinone and related hydroxy metabolites. However, hydroquinone is converted in the bone marrow by myeloperoxidase to benzoquinones, which are potent hematotoxic and genotoxic compounds (Gut *et al.*, 1996). Hydroquinone can be converted by NADPH: quinone oxidoreductase (NQO1) back to less toxic hydroxy metabolites (Ross, 1996). Therefore, high CYP2E1 and low NQO1 activities are associated with increased susceptibility to hematological malignancy in benzene-exposed workers (Rothman *et al.*, 1997).

CYP2E1 has also been associated with metabolic activation of N-nitrosamines, which results in dealkylation and formation of a carbonium ion presumed to alkylate DNA and initiate malignancy (Yoo *et al.*, 1988). Nitrosamines are ubiquitous in our environment; they are found in some preserved foods and beverages, e.g. beer and whisky, in tobacco smoke and industrial environments. CYP2E1 activates N-nitrosodimethylamine (NDMA) into carcinogenic compounds at higher rates than any other CYP isozyme (Yang *et al.*, 1990). Dialkylnitrosamines are metabolized by different pathways and different CYPs, depending on their structures: CYP2E1 is involved in the dealkylation of nitrosamines with short alkyl chains (one to three carbons) through an α-hydroxylation pathway, which leads to the formation of very electrophilic and reactive compounds. N-Nitrosamines with long alkyl chains are preferentially hydroxylated on β to ω positions by CYP 2A6, 2C and 3A4. The balance β to ω/α hydroxylation inversely correlates with nitrosamine mutagenicity (Bellec *et al.*, 1996). On the other hand, dialkylnitrosamines are metabolized by CYP2E1 and other CYPs to undergo denitrosation (Yang *et al.*, 1990). Pretreatment of rats with ethanol or acetone enhanced NDMA-induced methylation of DNA both *in vitro* and *in vivo* (Hong and Yang, 1985) and CYP2E1 inducers potentiated NDMA-induced hepatotoxicity (Lorr *et al.*, 1984). When ethanol and NDMA are given concomitantly in rodents or in primates, extrahepatic organs are more exposed to nitrosamines because of the competition between nitrosamines and ethanol in the liver; this yields DNA adducts and tumor development in the digestive tract (Anderson *et al.*, 1995). However, rodents appear to be much more vulnerable to NDMA carcinogenicity than humans (Lewis *et al.*, 1997).

Conclusion

Chronic ethanol consumption leads to increased CYP2E1 activity. This enzyme is toxicologically important because it participates in the metabolism and bioactivation of many chemically diverse compounds including ethanol, drugs, industrial solvents, and carcinogens. As ethanol and xenobiotics share the same metabolic pathway, pharmacokinetic and/or toxic interactions can be expected. Therefore, ethanol consumption has to be taken into consideration when drugs are prescribed or in workers exposed to industrial solvents. Susceptibility to xenobiotics' toxicity can be greatly influenced by differences in the activity of this enzyme.

Acknowledgments

The University of Bretagne Occidentale (UBO), the Region Bretagne, the Institut de Recherches Scientifiques sur les Boissons (IREB), the Ligue contre le Cancer, and European Contract INCO ERB-IC18-CT98-0341 support the research in the author's laboratory.

References

Albano, E., Comoglio, A., Clot, P., Iannone, A., Tomasi, A., and Ingelman-Sundberg, M. (1995) Activation of alkylhydrazines to free radical intermediates by ethanol-inducible cytochrome P-4502E1 (CYP2E1), *Biochimica et Biophysica Acta*, **1243**: 414–420.

Albano, E., Tomasi, A., Persson, J.O., Terelius, Y., Goria-Gatti, L., Ingelman-Sundberg, M., and Dianzani, M. (1991) Role of ethanol-inducible cytochrome P450 (P450IIE1) in catalysing the free radical activation of aliphatic alcohols, *Biochemical Pharmacology*, **41**: 1895–1902.

Anderson, L.M., Chhabra, S.K., Nerurkar, P.V., Souliotis, V.L., and Kyrtopoulos, S.A. (1995) Alcohol-related cancer risk: a toxicokinetic hypothesis, *Alcohol*, 12: 97–104.

Badger, T.M., Huang, J., Ronis, M., and Lumpkin, C.K. (1993) Induction of cytochrome P450 2E1 during ethanol exposure occurs via transcription of the CYP2E1 gene when blood concentrations are high, *Biochemical and Biophysical Research Communications*, 190: 780–785.

Bellec, G., Dreano, Y., Lozac'h, P., Menez, J-F., and Berthou, F. (1996) Cytochrome P450 metabolic dealkylation of nine N-nitrosodialkylamines by human liver microsomes, *Carcinogenesis*, 17: 2029–2034.

Cederbaum, A.I. (1987) Microsomal generation of hydroxyl radicals: its role in microsomal ethanol oxidizing system (MEOS) activity and requirement for iron. In *Alcohol and the Cell* (ed. E. Rubin), pp. 35–49. New York: The New York Academy of Sciences.

Dupont, I., Berthou, F., Bodenez, P., Bardou, L.-G., Guirriec, C., Stephan, N., Dreano, Y., and Lucas, D. (1999) Involvement of cytochrome P450 2E1 and 3A4 in the 5-hydroxylation of salicylate in humans, *Drug Metabolism and Disposition*, 27: 322–326.

Dupont, I., Bodenez, P., Berthou, F., Simon, B., Bardou, L.G., and Lucas, D. (2000) Cytochrome P450 2E1 activity and oxidative stress in alcoholic patients, *Alcohol and Alcoholism*, 35: 98–103.

Dupont, I., Lucas, D., Clot, P., Seccia, M., Menez, C., and Albano, E. (1998) Cytochrome P450 inducibility and hydroxyethyl radical formation among alcoholics, *Journal of Hepatology*, 28: 564–571.

Eliasson, E. and Kenna, J.G. (1996) Cytochrome P450 2E1 is a cell surface autoantigen in halothane hepatitis, *Molecular Pharmacology*, 50: 573–582.

Ferrara, R., Tolando, R., King, L.J., and Manno, M. (1997) Cytochrome P450 inactivation during reductive metabolism of 1,1-dichloro-2,2,2-trifluoroethane (HCFC-123) by phenobarbital and pyridine-induced rat liver microsomes, *Toxicology and Applied Pharmacology*, 143: 420–428.

Finnstrom, N., Thorn, M., Loof, L., and Rane, A. (2001) Independent patterns of cytochrome P450 gene expression in liver and blood in patients with suspected liver disease, *European Journal of Clinical Pharmacology*, 57: 403–409.

French, S.W., Mayer, R.J., Bardag-Gorce, F., Ingelman-Sundberg, M., Rouach, H., Neve, E., and Higashitsuji, H. (2001) The ubiquitin-proteasome 26s pathway in liver cell protein turnover: effect of ethanol and drugs, *Alcoholism: Clinical and Experimental Research*, 25 (Suppl. 1): 225S–229S.

Frye, R.F. and Branch, R.A. (2002) Effect of chronic disulfiram administration on the activities of CYP1A2, CYP2C19, CYP2D6, CYP2E1 and N-acetyltransferase in healthy human subjects, *British Journal of Clinical Pharmacology*, 53: 155–162.

Gannett, P.M., Iversen, P., and Lawson, T. (1990) The mechanism of inhibition of cytochrome P-450IIE1 by dihydrocapsaicin, *Bioorganic Chemistry*, 18: 185–198.

Garte, S., Gaspari, L., Alexandrie, A.K., Ambrosone, C., Autrup, H., Autrup, J.L., Baranova, H., Bathum, L., Benhamou, S., Boffetta, P. *et al.* (2001) Metabolic gene polymorphism frequencies in control populations, *Cancer Epidemiology, Biomarkers & Prevention*, 10: 1239–1248.

Gebhardt, A.C., Lucas, D., Menez, J-F., and Seitz, H.K. (1997) Chlormethiazole inhibition of cytochrome P450 2E1 as assessed by chlorzoxazone hydroxylation in humans, *Hepatology*, 26: 957–961.

Girre, C., Hispard, E., Palombo, S., N'guyen, C., and Dally, S. (1993) Increased metabolism of acetaminophen in chronically alcoholic patients, *Alcoholism: Clinical and Experimental Research*, 17: 170–173.

Guengerich, F.P., Kim, D.H., and Iwasaki, M. (1991) Role of human P-450 IIE1 in the oxidation of many low molecular weight cancer suspects, *Chemical Research in Toxicology*, **4**: 168–179.

Guengerich, F.P. and Turvy, C.G. (1991) Comparison of levels of several human microsomal P-450 enzymes and epoxide hydrolase in normal and disease states using immunochemical analysis of surgical liver samples, *Journal of Pharmacology and Experimental Therapeutics*, **256**: 1189–1194.

Gut, J., Christen, U., and Huwyler, J. (1993) Mechanisms of halothane toxicity: novel insights, *Pharmacology & Therapeutics*, **58**: 133–155.

Gut, I., Nedelcheva, V., Soucek, P., Stopka, P., Vodicka, P., Gelboin, H.V., and Ingelman-Sundberg, M. (1996) The role of CYP2E1 and 2B1 in metabolic activation of benzene derivatives, *Archives of Toxicology*, **71**: 45–56.

Halmes, N.C., Samokyszyn, V.M., and Pumford, N.R. (1997) Covalent binding and inhibition of cytochrome P4502E1 by trichloroethylene, *Xenobiotica*, **27**: 101–110.

Haufroid, V., Toubeau, F., Clippe, A., Buysschaert, M., Gala, J.-L., and Lison, D. (2001) Real-time quantification of cytochrome P4502E1 mRNA in human peripheral blood lymphocytes by reverse trancription-PCR: method and practical application, *Clinical Chemistry*, **47**: 1126–1129.

Hayashi, S., Watanabe, J., and Kaname, K. (1991) Genetic polymorphism in the 5′-flanking region change transcriptional regulation of the human cytochrome P450 IIE1 gene, *Journal of Biochemistry*, **110**: 559–565.

Hazai, E., Vereczkey, L., and Monostory, K. (2002) Reduction of toxic metabolite formation of acetaminophen, *Biochemical and Biophysical Research Communications*, **291**: 1089–1094.

Hirvonen, A., Husgafvel-Pursiainen, K., Anttila, S., Karjailainen, A., and Vainio, H. (1993) The human CYP2E1 gene and lung cancer: *Dra* I and *Rsa* I restriction fragment length polymorphisms in a Finnish study population, *Carcinogenesis*, **14**: 85–88.

Holtzman, J.L. (1995) The role of covalent binding to microsomal proteins in the hepatotoxicity of acetaminophen, *Drug Metabolism Reviews*, **27**: 277–297.

Hong, J., Pang, J., Gonzalez, F.J., Gelboin, H.V., and Yang, C.S. (1987) The induction of a specific form of cytochrome P-450 (P-450j) by fasting, *Biochemical and Biophysical Research Communications*, **142**: 1077–1083.

Hong, J. and Yang, C.S. (1985) The nature of microsomal N-nitrosodimethylamine demethylase and its role in carcinogen activation, *Carcinogenesis*, **6**: 1805–1809.

Ingelman-Sundberg, M., Johansson, I., Pentilla, K.E., Glaumann, H., and Lindros, K.O. (1988) Centrilobular expression of ethanol-inducible cytochrome P450 (IIE1) in rat liver, *Biochemical and Biophysical Research Communications*, **157**: 55–60.

Ioannides, C. (ed.) (1996) *Cytochromes P450, Metabolic and Toxicological Aspects*. Boca Raton, FL: CRC Press.

Ioannides, C. (1999) Effect of diet and nutrition on the expression of cytochromes P450, *Xenobiotica*, **29**: 109–154.

Johnston, S.C. and Pelletier, L.L. Jr (1997) Enhanced hepatotoxicity of acetaminophen in the alcoholic patient. Two case reports and a review of the literature, *Medicine* (Baltimore), **76**: 185–191.

Kedderis, G.L., Batra, R., and Koop, D.R. (1993) Epoxidation of acrylonitrile by rat and human cytochromes P450, *Chemical Research in Toxicology*, **6**: 866–871.

Kharash, E.D., Hankins, D.C., Jubert, C., Thummel, K.E., and Taraday, J.K. (1999) Lack of single-dose disulfiram effects on cytochrome P-450 2C9, 2C19, 2D6 and 3A4 activities: evidence for specificity toward P-450 2E1, *Drug Metabolism and Disposition*, 27: 717–723.

Kharash, E.D., Hankins, D., Mautz, D., and Thummel, K.E. (1996) Identification of the enzyme responsible for oxidative halothane metabolism: implications for prevention of halothane hepatitis, *Lancet*, 347: 1367–1371.

Kim, S.G., Kwak, J.Y., Lee, J.W., Novak, R.F., Park, S.S., and Kim, N.D. (1994) Malotilate, a hepatoprotectant, suppresses CYP2E1 expression in rats, *Biochemical and Biophysical Research Communications*, 200: 1414–1420.

Koop, D.R. and Tierney, D.J. (1990) Multiple mechanisms in the regulation of ethanol-inducible cytochrome P450 IIE1, *Bioassays*, 12: 429–435.

Korourian, S., Hakkak, R., Ronis, M.J., Shelnutt, S.R., Waldron, J., Ingelman-Sundberg, M., and Badger, T.M. (1999) Diet and risk of ethanol-induced hepatotoxicity: carbohydrate–fat relationships in rats, *Toxicological Sciences*, 47: 110–117.

Kurata, N., Nishimura, Y., Iwase, M., Fisher, N.E., Tang, B.K., Inaba, T., and Yasuhara, H. (1998) Trimethadione metabolism by human liver cytochrome P450: evidence for the involvement of CYP2E1, *Xenobiotica*, 28: 1041–1047.

Le Marchand, L., Wilkinson, G.R., and Wilkens, L.R. (1999) Genetic and dietary predictors of CYP2E1 activity: a phenotyping study in Hawaii Japanese using chlorzoxazone, *Cancer Epidemiology, Biomarkers & Prevention*, 8: 495–500.

Leclercq, I., Desager, J.-P., and Horsmans, Y. (1998) Inhibition of chlorzoxazone metabolism, a clinical probe for CYP2E1, by a single ingestion of watercress, *Clinical Pharmacology and Therapeutics*, 642: 144–149.

Leclercq, I., Hormans, Y., Desager, J.-P., Pauwels, S., and Geubel, A.P. (1999) Dietary restriction of energy and sugar results in a reduction in human cytochrome P450 2E1 activity, *British Journal of Nutrition*, 82: 257–262.

Lewis, D.F.V., Brantom, P.G., Ioannides, C., Walker, R., and Parke, D.V. (1997) Nitrosamine carcinogenesis: rodent assays, quantitative structure activity relationships, and human risk assessment, *Drug Metabolism Reviews*, 29: 1055–1078.

Lieber, C.S. (1991) Hepatic, metabolic and toxic effects of ethanol: 1991 update, *Alcoholism: Clinical and Experimental Research*, 15: 573–592.

Lieber, C.S. (1997) Cytochrome P-4502E1: its physiological and pathological role, *Physiological Reviews*, 77: 517–544.

Lieber, C.S. (1999) Microsomal ethanol-oxidizing system (MEOS): the first 30 years (1968–1998) – a review, *Alcoholism: Clinical and Experimental Research*, 23: 991–1007.

Lorr, N.A., Miller, K.W., Chung, H.R., and Yang, C.S. (1984) Potentiation of the hepatotoxicity of N-nitrosodimethylamine by fasting, diabetes, acetone, and isopropanol, *Toxicology and Applied Pharmacology*, 73: 423–431.

Lucas, D., Berthou, F., Dreano, Y., Lozac'h, P., Volant, A., and Menez, J.-F. (1993) Comparison of levels of cytochromes P450, CYP1A2, CYP2E1 and their related monooxygenase activities in human surgical liver samples, *Alcoholism: Clinical and Experimental Research*, 17: 900–905.

Lucas, D., Berthou, F., and Ménez, J.-F. (1996) Chlorzoxazone: *in vitro* and *in vivo* substrate probe for liver CYP2E1, *Methods in Enzymology*, 272: 115–123.

Lucas, D., Ferrara, R., Gonzalez, E., Bodenez, P., Albores, A., Manno, M., and Berthou, F. (1999) Chlorzoxazone, a selective probe for phenotyping CYP2E1 in humans, *Pharmacogenetics*, 9: 377–388.

Lucas, D., Menez, C., Girre, C., Berthou, F., Bodenez, P., Joannet, I., Hispard, E., Bardou, L.G., and Menez, J-F. (1995a) Cytochrome P4502E1 genotype and chlorzoxazone metabolism in healthy and alcoholic caucasian subjects, *Pharmacogenetics*, 5: 298–304.

Lucas, D., Menez, C., Girre, C., Bodenez, P., Hispard, E., and Menez, J-F. (1995b) Decrease in cytochrome P4502E1 as assessed by the rate of chlorzoxazone hydroxylation in alcoholics during the withdrawal phase, *Alcoholism: Clinical and Experimental Research*, **19**: 362–366.

McCarver, D.G., Byun, R., Hines, R.N., Hichme, M., and Wegenek, W. (1998) A genetic polymorphism in the regulatory sequences of human CYP2E1: association with increased chlorzoxazone hydroxylation in the presence of obesity and ethanol intake, *Toxicology and Applied Pharmacology*, **152**: 276–281.

McCay, P.B., Lai, E.K., Poyer, J.L., Dubose, C.M., and Janzen, E.G. (1984) Oxygen- and carbon-centered free radical formation during carbon tetrachloride metabolism. Observation of lipid radicals *in vivo* and *in vitro*, *Journal of Biological Chemistry*, **259**: 2135–2143.

Manno, M., Rezzadore, M., Grossi, M., and Sbrana, C. (1996) Potentiation of occupational carbon tetrachloride toxicity by ethanol abuse, *Human & Experimental Toxicology*, **15**: 294–300.

Mansuy, D. (1998) The great diversity of reactions catalyzed by cytochromes P450, *Comparative Biochemistry and Physiology*, **121**: 5–14.

Manyike, P.T., Kharash, E.D., Kalhorn, T.F., and Slattery, J.Y. (2000) Contribution of CYP2E1 and CYP3A to acetaminophen reactive metabolite formation, *Clinical Pharmacology and Therapeutics*, **67**: 275–282.

Nedelcheva, V., Gut, Y., Soucek, P., Tichavska, B., Tynkova, L., Mraz, J., Guengerich, F.P., and Ingelman-Sundberg, M. (1999) Metabolism of benzene in human liver microsomes: individual variations in relation to CYP2E1 expression, *Archives of Toxicology*, **73**: 33–40.

Nelson, D.R., Koymans, L., Kamataki, T., Stegeman, J.J., Feyereisen, R., Waxman, D.J., Waterman, M.R., Gotoh, O., Coon, M.J., Estabrook, R.W., Gunsalus, I.C., and Nebert, D.W. (1996) P450 superfamily: update on new sequences, gene mapping, accession numbers, and nomenclature, *Pharmacogenetics*, **6**: 1–42.

Nordmann, R., Ribiere, C., and Rouach, H. (1992) Implication of free radical mechanisms in ethanol-induced cellular injury, *Free Radical Biology and Medicine*, **12**: 219–240.

Novak, R.F. and Woodcroft, K.J. (2000) The alcohol-inducible form of cytochrome P450 (CYP2E1): role in toxicology and regulation of expression, *Archives of Pharmacal Research*, **23**: 267–282.

Oneta, C.M., Lieber, C.S., Li, J., Ruttimann, S., Schmid, B., Lattmann, J., Rosman, A.S., and Seitz, H.K. (2002) Dynamics of cytochrome P4502E1 activity in man: induction by ethanol and disappearance during withdrawal phase, *Journal of Hepatology*, **36**: 47–52.

O'Shea, D., Davis, S.N., Kim, R.B., and Wilkinson, G.R. (1994) Effect of fasting and obesity in humans on the 6-hydroxylation of chlorzoxazone: a putative probe of CYP2E1 activity, *Clinical Pharmacology and Therapeutics*, **56**: 359–367.

Parke, D.V., Ioannides, C., and Lewis, D.F. (1991) The role of the cytochromes P450 in the detoxication and activation of drugs and other chemicals, *Canadian Journal of Physiology and Pharmacology*, **69**: 537–549.

Perrot, N., Nalpas, B., Yang, C.S., and Beaune, P.H. (1989) Modulation of cytochrome P450 isozymes in human liver by ethanol and drug intake, *European Journal of Clinical Investigation*, **19**: 549–555.

Peter, R., Boker, R., Beaune, P.H., Iwasaki, M., Guengerich, F.P., and Yang, C.S. (1990) Hydroxylation of chlorzoxazone as a specific probe for human liver cytochrome P450 IIE1, *Chemical Research in Toxicology*, **3**: 566–573.

Petersen, D.R., Atkinson, N., and Hjelle, J.J. (1982) Increase in hepatic microsomal ethanol oxidation by a single dose of ethanol, *Journal of Pharmacology and Experimental Therapeutics*, **221**: 275–281.

Plee-Gautier, E., Foresto, F., Ferrara, R., Bodénez, P., Simon, B., Manno, M., Berthou, F., and Lucas, D. (2001) Genetic repeat polymorphism in the regulating region of CYP2E1: frequency and relationship with enzymatic activity in alcoholics, *Alcoholism: Clinical and Experimental Research*, **25**: 800–805.

Poupon, J., Lucas, D., and Berthou, F. (2002) Oxidation of ethanol into acetaldehyde, hydroxyethyl radical (HER) and acetic acid by CYP2E1 in rat liver microsomes, *Alcoholism: Clinical and Experimental Research*, **26** (suppl.): 185A.

Powell, H., Kitteringham, N.R., Pirmohamed, M., Smith, D.A., and Park, B.K. (1998) Expression of cytochrome P4502E1: assessment by mRNA, genotype and phenotype, *Pharmacogenetics*, **8**: 411–421.

Raucy, J.L., Curley, G., and Carpenter, S.P. (1995) Use of lymphocytes for assessing ethanol-mediated alterations in the expression of hepatic cytochrome P4502E1, *Alcoholism: Clinical and Experimental Research*, **19**: 1369–1375.

Raucy, J.L., Kraner, J.C., and Lasker, J.M. (1993) Bioactivation of halogenated hydrocarbons by cytochrome P450 2E1, *Critical Reviews in Toxicology*, **23**: 1–20.

Raucy, J.L., Schultz, E.D., Kearins, M.C., Arora, S., Johnston, D.E., Omdahl, J.L., Eckmann, L., and Carpenter, S.P. (1999) CYP2E1 expression in human lymphocytes from various ethnic populations, *Alcoholism: Clinical and Experimental Research*, **23**: 1868–1874.

Reinke, L.A., Moore, D.R., and McCay, P.B. (1997) Mechanisms for metabolism of ethanol to 1-hydroxyethyl radicals in rat liver microsomes, *Archives of Biochemistry and Biophysics*, **348**: 9–14.

Riihimaki, V., Savolainen, K., Pfaffli, P., Pekeri, K., Sippel, H.W., and Laine, A. (1982) Metabolic interaction between m-xylene and ethanol, *Archives of Toxicology*, **49**: 253–263.

Roberts, B.J., Shoaf, S.E., and Song, B.J. (1995a) Rapid changes in cytochrome P4502E1 (CYP2E1) activity and other P450 isozymes following ethanol withdrawal in rats, *Biochemical Pharmacology*, **49**: 1665–1673.

Roberts, B.J., Song, B.J., Soh, Y., Park, S.S., and Shoaf, S.E. (1995b) Ethanol induces CYP2E1 by protein stabilization, *Journal of Biological Chemistry*, **270**: 29632–29635.

Rodriguez-Antona, C., Donato, T., Pareja, E., Gomez-Lechon, M.-J., and Castell, J.V. (2001) Cytochrome P-450 mRNA expression in human liver and its relationship with enzymes activity, *Archives of Biochemistry and Biophysics*, **393**: 308–315.

Ronis, M.J., Huang, J., Crouch, J., Mercado, C., Irby, D., Valentine, C.R., Lumpkin, C.K., Ingelman-Sundberg, M., and Badger, T.M. (1993) Cytochrome P450 CYP2E1 induction during chronic alcohol exposure occurs by a two-step mechanism associated with blood alcohol concentrations in rats, *Journal of Pharmacology and Experimental Therapeutics*, **264**: 944–950.

Ronis, M.J., Lindros, K.O., and Ingelman-Sundberg, M. (1996) The CYP2E subfamily. In *Cytochromes P450: Metabolic and Toxicological Aspects* (ed. C. Ioannides), pp. 211–219. Boca Raton, FL: CRC Press.

Ross, D. (1996) Metabolic basis of benzene toxicity, *European Journal of Haematology*, **60** (Suppl.): 111–118.

Rothman, N., Smith, M.T., Hayes, R.B., Traver, R.D., Hoener, B.-A., Campleman, S., Li, G.-L., Domeseci, M., Linet, M., Zhang, L., Xi, L., Walchoder, S., Lu, W., Meyer, K.B.,

Titenko-Holland, N., Stewart, J.T., Yin, S., and Ross, D. (1997) Benzene poisoning, a risk factor for haematological malignancy, is associated with the NQO1 609 C→T mutation and rapid fractional excretion of chlorzoxazone, *Cancer Research*, **57**: 2839–2842.

Salmela, K.S., Kessova, I.G., Tsyrlov, I.B., and Lieber, C.S. (1998) Respective roles of human cytochrome P450 2E1, 1A2 and 3A4 in the hepatic microsomal ethanol oxidizing system, *Alcoholism: Clinical and Experimental Research*, **22**: 2125–2132.

Sato, C., Matsuda, Y., and Lieber, C.S. (1981) Increased hepatotoxicity of acetaminophen after chronic ethanol consumption in the rat, *Gastroenterology*, **80**: 140–148.

Seeff, L.B., Cuccherini, B.A., Zimmerman, H.J., Adler, E., and Benjamin, S.B. (1986) Acetaminophen hepatotoxicity in alcoholics. A therapeutic misadventure, *Annals of Internal Medicine*, **104**: 399–404.

Soucek, P., Tichavska, B., and Gut, I. (1994) Cytochrome P450 destruction and radical scavenging by benzene and its metabolites. Evidence for the key role of quinones, *Biochemical Pharmacology*, **47**: 2233–2242.

Stoyanovski, D.A. and Cederbaum, A.I. (1998) ESR and HPLC-EC analysis of ethanol oxidation to 1-hydroxyethyl radical: rapid reduction and quantification of POBN and PBN nitroxides, *Free Radical Biology & Medicine*, **25**: 536–545.

Streetman, D.S., Bertino, J.S. Jr, and Nafziger, A.N. (2000) Phenotyping of drug metabolizing enzymes in adults: a review of *in-vivo* cytochrome P450 phenotyping probes, *Pharmacogenetics*, **10**: 187–216.

Takahashi, H., Johansson, I., French, S.W., and Ingelman-Sundberg, M. (1992) Effects of dietary fat consumption on activities of the microsomal ethanol oxidizing system and ethanol-inducible cytochrome P450 in the liver of rats chronically fed ethanol, *Pharmacology & Toxicology*, **70**: 347–352.

Takahashi, H., Lasker, J.M., Rosman, A.S., and Lieber, C.S. (1993) Induction of P4502E1 in the human liver by ethanol is caused by a corresponding increase in encoding messenger RNA, *Hepatology*, **17**: 236–245.

Tassaneeyakul, W., Veronese, M.E., Birkett, D.J., Gonzales, F.J., and Miners, J.O. (1993) Validation of 4-nitrophenol as an *in vitro* substrate for human liver CYP2E1 using cDNA expression and microsomal kinetic techniques, *Biochemical Pharmacology*, **46**: 1975–1981.

Vermeulen, N.P.E. (1996) Role of metabolism in chemical toxicity. In *Cytochromes P450: Metabolic and Toxicological Aspects* (ed. C. Ioannides), pp. 29–53. Boca Raton, FL: CRC Press.

Wong, N.A.C., Rae, F., Simpson, K.J., Murray, G.D., and Harrison, D.J. (2000) Genetic polymorphism of cytochrome P4502E1 and susceptibility to alcoholic liver disease and hepatocellular carcinoma in a white population: a study and literature review, including meta-analysis, *Journal of Clinical Pathology: Molecular Pathology*, **53**: 88–93.

Yang, C.S., Yoo, J-S., Ishizaki, H., and Hong, J. (1990) Cytochrome P450 IIE1: roles in nitrosamine metabolism and mechanisms of regulation, *Drug Metabolism Reviews*, **22**: 147–159.

Yano, H., Tsutsumi, M., Fukura, M., Chen, W.-B., Shimanaka, K., Tsuchishima, M., Takase, S., Imaoka, S., and Funae, Y. (2001) Study of cytochrome P4502E1 mRNA level of mononuclear cells in patients with alcoholic liver disease, *Alcoholism: Clinical and Experimental Research*, **25** (Suppl.): 2S–6S.

Yoo, J.S.H., Guengerich, F.P., and Yang, C.S. (1988) Metabolism of N-nitrosodialkylamines by human liver microsomes, *Cancer Research*, **48**: 1499–1504.

Yoo, J.S.H., Ning, S.M., Pantuck, C.B., Pantuck, E.J., and Yang, C.S. (1991) Regulation of hepatic microsomal cytochrome P450IIE1 level by dietary lipids and carbohydrates in rats, *Journal of Nutrition*, **121**: 959–961.

Zerilli, A., Lucas, D., Amet, Y., Beauge, F., Volant, A., Floch, H.H., Berthou, F., and Menez, J.F. (1995) Cytochrome P450 2E1 in rat liver, kidney and lung microsomes after chronic administration of ethanol either orally or by inhalation, *Alcohol and Alcoholism*, **30**: 357–365.

15 Dietary factors influencing apoptosis in the intestine

Patricia M. Heavey and Ian R. Rowland

Summary

The functions of the large intestine include microbial fermentation, formation and storage of feces, and recovery of water and electrolytes. It is well recognized that the maintenance of these functions plays an important role in human health. Cell populations in the intestinal mucosa are normally maintained in equilibrium by balancing cell proliferation and apoptosis. Apoptosis, or programmed cell death, is an intrinsic mechanism of cell suicide, is associated with the removal of damaged cells, and is considered a protective effect. It is widely accepted that the accumulation of mutations in specific genes controlling cell division, apoptosis and DNA repair may result in carcinogenesis. Dysregulation of either proliferation or apoptosis may contribute to an increase in neoplastic cells. Certain foods and nutrients have been identified which are thought to exert an effect on apoptosis. In particular there has been much focus on the pro-apoptotic effects of the short-chain fatty acid (SCFA) butyrate, prebiotics and other bioactive food components as well as the nonsteroidal anti-inflammatory drugs (NSAIDs).

Introduction

Colorectal cancer (CRC) is the second most common cause of death from malignant neoplasia in Europe with 190 000 new cases per year, affecting 6% of men and women by the age of 65 (Bingham, 1996). Within a given population there will be individuals whose genetic background increases their susceptibility to colorectal cancer. However, it would appear that environmental factors, which include diet, lifestyle, cultural and social practices, all participate in the etiology of colorectal cancer. The importance of environmental factors is demonstrated by the high incidence of colorectal cancer in migrant groups who move from poor countries to those that are more affluent. Several studies have illustrated that regardless of the incidence of CRC in the migrants' original country, their risk of the disease becomes similar to that of the native population (Buell and Dunn, 1965; Haenszel, 1961; Pisa et al., 2000).

Epidemiological studies have highlighted certain foods, nutrients and lifestyle factors that may play a role in the development or prevention of colorectal cancer. The major risk factors that have been identified for colorectal neoplasia include positive family history, meat, smoking, and alcohol; while protective factors include vegetables, calcium, hormone replacement therapy (HRT), folate, nonsteroidal anti-inflammatory drugs (NSAIDS), and physical activity. For the purpose of this review, we will focus primarily on nutrients and foods that are thought to exert an effect on apoptosis. The research reported in the literature has centered on the pro-apoptotic effects of the short chain fatty acid (SCFA) butyrate, prebiotics and other bioactive food components as well as the non-steroidal anti-inflammatory drugs (NSAIDs). Since diet is associated with 80% of colorectal cancer cases (Willett, 1995) it is important to comprehend the mechanisms and underlying molecular basis of these interactions in order to provide a link between epidemiological studies and the risk of colorectal cancer. Changes in the balance of cell proliferation and apoptosis in the colonic mucosa in response to changes in the diet are being investigated in both *in vitro* and *in vivo* models of the human intestine.

The intestinal mucosa of rodents and other mammals is renewed every two to three days (Goodlad and Wright, 1990). In humans, the stem cells of the colonic mucosa generate approximately 10^7 new cells every hour (Potten *et al.*, 1979). Maintenance of the architecture of the colonic mucosa, and in particular of mucosal crypts, is the consequence of the balance of a number of factors. In normal adult tissues, proliferation, apoptosis and DNA repair are in equilibrium and this ensures a steady state of healthy cells. The passage from normal epithelium to carcinoma is characterized by one or more genetic alterations that change how the cell functions. This involves the deregulation of specific genes that control cell division, apoptosis, and DNA repair. These include oncogenes, suppressor genes and mismatch repair (MMR) genes. The mechanism of self-destruction within cells is referred to as apoptosis or programmed cell death (PCD). It is associated with the removal of damaged cells and is considered a protective event.

Microarchitecture of the large intestine

The intestinal mucosa provides an important barrier between the host and its environment. Through this mucosal barrier we acquire water, nutrients and other bioactive compounds, while combating toxins and infective agents. These duties are carried out by cells produced in the crypts. The surface of the large intestine is characterized by crypts (Figure 15.1), which are about 50 cells deep. Replication occurs in the stem cells located in the lowest third of the crypt. This location combined with the upward pressure exerted in the crypt ensures protection from the potentially genotoxic compounds found in the luminal contents. The replicating cells push upward to the surface of the crypt and in doing so proliferate and differentiate. At the top of the crypt the cells undergo apoptosis and so any damage induced by the luminal contents will have no influence on the integrity of the crypt.

Since it is widely accepted that tumors arise from stem cells, it has been assumed that the first mutation would most probably be a consequence of a

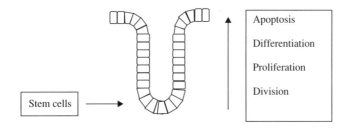

Figure 15.1 The colonic mucosal crypt.

blood-borne mutagen. This would result in replicating abnormal cells producing a polyp at the top of the crypt, that would be exposed to the genotoxic components of the luminal stream and consequently increase the likelihood of further mutations. This process is at present circumstantial and has been contradicted by the top-down morphogenesis of colorectal cancer put forward by Shih *et al.* (2001). This group examined the molecular characteristics of cells from both the top and bottom of the same crypt in small colorectal adenomas. They observed that the dysplastic cells at the top of the crypts frequently exhibited genetic alterations of adenomatous polyposis coli (APC) and neoplasia-associated patterns of gene expression. The cells at the bottom of the same crypt did not display these alterations. Shih and coworkers propose that the development of adenomatous polyps proceeds through a top-down mechanism. Those cells that have been genetically altered would spread laterally and downward to form new crypts that would eventually replace the pre-existing normal crypts.

Molecular pathways involved in colorectal cancer

Our understanding of the molecular basis of colorectal cancer has been greatly assisted by the study of two inherited forms of the disease, familial adenomatous polyposis (FAP) and hereditary non-polyposis colorectal cancer (HNPCC). FAP is a rare autosomal dominant syndrome (Veale, 1965) which is caused by an inherited mutation in the APC gene. This disease is characterized by the development of numerous polyps that usually begin in childhood, which will progress to malignant cancer by the fourth decade if left untreated. The majority of germline mutations result in a truncated protein product with abnormal function. There will also be an additional somatic mutation or loss of heterozygosity (LOH) at this locus in colorectal tumors from FAP patients. These inherited highly penetrant APC mutations account for only 1% of CRC cases. Loss of the tumor suppressor APC gene has also been identified as one of the initial events in the colorectal cancer pathway, with an estimated 80% of sporadic colon tumors showing acquired mutations in this gene (Powell *et al.*, 1992). There are at least five to seven major molecular alterations which need to occur for a normal epithelial cell to proceed to carcinoma and this is referred to as the

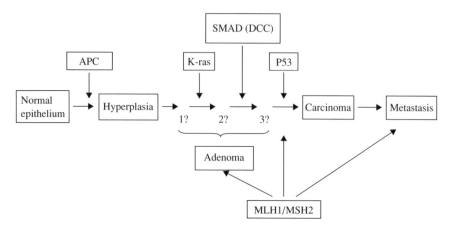

Figure 15.2 Genetic changes during colon carcinogenesis.

adenoma–carcinoma sequence (Fearon and Vogelstein, 1990). This process is now accepted as central to the majority of cancers and has been extensively studied in CRC. Several genes have been identified including the APC suppressor gene, k-ras oncogene, 18q and p53 suppressor genes, and genes involved in methylation pathways (Figure 15.2).

APC is located on chromosome 5q and it codes for a 2843-amino acid protein which is important in cell adhesion, signal transduction, and transcriptional activation. It is referred to as the housekeeping gene and is important in cell adhesion as well as in the Wg/wnt signaling pathway. It is also involved in proliferation via β catenin/Tdf and in motility via interaction with the cytoskeleton. APC mutations create all the conditions – abnormalities of adhesion, migration, and replication – to grow a polyp. One APC mutation usually results in a truncated protein while the other is either a similar mutation or a loss of heterozygosity (LOH). A large percentage (~60%) of APC somatic mutations occur between codons 1286 and 1513, referred to as the mutation cluster region (MCR). Mutations within this region are associated with allelic loss (LOH), while tumors with non-MCR mutations are associated with truncating mutations (Rowan *et al.*, 2000).

Ki-ras is a proto-oncogene whose primary function is the activation of signal transduction. Mutations in this gene were among the first to be associated with the pathogenesis of colon cancer (Vogelstein *et al.*, 1988) and it has found in 30–50% of adenomas and carcinomas (Bos *et al.*, 1987).

The long arm of chromosome 18 (18q) has also been implicated in the CRC pathway. LOH affecting 18q increased from zero in normal tissue to 13% in small adenomas, 47% in larger ones, and 73% in carcinomas (Vogelstein *et al.*, 1988). However, it is still uncertain what gene(s) are involved. DCC (deleted in colorectal cancer), SMAD4/DPC4, and MADR2 have all been linked to CRC. DCC was considered to be a cell adhesion molecule while MADR2 and

SMAD4 are understood to be involved in intracellular pathways responsive to transforming growth factor-beta (TGF-β), which is a negative growth signal. The long arm of chromosome 18 and these genes continue to be studied.

The P53 tumor repressor gene exhibits molecular abnormalities observed in a wide range of human cancers, and is associated with the transition from adenoma to carcinoma in CRC (Cho and Vogelstein, 1992). P53 is located on 17p and codes for a protein consisting of 393 amino acids. The p53 repressor protein is an important factor in integrating responses from the DNA synthesis, repair and apoptosis pathways and it also acts as a transcription factor for several genes. Due to the protein's diverse functions, p53 is frequently referred to as the "Guardian of the Genome". Mutations in p53 are mostly mis-sense mutations, resulting in loss of function and increased quantity or over-expression of the p53 protein (Greenblatt *et al.*, 1994).

Acquired or inherited mutations of DNA damage repair genes also play a role in predisposing colorectal epithelial cells to mutations. Repair of damaged DNA is an important defense mechanism that prevents most people from developing cancer. Defects in DNA repair processes have been identified in a subtype of inherited colorectal cancer, hereditary non-polyposis colon cancer (HNPCC). HNPCC is also an inherited autosomal dominant syndrome (Lynch and Lynch, 1985), but unlike FAP it is not easily distinguishable from sporadic CRC as there is no extensive polyposis. It is the most common form of hereditary CRC, accounting for 5–8% of cases (Lynch and de la Chapelle, 1999). Patients with this disease carry a mutation in genes coding for enzymes involved in mismatch repair (Salahshor *et al.*, 1999). Repair of damaged DNA is an important defense mechanism that prevents most people from developing cancer. To date, five genes have been identified that when mutated are linked to HNPCC. These genes, referred to as the mismatch repair (MMR) genes, include hMSH2 on chromosome 2, hMLH1 on chromosome 3, hPMS1 on chromosome 2, and hPMS2 on chromosome 7. Defects in mismatch repair genes also account for between 10% and 15% of sporadic colon cancers (Peltomaki *et al.*, 1993). Throughout the cell cycle somatic mutations arise in a variety of ways which may result in base–base mismatches and insertion–deletion loops. Stretches of re-petitive DNA units are particularly susceptible to insertion–deletion loops and, because of this defect, microsatellite instability is frequently observed. This genetic instability has been shown to lead to mutations in transforming growth factor-β1 (TGF-β1) (Markowitz *et al.*, 1995). TGF-β is a cytokine involved in controlling cell cycle progression, cell differentiation and morphogenesis (Massague and Polyak, 1995) and exerts various effects depending on concen-tration and cell type involved. It has been demonstrated that TGF-β can both inhibit (Cerwenka *et al.*, 1996) and induce apoptosis (Oberhammer *et al.*, 1992). The TGF-β type II receptor is considered a colon cancer suppressor gene that is also inactivated by mutation in 90% of human colon cancers arising via the microsatellite instability pathway. Grady *et al.* (1998) showed that these muta-tions were a late event in this form of colon cancer and correlated with the progression of adenoma to carcinoma.

The cell cycle and apoptosis

Apoptosis is regulated by inhibitors and activators of the cell cycle. Loss of these internal controls (checkpoints) can initiate apoptosis. The cell cycle comprises four phases: G1, S, G2, and M. After cell division the cell enters G1 and at a point called the restriction point, the cell is committed to proceed through the cell cycle. During the S phase, DNA replication takes place and this is followed by preparation of the chromatin in the G2 phase. Eventually the cells undergo mitosis. The cell cycle progression is regulated by the cyclin-dependent kinases (CDKs). CDKs are controlled by a series of complex phosphorylation and dephosphorylation events. Other proteins also regulate CDK–cyclin activity, namely the cyclin-dependent kinase inhibitors (CDKIs). They inhibit kinase activity by binding to either the CDK or the CDK–cyclin complex. P21 and p16 have been identified in mammalian cells as CDK–cyclin kinase inhibitors. P21 expression is regulated by the tumor suppressor gene p53 when there is DNA damage. The tumor suppressor genes, Rb (retinoblastoma protein) and p53 act as negative regulators of cell growth. Rb exerts its effect in the G1 phase whereas p53 functions in two pathways including G1/S cell cycle arrest following DNA damage and also apoptosis.

Apoptosis

The term "apoptosis" was introduced into modern scientific literature by Kerr *et al.* in 1972 to describe a form of cell death that was distinct from necrosis (Table 15.1). Necrosis is a non-programmed, non-physiological form of cell death that is induced by extremes in the external environment such as hypoxia, hypothermia, and certain cytotoxic agents. It results in the cellular metabolic collapse of the cell with the membrane of the cell rupturing and releasing cytoplasmic contents including the lysosomal enzymes into the extracellular fluid, which generates an inflammatory response. Local inflammation ensues, causing further cell damage.

Apoptosis, however, is a genetically programmed mode of cell death that is regulated by many genes, including oncogenes and oncosuppressor genes, which may be mutated, delayed or abnormally expressed in neoplasms, thus altering tumor cell susceptibility to apoptosis (Arends, 1995). Table 15.1 compares the morphological and biochemical differences between apoptosis and necrosis. Once initiated, apoptosis leads to a cascade of biochemical and morphological actions that results in irreversible degradation of the genomic DNA and disintegration of the cells. It is a localized event affecting individual cells and is characterized by membrane inversion and exposure of phosphatidylserine residues, blebbing (referred to as zeiosis), fragmentation of the nucleus, chromatin condensation, and DNA degradation. This is followed by the deterioration of the entire cell into many intact fragments. These "apoptotic bodies" are then phagocytosed by neighboring or immune cells.

Table 15.1 Morphological and biochemical differences between apoptosis and necrosis

Morphological differences

Apoptosis	*Necrosis*
Single cells deleted	Death of cell groups
Membrane blebbing	Loss of membrane integrity
Cell shrinkage	Cells swell and lyze
No inflammatory response	Significant inflammatory response
Phagocytosis by adjacent normal cells	Phagocytosis by macrophages
Lysosomes intact	Lysosomal leakage
Chromatin condenses	Indistinct aggregation of chromatin

Biochemical differences

Apoptosis	*Necrosis*
Induced by physiological stimuli disturbances	Evoked by nonphysiological disturbances
Tightly regulated process	Loss of ion homeostasis
Requires energy	Does not require energy
Entails macromolecular synthesis	No requirements for protein or nucleic acid synthesis
De novo gene transcription	No new gene transcription
Nonrandom oligonucleosomal length fragmentation of DNA	Random digestion of DNA

This form of programmed cell death is an essential component of normal development and is necessary for maintaining tissue homeostasis. Dysregulation of apoptosis may result in many diseases including cancer, AIDS, Alzheimer's disease, Parkinson's disease, and heart disease.

The initiation and regulation of apoptosis involves several pathways and has yet to be fully elucidated (Figure 15.3). The following is a brief overview of some of the major steps in this pathway. There are two different mechanisms by which apoptosis may be induced in a cell. The first is generated by signals arising within the mitochondria, referred to as the "intrinsic pathway"; the other is triggered by death activators binding to receptors at the cell surface (extrinsic pathway). In both pathways, a family of proteases called caspases (cysteine aspartyl-specific proteases) are triggered and cleave cellular substrates, resulting in biochemical and morphological changes characteristic of apoptosis.

Several caspases are now known as being key regulators and effectors of the apoptotic response in a number of species. In humans, 14 proteolytic enzymes (caspases 1–14) have been identified. The caspases are initially expressed in the cell as zymogens which are inactive. Initiation of the pathway requires dimerization of the caspases, triggering a signaling cascade that advances and augments the intracellular death signal and mediates an elaborate range of intracellular events. Dimerization is induced at the cell surface when death-inducing receptors at the cell surface (e.g. FAS/APO1/CD95 and the tumor

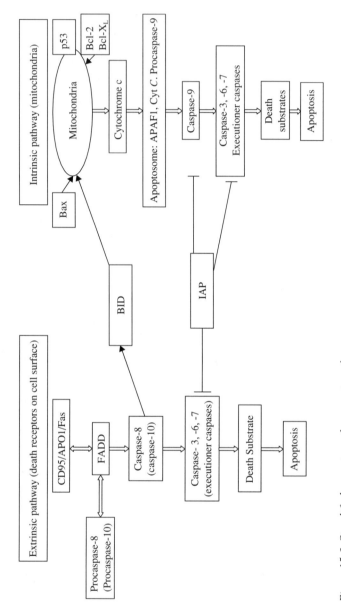

Figure 15.3 Simplified overview of apoptosis pathways.

necrosis factor (TNF) family or the mitochondria activate caspase-8 and/or caspase-10 monomers. These death domains attract the intracellular adaptor protein Fas-associated death domain protein (FADD). The caspases that are recruited to this death-inducing signaling complex (DISC) are caspase-8 and caspase-10. In some cells the amount of active caspase-8 is sufficient to induce apoptosis directly, but in other cells the amount is too small and the mitochondria are used to amplify the apoptotic signal. Activation of the mitochondria is mediated by the Bcl2 family member BID. The Bcl-2 family of proteins regulates the integrity of the outer mitochondria membrane barrier. This family of proteins has both pro- and anti-apoptotic members. The pro-apoptotic members induce the release of cytochrome c from the mitochondria whereas the anti-apoptotic members counteract the pro-apoptotic members and prevent the release of cytochrome c from the mitochondria. Overexpression of Bcl-2 has been implicated in a variety of cancers including colorectal cancer.

Dimerization also occurs when the caspase-9 binding protein, Apaf-1, is cleaved. Cleavage of Apaf-1 is initiated by binding of cytochrome c. In healthy cells, Apaf-1 is located outside the mitochondria and cytochrome c is within the mitochondrial intermembrane space. Segregation of the two prevents caspase activation. When the membrane barrier is breached, cytochrome c is released and caspases are activated. Bax, which is a pro-apoptotic protein, facilitates the release of cytochrome c from the mitochondrial inner membrane.

Once these caspases are activated they in turn activate caspase-3, caspase-6, and caspase-7 referred to as the "executioner" caspases. These active executioner caspases cleave cellular substrates, resulting in the biochemical and morphological changes associated with apoptosis.

Measurement of apoptosis – practical aspects

As discussed in the previous section, several molecular and biochemical events occur that are unique to apoptosis, many of which are used as markers to identify this mode of cell death. Several methods have been employed to assess apoptosis, including DNA ladder formation by gel electrophoresis, morphological examination by electron microscopy, and the more recent use of flow cytometry.

Features of apoptosis such as condensation of nuclear chromatin may be identified with fluorescent or light-absorbing dyes (Figure 15.4). Nucleosomal and oligonucleosomal DNA fragments which are products of DNA degradation generate a characteristic "ladder" pattern and are identified using agarose gel electrophoresis. Changes in morphology of the dying cell can also be detected by analysis of a light scatter signal by flow cytometry.

Endonucleolytic DNA cleavage results in extensive DNA breakage. Cleavage of the DNA may yield double-stranded as well as single-stranded "nicks" in the DNA. These DNA strand breaks can be detected by enzymatic labeling of the free 3′-OH termini with modified nucleotides. This is referred to as the TUNEL enzymatic labeling assay, which is very specific for apoptosis (Gold *et al.*, 1994).

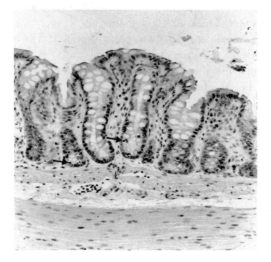

Figure 15.4 Apoptotic bodies identified by H & E staining (Hambly *et al.*, 2002; reproduced by permission of *Food and Chemical Toxicology*, 2002).

More recently, a new method was introduced in which BrdUTP, incorporated by TdT, is used as the marker of DNA strand breaks (Li and Darzynkiewicz, 1995). This approach employing TdT appears to be the most specific in terms of positive identification of apoptotic cells. It is generally considered that in experimental studies of apoptosis at least two methods of assessment should be used, usually H & E staining and TUNEL.

Apoptosis and diet

A variety of compounds either found in or derived from the diet have been shown to modulate apoptosis both *in vitro* and *in vivo*. Those compounds that initiate apoptotic pathways could potentially protect against cancer through the elimination of precancerous cells whereas compounds inhibiting apoptosis could promote tumorogenesis. One of the most publicized areas has been the role of butyric acid in apoptosis.

Dietary carbohydrates and butyrate

Early epidemiology studies support the hypothesis that dietary fiber reduces the risk of CRC in humans (Burkitt, 1969; Higginson and Oettle, 1960). A meta-analysis, which included 16 case–control studies, reported that those with the highest consumption of fiber had a 40% reduction in risk of CRC (Trock *et al.*, 1990). Fiber exerts several effects in the digestive tract, but the precise mechanisms for its protective role are still not clearly understood. Beneficial effects suggested include its ability to dilute fecal contents, increase transit time, and increase stool weights (Cummings, 1981), but there is considerable evidence to implicate fermentation products, especially short-chain fatty acids (SCFAs), in proactive effects.

A wide range of dietary carbohydrates as well as endogenously-produced mucins reach the colon and are hydrolyzed by gut bacterial enzymes to produce the SCFAs acetate, propionate and butyrate. These SCFAs provide an energy source for the intestinal cells and are also thought to confer beneficial effects on the host. SCFAs decrease colonic and fecal pH and this acidic environment is thought to be beneficial to the host (Silvi *et al.*, 1999). The pattern of SCFA production, in particular the proportion of butyric acid generated, varies considerably depending on the carbohydrate substrate. For example, pectin is fermented mainly to acetic acid whereas wheat bran stimulates butyrate production (Edwards and Rowland, 1991). Recently, interest has focused on dietary starch, which *in vitro* generates large amounts of butyric acid. Epidemiological studies reveal an inverse relationship between starch intake and CRC risk (Bingham, 1996). Although the majority of starches are hydrolyzed by amylase in the small intestine, some, termed resistant starch (RS), are less readily broken down and so reach the colon relatively intact (Rowland, 2000). The various effects of RS on gut microflora composition and metabolism, including the stimulation of butyrate formation, are likely mechanisms responsible for the changes in gut mucosal functions related to colon cancer risk.

Butyrate has been found at concentrations of up to 20mM in the intestine (Cummings, 1981) and its oxidation accounts for more than 70% of the oxygen consumption by the human colonic tissue (Roediger, 1990), implying that butyrate is the principal energy substrate of the colonocyte. This SCFA is of specific interest since it has been shown to induce apoptosis in colon adenoma and colon cell lines. *In vitro* studies have shown that increased butyrate supply to colon cells induces growth of the gut epithelium whereas reduced butyrate supply causes gut atrophy and functional impairments (Cummings, 1981; Roediger, 1990; Scheppach, 1994). Hague *et al.* (1995) also demonstrated that the three major SCFAs (acetate, propionate, and butyrate) all induced apoptosis in adenoma and carcinoma cell lines, with butyrate being the most effective.

Sodium butyrate (NaB) has been observed to induce apoptosis and to alter the resistance of colonic tumor cells to apoptosis (Archer, 1998; Smith *et al.*, 1998; Velàzquez *et al.*, 1996). Butyrate is thought to act at the gene level by increasing the accessibility of DNA to a number of transcription factors (Bordonaro *et al.*, 2002; Hassig *et al.*, 1997).

The mechanism by which butyrate induces apoptosis is caspase-dependent (Chai *et al.*, 2000) and is thought to involve signal transduction via the Fas-ligand death receptor (Chapkin *et al.*, 2000). Heerdt *et al.* (1997) further demonstrated that butyrate induces a pathway that enhances mitochondrial function which results in initiation of growth arrest and apoptosis of colonic epithelial cells. It has been suggested that butyrate may protect against cancer not only of the large intestine but also of the breast (Heerdt *et al.*, 1999) and prostate (Ellerhorst *et al.*, 1999).

The protective effect of butyrate may also be mediated through reactive oxygen species. Rosignoli *et al.* (2001) demonstrated a protective effect of butyrate on hydrogen peroxide-induced DNA damage in both isolated human colonocytes and HT29 tumor cells.

There is also increasing evidence to suggest that butyrate exerts a pro-apoptotic effect through the inhibition of the enzyme histone deacetylase. This enzyme is involved in transcription, which is one of the first steps in cell division. Histone deacetylase inhibitors cause growth arrest and apoptosis of cancer cells by both p21-dependent and -independent pathways (Richon *et al.*, 2000). There is also evidence that diets rich in fiber (wheat bran) promote histone acetylation of rat colonic epithelial cells *in vivo* (Boffa *et al.*, 1992).

The beneficial effects of butyrate have been demonstrated successfully in the majority of *in vitro* studies; however, there have been conflicting views, in particular from *in vivo* studies (Hardman and Cameron, 1995; Ishizuka *et al.*, 1997; Nigro *et al.*, 1979). Several colorectal carcinogens are used to study the effects of different dietary compounds on apoptosis in animal models. These include azoxymethane, PhIP and the commonly used 1,2-dimethylhydrazine (DMH).

Butyrate fed in the form of gastro-resistant pellets did not have an effect on apoptosis in chemically induced colon carcinogenesis in rats, nor did it affect the expression of p21^{CIP}, a cell cycle-related protein (Caderni *et al.*, 2001).

It has been hypothesized that the ingestion of indigestible carbohydrates (including resistant starch) resulting in the production of butyrate in the large intestine may be beneficial in terms of reducing risk factors for colorectal cancer (Bird, 2000). Butyrate has been implicated in the protective effect of fiber in rodents (McIntyre *et al.*, 1993).

Jenab and Thompson (2000) treated five groups of male Fisher rats with azoxymethane. The rats were maintained on either a basal control diet or a control diet supplemented with 25% wheat bran, 25% dephytinized wheat bran, 25% dephytinized wheat bran with 1% phytic acid, or 1% phytic acid for 100 days. The rate of apoptosis and cell differentiation increased in the whole crypt and the top 40% of the crypt in rats fed the wheat bran, dephytinized wheat bran and phytic acid diets. These diets also significantly increased apoptosis in the bottom 60% of the crypt, while all treatments significantly increased differentiation in the bottom 60% of the crypt compared to the controls. The authors concluded that wheat bran can favorably increase apoptosis and differentiation due to its dietary fiber and phytic acid content. Phytic acid showed similar results when added to a low fiber diet.

Prebiotics

Attempts to modify the composition of the gut microflora by altering the diet have in general been unsuccessful (Marteau *et al.*, 1990), although recently non-digestible oligosaccharides have been shown to exert some effects (Gibson *et al.*, 1995; Rowland and Tanaka, 1993). These dietary carbohydrates and in particular oligosaccharides are of current interest due to their bifidogenic effect within the large intestine (Crittenden and Playne, 1996). Oligosaccharides are currently being added to foods and have been described as prebiotics. Prebiotics are defined as non-digestible food ingredients that beneficially affect the host by selectively stimulating the growth and/or activity of one or a limited number of bacteria in the colon and thus improve host health (Gibson and Roberfroid, 1995). Non-digestible oligosaccharides are found in a variety of foods such as garlic, onions, and soybeans. Many non-digestible oligosaccharides, including inulin, galactooligosaccharide (TOS), and oligofructose (OF), reach the large intestine intact and are known to be fermented to SCFAs. This results in increased growth of bifidobacteria and/or lactobacilli accompanied by enhanced production of butyrate (Kleessen *et al.*, 2001).

Oligofructose and inulin both significantly increased apoptosis in rat colon tissue ($p < 0.05$) compared with controls (Hughes and Rowland, 2001). This study was carried out to determine the effects of two prebiotics, chicory frutans-oligofructose and long chain inulin, on apoptosis. After a stock diet for one week, three groups of six animals were fed one of three diets: basal, basal with oligofructose (5% w/w), or basal with long chain inulin (5% w/w) for three weeks. All animals were dosed with 1,2-dimethylhydrazine and killed 24 h later. The mean number of apoptotic cells per crypt was significantly higher in the rats fed oligofructose ($p = 0.049$) and long chain inulin ($p = 0.017$) compared to animals fed the basal diet. This study was the first to demonstrate the significant effect of chicory frutans on apoptosis and the authors concluded that these prebiotics may have cancer-preventing properties. These results are consistent with studies on induction of preneoplastic lesions in rats. These precancerous lesions are referred to as aberrant crypt foci (ACF) and are the earliest lesions to appear in the colonic mucosa of patients with adenomas or carcinoma. They also appear in animal models after treatment with carcinogens. Rowland *et al.* (1998) found that *Bifidobacterium longum* and inulin were effective in reducing the incidence of ACFs in rats when given after initiation events, suggesting that elimination of damaged cells by apoptosis could be a possible mechanism.

Western-style diets

Risio *et al.* (1996) found that mice fed a Western-style diet (high fat, low calcium, and low vitamin D) without any chemical carcinogen for two years induced colonic neoplasia. During the first four months of feeding increased cell division was observed in the animals on the Western-style diet. A significant increase of apoptotic cells was also observed during this period and may be interpreted as a homeostatic response. However, during the middle of the lifespan of the mice there was a dramatic depletion in apoptotic cells in the mid-region of the crypt and this was attributed to an impairment of the apoptotic process. Other studies examining the impact of high- and low-risk diets in animal models have also been reported in the literature. Hambly *et al.* (2002) reported a significant dose-dependent induction of apoptosis in the colonic crypts by the carcinogen 1,2-dimethylhydrazine (DMH) of rats fed a diet containing low-risk factors for colon cancer (low fat content, high calcium, and high non-digestible carbohydrate) compared with rats fed a high-risk diet (high fat, low calcium, low non-digestible carbohydrate).

Fatty acids

There has been much controversy in recent years regarding the relationship between fat intake and carcinogenesis. However, it would appear that the effect is determined by the fatty acid composition of the diet. The n-3 polyunsaturated fatty acids (PUFAs) such as EPA (eicosapentaenoic acid) and DHA (docosahexaenoic acid) appear to confer a mild protective effect, monounsaturated fatty acids offer no effect, and the PUFAs of the n-6 series may induce tumorogenesis in rodents (Fay *et al.*, 1997). Latham *et al.* (1999) demonstrated that n-3 polyunsaturated fatty acids protected against aberrant crypt foci promotion and induced apoptosis in rats. EPA also induced apoptosis in HT29 colorectal adenocarcinoma cells *in vivo* (Latham *et al.*, 2001). It is thought that n-3 polyunsaturated fatty acids are cyclooxygenase inhibitors (Chen *et al.*, 1994; Singh *et al.*, 1997). Other mechanisms that have been put forward include a direct event on the cells and by activation of the cascade through cytochrome c release combined with mitochondrial membrane depolarization (Arita *et al.*, 2001).

Isoflavonoids

The water-soluble flavonoids are polyphenolic compounds possessing 15 carbon atoms and two benzene rings joined by a linear three-carbon chain. They are biologically active phytochemicals characterized by weak estrogenic activity and are found almost exclusively in soybeans and soya products. It has been suggested that isoflavones may be protective against hormone-related cancers (Messina and Barnes, 1991; Miksicek, 1995) and also colorectal cancer. Although CRC is not considered to be a hormone-related cancer, the human gut is known to contain estrogen receptors (Erβ) (Enmark and Gustafsson, 1999) and there is some evidence to suggest that these play a role in tumor development. In addition, hormone replacement therapy (HRT) is associated with a modest decrease in colon cancer risk (Folsom *et al.*, 1995). It would appear that HRT may decrease the risk of CRC among recent postmenopausal HRT users (Crandall, 1999; Franceschi and La Vecchia, 1998; Nanda *et al.*, 1999). It is hypothesized that HRT may increase endogenous estrogen levels which would be declining in postmenopausal women and therefore inhibit estrogen receptor (ER) hypermethylation. Several anticarcinogenic effects of isoflavonoids have been postulated, including a role in apoptosis (Kyle *et al.*, 1997). They have also been shown to influence intracellular enzymes, protein synthesis, growth factor action, and malignant cell proliferation (Adlercreutz *et al.*, 1995).

The isoflavonoid genistein inhibits mitosis and increases apoptosis in a variety of tumor cell lines *in vitro* (Table 15.2) (Messina *et al.*, 1994; Molteni *et al.*,

Table 15.2 Response of different cell lines to the effects of isoflavonoids

Cancer	Cell line	Compound	Effect or result	Reference
Colon	HT29 Caco-2 Rat non-transformed intestinal Crypt cells (IEC-6)	Genistein or quercetin	Effect was dose dependent for each and chromatin condensation observed in all cell lines – indicator of apoptosis	Kuo (1996)
Prostate	LNCaP	Genistein/daidzein	Genestein most effective – inhibits growth, suppresses DNA synthesis, induces apoptosis	Onozzawa et al. (1998)
Bladder	HT-1376, UM-UC-3, RT-4, J82, TCCSUP	Genistein/genistin/ daidzein/biochanin A	Growth inhibition All induce G2-M cell cycle arrest Some DNA fragmentation	Zhou et al. (1998)
Lung	H460 non-small-cell lung cancer	Genistein	Induces apoptosis P53 pathway	Lian et al. (1999)
Breast	Normal (MCF10A, MCF12A) Malignant (MCF10CA1a, MDA-MB-231)	Genistein	$\uparrow$ G(2) arrest and apoptosis in malignant cells. P21 may play role	Upadhyay et al. (2001)

1995). In a study conducted by Gee *et al.* (2000), genistein or soya protein isolates were fed to rats before they were treated with DMH. Neither the genistein nor the soya protein had a significant effect on mitosis or apoptosis in the rat *in vivo*. However, both promoted the induction of aberrant crypt foci in the distal colon when fed immediately before treatment with DMH.

Glucosinolates

There is strong evidence for a protective effect of vegetables against CRC risk (Franceschi, 1999). Epidemiological evidence suggesting that intake of cruciferous vegetables has an inverse relationship with risk of colorectal cancer has focussed attention on the glucosinolates and their derivatives, isothiocynates, present in these vegetables. A cohort study conducted in the Netherlands on diet and cancer showed no statistically significant associations with total vegetable intake or total fruit intake. However, brassica vegetables and green leafy vegetables showed inverse associations for both men and women (Voorrips *et al.*, 2000). In a randomly assigned cross-over study, consumption of Brussels sprouts increased intestinal glutathione S-transferases – a phase II detoxification enzyme (Nijhoff *et al.*, 1995).

The brassica family includes dark leafy green vegetables, broccoli, Brussels sprouts, and cabbage. The glucosinolates are converted to isothiocyanates by plant myrosinases and the gut microflora (Figure 15.5). Glucosinolates have been shown to exhibit chemopreventive activity by upregulating certain mammalian (hepatic and gut mucosa) enzymes involved in the detoxification of xenobiotic compounds. Of particular interest are the glutathione S-transferases (GSTs) (Nastruzzi *et al.*, 2000; Steinkellner *et al.*, 2001). Dietary components that induce elevated levels of GSTs are thought to be protective agents.

Although induction of GST appears to be an important mechanism of protective action of ITC, there is also evidence from *in vitro* and *in vivo* studies that apoptosis may also be involved.

In vitro studies have demonstrated that dietary isothiocyanates from cruciferous vegetables can stimulate apoptosis in a variety of human colon cell lines (Bonnesen *et al.*, 2001). Refer to Table 15.3 for a summary of the effect of

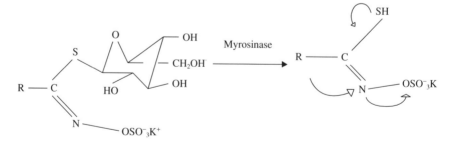

Figure 15.5 Formation of isothiocyanates from glucosinolates.

Table 15.3 Response of different cell lines to the effects of different isothiocyanates

Cancer	Cell line	Compound	Effect/Result	Reference
Liver	HeLa	Phenethyl isothiocyanate Phenylmethyl isothiocyanate Phenylbutyl isothiocyanate Phenylhexyl isothiocyanate	↑ apoptosis Caspase-3 dependent mechanism	Yu et al. (1998)
		Phenyl isothiocyanate	No effect	
Leukemia	HL60 (p53−) HL-1 (p53+)	Phenethyl isothiocyanate Allyl isothiocyanate	Both ↑ apoptosis. Critical role for caspase 8, supporting role for caspase 3 Not necessarily p53 dependent	Xu and Thornalley (2000)
Colon	CaCO$_2$ LS-174	Sulforaphane Benzyl isothiocyanate	Both ↑ apoptosis in each cell line	Bonneson et al. (2001)
Leukemia	Jurkat T-cells	Sulforaphane	G(2)M-phase arrest ↑ apoptosis ↑ p53 and bax expression Necrosis after prolonged exposure	Fimognari et al. (2002)

isothiocyanates on various cell lines. Apoptosis was also induced in rat liver epithelial RL34 cells by a cancer chemopreventive compound, benzyl isothiocyanate (BITC) (Nakamura *et al.*, 2002). The authors suggested that BITC induces apoptosis through a mitochondrial redox-sensitive mechanism.

Similar results have been observed *in vivo* by Smith *et al.* (1998). This group fed rats a diet rich in sinigrin (a glucosinolate precurser of allyl isothiocyanate). 48 h after treatment with DMH they observed suppressed mitosis and an increase level of apoptosis in the colorectal crypts of the treated rats. This effect was not observed in the control rats. In a second experiment rats were given sinigrin 22 h after treatment with DMH. Apoptosis was again significantly higher in the DMH-treated rats given sinigrin when compared with controls. Numbers of aberrant crypt foci (ACF) were also determined (22 days after treatment with DMH) and were significantly lower in the control rats.

Bile acids

Bile acids are derivatives of cholesterol, which are synthesized in the liver and excreted into the digestive tract where they assist in the absorption of dietary fats. The bile acids are normally reabsorbed from the ileum and returned to the liver. However, those bile acids that either escape absorption or amass through high-fat diets accumulate in the feces, where the enteric bacteria metabolize them to produce secondary bile acids (Hill *et al.*, 1971). Fecal bile acid concentrations appear to be consistently higher in those people at high risk of colorectal cancer (Kishida *et al.*, 1997). Bile acids including cholic acid (CA), lithocholic acid (LCA), deoxycholic acid (DCA), and chenodeoxycholic acid (CDCA) have been implicated as tumor promoters both *in vitro* (McMillan *et al.*, 2000) and *in vivo* (Baijal *et al.*, 1998). In *in vitro* studies using colon cells, bile acids, particularly secondary bile acids, are cytotoxic (Haza *et al.*, 2000). This cytotoxicity is considered to be responsible for the stimulation of cell proliferation seen after exposure to bile acids *in vitro* (Milovic *et al.*, 2002). Effects of bile acids on apoptosis in cultured colon cells are variable, possibly reflecting the wide range of cell lines, type of bile acid (primary, secondary, free and sodium salt), and concentrations used. Table 15.4 is a summary of the effects of bile acids in several *in vitro* studies. A number of studies found that apoptosis was increased after exposure to bile acids, particularly the secondary bile acid DCA, although most of these studies used relatively high concentrations. McMillan *et al.* (2000) demonstrated that at levels found in the colon the bile acids deoxycholic acid (DCA) and chenodeoxycholic acid (CDCA) modestly increased cell proliferation and decreased spontaneous apoptosis in AA/C1 adenoma cells. The bile acids also significantly inhibited the induction of apoptosis by butyrate in the same cell line, although this was overcome by increasing the concentration of sodium butyrate. However, Marchetti *et al.* (1997) demonstrated that the bile acid DCA was able to induce apoptosis in the HT-29 colonic tumor cell line and that this was directly related to calcium ion concentration. Interestingly, DCA induced a much higher level of apoptosis than the

Table 15.4 Response of different cell lines to the effects of bile acids

Cancer	Cell line	Compound	Effect/Result	Reference
Colon	RG/C2, PC/JW/FI AA/C1	Sodium deoxycholate Sodium deoxycholate	0.5 mM ↑ apoptosis 0.5 mM no effect	Hague et al. (1995)
Colon	HT-29	DCA	500 µM ↑ apoptosis	Marchetti et al. (1997)
Colon	HCT116, HT29	DCA CDCA UDCA CA	500 µM ↑ apoptosis 500 µM ↑ apoptosis 500 µM inhibits growth/blocked cells in G1 phase 500 µM no effect	Martinez et al. (1998)
Colon	AA/C1	DCA CDCA	10 µM ↑ proliferation, ↓ apoptosis 10 µM ↑ proliferation, ↓ apoptosis	McMillan et al. (2000)
Colon	HT29, Caco2	DCA	≤20 µM ↑ proliferation >100 µM ↑ apoptosis	Milovic et al. (2002)

SCFAs butyrate and propionate. In a recent study, concentrations of ≤ 20 μM DCA induced proliferation in both HT29 and Caco2 colon cancer cell lines. However, concentrations >100 μM DCA increased apoptosis (Milovic *et al.*, 2002). Interestingly, an *in vivo* study by Kozoni *et al.* (2000) found that lithocholic acid (LCA) suppressed apoptosis in a 1,2-dimethylhydrazine (DHM)-induced murine carcinogenesis model. Overall, it would appear that bile acids may participate in the etiology of colorectal cancer by altering the balance between cell proliferation and apoptosis in the colon.

Conclusion

It is well recognized that environmental and dietary factors both contribute to the etiology and progression of colorectal cancer. Our knowledge of the effects of different components of the diet on epithelial cell proliferation and apoptosis is increasing. Our understanding of diet in this fine balance between proliferation and apoptosis is imperative to future guidelines for cancer prevention as well as the development of new strategies for anticancer treatments.

References

Adlercreutz, H., Goldin, B.R., Gorbach, S.L., Hockerstedt, K.A.V., Watanabe, S., Hamalainen, E.K., Markkanen, M.H., Makela, T.H., Wahala, K.T., Tase, T.A., and Fotsis, T. (1995) Soybean phyto-oestrogen intake and cancer risk, *Journal of Nutrition*, **125**: S757–S770.

Archer, S., Meng, S., Shei, A., and Hodin, R.A. (1998) P21WAFI is required for butyrate-mediated growth inhibition of human colon cancer cells, *Proceedings of the National Academy of Sciences, USA*, **95**: 6791–6796.

Arends, M.J. (1995) How do cancer cells die? Apoptosis and its role in neoplastic progression. In *The Biology of Gynaecological Cancer* (eds R. Leake, M. Gore and R.H. Ward), pp. 73–91. London: RCOG Press.

Arita, K., Kobuchi, H., Utsumi, T., Takehara, Y., Akiyama, J., Horton, A.A., and Utsumi, K. (2001) Mechanism of apoptosis in HL-60 cells induced by n-3 and n-6 polyunsaturated fatty acids, *Biochemical Pharmacology*, **62**: 821–828.

Baijal, P.K., Clow, E.P., Fitzpatrick, D.W., and Bird, R.P. (1998) Tumor-enhancing effects of cholic acid are exerted on the early stages of colon carcinogenesis via induction of aberrant crypt foci with an enhanced growth phenotype, *Canadian Journal of Physiology and Pharmacology*, **76**: 1095–1102.

Bingham, S.A. (1996) Epidemiology and mechanisms relating to risk of colorectal cancer, *Nutrition Research Reviews*, **9**: 197–239.

Bird, A.R., Brown, I.L., and Topping, D.L. (2000) Starches, resistant starches, the gut microflora and human health, *Current Issues in Intestinal Microbiology*, **1**: 25–37.

Boffa, L.C., Lupton, J.R., Mariani, M.R., Ceppi, M., Newmark, H.L., Scalmati, A., and Lipkin, M. (1992) Modulation of colonic epithelial cell proliferation, histone acetylation, and luminal short chain fatty acids by variation of dietary fiber (wheat bran) in rats, *Cancer Research*, **52**: 5906–5912.

Bonnesen, C., Eggleston, I.M., and Hayes, J.D. (2001) Dietary indoles and isothiocyanates that are generated from cruciferous vegetables can both stimulate apoptosis and confer protection against DNA damage in human colon cell lines, *Cancer Research*, **61**: 6120–6130.

Bordonaro, M., Lazarova, D.L., Augenlicht, L.H., and Sartorelli, A.C. (2002) Cell type-and promoter-dependent modulation of the Wnt signalling pathway by sodium butyrate, *International Journal of Cancer*, **97**: 42–51.

Bos, J.L., Fearon, E.R., Hamilton, E.R., Verlaande Vries, M., Vander, E.A.J., and Vogelstein, B. (1987) Prevalence of *ras* mutations in human colorectal cancers, *Nature*, **327**: 293–297.

Buell, P. and Dunn, J.E. (1965) Cancer mortality among Japanese issii and nisei of California, *Cancer*, **18**: 656–664.

Burkitt, D.P. (1969) Related disease, related cause?, *Lancet*, **2**: 1229–1231.

Caderni, G., Luceri, C., De Filippo, C., Salvadori, M., Giannini, A., Tessitore, L., and Dolara, P. (2001) Slow-release pellets of sodium butyrate do not modify azoxymethane (AOM)-induced intestinal carcinogenesis in F344 rats, *Carcinogenesis*, **22**: 525–527.

Cerwenka, A., Kovar, H., Majdic, O., and Holter, W. (1996) Fas- and activation-induced apoptosis are reduced in human T cells preactivated in the presence of TGF-beta 1, *Journal of Immunology*, **156**: 459–464.

Chai, F., Evdokiou, A., Young, G.P., and Zalewski, P.D. (2000) Involvement of p21 (Waf1/Cip1) and its cleavage by DEVD-caspase during apoptosis of colorectal cancer cells induced by buytrate, *Carcinogenesis*, **21**: 7–14.

Chapkin, R.S., Fan, Y., and Lupton, J.R (2000) Effect of diet on colonic programmed cell death: molecular mechanism of action, *Toxicology Letters*, **112–113**: 411–414.

Chen, L.Y., Lawson, D.L., and Mehta, J.L. (1994) Reduction in human neutrophil superoxide anion generation by n-3 polyunsaturated fatty acids: role of cyclooxygenase products and endothelium-derived relaxing factor, *Thrombosis Research*, **76**: 317–322.

Cho, K.R. and Vogelstein, B. (1992) Suppressor gene alterations in the colorectal adenoma–carcinoma sequence, *Journal of Cellular Biochemistry*, **16G**: 137–141.

Crandall, C.J. (1999) Estrogen replacement therapy and colon cancer: a clinical review, *Journal of Women's Health and Gender-Based Medicine*, **8**: 1155–1166.

Crittenden, R.G. and Playne, M.J. (1996) Production, properties and applications of food grade oligosaccharides, *Trends in Food Science and Technology*, **7**: 353–361.

Cummings, J. (1981) Short chain fatty acids in the human colon, *Gut*, **22**: 763–779.

Edwards, C.A. and Rowland, I.R. (1991) Bacterial fermentation in the colon and its measurement. In *Dietary Fibre, a Component of Food, Nutritional Function in Health and Disease* (eds T. Schweizer and C.A. Edwards), pp. 119–136. Brussels: ILSI Europe.

Ellerhorst, J., Nguyen, T., Cooper, D.N.W., Estroy, Y., Lotan, D., and Lotan, R. (1999) Induction of differentiation and apoptosis in the prostate cancer cell line LNCaP by sodium butyrate and galectin-1, *International Journal of Oncology*, **14**: 225–232.

Enmark, E. and Gustafsson, J.A. (1999) Oestrogen receptors – an overview, *Journal of Internal Medicine*, **246**: 133–138.

Fay, M.P., Freedman, L.S., Clifford, C.K., and Midthune, D.N. (1997) Effects of different types of fat on the development of mammary tumours in rodents: a review, *Cancer Research*, **57**: 3979–3988.

Fearon, E.R. and Vogelstein, B. (1990) A genetic model for colorectal tumorgenesis, *Cell*, **61**: 759–767.

Fimognari, C., Nusse, M., Cesari, R., Lori, R., Cantelli-Forti, G., and Hrelia, P. (2002) Growth inhibition, cell cycle arrest and apoptosis in human T-cell leukaemia by the isothiocyanate sulforaphane, *Carcinogenesis*, **23**: 581–586.

Folsom, A.R., Mink, P.J., Sellers, T.A., Hong, C.P., Zheng, W., and Potter, J.D. (1995) Hormonal replacement therapy and morbidity and mortality in a prospective-study of postmenopausal women, *American Journal of Public Health*, **85**: 1128–1132.

Franceschi, S. (1999) Nutrient and food groups and large bowel cancer in Europe, *European Journal of Cancer Prevention*, **8**: S49–S52.

Franceschi, S. and La Vecchia, C. (1998) Colorectal cancer and hormone replacement therapy: an unexpected finding, *European Journal of Cancer Prevention*, **7**: 427–438.

Gee, J.M., Noteborn, H.P., Polley, A.C., and Johnson, I.T. (2000) Increased induction of aberrant crypt foci by 1,2-dimethylhydrazine in rats fed diets containing purified genistein or genistein-rich soya protein, *Carcinogenesis*, **21**: 2255–2259.

Gibson, G.R., Beatty, E.R., Wang, X., and Cummings, J.H. (1995) Selective stimulation of Bifidobacteria in the human colon by oligofructose and inulin, *Gastroenterology*, **108**: 975–982.

Gibson, G.R. and Roberfroid, M.B. (1995) Dietary modulation of the human colonic microbiota: introducing the concept of prebiotics, *Journal of Nutrition*, **125**: 1401–1412.

Gold, R., Schmied, M., Giegench, G., Breitschopf, H., Hartung, H.P., Toyka, K.V., and Lassman, H. (1994) Differentiation between cellular apoptosis and necrosis by the combined use of *in situ* tailing and nick translation techniques, *Laboratory Techniques*, **71**: 219–225.

Goodlad, R.A. and Wright, N.A. (1990) Changes in intestinal cell proliferation, absorptive capacity and structure in young, adult and old rats, *Journal of Anatomy*, **173**: 109–118.

Grady, W.H., Rajput, A., Myeroff, L., Liu, D.F., Kwon, K., Willis, J., and Markowitz, S. (1998) Mutation of the Type II transforming growth factor-beta receptor is coincident with the transformation of human colon adenomas to malignant carcinomas, *Cancer Research*, **58**: 3101–3104.

Greenblatt, M.S., Bennett, W.P., Hollstein, M., and Harris, C.C. (1994) Mutations in the p53 tumor-suppressor gene: clues to cancer aetiology and molecular pathogenesis, *Cancer Research*, **54**: 4855–4878.

Hague, A., Elder, D.J.E., Hicks, D.J., and Paraskeva, C. (1995) Apoptosis in colorectal tumour cells: induction by the short chain fatty acids butyrate, propionate and acetate and by the bile salt deoxycholate, *International Journal of Cancer*, **60**: 400–406.

Haenszel, W. (1961) Cancer mortality among the foreign born in the U.S., *Journal of the National Cancer Institute USA*, **26**: 37–132.

Hambly, R.J., Saunders, M., Rijken, P.J., and Rowland, I.R. (2002) Influence of dietary components associated with high or low risk of colon cancer on apoptosis in the rat colon, *Food and Chemical Toxicology*, **40**: 801–808.

Hardman, W.E. and Cameron, I.L. (1995) Site-specific reduction of colon cancer incidence, without a concomitant reduction in cryptal cell proliferation, in 1,2-dimethylhydrazine-treated rats by diets containing 10% pectin with 5% or 20% corn oil, *Carcinogenesis*, **16**: 1425–1431.

Hassig, C.A., Tong, J.K., and Schreiber, S.L. (1997) Fibre-derived butyrate and the prevention of colon cancer, *Chemistry and Biology*, **4**: 783–789.

Haza, A.I., Glinghammer, B., Grandien, A., and Rafter, J. (2000) Effect of colonic luminal components on induction of apoptosis in human colonic cell lines, *Nutrition and Cancer*, **32**: 29–34.

Heerdt, B.G., Houston, M.A., Anthony, G.M., and Augenlicht, L.H. (1999) Initiation of growth arrest and apoptosis of MCF-7 mammary carcinoma cells by tributyrin, a triglyceride analogue of the short-chain fatty acid butyrate, is associated with mitochondrial activity, *Cancer Research*, **59**: 1584–1591.

Heerdt, B.G., Houston, M.A., and Augenlicht, L.H. (1997) Short-chain fatty acid-initiated cell cycle arrest and apoptosis of colonic epithelial cells is linked to mitochondrial function, *Cell Growth and Differentiation*, 8: 523–532.

Higginson, J. and Oettle, A.G. (1960) Cancer incidence in Bantu and "Cape coloured" races of South Africa: report of a cancer survey of the Transvaal (1953–1955), *Journal of the National Cancer Institute USA*, 24: 589–671.

Hill, M.J., Draser, B.S., Hawksworth, G., Aries, V., Crowther, J.S., and Williams, R.E. (1971) Bacteria and aetiology of cancer of large bowel, *Lancet*, 1: 95–100.

Hughes, R. and Rowland, I.R. (2001) Stimulation of apoptosis by two prebiotic chicory fructans in the rat colon, *Carcinogenesis*, 22: 43–47.

Ishizuka, S., Sonoyama, K., and Kassai, T. (1997) Changes in the number and apoptosis of epithelial cells in the colorectum of wheat bran-fed rats soon after administering 1,2-dimethylhydrazine, *Bioscience, Biotechnology and Biochemistry*, 61: 1337–1341.

Jenab, M. and Thompson, L.U. (2000) Phytic acid in wheat bran affects colon morphology, cell differentiation and apoptosis, *Carcinogenesis*, 21: 1547–1552.

Kerr, J.F., Wyllie, A.H., and Currie, A.R. (1972) Apoptosis: a basic biological phenomenon with wide-ranging implications in tissue kinetics, *British Journal of Cancer*, 26: 239–257.

Kishida, T., Taguchi, F., Feng, L., Tatsuguchi, A., Sato, J., and Fujimori, S. (1997) Analysis of bile acids in colon residual liquid or faecal material in patients with colorectal neoplasia and control subjects, *Journal of Gastroenterology*, 32: 306–311.

Kleessen, B., Hartmann, L., and Blaut, M. (2001) Oligofructose and long-chain inulin: influence on the gut microbial ecology of rats associated with a human faecal flora, *British Journal of Nutrition*, 86: 291–300.

Kozoni, V., Tsioulias, G., Shiff, S., and Rigas, B. (2000) The effect of lithocholic acid on proliferation and apoptosis during the early stages of colon carcinogenesis: differential effect on apoptosis in the presence of a colon carcinogen, *Carcinogenesis*, 21: 999–1005.

Kuo, S.M. (1996) Antiproliferative potency of structurally distinct dietary flavonoids on human colon cancer cells, *Cancer Letters*, 110: 41–48.

Kyle, E., Neckers, L., Takimoto, C., Curt, G., and Brefan, R. (1997) Genistein induced apoptosis of prostate cancer cells is preceded by a specific decrease in focal adhesion kinase activity, *Molecular Pharmacology*, 51: 193–200.

Latham, P., Lund, E.K., Brown, J.C., and Johnson, I.T. (2001) Effects of cellular redox balance on induction of apoptosis by eicosapentaenoic acid in HT29 colorectal adenocarcinoma cells and rat colon *in vivo*, *Gut*, 49: 97–105.

Latham, P., Lund, E.K., and Johnson, I.T. (1999) Dietary n-3 PUFA increases the apoptotic response to 1,2-dimethylhydrazine, reduces mitosis and suppresses the induction of carcinogenesis in the rat colon, *Carcinogenesis*, 20: 645–650.

Li, X. and Darzynkiewicz, Z. (1995) Labelling DNA strand breaks with brduTP. Detection of apoptosis and cell proliferation, *Cell Proliferation*, 28: 571–579.

Lian, F., Li, Y., Bhuiyan, M., and Sarkar, F.H. (1999) p53-independent apoptosis induced by genistein in lung cancer cells, *Nutrition and Cancer*, 33: 125–131.

Lynch, H.T. and de la Chapelle, A. (1999) Genetic susceptibility to non-polyposis colorectal cancer, *Journal of Medical Genetics*, 36: 801–818.

Lynch, H.T. and Lynch, J.F. (1985) Hereditary non-polyposis colorectal cancer (Lynch Syndrome I and II): a common genotype linked to oncogenes?, *Medical Hypotheses*, 18: 19–28.

McIntyre, A., Gibson, P.R., and Young, G.P. (1993) Butyrate production from dietary fibre and protection against large bowel cancer in a rat model, *Gut*, **34**: 386–391.

McMillan, L., Butcher, S., Wallis, Y., Neoptolemos, J.P., and Lord, J.M. (2000) Bile acids reduce the apoptosis-inducing effects of sodium butyrate on human colon adenoma (AA/C1) cells: implications for colon carcinogenesis, *Biochemical and Biophysical Research Communications*, **273**: 45–49.

Marchetti, C., Migliorati, G., Moraca, R., Riccardi, C., Nicoletti, I., Fabiani, R., Mastrandrea, V., and Morozzi, G. (1997) Deoxycholic acid and SCFA-induced apoptosis in the human tumor cell line HT-29 and possible mechanisms, *Cancer Letters*, **114**: 97–99.

Markowitz, S., Wang, J., Myeroff, L., Parsons, R., Sun, L., Lutterbaugh, J., Fan, R.S., Zborowska, E., Kinzler, K.W., and Vogelstein, B. (1995) Inactivation of the type II TGF-beta receptor in colon cancer cells with microsatellite instability, *Science*, **2685**: 1336–1338.

Marteau, P., Pochard, P., Flouie, B., Pellier, P., Santos, L., Desjeux, J.F., and Rambaud, J.C. (1990) Effect of chronic ingestion of a fermented dairy product containing *Lactobacillus acidophilus* and *Bifidobacterium bifidum* on metabolic activities of the colonic flora in humans, *American Journal of Clinical Nutrition*, **52**: 685–688.

Martinez, J.D., Stratagoules, E.D., LaRue, J.M., Powell, A.A., Gause, P.R., Craven, M.T., Payne, C.M., Powell, M.B., Gerner, E.W., and Earnest, D.L. (1998) Different bile acids exhibit distinct biological effects: the tumour promoter deoxycholic acid induces apoptosis and the chemopreventive agent ursodeoxycholic acid inhibits cell proliferation, *Nutrition and Cancer*, **31**: 111–118.

Massague, J. and Polyak, K. (1995) Mammalian antiproliferative signals and their targets, *Current Opinion in Genetics and Development*, **5**: 91–96.

Messina, M.J. and Barnes, S. (1991) The role of soy products in reducing risk of cancer, *Journal of the National Cancer Institute USA*, **83**: 541–546.

Messina, M.J., Persky, V., Setchell, K.D.R., and Barnes, S. (1994) Soy intake and cancer risk: a review of the *in vitro* and *in vivo* data, *Nutrition and Cancer*, **21**: 113–131.

Miksicek, R.J. (1995) Estrogenic flavonoids; structural requirements for biological activity, *Proceedings of the Society for Experimental Biology and Medicine*, **208**: 44–50.

Milovic, V., Teller, I.C., Faust, D., Caspary, W.F., and Stein, J. (2002) Effects of deoxycholate on human colon cancer cells: apoptosis or proliferation, *European Journal of Clinical Investigation*, **32**: 29–34.

Molteni, A., Brizio-Molteni, L., and Persky, V. (1995) *In vitro* hormonal effects of soybean isoflavones, *Journal of Nutrition*, **125**: S751–S756.

Nakamura, Y., Kawakami, M., Yoshihiro, A., Miyoshi, N., Ohigashi, H., Kawai, K., Osawa, T., and Uchida, K. (2002) Involvement of the mitochondrial death pathway in chemopreventive benzyl isothiocyanate induced apoptosis, *Journal of Biological Chemistry*, **277**: 8492–8499.

Nanda, K., Bastian, L.A., Hasselblad, V., and Simel, D.L. (1999) Hormone replacement therapy and the risk of colorectal cancer: a meta-analysis, *Obstetrics and Gynecology*, **93**: 880–888.

Nastruzzi, C., Cortesi, R., Esposito, E., Menegatti, E., Leoni, O., Iori, R., and Palmieri, S. (2000) *In vitro* antiproliferative activity of isothiocyanates and nitriles generated by myrosinase-mediated hydrolysis of glucosinolates from seeds of cruciferous vegetables, *Journal of Agricultural and Food Chemistry*, **48**: 3572–3575.

Nigro, N.D., Bull, A.W., Klopfer, B.A., Paks, M.S., and Campbell, R.L. (1979) Effects of dietary fibre on azoxymethane-induced intestinal carcinogenesis in rats, *Journal of the National Cancer Institute USA*, **62**: 1097–1102.

Nijhoff, W.A., Grubben, M.J., Nagengast, F.M., Jansen, J.B., Verhagen, H., van Poppel, G., and Peters, W.H. (1995) Effects of consumption of Brussels sprouts on intestinal and lymphocytic glutathione S-transferases in humans, *Carcinogenesis*, **16**: 2125–2128.

Oberhammer, F.A., Pavelka, M., Sharma, S., Tiefenbacher, R., Purchio, A.F., Bursch, W., and Schulte-Hermann, R. (1992) Induction of apoptosis in cultured hepatocytes and in regressing liver by transforming growth factor beta 1, *Proceedings of the National Academy of Sciences USA*, **89**: 5408–5412.

Onozzawa, M., Fukuda, K., Ohtani, M., Akaza, H., Sugimura, T., and Wakabayashi, K. (1998) Effects of soybean isoflavones on cell growth and apoptosis of the human prostatic cancer cell line LNCaP, *Japanese Journal of Clinical Oncology*, **28**: 360–363.

Peltomaki, P., Aaltonen, L.A., Sistonen, P., Pylkkanen, L., Mecklin, J.P., Jarvinen, H., Green, J.S., Jass, J.R., Weber, J.L., and Leach, F.S. (1993) Genetic mapping of a locus predisposing to human colorectal cancer, *Science*, **260**: 810–812.

Pisa, F.E., Barbone, F., Montella, M., Talamini, R., La Vecchia, C., and Franceschi, S. (2000) Migration, socio-economic status and the risk of colorectal cancer in Italy, *European Journal of Cancer Prevention*, **9**: 409–416.

Potten, C.S., Schofield, R., and Lajtha, L.G.A. (1979) A comparison of cell replacement in bone marrow, testis and three regions of surface epithelium, *Biochimica et Biophysica Acta*, **560**: 281–299.

Powell, S.M., Zilz, N., Beazer-Barclay, Y., Bryan, T.M., Hamilton, S.R., Thibodeau, S.N., Vogelstein, B., and Kinzler, K. (1992) APC mutations occur early during colorectal tumorigenesis, *Nature*, **359**: 235–237.

Richon, V.M., Sandhoff, T.W., Rifkind, R.A., and Marks, P.A. (2000) Histone deacetylase inhibitors selectively induces p21 super (WAF1) expression and gene associated histone acetylation, *Proceedings of the National Academy of Sciences USA*, **97**: 10014–10019.

Risio, M., Lipkin, M., Newmark, H., Yang, K., Rossini, F.P., Steele, W.E., Boone, C.W., and Kelloff, G.J. (1996) Apoptosis, cell replication and western-style diet induced tumorigenesis in mouse colon, *Cancer Research*, **56**: 4910–4916.

Roediger, W.E. (1990) The starved colon – diminished mucosal nutrition, diminished absorption, and colitis, *Diseases of the Colon and Rectum*, **33**: 858–862.

Rosignoli, P., Fabiani, R., De Bartolomeo, A., Spinozzi, F., Agea, E., Pelli, M.A., and Morozzi, G. (2001) Protective activity of butyrate on hydrogen peroxide-induced DNA damage in isolated human colonocytes and HT29 tumour cells, *Carcinogenesis*, **22**: 1675–1680.

Rowan, A.J., Lamlum, H., Ilyas, M., Wheeler, J., Straub, J., Papadopoulou, A., Bichnell, D., Bodmer, W.F., and Tomlinson, I.P. (2000) APC mutations in sporadic colorectal tumors: a mutational "hotspot" and interdependence of the "two hits", *Proceedings of the National Academy of Sciences USA*, **97**: 3352–3357.

Rowland, I.R. (2000) Non-digestible carbohydrates and gut function: implications for carcinogenesis. In *Advanced Dietary Fibre Technology* (eds B.V. McCleary and L. Prosky). London: Blackwell Science.

Rowland, I.R. Rumney, C.J., Coutts, J.T., and Lievense, L.C. (1998) Effect of *Bifidobacterium longum* and inulin on gut bacterial metabolism and carcinogen-induced aberrant crypt foci in rats, *Carcinogenesis*, **19**: 281–285.

Rowland, I.R. and Tanaka, R. (1993) The effects of transgalactosylated oligosaccharides on gut flora metabolism in rats associated with a human faecal microflora, *Journal of Applied Bacteriology*, **74**: 667–674.

Salahshor, S., Kressner, U., Pahlman, L., Glimelius, B., Lindmark, G., and Lindblom, A. (1999) Colorectal cancer with and without microsatellite instability involves different genes, *Genes, Chromosomes and Cancer*, **26**: 247–252.

Scheppach, W. (1994) Effects of short chain fatty acids on gut morphology and function, *Gut* (Suppl. 1): S35–S38.

Shih, M., Wang, T.L., Traverso, G., Romans, K., Hamilton, S.R., Ben-Sasson, S., Kinzler, K.W., and Vogelstein, B. (2001) Top-down morphogenesis of colorectal tumors, *Proceedings of the National Academy of Sciences USA*, **98**: 2640–2645.

Silvi, S., Rumney, C.J., Cresci, A., and Rowland, I.R. (1999) Resistant starch modifies gut microflora and microbial metabolism in human flora-associated rats innoculated with faeces from Italian and UK donors, *Journal of Applied Microbiology*, **86**: 521–530.

Singh, J., Hamid, R., and Reddy, B.S. (1997) Dietary fat and colon cancer: modulation of cyclooxygenase-2 by types and amount of dietary fat during the postinitiation stage of colon carcinogenesis, *Cancer Research*, **57**: 3465–3470.

Smith, J.G., Yokoyama, W.H., and German, B.G. (1998) Butyric acid from the diet: actions at the level of gene expression, *Clinical Reviews in Food Science*, **38**: 259–297.

Smith, T.K., Lund, E.K., and Johnson, I.T. (1998) Inhibition of dimethylhydrazine-induced aberrant crypt foci and induction of apoptosis in rat colon following oral administration of the glucosinolate sinigrin, *Carcinogenesis*, **19**: 267–273.

Steinkellner, H., Rabot, S., Freywald, C., Nobis, E., Scharf, G., Chabicovsky, M., Knasmuller, S., and Kassie, F. (2001) Effects of cruciferous vegetables and their constituents on drug metabolizing enzymes involved in the bioactivation of DNA-reactive dietary carcinogens, *Mutation Research*, **480–481**: 285–297.

Trock, B., Lanza, E., and Greenwald, P. (1990) Dietary fiber, vegetables, and colon cancer; critical review and meta-analysis of the epidemiologic evidence, *Journal of the National Cancer Institute USA*, **82**: 650–661.

Upadhyay, S., Neburi, M., Chinni, S.R., Alhassan, S., Miller, F., and Sarkar, F.H. (2001) Differential sensitivity of normal and malignant breast epithelial cells to genistein is partly mediated by p21 (WAF1), *Clinical Cancer Research*, **7**: 1782–1789.

Veale, A.M.O. (1965) Intestinal polyposis, *Eugenics Laboratory Memoirs*, Series 40. London: Cambridge University Press.

Velàzquez, O.C., Howard, M., and Rombeau, J.L. (1996) Butyrate and the colonocyte. Implications for neoplasia, *Digestive Disease and Sciences*, **41**: 727–739.

Vogelstein, B.E.R., Fearon, S.R., Hamilton, S.E., Kern, A.C., Preisinger, M., Lepper, Y., Nakamura, R., White, A., Smits, M.M., and Bos, J.L. (1988) Genetic alterations during colorectal tumor development, *New England Journal of Medicine*, **319**: 525–532.

Voorrips, L.E., Goldbohm, R.A., van Poppel, G., Sturmans, F., Hermus, R.J., and van den Brandt, P.A. (2000) Vegetable and fruit consumption and risks of colon and rectal cancer in a prospective cohort study: The Netherlands Cohort Study on Diet and Cancer, *American Journal of Epidemiology*, **152**: 1081–1092.

Willett, W.C. (1995) Diet, Nutrition and avoidable cancer, *Environmental Health Perspectives*, **103**: 165–170.

Xu, K. and Thornalley, P.J. (2000) Studies on the mechanism of the inhibition of human leukaemia cell growth by dietary isothiocyanates and their cysteine adducts *in vitro*, *Biochemical Pharmacology*, **60**: 221–231.

Yu, R., Mandlekar, S., Harvey, K.J., Ucker, D.S., and Kong, A.N. (1998) Chemopreventive isothiocyantes induce apoptosis and caspase-3 like protease activity, *Cancer Research*, **58**: 402–408.

Zhou, J.R., Mukherjee, P., Gugger, E.T., Tanaka, T., Blackburn, G.L., and Clinton, S.K. (1998) Inhibition of murine bladder tumorigenesis by soy isoflavones via alterations in the cell cycle, apoptosis and angiogenesis, *Cancer Research*, **58**: 5231–5238.

16 Free radicals as toxic agents: nutritional aspects

David Mantle, Richard M. Wilkins, and Victor R. Preedy

Summary

Free radicals are highly reactive chemical species formed in all cells as unwanted byproducts of metabolism, and as such can be regarded as "toxic agents" with regard to their potential for initiating intracellular damage. Cells are protected from such oxidative damage by a variety of endogenous and exogenous antioxidant enzymes and chemical compounds. An imbalance in oxidant/antioxidant levels ("oxidative stress") has been implicated in the pathogenesis of a variety of human disorders. In this chapter, we review recent evidence for the involvement of oxidative stress in the pathogenesis of neurodegenerative diseases (motor neuron disease, Parkinson's disease, and Alzheimer's dementia), muscle disease, and aging, together with evidence for the beneficial role of nutritional antioxidants in the prevention and treatment of these disorders.

Background and definitions

Free radicals are highly reactive, transient chemical species characterized by the presence of unpaired electrons (conventionally denoted by a point suffix: $^{\bullet}$). In biological systems, free radicals may be centered on oxygen, carbon or sulfur atoms. Most research has focused on oxygen centered radicals, with the hydroxyl ($OH^{\bullet}$) and superoxide ($O_2^{-\bullet}$) radicals considered to be the most physiologically important primary tissue damaging free radical species. Other important radicals derived from these primary species include the peralkoxyl ($RO_2^{\bullet}$) and alkoxyl ($RO^{\bullet}$) species. Hydrogen peroxide is also capable of inducing tissue damage directly, but is not classed as a free radical since it does not contain unpaired electrons; these species ($OH^{\bullet}$, $O_2^{-\bullet}$, $RO_2^{\bullet}$, $RO^{\bullet}$, H_2O_2) are therefore conveniently classed as reactive oxygen species (ROS) (Cheeseman and Slater, 1993).

In relatively few instances, free radicals may perform beneficial functions, e.g. $O_2^{-\bullet}$ generation during phagocytic activation, $NO^{\bullet}$ in the regulation of vascular tone. In general, however, free radicals are unwanted byproducts of normal aerobic cellular metabolism, with the potential to damage the various intracellular organelles and components (nucleic acids, lipids, and proteins) on which normal cell function depends. Free radical reactions are characterized by induction, propagation, and termination phases (of particular importance in the peroxidation of the lipid components of cell membranes). The $OH^\bullet$ radical is the most oxidizing (reactive) free radical species (estimated half-life in the nanosecond range) found in biological systems, reacting indiscriminately with most biomolecular targets at near diffusion controlled rates, and capable of causing extensive damage within a small radius of the site of production. In comparison to $OH^\bullet$, $O_2^{-\bullet}$ is a less damaging free radical species, with the potential for greater discrimination in biomolecular targeting (half-life $\sim$10 μs); $O_2^{-\bullet}$ can also react rapidly with $NO^\bullet$ to form peroxynitrite, a potentially damaging species which can generate $OH^\bullet$ radicals. Hydrogen peroxide has the capacity to oxidize intracellular components directly, although it is a relatively unreactive species compared to the above (half-life in the order of minutes), and is able to diffuse between and within cells, and to cross cell membranes. The main significance of H_2O_2 is as a source of $OH^\bullet$, via reaction with transition metal ions (as described in the following section). Nucleic acids, lipids, and proteins are attacked by $OH^\bullet$, whereas $O_2^{-\bullet}$ and H_2O_2 do not attack DNA or initiate lipid peroxidation. Proteins are susceptible to attack by all ROS species, either by oxidation of essential –SH groups or by other chemical modifications of the constituent amino acids.

Sources of ROS

The principal source of ROS generation *in vivo* results from leakage of electrons from the mitochondrial respiratory chain (i.e. from intermediate electron carriers onto molecular oxygen) during oxidative metabolism to generate ATP. It has been estimated that 3–5% of total electron flux results in the formation of ROS, which in a typical human (even at rest) corresponds to the production of approximately 2 kg of $O_2^{-\bullet}$ per annum. An additional source of $O_2^{-\bullet}$ generation results from the action of specific enzymes (principally oxidases) during the metabolism of purines (xanthine oxidases), catecholamines (monoamine oxidase), prostanoids (lipoxygenase), and xenobiotics (cytochrome P450). The generation of ROS via the above reactions may be exacerbated by such factors as failure of Ca^{2+} homeostasis, following trauma or ischemia. The main source of $OH^\bullet$ generation results from the interaction of H_2O_2 with transition metal ions (normally sequestered by binding proteins *in vivo*) such as Fe^{2+} or Cu^{2+} (Fenton reaction), as well as via the Fe^{2+} catalyzed reaction between H_2O_2 and $O_2^{-\bullet}$ (Haber-Weiss reaction). Hydroxyl radicals are also generated from peroxynitrite (which rapidly disproportionates at physiological pH), which is in turn rapidly formed via reaction between $NO^\bullet$ and $O_2^{-\bullet}$ under appropriate stoichiometric conditions. Hydrogen peroxide is formed via the dismutation of $O_2^{-\bullet}$ catalyzed by the enzyme superoxide dismutase, and is also produced via the action of several other oxidase enzymes (e.g. amino acid oxidases). Nitric oxide ($NO^\bullet$) is synthesized from the amino acid L-arginine by the enzyme nitric oxide synthase in endothelial cells (as a regulator of vascular tone), as well as in many other cell types (where it may act as a second messenger, readily diffusing through cell membranes). The total body generation of NO$^•$ is appreciable, of the order of 1 mmol/day based on quantitation of NO$_2$ and NO$_3$ (end products of NO$^•$ oxidation) in plasma (Wennmalm *et al.*, 1994). As well as the above, activated phagocytes are capable of generating O$_2^{-•}$, H$_2$O$_2$ and NO$^•$ species (as well as hypochlorous acid, HOCl), all of which may contribute to tissue injury during inflammation. In addition, ROS may amplify the inflammation process by upregulation of various species involved in the inflammatory response, particularly via activation of the nuclear transcription factor NFkβ, which in turn upregulates pro-inflammatory cytokines and leukocyte adhesion molecules. There is evidence that NO$^•$ may act as a messenger for cell fusion in chick embryonic myoblasts, and that NFkβ dependent expression of NOS is an important step in myoblast membrane fusion (Lee *et al.*, 1997).

Antioxidants

Cells are protected from free radical induced damage by a variety of endogenous radical scavenging proteins, enzymes, and chemical (water or lipid soluble) compounds. These include metal ion sequestering proteins such as transferrin (Fe^{2+}) or ceruloplasmin (Cu^{2+}), and ROS metabolizing enzymes such as superoxide dismutase (O$_2^{-•}$), catalase and glutathione peroxidase (H$_2$O$_2$); the glutathione peroxidase seleno-enzyme forms part of a self-regenerating cycle involving reduced/oxidized glutathione and the enzyme glutathione reductase. Glutathione peroxidase and superoxide dismutase occur in both mitochondrial and cytoplasmic isoforms. As well as biothiols such as glutathione, other important antioxidant compounds include α-tocopherol (vitamin E), ascorbic acid (vitamin C), uric acid, and the histidine-containing dipeptides carnosine and anserine. In addition to the above, a number of plant-derived dietary antioxidant compounds such as carotenoids and flavonoids have been identified. There are also a number of enzymic mechanisms to salvage and repair oxidative damage to nucleic acids and proteins; these may be of particular importance in counteracting oxidative damage caused by the OH$^•$ radical, which may not be efficiently scavenged by antioxidants, due to the high reactivity of OH$^•$ with potential biomolecular targets.

Measurement of ROS

Because of their high reactivity (second-order rate constants approx. 10^6–10^9/mol^{-1} per s) and short half lives (10^{-9}–10^{-4} s), direct analysis of ROS (especially in humans) is extremely difficult. The only technique capable of direct analysis of ROS is that of electron spin resonance (ESR) spectroscopy, which is normally used in conjunction with chemical compounds (typically nitrone derivatives) known as spin trapping agents, which produce longer lived radicals with distinctive ESR spectra. Thus phenyl-N-tert-butylnitrone (PBN) and 5,5-dimethyl-1-pyroline-N-oxide (DMPO) are used in the identification and quantification of OH$^•$ and O$_2^{-•}$ respectively. Because of the low steady state concentrations of ROS formed in tissues, this technique suffers from relatively poor sensitivity, and there are also ethical considerations precluding the administration of potentially toxic spin trapping agents to patients. An alternative approach has been to measure OH$^{\bullet}$ levels *in vivo*, based on reaction with salicylate, which is less toxic than other spin traps, and reacts rapidly with OH$^{\bullet}$ to form stable products. One of the main products formed is dihydroxybenzoic acid (DHBA), which does not occur endogenously in biological systems, and which can be quantitated via high performance liquid chromatography (HPLC) with electrochemical detection.

Another approach to quantification of ROS is based on the indirect analysis of ROS damage products in tissues, resulting from oxidative attack on nucleic acids, lipids and proteins. Oxidative damage to DNA is typically quantified by measurement of the marker 8-OH-guanosine in tissues or urine via HPLC (with electrochemical detection). Malondialdehyde and 4-hydroxynonenol (end-products of the peroxidation of polyunsaturated fatty acids) are used as markers to assess ROS induced lipid peroxidation. The most common assay procedure for measurement of these compounds has relied on the derivitization reaction obtained by boiling the sample with acidified thiobariburic acid, the methodology of which is now known to be subject to formation of artifacts (Marshall *et al.*, 1985). Quantification of lipid peroxidation via measurement of diene conjugation in tissues/urine is regarded as a similarly non-specific and unreliable methodology. Lipid peroxides are now quantified via HPLC (with electrochemical detection), either directly or following reaction with thiobarbituric acid.

The measurement of oxidized nucleic acids has been of particular value in investigating the role of ROS in malignant disease (Shigenaga *et al.*, 1990), and lipid peroxidation in the pathogenesis of cardiovascular disease and degenerative disorders of the CNS (Hall *et al.*, 1990). Oxidative damage by ROS on proteins induces a variety of structural modifications, the most extensively studied being the formation of carbonyl groups in amino acid residues (especially proline, arginine, lysine, and threosine), which can be quantified via reaction with 2,4-dinitrophenylhydrazine to form a yellow protein hydrazone adduct. The quantification of carbonyl groups by this method is considered to be a reliable hallmark of oxidative damage to proteins, provided appropriate practical precautions (e.g. removal of nucleic acids from samples) are taken. Protein carbonyl levels can be measured by a colorimetric assay procedure (for determination of total protein oxidation) (Reznick and Packer, 1994), or via immunoblotting analysis using commercially available monoclonal antibodies to dinitrophenylhydrazine (for identification of oxidative damage to individual proteins) (Levine *et al.*, 1994).

Levels of NO$^{\bullet}$ have been determined by both direct (electrochemical, ESR spectroscopy) and indirect (measurement of NO$_2$ or NO$_3$ oxidation product levels) methods. Oxidative damage to proteins by NO$^{\bullet}$ results in the formation of nitrotyrosine, which can be quantified by HPLC (with electrochemical detection), or immunologically using commercial antibodies against nitrotyrosine. In addition, nitric oxide synthase can be measured via analysis of mRNA (Northern blotting, *in situ* hybridization, polymerase chain reaction), DNA analysis (Southern blotting, polymerase chain reaction), or protein analysis (Western blotting, immunocytochemistry). Another indirect method of quantifying ROS activity is by measurement of changes in tissue antioxidant levels, either as total antioxidant capacity or as the activity of individual antioxidant enzymes or chemical compounds. Decreases in antioxidant levels, for example following surgically induced ischemia reperfusion injury, have been interpreted as an indirect measure of ROS production (Khaira *et al.*, 1996). Alternatively, moderate increases in ROS generation may result in adaptive increases in antioxidant levels (e.g. following exercise training).

Cellular damage resulting from an imbalance between the free radical generating and scavenging systems described above ("oxidative stress") has been implicated in the pathogenesis of a variety of disorders, some examples of which are reviewed in the following sections.

Neurodegenerative disorders and oxidative stress

There is evidence for the role of oxidative stress in the pathogenesis of CNS disorders, based on increased tissue levels of free radical damage markers, and/or altered levels of endogenous antioxidants. In particular, a number of factors contribute to making the brain particularly vulnerable to free radical induced damage compared to other organs, including the inability of neurons to regenerate after injury, increased tissue fatty acid content, increased tissue oxygen requirement and reliance on oxidative metabolism, high oxidase enzyme activities, decreased antioxidant levels, etc. (Tabet *et al.*, 2000).

Motor neuron disease

There is evidence that oxidative stress is an important factor in the pathogenesis of motor neuron disease (MND). MND is one of the most common neurodegenerative disorders, with an incidence of 1–2/100 000, primarily affecting the middle-aged and elderly, with an average age of onset of 55 years of age. MND is sporadic in about 90% of cases, with the other 10% of cases being inherited in an autosomal dominant manner (familial MND). MND is characterized by progressive injury and cell death of the lower motor neuron groups in spinal cord and brainstem, and upper motor neurons in the motor cortex, manifest clinically as motor dysfunction and muscle wasting. Point mutations in the antioxidant enzyme CuZn superoxide dismutase (SOD 1) have been found in some cases with the familial form of MND, although how mutations of this ubiquitously occurring enzyme may cause the relatively selective death of specific groups of motor neurons remains unclear (a toxic gain of function, rather than a loss of function, is suspected). Work has been undertaken to elucidate this problem, using cultured cells which express mutant SOD 1 protein, or transgenic mice models which express mutant SOD 1; both these cell culture (Cha *et al.*, 2000) and transgenic mouse (Andrus *et al.*, 1998; Cha *et al.*, 2000) models are characterized by increased levels of oxidative damage markers (protein carbonyl, lipid peroxide, nitrotyrosine) and/or altered antioxidant (glutathione, glutathione peroxidase) levels. There is also evidence for free radical mediated neuronal damage in the sporadic form of MND. Studies of human postmortem CNS tissues have shown increased levels of oxidative damage markers (protein carbonyl and/or 8-hydroxyguanosine) (Ferrante et al., 1997; Shaw, 1995), or altered levels of intracellular antioxidants (Ince et al., 1994; Shaw et al., 1997) which have been interpreted as an attempted compensatory response to oxidative stress. In addition, increased levels of 4-hydroxynonenol and 3-nitrotyrosine have been reported in CSF (cerebrospinal fluid) from MND patients (Smith et al., 1998; Tohgi et al., 1999). It is likely therefore that the mechanism underlying MND involves a complex interplay between oxidative stress and an imbalance in glutamatergic excitatory control in motor neurons, resulting in damage to intracellular proteins (neurofilaments) and organelle (mitochiondria) targets, resulting in protein aggregation, apoptosis, etc.

Nutritional aspects of motor neuron disease

Dietary components have been suspected as risk factors in the development of MND, but there is relatively little data, particularly in humans, to confirm this hypothesis. A case–control study of >100 MND patients in the USA did not find evidence linking dietary antioxidant intake with risk of disease, although a modest protective effect with lycopene was noted (Longnecker et al., 2000). Nutritional factors, particularly a deficiency of vitamin E, have been identified as risk factors for the development of equine motor neuron disease (De la Rua-Domenech et al., 1997). No large-scale therapeutic trials of antioxidants in MND patients have been reported to date. An under-powered trial of N-acetyl-cysteine therapy in 110 patients showed a trend towards improved survival in limb affected disease, which just failed to reach statistical significance (Louwerse et al., 1995). Using the SOD 1 transgenic mouse model, dietary supplementation with vitamin E was found to delay the onset of disease, but did not prolong overall survival, Using the same mouse model, Ferrante et al. (2001) reported that dietary administration of a standardized extract of Ginkgo biloba (EGb 761) with known antioxidant activity significantly improved motor performance and survival, and protected against loss of spinal cord anterior horn neurons.

Parkinson's disease

Parkinson's disease (PD) is the second most common neurodegenerative disorder, affecting 1% of the population over 65 years of age. Clinical manifestations include bradykinesia, rest tremor, rigidity, gait abnormalities, and postural instability. PD is characterized pathologically by the selective loss of dopaminergic neurons from the substantia nigra of the brain, with treatment currently via dopamine replacement therapy (as the precursor L-dopa). The reason for the loss of dopaminergic neurons in PD is unknown, although oxidative stress and mitochondrial dysfunction have been implicated in the most common, sporadic form of PD. Thus postmortem studies in human tissue (substantia nigra) have shown increased levels of Fe^{2+} and lipid peroxidation products, reduced levels of glutathione antioxidant, and altered mitochondrial complex 1 activity (Zhang *et al.*, 2000). Defective respiratory chain and dopamine metabolism is also thought to contribute to free radical production (Jenner and Olanow, 1996). The discovery that a synthetic heroin analogue, 1-methyl-4-phenyl-1,2,3,6 tetrahydrapyridine (MPTP) can selectively damage neurons in the nigrostriatal dopaminergic pathway and produce Parkinson-like disease in humans and in animals (primates, mice) has provided a useful model system for investigating the pathogenesis of PD (Langston, 1996). In the CNS, MPTP is oxidized by monoamine oxidase B to MPP+, which is selectively taken up (by active transport) by dopaminergic neurons, where it enters the mitochondria and inhibits complex I formation; this in turn results in increased $O_2^{-•}$ production, and reaction of the latter with $NO^•$ to form the highly damaging oxidizing species peroxynitrite. Consistent with the above is the observation that NO synthetase inhibitors are protective against MPTP induced toxicity in mouse models, and mice lacking glutathione peroxidase are more vulnerable to MPTP toxicity. The downstream targets of peroxynitrite have still to be identified, although the proteins alpha synuclein and parkin (implicated in familial forms of PD) have been suggested.

Nutritional aspects of Parkinson's disease

With regard to the possible nutritional links between oxidative stress and PD, there have been a number of reports indicating that dietary antioxidant intake does not influence the risk of developing PD. For example, in a German case–control study of 342 PD patients, Hellenbrand *et al.* (1996) found no significant difference in those patients with vitamin E and beta-carotene intake compared to controls. In a case–control study of 110 PD patients reported by Logroscino *et al.* (1996), no correlation was found between the incidence of PD and intake of antioxidants (including antioxidant supplements), although an increased consumption of fat among PD patients was noted, consistent with the hypothesis that oxidative stress and lipid peroxidation are important in the pathogenesis of PD. There was no correlation between long-term (i.e. 20 year) dietary intake of antioxidants (especially vitamin E, carotenoids) in 57 PD cases compared to controls (Scheider *et al.*, 1997) and a review of the literature (Jimenez-Jimenez *et al.*, 1999) found no evidence for a link between pre-morbid dietary antioxidant consumption (especially vitamin E) and risk of developing PD. A Spanish case–control study of 79 patients with PD reported reduced levels of glutathione in plasma, although levels of lipid peroxidation products and dietary antioxidant intake markers (beta-carotene, lycopene) were similar to controls (Larumbe *et al.*, 2001). However, a case–control study by Morens *et al.* (1996) of 84 PD patients showed that the risk of PD was significantly reduced with increasing dietary consumption of legume vegetables, although this phenomenon was not necessarily related to the high legume vitamin E content. In addition, dietary folate deficiency, with associated increased plasma levels of homocysteine (which promotes oxidative stress) sensitized mice to MPTP-induced PD-like disease (Duan et al., 2002), suggesting that dietary folate deficiency/increased plasma homocysteine may sensitize dopaminergic neurons to environmental toxins, thereby influencing the risk of PD in humans.

Alzheimer's disease

Alzheimer's disease (AD) is a disorder characterized by progressive impairment of memory and other higher cognitive functions, and personality and behavioral problems. AD is the most common form of dementia, affecting approximately 5% of the population over 65 years, and 25% of the population over 80 years of age. AD is characterized pathologically by loss of neurons from selective brain regions, accompanied by formation of characteristic deposits (plaques and tangles) which are a hallmark in the pathological diagnosis of this disease. Progress in the elucidation of the nature of these deposits and their role in the disease process have been made only relatively recently. There is increasing evidence for the role of free radical induced oxidative stress in the pathogenesis of AD. This includes increased levels of biomarkers of oxidative damage to nucleic acids, lipids, and proteins in postmortem brain tissue; for example, increased levels of lipid peroxidation (determined as thiobarbituric acid reactive substances) in AD frontal and temporal cortex (Marcus et al., 1998), F2 and F4 isoprostanes (peroxidation products of arachidonic acid) in AD frontal/temporal lobes (Pratico, 2002) or cortical regions (Nourooz-Zadeh et al., 1999), and 4-hydroxynonenol in AD amyglada, hippocampus and hippocampus gyras (Markesbery and Lovell, 1998). Increased levels of protein carbonyl and 8-hydroxyguanine in various brain regions have also been reported (Lyras et al., 1997). Tabet et al. (2000) have proposed that the potential reciprocal synergistic interaction between oxidative stress and other factors implicated in AD (beta amyloidosis, mitochondrial dysfunction, generation of inflammatory cytokines, etc.) should be considered in the pathogenesis and treatment of this disorder. Levels of antioxidant enzymes or compounds in brain tissue have been variously reported to be increased (Lovell et al., 1995), decreased (Gsell et al., 1995; Gu et al., 1998), or unchanged (Hayn et al., 1996; Makar et al., 1995) in AD, and both increased or decreased antioxidant levels have been interpreted as evidence of oxidative stress in this disorder (Tabet et al., 2000). Similarly, comparison of antioxidant levels in peripheral tissues from AD cases (versus controls) has shown reduced levels of superoxide dismutase in plasma or red cells (Ihara et al., 1997; Snaedal et al., 1998), unchanged activity of superoxide dismutase, glutathione reductase and glutathione peroxidase in red cells (Ceballos-Picot et al., 1996), and increased superoxide dismutase activity in skin fibroblasts (Urakami et al., 1995). Differences in the levels of the various antioxidants in blood or brain outlined above may have resulted from methodological differences between laboratories, or reflected variations in antioxidant levels in different stages of the disease, which may not have been taken into consideration in selection of patients. In addition, most studies do not take account of the precise dietary intake of subjects and controls, and the possible effect on antioxidant levels.

Nutritional aspects of Alzheimer's disease

In terms of the nutritional link between oxidative stress and cognitive dysfunction, a lower intake of vitamin A was associated with impaired cognitive functions measured by Mini Mental State examination (Jama et al., 1996). Vitamin C intake and plasma levels were shown to be lower in patients with cognitive impairment, and with cerebrovascular disease, while high intake of vitamin C was protective against both (Gale et al., 1996). Levels of vitamins A and C correlate significantly with recall, recognition, vocabulary, and semantic memory, but not with primary or working memory (Perrig et al., 1997). A direct relationship has been shown between blood levels of antioxidant vitamins and cognitive functions (Lethem and Orrell, 1997). Most investigators have reported a deficiency in dietary antioxidants, such as vitamin C (Deschamps et al., 2001; Gonzalez-Gross et al., 2001) or vitamin E (Jimenez-Jimenez et al., 1997; Tohgi et al., 1994; Zaman et al., 1992), in AD. A population-based prospective cohort study of >5000 Dutch participants demonstrated a reduced risk of AD with high dietary intake of vitamins C and E (Engelhart et al., 2002). A prospective study of >1300 elderly cases has reported a reduced risk of AD with increasing dietary intake of antioxidant flavonoids (Commenges et al., 2000). Vitamin E (2000 IU daily) supplements given to moderately severe AD cases appear to slow progression of the disease (Sano et al., 1997).

Pathological muscle

There is increasing evidence that free radicals are produced during strenuous skeletal muscle contraction (resulting from increased oxygen consumption and mitochondrial electron transport flux) and that they may contribute to the development of muscle fatigue via modulation of contractile function. Data supporting this hypothesis include:

1   direct (electron spin resonance spectroscopy) and indirect (markers of lipid or protein oxidation, or altered antioxidant capacity) evidence for increased free radical production in contracting muscle
2   evidence that free radical scavenging compounds reduce the development of muscle fatigue
3   evidence that pharmacological or dietary depletion of muscle antioxidant capacity increases the degree of muscle fatigue after exercise.

Much of the research in this area has utilized rat diaphragm muscle (*in vivo* or *in vitro*) as a model system for electrophysiological or biochemical studies. Trained individuals (human or animal) have an advantage, compared to untrained individuals, in resisting the effect of oxidative stress-induced muscle fatigue, resulting from adaptive increases in the overall antioxidant capacity and/or specific antioxidant enzymes (Dekkers et al., 1996). In humans, jump training resulted in increased levels of antioxidant enzymes in muscle tissue (but not in blood), with a corresponding decrease in muscle-derived creatine kinase efflux (a biomarker of muscle damage), compared with untrained controls (Ortenblad et al., 1997). Intermittent sprint cycle training, over several weeks, was shown (via muscle biopsy) to increase the levels of muscle antioxidant enzymes (Hellsten et al., 1997). Although participation in events such as long-distance triathalons would be expected to generate free radicals (because of the large consumption of oxygen), there was no evidence for oxidative damage in muscle tissue in trained athletes after competition (Margaritis et al., 1997). Manipulation of endogenous or dietary antioxidants may reduce exercise-induced fatigue and muscle damage associated with free radical generation (Sen et al., 1995). For example, supplementation with vitamin E reduced muscle membrane damage (assessed via creatine kinase efflux) resulting from increased free radical generation associated with high-intensity resistance exercise in weight trained males, compared to placebo (McBride et al., 1998).

The hereditary muscular dystrophies are Xp21-linked degenerative disorders of human skeletal muscle, manifesting as more severe (Duchenne) and less severe (Becker) clinical phenotypes. These disorders result from genetic mutations causing altered expression of dystrophin, a 427 kDa protein which links actin filaments within the muscle cell to a complex of plasma membrane associated glycoproteins (Ervasti and Campbell, 1993). While the absence of dystrophin is generally believed to weaken the muscle cell membrane, resulting in contractile-induced cellular damage, the precise mechanism responsible for necrosis and muscle wasting is unknown. A potential role for free radicals in this process was first indicated following the recognition of a form of muscular dystrophy in animals induced by a nutritional deficiency of vitamin A and/or selenium (Bradley and Fell, 1980); these include the so-called white muscle disease of commercial importance in farm animals. Myopathies resulting from combined selenium and vitamin E deficiency are usually more severe than that occurring with either of these factors alone (e.g. Hill et al., 2001). More recently, using myotube cultures from normal or dystrophin deficient (mdx) mice, the susceptibility of cells to different metabolic stresses *in vitro* has been evaluated. Dystrophin deficient cells were more susceptible to free radical induced injury than normal cells, but the two populations were equally susceptible to other forms of metabolic stress. This differential response appeared to be specifically related to dystrophin expression, since undifferentiated myoblasts (which do not express dystrophin) from normal and mdx mice were equally sensitive to oxidative stress (Rando et al., 1998). In addition, mdx mice have significantly increased levels of the OH$^•$ tissue damage biomarker o-tyrosine compared to controls (although mitochondrial enzyme activities measured in muscle homogenates were not impaired) (Hauser et al., 1995). Therefore the absence of dystrophin appears to render muscle specifically more susceptible to free radical induced injury. Further data to support the hypothesis for free radical involvement in muscle cell damage in muscular dystrophy have been obtained from studies in humans. The levels of protein carbonyl in quadriceps muscle biopsies were significantly increased in tissue from Duchenne cases compared to controls, indicating that cellular proteins in the latter muscle tissue are present in a quantitatively more oxidized state (Haycock et al., 1996). A subsequent study based on immunoblotting analysis of muscle biopsy tissue from Duchenne and Becker cases showed a heavily oxidized protein species (provisionally identified as myosin) which was absent in control tissue (Haycock et al., 1998). The question as to why myosin should be particularly susceptible to free radical-induced oxidative damage in dystrophic muscle, and the role such damage might play in the disease process, has still to be determined. In this regard, the finding of the absence of nitric oxide synthase (NOS, which is normally associated with dystrophin) in Duchenne or mdx muscles is of note. Investigations using NONOates (as physiologically relevant sources of $NO^•$) suggest that these may have a protective function against the damaging action of free radicals, i.e. $NO^•$ at low concentration protects against toxicity of $O_2^{-•}$, H_2O_2 and alkyl peroxides in cultured cells (Wink et al., 1995). Similarly, the $NO^•$ releasing drug C87-375 prevents $O_2^{-•}$ formation during stretch-induced programmed myocyte cell death (Cheng et al., 1995). It is possible, therefore, that $NO^•$ may have a role in preventing oxidative damage in normal muscle, and the absence of dystrophin and NOS in dystrophic muscle results in oxidative tissue damage.

Nutritional aspects of pathological muscle

Over the past 30 years, a number of therapeutic trials of antioxidants have been carried out in muscular dystrophy patients, including vitamin E and/or selenium (Edwards et al., 1984; Jackson et al., 1989), allopurinol (Griffiths et al., 1985), coenzyme Q10 (Folkers and Simonsen, 1995) and superoxide dismutase (Stern et al., 1982). No beneficial effects were demonstrated in any of the above trials, controlled in accordance with the recommendations of Dubowitz and Heckmatt (1980). In particular, exogenous administration of superoxide dismutase or catalase (orally or injected) was unlikely to prove of benefit, given the lack of absorption from the gut (Greenwald, 1990), and circulatory half lives of 8 and 20 min respectively (although conjugation with polyethylene glycol or albumin has been shown to increase the bioavailability of these enzymes; Radak et al., 1996). It is of note that 21-aminosteroid related compounds (lazeroids) have been shown to promote myogenesis in cultured cells via scavenging of free radicals (Vernier et al., 1995). Both vitamin E derived U83836E and glucocorticoid derived U74389P enhanced myogenesis of dystrophin-deficient cultures, and the potential of these compounds in the treatment of Duchenne and Becker muscular dystrophies remains to be determined. Relatively little information is available regarding the influence of nutritional antioxidants on the course of the hereditary muscular dystrophies. However, wheat kernel ingestion by mdx mice prevented development of muscle weakness, whereas dietary supplementation with vitamin E was less effective, indicating that a component of the wheat kernels (other than alpha tocopherol) may prevent muscle wasting in this disorder (Hubner *et al.*, 1996). Of particular note is the recent finding that dietary supplementation with 0.01–0.05% green tea extract (which has known antioxidant activity) significantly and dose dependently delayed or reduced necrosis in some muscle types in mdx mice (Buetler *et al.*, 2002).

Aging

It is generally recognized that aging is a complex, multifactorial process resulting in a generalized decline in physiological systems (immune function, endocrine function, etc.). Among the many theories of aging which have been proposed, it is now believed that free radical damage to cellular components is a major contributor to the aging process. Oxidative stress results from a time-dependent shift in the oxidant/antioxidant balance, the rate of which may be modified by genetic or environmental factors. Free radical-mediated damage to mitochondria results in mitochondrial DNA mutations, leading to a progressive reduction in cellular energy supply, and consequential physiological decline, characterized by the inactivation of key enzymes and accumulation of oxidized proteins. The only factor definitively shown to affect longevity is calorific restriction, which increases lifespan in many species, presumably as a result of reduced free radical flux associated with reduced cellular respiration (Merker *et al.*, 2001).

Nutritional aspects of aging

In nutritional terms, the elderly are particularly at risk from dietary deficiencies and malnutrition. Epidemiological data strongly indicate that high intakes of fruit and vegetables are associated with a reduced risk of a variety of age-associated degenerative diseases. In this regard, particular attention has focused on antioxidant components including antioxidant vitamins (e.g. vitamins C and E) and/or antioxidant compounds (e.g. flavonoids, carotenoids) (Weisburger, 1999). Thus, the traditional Mediterranean diet, based on a high consumption of fruit, vegetables and olive oil is associated with longer survival and a reduced risk of cancer and cardiovascular disease; these protective effects are thought to result from the high intake of antioxidant flavonoids from fruit and vegetables, and antioxidant phenolic compounds from olive oil (Owen *et al.*, 2000; Trichopoulou and Vasilopoulou, 2000). Dietary supplementation with vitamin E reduced the risk of cardiovascular disease (Losonczy *et al.*, 1996) and improved immune function (Meydani, 2000; Serafini, 2000) in elderly subjects. Increasing the dietary intake of fruit and vegetables (e.g. blueberry, spinach) with a high content of antioxidant compounds (especially anthocyanins) has been shown to retard or reverse age-related decline in brain function (cognitive or motor performance) in rats (Galli *et al.*, 2002). While there is evidence for the beneficial action of antioxidants in promoting longevity by reducing the risk of life-threatening diseases in man, the question as to whether antioxidants may increase maximum lifespan remains equivocal. However, it is of note that in model systems for studying aging based on *Caenorabdus elegans* or *Drosophila melanogaster*, mutants with greatly increased lifespans (relative to the wild-type strains) have increased activities of antioxidant enzymes such as superoxide dismutase or catalase (Knight, 2000; Lindsay, 1999).

Conclusion

In this chapter we have reviewed recent evidence from animal model and human (epidemiological, intervention, etc.) studies for the role of oxidative stress and antioxidants in the pathogenesis of a variety of disorders. The balance of such studies shows a clear benefit for the role of nutritional antioxidants in the prevention and/or treatment of such diseases.

References

Andrus, P.K., Fleck, T.J., Gurney, M.E., and Hall, E.D. (1998) Protein oxidative damage in a transgenic mouse model of familial amyotrophic lateral sclerosis, *Journal of Neurochemistry*, **71**: 2041–2048.

Bradley, R. and Fell, B.F. (1980) Myopathies in animals. In: *Disorders of Voluntary Muscle* (ed. J.N. Walton), 3rd edn, pp. 824–872. London: Churchill Livingstone.

Buetler, T.M., Renard, M., Offord, E.A., Schneider, H., and Ruegg, U.T. (2002) Green tea extract decreases muscle necrosis in mdx mice and protects against reactive oxygen species, *American Journal of Clinical Nutrition*, **75**: 749–753.

Ceballos-Picot, I., Merad-Boudia, M., Nicole, A., Thevenin, M., Hellier, G., Legrain, S., and Berr, C. (1996) Peripheral antioxidant enzyme activities and selenium in elderly subjects and in dementia of Alzheimer's type – place of the extracellular glutathione peroxidase, *Free Radical Biology and Medicine*, **20**: 579–587.

Cha, C.I., Chung, Y.H., Shin, C.M., Shin, D.H., Kim, Y.S., Gurney, M.E., and Lee, K.W. (2000) Immunocytochemical study on the distribution of nitrotyrosine in the brain of the transgenic mice expressing a human Cu/Zn SOD mutation, *Brain Research*, **853**: 156–161.

Cheeseman, K.H. and Slater, T.F. (1993) An introduction to free radical biochemistry, *British Medical Bulletin*, **49**: 481–493.

Cheng, W., Li, B., Kajstura, J., Li, P., Wolin, M.S., Sonnenblick, E.H., Hintze, T.H., Olivetti, G., and Anversa, P. (1995) Stretch-induced programmed myocyte cell death, *Journal of Clinical Investigation*, **96**: 2247–2259.

Commenges, D., Scotet, V., Renaud, S., Jacqmin-Gadda, H., Barberger-Gateau, P., and Dartigues, J.F. (2000) Intake of flavonoids and risk of dementia, *European Journal of Epidemiology*, **16**: 357–363.

Dekkers, J.C., van Doornen, L.J., and Kemper, H.C. (1996) The role of antioxidant vitamins and enzymes in the prevention of exercise-induced muscle damage, *Sports Medicine*, **21**: 213–238.

De la Rua-Domenech, R., Mohammed, H.O., Cummings, J.F., Divers, T.J., De Lahunta, A., and Summers, B.A. (1997) Association between plasma vitamin E concentration and the risk of equine motor neuron disease, *Veterinary Journal*, **154**: 203–213.

Deschamps, V., Barberger-Gateau, P., Peuchant, E., and Orgogozo, J.M. (2001) Nutritional factors in cerebral aging and dementia: epidemiological arguments for a role of oxidative stress, *Neuroepidemiology*, **20**: 7–15.

Duan, W., Ladenheim, B., Cutler, R.G., Kruman, I.I., Cadet, J.L., and Mattson, M.P. (2002) Dietary folate deficiency and elevated homocysteine levels endanger dopaminergic neurons in models of Parkinson's disease, *Journal of Neurochemistry*, **80**: 101–110.

Dubowitz, V. and Heckmatt, J. (1980) Management of muscular dystrophy. Pharmacological and physical aspects, *British Medical Bulletin*, **36**: 139–144.

Edwards, R.H., Jones, D.A., and Jackson, M.J. (1984) An approach to treatment trials in muscular dystrophy with particular reference to agents influencing free radical damage, *Medical Biology*, **62**: 143–147.

Engelhart, M.J., Geerlings, M.I., Ruitenberg, A., van Swieten, J.C., Hofman, A., Witteman, J.C., and Breteler, M.M. (2002) Dietary intake of antioxidants and risk of Alzheimer disease, *Journal of the American Medical Association*, **287**(24): 3223–3229.

Ervasti, J.M. and Campbell, K.P. (1993) A role for the dystrophin–glycoprotein complex as a transmembrane linker between laminin and actin, *Journal of Cell Biology*, **122**: 809–823.

Ferrante, R.J., Browne, S.E., Shinobu, L.A., Bowling, A.C., Baik, M.J., MacGarvey, U., Kowall, N.W., Brown, R.H. Jr, and Beal, M.F. (1997) Evidence of increased oxidative damage in both sporadic and familial amyotrophic lateral sclerosis, *Journal of Neurochemistry*, **69**: 2064–2074.

Ferrante, R.J., Klein, A.M., Dedeoglu, A., and Beal, M.F. (2001) Therapeutic efficacy of EGb761 (Gingko biloba extract) in a transgenic mouse model of amyotrophic lateral sclerosis, *Journal of Molecular Neuroscience*, **17**: 89–96.

Folkers, K. and Simonsen, R. (1995) Two successful double-blind trials with coenzyme Q10 (vitamin Q10) on muscular dystrophies and neurogenic atrophies, *Biochimica et Biophysica Acta*, **1271**: 281–286.

Gale, C.R., Martyn, C.N., and Cooper, C. (1996) Cognitive impairment and mortality in a cohort of elderly people, *British Medical Journal*, **312**: 608–611.

Galli, R.L., Shukitt-Hale, B., Youdim, K.A., and Joseph, J.A. (2002) Fruit polyphenolics and brain aging: nutritional interventions targeting age-related neuronal and behavioral deficits, *Annals of the New York Academy of Science*, **959**: 128–132.

Gonzalez-Gross, M., Marcos, A., and Pietrzik, K. (2001) Nutrition and cognitive impairment in the elderly, *British Journal of Nutrition*, **86**: 313–321.

Greenwald, R.A. (1990) Superoxide dismutase and catalase as therapeutic agents for human diseases. A critical review, *Free Radical Biology and Medicine*, **8**: 201–209.

Griffiths, R.D., Cady, E.B., Edwards, R.H., and Wilkie, D.R. (1985) Muscle energy metabolism in Duchenne dystrophy studied by 31P-NMR: controlled trials show no effect of allopurinol or ribose, *Muscle and Nerve*, **8**: 760–767.

Gsell, W., Conrad, R., Hickethier, M., Sofic, E., Frolich, L., Wichart, I., Jellinger, K., Moll, G., Ransmayr, G., Beckmann, H., et al. (1995) Decreased catalase activity but unchanged superoxide dismutase activity in brains of patients with dementia of Alzheimer type, *Journal of Neurochemistry*, **64**: 1216–1223.

Gu, M., Owen, A.D., Toffa, S.E., Cooper, J.M., Dexter, D.T., Jenner, P., Marsden, C.D., and Schapira, A.H. (1998) Mitochondrial function, GSH and iron in neurodegeneration and Lewy body diseases, *Journal of Neurological Science*, **158**: 24–29.

Hall, E.D., Braughler, J.M., and McCall, J.M. (1990) Role of oxygen radicals in stroke: effects of the 21-aminosteroids (lazaroids). A novel class of antioxidants, *Progress in Clinical Biology Research*, **361**: 351–362.

Hauser, E., Hoger, H., Bittner, R., Widhalm, K., Herkner, K., and Lubec, G. (1995) Oxyradical damage and mitochondrial enzyme activities in the mdx mouse, *Neuropediatrics*, **26**: 260–262.

Hayn, M., Kremser, K., Singewald, N., Cairns, N., Nemethova, M., Lubec, B., and Lubec, G. (1996) Evidence against the involvement of reactive oxygen species in the pathogenesis of neuronal death in Down's syndrome and Alzheimer's disease, *Life Sciences*, **59**: 537–544.

Haycock, J.W., MacNeil, S., Jones, P., Harris, J.B., and Mantle, D. (1996) Oxidative damage to muscle protein in Duchenne muscular dystrophy, *Neuroreport*, **8**: 357–361.

Haycock, J.W., MacNeil, S. and Mantle, D. (1998) 'Differential protein oxidation in Duchenne and Becker muscular dystrophy, *Neuroreport*, **9**: 2201–2207.

Hellenbrand, W., Boeing, H., Robra, B.P., Seidler, A., Vieregge, P., Nischan, P., Joerg, J., Oertel, W.H., Schneider, E., and Ulm, G. (1996) Diet and Parkinson's disease. II: A possible role for the past intake of specific nutrients. Results from a self-administered food-frequency questionnaire in a case–control study, *Neurology*, **47**: 644–650.

Hellsten, Y., Tullson, P.C., Richter, E.A., and Bangsbo, J. (1997) Oxidation of urate in human skeletal muscle during exercise, *Free Radical Biology and Medicine*, **22**: 169–174.

Hill, K.E., Motley, A.K., Li, X., May, J.M., and Burk, R.F. (2001) Combined selenium and vitamin E deficiency causes fatal myopathy in guinea pigs, *Journal of Nutrition*, **131**: 1798–1802.

Hubner, C., Lehr, H.A., Bodlaj, R., Finckh, B., Oexle, K., Marklund, S.L., Freudenberg, K., Kontush, A., Speer, A., Terwolbeck, K., Voit, T., and Kohlschutter, A. (1996) Wheat kernel ingestion protects from progression of muscle weakness in mdx mice, an animal model of Duchenne muscular dystrophy, *Pediatric Research*, **40**: 444–449.

Ihara, Y., Hayabara, T., Sasaki, K., Fujisawa, Y., Kawada, R., Yamamoto, T., Nakashima, Y., Yoshimune, S., Kawai, M., Kibata, M., and Kuroda, S. (1997) Free radicals and superoxide dismutase in blood of patients with Alzheimer's disease and vascular dementia, *Journal of Neurological Science*, **153**: 76–81.

Ince, P.G., Shaw, P.J., Candy, J.M., Mantle, D., Tandon, L., Ehmann, W.D., and Markesbery, W.R. (1994) 'Iron, selenium and glutathione peroxidase activity are elevated in sporadic motor neuron disease, *Neuroscience Letters*, **182**: 87–90.

Jackson, M.J., Coakley, J., Stokes, M., Edwards, R.H., and Oster, O. (1989) Selenium metabolism and supplementation in patients with muscular dystrophy, *Neurology*, **39**: 655–659.

Jama, J.W., Launer, L.J., Witteman, J.C., den Breeijen, J.H., Breteler, M.M., Grobbee, D.E., and Hofman, A. (1996) Dietary antioxidants and cognitive function in a population-based sample of older persons. The Rotterdam Study, *American Journal of Epidemiology*, **144**: 275–280.

Jenner, P. and Olanow, C.W. (1996) Oxidative stress and the pathogenesis of Parkinson's disease, *Neurology*, **47**: S161–S170.

Jimenez-Jimenez, F.J., Ayuso-Peralta, L., Molina, J.A., and Cabrera-Valdivia, F. (1999) Do antioxidants in the diet affect the risk of developing Parkinson disease?, *Reviews in Neurology*, **29**: 741–744 (in Spanish).

Jimenez-Jimenez, F.J., de Bustos, F., Molina, J.A., Benito-Leon, J., Tallon-Barranco, A., Gasalla, T., Orti-Pareja, M., Guillamon, F., Rubio, J.C., Arenas, J., and Enriquez-de-Salamanca, R. (1997) Cerebrospinal fluid levels of alpha-tocopherol (vitamin E) in Alzheimer's disease, *Journal of Neural Transmission*, **104**: 703–710.

Khaira, H.S., Maxwell, S.R., Thomason, H., Thorpe, G.H., Green, M.A., and Shearman, C.P. (1996) Antioxidant depletion during aortic aneurysm repair, *British Journal of Surgery*, **83**: 401–403.

Knight, J.A. (2000) The biochemistry of aging, *Advances in Clinical Chemistry*, **35**: 1–62.

Langston, J.W. (1996) The etiology of Parkinson's disease with emphasis on the MPTP story, *Neurology*, **47**: S153–S160.

Larumbe, J.R., Ferrer, J.V., Vines. J.J., and Fraile, P. (2001) Case control study of markers of oxidative stress and metabolism of blood iron in Parkinson's disease, *Revista Española de Salud Publica*, **75**: 45–53.

Lee, H.S., Jeong, J.Y., Kim, B.C., Kim, Y.S., Zhang, Y.Z., and Chung, H.K. (1997) Dietary antioxidant inhibits lipoprotein oxidation and renal injury in experimental focal segmental glomerulosclerosis, *Kidney International*, **51**: 1151–1159.

Lethem, R. and Orrell, M. (1997) Antioxidants and dementia, *Lancet*, **349**(9060): 1189–1190.

Levine, R.L., Williams, J.A., Stadtman, E.R., and Shacter, E. (1994) Carbonyl assays for determination of oxidatively modified proteins, *Methods in Enzymology*, **233**: 346–357.

Lindsay, D.G. (1999) Diet and ageing: the possible relation to reactive oxygen species, *Journal of Nutrition, Health and Aging*, **3**: 84–91.

Logroscino, G., Marder, K., Cote, L., Tang, M.X., Shea, S., and Mayeux, R. (1996) Dietary lipids and antioxidants in Parkinson's disease: a population-based, case–control study, *Annals of Neurology*, **39**: 89–94.

Longnecker, M.P., Kamel, F., Umbach, D.M., Munsat, T.L., Shefner, J.M., Lansdell, L.W., and Sandler, D.P. (2000) Dietary intake of calcium, magnesium and antioxidants in relation to risk of amyotrophic lateral sclerosis, *Neuroepidemiology*, **19**: 210–216.

Losonczy, K.G., Harris, T.B., and Havlik, R.J. (1996) Vitamin E and vitamin C supplement use and risk of all-cause and coronary heart disease mortality in older persons: the Established Populations for Epidemiologic Studies of the Elderly, *American Journal of Clinical Nutrition*, **64**: 190–196.

Louwerse, E.S., Weverling, G.J., Bossuyt, P.M., Meyjes, F.E., and de Jong, J.M. (1995) Randomized, double-blind, controlled trial of acetylcysteine in amyotrophic lateral sclerosis, *Archives of Neurology*, **52**: 559–564.

Lovell, M.A., Ehmann, W.D., Butler, S.M., and Markesbery, W.R. (1995) Elevated thiobarbituric acid-reactive substances and antioxidant enzyme activity in the brain in Alzheimer's disease, *Neurology*, **45**: 1594–1601.

Lyras, L., Cairns, N.J., Jenner, A., Jenner, P., and Halliwell, B. (1997) An assessment of oxidative damage to proteins, lipids, and DNA in brain from patients with Alzheimer's disease, *Journal of Neurochemistry*, **68**: 2061–2069.

McBride, J.M., Kraemer, W.J., Triplett-McBride, T., and Sebastianelli, W. (1998) Effect of resistance exercise on free radical production, *Medicine and Science in Sports and Exercise*, **30**: 67–72.

Makar, T.K., Cooper, A.J., Tofel-Grehl, B., Thaler, H.T., and Blass, J.P. (1995) Carnitine, carnitine acetyltransferase, and glutathione in Alzheimer brain, *Neurochemical Research*, **20**: 705–711.

Marcus, D.L., Thomas, C., Rodriguez, C., Simberkoff, K., Tsai, J.S., Strafaci, J.A., and Freedman, M.L. (1998) Increased peroxidation and reduced antioxidant enzyme activity in Alzheimer's disease, *Experimental Neurology*, **150**: 40–44.

Margaritis, I., Tessier, F., Richard, M.J., and Marconnet, P. (1997) No evidence of oxidative stress after a triathlon race in highly trained competitors, *International Journal of Sports Medicine*, **18**: 186–190.

Markesbery, W.R. and Lovell, M.A. (1998) Four-hydroxynonenal, a product of lipid peroxidation, is increased in the brain in Alzheimer's disease, *Neurobiology and Aging*, **19**: 33–36.

Marshall, P.J., Warso, M.A., and Lands, W.E. (1985) Selective microdetermination of lipid hydroperoxides, *Analytical Biochemistry*, **145**: 192–199.

Merker, K., Stolzing, A., and Grune, T. (2001) Proteolysis, caloric restriction and aging, *Mechanisms of Ageing and Development*, **122**: 595–615.

Meydani, M. (2000) Effect of functional food ingredients: vitamin E modulation of cardiovascular diseases and immune status in the elderly, *American Journal of Clinical Nutrition*, **71**(Suppl. 6): 1665S–1668S; discussion 1674S–1675S.

Morens, D.M., Grandinetti, A., Waslien, C.I., Park, C.B., Ross, G.W., and White, L.R. (1996) Case–control study of idiopathic Parkinson's disease and dietary vitamin E intake, *Neurology*, **46**: 1270–1274.

Nourooz-Zadeh, J., Liu, E.H., Yhlen, B., Anggard, E.E., and Halliwell, B. (1999) F4-isoprostanes as specific marker of docosahaenoic acid peroxidation in Alzheimer's disease, *Journal of Neurochemistry*, **72**: 734–740.

Ortenblad, N., Madsen, K., and Djurhuus, M.S. (1997) Antioxidant status and lipid peroxidation after short-term maximal exercise in trained and untrained humans, *American Journal of Physiology*, **272**: R1258–R1263.

Owen, R.W., Giacosa, A., Hull, W.E., Haubner, R., Wurtele, G., Spiegelhalder, B., and Bartsch, H. (2000) Olive-oil consumption and health: the possible role of antioxidants, *Lancet Oncology*, 107–112.

Perrig, W.J., Perrig, P., and Stahelin, H.B. (1997) The relation between antioxidants and memory performance in the old and very old, *Journal of the American Geriatric Society*, **45**: 718–724.

Pratico, D. (2002) Alzheimer's disease and oxygen radicals: new insights, *Biochemical Pharmacology*, **63**: 563–567.

Radak, Z., Asano, K., Inoue, M., Kizaki, T., Oh-Ishi, S., Suzuki, K., Taniguchi, N., and Ohno, H. (1996) Superoxide dismutase derivative prevents oxidative damage in liver and kidney of rats induced by exhausting exercise, *European Journal of Applied Physiology and Occupational Physiology*, **72**: 189–194.

Rando, T.A., Disatnik, M.H., Yu, Y., and Franco, A. (1998) Muscle cells from mdx mice have an increased susceptibility to oxidative stress, *Neuromuscular Disorders*, **8**: 14–21.

Reznick, A.Z. and Packer, L. (1994) Oxidative damage to proteins: spectrophotometric method for carbonyl assay, *Methods in Enzymology*, **233**: 357–363.

Sano, M., Ernesto, C., Thomas, R.G., Klauber, M.R., Schafer, K., Grundman, M., Woodbury, P., Growdon, J., Cotman, C.W., Pfeiffer, E., Schneider, L.S., and Thal, L.J. (1997) A controlled trial of selegiline, alpha-tocopherol, or both as treatment for Alzheimer's disease. The Alzheimer's Disease Cooperative Study, *New England Journal of Medicine*, **336**: 1216–1222.

Scheider, W.L., Hershey, L.A., Vena, J.E., Holmlund, T., Marshall, J.R., and Freudenheim, J. (1997) Dietary antioxidants and other dietary factors in the etiology of Parkinson's disease, *Movement Disorders*, **12**: 190–196.

Sen, C.K., Kolosova, I., Hanninen, O., and Orlov, S.N. (1995) Inward potassium transport systems in skeletal muscle derived cells are highly sensitive to oxidant exposure, *Free Radical Biology and Medicine*, **18**: 795–800.

Serafini, M. (2000) Dietary vitamin E and T cell-mediated function in the elderly: effectiveness and mechanism of action, *International Journal of Developments in Neuroscience*, **18**: 401–410.

Shaw, P.J., Ince, P.G., Falkous, G., and Mantle, D. (1995) Oxidative damage to protein in sporadic motor neuron disease spinal cord, *Annals of Neurology*, **38**: 691–695.

Shaw, P.J., Chinnery, R.M., Thagesen, H., Borthwick, G.M., and Ince, P.G. (1997) Immunocytochemical study of the distribution of the free radical scavenging enzymes Cu/Zn superoxide dismutase (SOD1); MN superoxide dismutase (MN SOD) and catalase in the normal human spinal cord and in motor neuron disease, *Journal of Neurological Science*, **147**: 115–125.

Shigenaga, M.K., Park, J.W., Cundy, K.C., Gimeno, C.J., and Ames, B.N. (1990) In vivo oxidative DNA damage: measurement of 8-hydroxy-2′-deoxyguanosine in DNA and urine by high-performance liquid chromatography with electrochemical detection, *Methods in Enzymology*, **186**: 521–530.

Smith, R.G., Henry, Y.K., Mattson, M.P., and Appel, S.H. (1998) Presence of 4-hydroxynonenal in cerebrospinal fluid of patients with sporadic amyotrophic lateral sclerosis, *Annals of Neurology*, **44**: 696–699.

Snaedal, J., Kristinsson, J., Gunnarsdottir, S., Olafsdottir, J., Baldvinsson, M., and Johannesson, T. (1998) Copper, ceruloplasmin and superoxide dismutase in patients with Alzheimer's disease: a case–control study, *Dementia and Geriatric Cognitive Disorders*, **9**: 239–242.

Stern, L.Z., Ringel, S.P., Ziter, F.A., Menander-Huber, K.B., Ionasescu, V., Pellegrino, R.J., and Snyder, R.D. (1982) Drug trial of superoxide dismutase in Duchenne's muscular dystrophy, *Archives of Neurology*, **39**: 342–346.

Tabet, N., Mantle, D., and Orrell, M. (2000) Free radicals as mediators of toxicity in Alzheimer's disease: a review and hypothesis, *Adverse Drug Reactions and Toxicology Reviews*, **19**: 127–152.

Tohgi, H., Abe, T., Nakanishi, M., Hamato, F., Sasaki, K., and Takahashi, S. (1994) Concentrations of alpha-tocopherol and its quinone derivative in cerebrospinal fluid from patients with vascular dementia of the Binswanger type and Alzheimer type dementia, *Neuroscience Letters*, **6**: 73–76.

Tohgi, H., Abe, T., Yamazaki, K., Murata, T., and Isobe, C. (1999) Remarkable increase in CSF 3-nitrotyrosine in patients with sporadic amyotrophic lateral scleritis, *Annals of Neurology*, **46**: 129–131.

Trichopoulou, A. and Vasilopoulou, E. (2000) Mediterranean diet and longevity, *British Journal of Nutrition*, **84**(Suppl. 2): S205–S209.

Urakami, K., Sato, K., Okada, A., Mura, T., Shimomura, T., Takenaka, T., Wakutani, Y., Oshima, T., Adachi, Y., Takahashi, K., *et al.* (1995) Cu, Zn superoxide dismutase in patients with dementia of the Alzheimer type, *Acta Neurological Scandinavia*, **91**: 165–168.

Vernier, A., Metzinger, L., Warter, J.M., Poindron, P., and Passaquin, A.C. (1995) Antioxidant lazaroids enhance differentiation of C2 skeletal muscle cells, *Neuroscience Letters*, **186**: 177–180.

Weisburger, J.H. (1999) Mechanisms of action of antioxidants as exemplified in vegetables, tomatoes and tea, *Food Chemistry and Toxicology*, **37**: 943–948.

Wennmalm, A., Benthin, G., Edlund, A., Kieler-Jensen, N., Lundin, S., Petersson, A.S., and Waagstein, F. (1994) Nitric oxide synthesis and metabolism in man, *Annals of the New York Academy of Science*, **714**, 158–164.

Wink, D.A., Cook, J.A., Pacelli, R., Liebmann, J., Krishna, M.C., and Mitchell, J.B. (1995) Nitric oxide (NO) protects against cellular damage by reactive oxygen species, *Toxicology Letters*, **82–83**: 221–226.

Zaman, Z., Roche, S., Fielden, P., Frost, P.G., Niriella, D.C., and Cayley, A.C. (1992) Plasma concentrations of vitamins A and E and carotenoids in Alzheimer's disease, *Age and Ageing*, **21**: 91–94.

Zhang, Y., Gao, J., Chung, K.K., Huang, H., Dawson, V.L., and Dawson, T.M. (2000) Parkin functions as an E2-dependent ubiquitin-protein ligase and promotes the degradation of the synaptic vesicle-associated protein, CDCrel-1, *Proceedings of the National Academy of Science USA*, **97**: 13354–13359.

17 Ethylene oxide in the food supply: an assessment of health risks

Jefferson Fowles

Introduction

Ethylene oxide (ETO) is considered by the International Agency for Research on Cancer (IARC) to be a known genotoxic human carcinogen (IARC, 1994). However, ETO is introduced into the food supply in trace quantities through fumigation in some countries to sterilize commodities that may have pathogenic bacterial contaminants. ETO is also formed from degradation of polymers, polysorbates and emulsifiers, as well as by endogenous gut microflora reactions involving ethylene. Due to its intrinsic cancer hazard, it is appropriate that attention be paid to minimizing consumer exposure to unnecessary ETO residues.

Hazard assessment

The status of ETO was upgraded by the IARC from Group 2A to Group 1 (*carcinogenic in humans*) in 1994 due to increasing epidemiological and occupational evidence of carcinogenicity and laboratory genetic toxicity studies showing that ETO was a genotoxic carcinogen capable of causing tumors in both animals and humans. The evidence of carcinogenicity in laboratory animals comes largely from inhalation studies (NTP, 1985a; Snellings *et al.*, 1984), but the designation by IARC is not qualified by the route of exposure. Furthermore, oral exposure data in laboratory animals have yielded stomach and systemic tumors (Dunkelberg, 1982). It has been assumed, for the purposes of some risk assessments, that ETO is a human carcinogen by ingestion (Fowles *et al.*, 2001). Structurally similar chemicals such as formaldehyde and propylene oxide are also probable human carcinogens. When comparing the potency of ETO in laboratory animals and human epidemiological studies, agencies have concluded that the potency of ETO was comparable in animals and humans (California Air Resources Board (CARB), 1987). The USEPA and the State of California have designated ETO a carcinogen and ETO air emissions by facilities are subject to tight regulatory controls.

Laboratory bioassays have shown lymphoid, mesothelial, subcutaneous, pituitary, and brain tumors to occur in rats exposed to ETO by inhalation (Lynch *et al.*, 1984; Snellings *et al.*, 1981, 1984), and stomach squamous cell carcinomas,

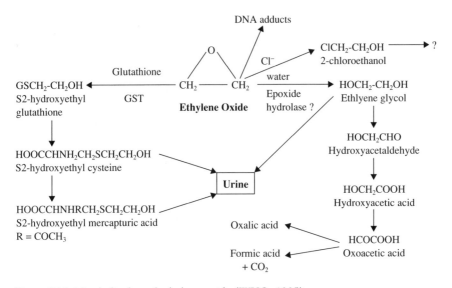

Figure 17.1 Metabolic fate of ethylene oxide (WHO, 1985).

fibrosarcomas, and systemic tumors upon oral exposure in rats (Dunkelberg, 1982). Inhalation studies in mice have shown a significantly elevated incidence of lung tumors in males and females as well as an increase in uterine and mammary tumors in females (NTP, 1986). Laboratory studies have shown that ETO is absorbed efficiently by animals upon inhalation (WHO, 1985). Studies on the oral absorption of ETO are not available and the kinetics of breakdown of ETO in the gastrointestinal tract are not known. The metabolic fate of ETO is illustrated in Figure 17.1. It is reasonable to assume that the stomach lining, as a point of first contact, would be a tissue at risk for developing cancer from ETO exposure.

A wide range of *in vitro* studies have demonstrated that ETO is a powerful mutagen in mammalian cells, as well as in bacteria, plants, and fungi (IARC, 1994; WHO, 1985).

Ethylene oxide also has a wide variety of non-cancer health effects in animals when inhaled in high concentrations, including reproductive and developmental toxicity (Weller *et al.*, 1999) and toxicity to various parts of the lung (CARB, 1987). These effects occur at levels many orders of magnitude higher than would be encountered from residues typically found in foods. The most critical effect from chronic exposure to low doses of ETO is cancer.

Epidemiological and toxicological evidence of carcinogenicity

Epidemiological studies have shown positive associations between ETO exposures and lymphatic and hematopoietic cancer incidence in hospital workers that sterilized hospital equipment with ETO (Bisanti *et al.*, 1993; Hogstedt *et al.*,

1986). Similar elevations in rates of these types of cancers are seen in chemical workers in manufacturing or otherwise using ETO (IARC, 1994).

Several epidemiological studies have reported an association between exposure to ETO and increased leukemia and stomach cancer risk (Hogstedt, 1988; Hogstedt *et al.*, 1979, 1986); however, other studies found no significant excesses in cancer risk (Bisanti *et al.*, 1993; Steenland *et al.*, 1991). In most studies, information about the extent of actual ETO exposure was limited. The most frequently reported association in exposed workers has been for lymphatic and hematopoietic cancer. A meta-analysis of ten distinct cohort studies of workers exposed to ETO found no association between exposure to ETO and increased risk of pancreatic or brain cancers. There was, however, a suggestive risk for non-Hodgkin's lymphoma and for stomach cancer (Shore *et al.*, 1993).

The largest study of US workers exposed to ETO at plants producing sterilized medical supplies and spices (Steenland *et al.*, 1991) found no increase in mortality from any cause of death; however, an increase in mortality from all hematopoietic neoplasms, concentrated in the subcategories lymphosarcoma, reticulosarcoma, and non-Hodgkin's lymphoma, was observed among males. An analysis of the exposure-response data from the study by Steenland *et al.* (1991) found a positive trend in risk with increasing cumulative exposure to ETO and mortality from lymphatic and hematopoietic neoplasms. This trend was strengthened when analysis was restricted to neoplasms of lymphoid cell origin (lymphocytic leukemia and non-Hodgkin's lymphoma combined). The relationship between cumulative exposure to ETO and leukemia was positive, but nonsignificant (Stayner *et al.*, 1993).

The evidence that ETO is a human carcinogen is supported by experimental studies in laboratory animals that have demonstrated that ETO is carcinogenic at multiple organ sites in rats and mice, likely due to its direct alkylating activity. Sites of tumor induction in rats included the hematopoietic system, brain, and mesothelium (Lynch *et al.*, 1984; Snellings *et al.*, 1984). An IARC evaluation (IARC, 1994) noted that ETO is associated with malignancies of the lymphatic and hematopoietic system in both humans and experimental animals, and concluded that ETO was carcinogenic to humans. No additional cancer studies of ETO in experimental animals have been reported since the IARC review.

DNA adducts of ETO exposure

The major DNA adduct of ETO is N7-(2-hydroxyethyl)guanine. Dose-related increases in this adduct, as well as smaller amounts of O6-(2-hydroxyethyl)guanine and N3-(2-hydroxyethyl)adenine, have been measured in rodents exposed to ETO (NTP, 1998). Background levels of hemoglobin and DNA adducts of ETO in humans and experimental animals have been suggested to arise from endogenous production of ethene (ethylene) by gut flora or metabolism of unsaturated dietary lipids (Ehrenberg and Tornqvist, 1995; Granath *et al.*, 1996).

Halohydrin breakdown products

Most of the ETO residues in foods react with available chloride or bromide to form 2-chloroethanol (ethylene chlorohydrin; ECH) or 2-bromoethanol (ethylene bromohydrin; EBH), the toxicity of both of which is not well characterized in terms of long-term studies of cancer risk. Other breakdown products include ethylene glycol, chloroacetaldehyde, and chloroacetic acid.

One long-term animal study on EBH used B6C3F1 mice (29/sex) exposed to 75 mg/kg per day in distilled drinking water for 1.5 years (Van Duuren *et al.*, 1985). Squamous papillomas of the stomach were found in 10 females and nine males. Two stomach papillomas were reported in the 95 control animals. No significant incidence of tumors was reported at any other site. A single long-term animal study on ECH exposed rats and mice for two years by the dermal route found no evidence of carcinogenicity (NTP, 1985b). However, only one study has been published on carcinogenicity of ECH by the oral route, in which four groups of six rats were given 0, 4, 8, or 16 mg/kg ECH in drinking water for two years without any apparent gross or histological effects (Johnson, 1967). This limited study would not be considered adequate for the purposes of assessing the carcinogenicity of ECH.

A comparison of the mutagenicity of ECH and ETO shows that, as an *in vitro* mutagen, ECH is approximately 20-fold less mutagenic than ETO at the same dose levels in bacteria (Pfeiffer and Dunkelberg, 1980). The NTP concluded that there was evidence of mutagenicity in bacterial and non-mammalian eukaryotes (NTP, 1985a). The evidence for mutagenicity of ECH in mammalian systems is less clear. No evidence was found of DNA damage in livers of mice injected intraperitoneally with high doses of ECH (Storer and Connolly, 1985). ECH tested positive for inducing unscheduled DNA synthesis in human fibroblasts (Stich *et al.*, 1976) and caused chromosomal aberrations in rat bone marrow cells (Isakova *et al.*, 1971). Similarly, reverse mutations and chromosome aberrations were reported in mammalian cells in the presence of the S9 fraction of liver homogenate (Ivett *et al.*, 1989; McGregor *et al.*, 1988). However, three studies of different aspects of mammalian mutagenicity were negative (Conan *et al.*, 1979; Epstein *et al.*, 1972; Sheu *et al.*, 1983). Under aqueous conditions or in the presence of liver metabolizing enzymes, ECH is oxidized to 2-chloroacetaldehyde and ultimately to 2-chloroacetic acid. The NTP has concluded that ECH is a weak mutagen but that its oxidized metabolic product, 2-chloroacetaldehyde, is a strong mutagen (NTP, 1985a).

There is some evidence that chlorohydrin exposure in occupational settings is carcinogenic. Significant increases in pancreatic, lymphopoietic and hematopoietic cancers were found in 278 workers assigned to ethylene and propylene chlorohydrin production units for a mean duration of 5.9 years, with a mean follow-up of 36.5 years (Benson and Teta, 1993). A subsequent study (Olsen *et al.*, 1997) found no significant increases in cancers in 1361 workers in a similar work setting, but the duration of exposure in this latter study included people with just 30 days' or more workplace experience.

Dose response assessment

Cancer potency

There are several studies available for calculation of a cancer potency factor (CPF) for ETO (Dunkelberg, 1982; NTP, 1986; Snellings *et al.*, 1984). The two-year inhalation study in rats (Snellings *et al.*, 1981, 1984) was used by the United States Environmental Protection Agency (USEPA) and the State of California to derive inhalation and oral CPFs for ETO (CARB, 1987). The two-year gavage study in rats (Dunkelberg, 1982) is the only study to assess effects of oral exposure to ETO. The data from the inhalation (Snellings *et al.*, 1984) and oral (Dunkelberg, 1982) studies are provided in Tables 17.1 and 17.2.

Table 17.1 Mononuclear cell leukemia in female Fischer-344 rats exposed to ETO by inhalation five days/week for 25 months (Snellings *et al.*, 1981, 1984)

Exposure Dose (rat)		Equivalent human lifetime dose (mg/kg per day)[b]	Leukemia incidence Reported by:		
(ppm)	(mg/kg per day)[a]		USEPA (1985)	WHO (1985)	Snellings et al. (1984)
0	0	0	22/186[c]	22/235[d]	11/115[e]
10	2.7	0.28 (0.46)	14/71	14/77	11/54
33	5.12	0.75 (0.86)	24/72	24/79	14/48
100	20.24	2.11 (3.42)	28/73	28/113	15/26

[a] Toxicokinetic studies indicated approximate dosages from inhaled concentrations of ETO. A time adjustment of 5/7 was applied to account for the 5 days/week exposure in the rat study.
[b] Equivalent human lifetime doses were calculated using the surface area adjustment: dose (human) = dose (animal)/[wt(h)/wt(a)]$^{1/3}$, using 70 kg for average human weight and 0.22 kg for an adult female rat. Doses using body weight to the $^{3}/_{4}$ power are shown in parentheses.
[c] Data analyzed by United States Environmental Protection Agency – negative tumor results at interim sacrifice (18 months) were not included in the analysis.
[d] Data reported by WHO include all observations, interim and final – including consideration of all negative findings at interim sacrifice as negative findings.
[e] The data in Snellings *et al.* (1984) contain only part of the total Bushy Run study.

Table 17.2 Stomach and forestomach tumors in rats exposed to ETO by oral gavage (Dunkelberg, 1982)

Exposure (mg/kg)	Incidence of rat stomach and forestomach tumors	Systemic tumors (mammary, uterine, ovary, lymphoid, pituitary, neural, s.c., intestine)[c]	Equivalent human lifetime dose (mg/kg per day)[a]
0	0/50	20/50	0
7.5	8/50[b]	28/50	0.51
30	31/50[b]	29/50[b]	2.03

[a] Equivalent human lifetime doses were calculated using the surface area adjustment: dose (human) = dose (animal)/[wt(h)/wt(a)]$^{1/4}$, using 70 kg for average human weight and 0.22 kg for an adult female rat. A time adjustment of 2/7 was applied to account for the 2 days/week exposure in the rat study.
[b] Significantly greater incidence than controls ($p < 0.05$, Fisher's Exact Test).
[c] s.c. = subcutaneous

Table 17.1 shows the mononuclear cell leukemia incidence in experimental rats reported by the USEPA (1985) and later by the State of California (CARB, 1987). Also included are the incidences reported by the World Health Organization (WHO, 1985), and by Snellings *et al.* (1984). The number of rats used in the cancer potency analyses varied depending on the assumptions made about the contribution of negative findings at the interim sacrifice. The USEPA and CARB chose not to include negative findings at interim sacrifice as indicating true negative results as these rats could have been at risk for developing tumors later in the study, whereas the WHO included all rats throughout the study in the denominator. All sources were in agreement that mononuclear cell leukemia in female rats was the most sensitive cancer endpoint with ETO inhalation.

The inhalation study in mice by NTP (1986) found a significant incidence of lung tumors, malignant lymphoma, uterine adenoma (females), and mammary gland adenosarcoma (females), but the sample groups were small in comparison to the studies in rats, and only two dose groups were studied in addition to controls. Therefore, the Snellings *et al.* study represented a more robust dose–response relationship.

The oral gavage studies in rats by Dunkelberg are the only long-term oral carcinogenicity studies for ETO. Ethylene oxide induced squamous cell carcinomas in the stomach and forestomach in rats at the doses used. Female rats (50 per group, plus 50 vehicle controls and 50 untreated rats) were gavaged twice per week for 150 weeks with ETO in salad oil. Doses of ETO were 0, 7.5, or 30 mg/kg. Treatments were temporarily suspended due to a pneumonia outbreak in the test animals. All animals were treated with antibiotics during the interruption period. There was a similar rate of mortality between treated and control groups at 104 weeks (30%).

The results of fitting the linear multistage model to these various data sets are shown in Table 17.3. The State of California (CARB, 1987) extensively reviewed the available literature in their derivation of the oral cancer potency value of 0.29 (mg/kg per day)$^{-1}$. The data used in their calculations came from the inhalation study (Snellings *et al.*, 1981). Later, the Cal/EPA revised the CPF to 0.31 (mg/kg per day)$^{-1}$.

Despite exposure through the inhalation route, the study in rats showed that the tumors were systemic in nature. Therefore, the cancer potency is likely to be relevant to other exposure routes, but would not reflect the potency toward portal of entry tumors for the oral route of exposure.

The data presented by WHO did not meet the chi-square test for goodness-of-fit criteria. As indicated in Table 17.3, the WHO compared the number of animals with tumors to the total number of animals in the study. A more statistically appropriate and health-protective assumption used by USEPA is to ignore negative cases at interim sacrifice times. This is because there is no guarantee these animals would not have had some incidence of tumors if they had been allowed to live out their lifespan or to the end of the 25 month study.

Table 17.3 Cancer potency values (q_1 and q_1^*) in (mg/kg per day)$^{-1}$ and other multistage model parameters derived from the tumor incidence data in Tables 17.1 and 17.2 (adapted from Fowles *et al.*, 2001).

Parameter	Mononuclear cell leukemia (inhalation)			Stomach tumors (oral) – ETO
	CARB (1987)	WHO (1985)	Snellings et al. (1984)	Dunkelberg (1982)
q_0	0.14	0.13	0.10	0
q_1	0.20	0.11	0.35	0.30
				0.73[b]
q_1^*	**0.29**[a]	**0.17**	**0.51**	**0.55**[c]
(95% UCL)	**(0.18)**			0.36[d]
p-value, chi-square goodness-of-fit test	0.16	0.005[e]	0.64	1.0

q_1^* values represent 95% upper confidence limits (UCL) of cancer potency factors in (mg/kg per day)$^{-1}$.

[a] This cancer potency value was derived by the California Air Resources Board in 1987 based on an earlier USEPA (1985) assessment. A revised value of 0.31 (mg/kg per day)$^{-1}$ is currently found on the Cal/EPA OEHHA website at http://www.oehha.org. The 0.18 value represents the same data using the body weight raised to the $^3/_4$ power for interspecies scaling, which is the currently accepted default.

[b] Cancer potency including carcinomas, fibrosarcomas, and *in situ* carcinomas of the forestomach and stomach.

[c] Cancer potency including carcinomas and fibrosarcomas of the stomach and forestomach. This is the value used as the oral cancer potency estimate for ETO in this risk assessment.

[d] Cancer potency from all systemic tumors distal to the stomach.

[e] The data presented in the WHO monograph do not meet goodness-of-fit requirements for the multistage model. This cancer potency factor was therefore not used in the risk assessment.

Exposure assessment

ETO in the food supply

Ethylene oxide occurs in the food supply as a result of fumigation/sterilization practices, degradation of polyethoxylated compounds (e.g. polysorbates), and from endogenous production of ethylene by gut microflora. The best quantified ETO residue data are from studies of fumigation practices, such as those for herbs and spices. However, there are indications that this is not the dominant source of overall ETO exposure for consumers. The prevailing view among the USEPA and the World Health Organisation (WHO) has been that the contribution of any cancer risk from the consumption of low levels of ETO residues in spices is unlikely to be significant due to the relatively small exposures involved (USEPA, 1996; WHO, 1985).

According to the NTP, most of the ingested ETO comes from the use of the food additive polyethylene glycol. Also, the use of ETO polymer is permitted in beer in the USA; however, the USFDA indicates that the compound is not at present used in this capacity. According to the NTP, the USEPA reported that small amounts of ETO, used as a fumigant, were found in some food commodities, such as cocoa, flour, dried fruits and vegetables, and fish. Other sources, however, list ETO as a fumigant for only three foods: spices, black walnuts, and copra (ATSDR, 1990).

Internationally, the issue of ETO exposures from food has been considered in a qualitative sense, but few risk assessments have been published. The WHO concluded that significant oral exposure of humans to ETO residues from fumigation is unlikely, due to the rapid disappearance of the residues through evaporation and the rapid formation of stable breakdown products (WHO, 1985). The NTP (1998) cited a report by the Agency for Toxic Substance and Disease Registry (ATSDR, 1990) that found there was no information indicating that ETO is a common contaminant in food. This appears to be an absence of information rather than a negative finding, as no studies were cited to support this conclusion.

The NTP (1985a) cited an USFDA communication that the "potential daily intake [of ETO] per person in the United States is estimated to be 10 micrograms" (1.6×10^{-4} mg/kg per day) (Modderman, 1986; cited in CARB, 1987). This estimate apparently included dietary intakes from all other sources, such as packaging materials (ETO polymers) and food additives (polysorbate emulsifiers). The worst case exposure estimate given was as high as 19 µg per person, which is about 1000-fold below the daily dose causing 16% added incidence of tumors in rats (Dunkelberg, 1982).

The European Union recently published an estimate of the intake of ETO from foods, using worst case scenario. They derived an estimate by assuming that 1 kg of food is consumed daily, all of which contains polysorbates as surfactants at the highest permitted use level of 5 g/kg of food. This would equate to an intake of 5 µg of ETO per day, assuming the polysorbates all contained ETO at the maximum permitted level of 1 µg/g of additive. It should be noted that there is likely to be significant loss of ETO from foods during cooking. Therefore, the potential intake of ETO from food additives in the EU would be unlikely to exceed 1 µg/day and would probably be much lower than that (EC, 2002).

It should be noted that while ETO fumigation is banned in the European Community, it has been clear from studies in New Zealand that the fumigation of herbs and spices takes place at or near the source of the product and not usually by the receiving country. Therefore, unless there is a monitoring programme in place, there is a possibility of residues occuring despite the ban.

ETO residues in herbs and spices

Data from the USEPA (1988, 1996) have shown that ETO levels decrease rapidly over the first few days and then more slowly to become non-detectable (at 0.1 ppm) by a period of about two months (Table 17.4). The study of retail spices (Fowles *et al.*, 2001) indicated that levels fell below 5 ppm in fumigated black peppercorns or ground pepper within 14 days. In the survey of retail samples in New Zealand, two of 31 (6.5%) samples known to be treated with ETO still had measurable levels of ETO (above 2 ppm) after an unknown length of time on the shelf (Fowles *et al.*, 2001). The vast bulk of the residues

Table 17.4 Ethylene oxide levels reported in fumigated spices (USEPA, 1988, 1996)

Spice	Concentration at time since fumigation (ppm)		
	4–7 days	*14 days*	*30 days*
Black pepper	51.1 (50.9)[a]	49.4 (42.7)	27.9 (59.3)
Cinnamon/cassia	122.9 (139.1)	23.5 (21.9)	0.43 (0.31)
Paprika	23.5 (22.3)	183.5 (123, 244)[b]	354
Chilli powder	80.2 (106.0)	33.0 (15.9)	3.2 (5.3)
Nutmeg	61.9 (37.5)	25.8 (32.4)	14.1 (30.1)

[a] Values are expressed as means. Standard deviations are given in parentheses.
[b] Only two values were available for paprika at 14 days; these values are given in parentheses. Only one sample was reported for paprika at 30 days. This single paprika sample was treated as an outlier. The limit of detection for ETO was 0.1–0.5 ppm.

found in fumigated spices, however, is in the form of ECH or EBH (Fowles *et al.*, 2001; USEPA, 1996).

An analysis of the USEPA data shows that, in general, residues decreased with time but were still detectable by 30 to 60 days. The greatest reduction in average ETO levels by 30 days was with cinnamon, and the slowest rate of reduction was for black pepper.

A significant proportion of spices off the shelf have shown levels of ECH above 5 ppm (Fowles *et al.*, 2001). These residues were found to be log-normally distributed, with an average value for ECH of 342 ppm, and a median of 140 ppm, and the 95% value was 2044 ppm.

ETO residues in other foods

According to IARC (1994), ETO residues were detected in the following food products sampled from Danish retail shops: herbs and spices (14–580 mg/kg), dairy (0.06–4.2 mg/kg), pickled fish (0.08–2.0 mg/kg), meat products (0.05–20 mg/kg), cocoa products (0.06–0.98 mg/kg), and black and herb teas (3–5 mg/kg; one sample contained 1800 mg/kg). No ETO residue was detected in a follow-up study of 59 honey samples (IARC, 1994).

Researchers concluded that the persistence or disappearance of ETO and its byproducts in fumigated commodities depends on the grain size, type of food aeration procedures, temperature, and storage and cooking conditions. Most fumigated commodities had levels of ETO below 1 ppm after 14 days in normal storage conditions (ATSDR, 1990).

Table 17.5 summarizes the reported exposures and effects of ethylene oxide in humans and laboratory animals. The estimates for human exposure to ETO in the non-occupationally exposed population are about 1/100 000 the doses seen to cause tumors in laboratory animals. This does not include endogenous production of ETO through gut microflora reactions.

Cooking reduces ETO residues in spices and other foods substantially. USEPA (1996) reports that at least 90% of ETO residues are converted to the non-carcinogenic ethylene glycol or 1,2-ethanediol upon cooking.

Table 17.5 Reported exposures and effects of ethylene oxide

Species	Exposure setting	Exposure range	Health effect	Reference
Human	Food consumption	0.014–0.27 µg/kg per day	7.7×10^{-6} to 1.5×10^{-4} Cancer risk estimate using $q_1^* = 0.55$ (mg/kg per day)$^{-1}$	EC, 2002; Fowles et al., 2001
Human	Ambient air (California EPA estimate for South Coast District)	0.026 µg/kg per day	Estimated 55 excess cancer cases per 7 million people	CARB, 1987
Human	Occupational (pharmaceutical industry)	7.8–78 µg/kg per day	NR**	Ehrenberg and Tornqvist, 1995
Human	Occupational	5–20 ppm	Cancer	Hogstedt et al., 1986
Human	Occupational	2900 µg/kg per day	Proteinuria	Currier et al., 1984
Rat	Experimental (inhalation)	0, 10, 33, or 100 ppm (17 000, 56 100, or 170 000 µg/kg per day)*	Multiple systemic tumors in all exposed groups	Snellings et al., 1984
Rat	Experimental (inhalation)	0, 10, 50, or 100 ppm (17 000, 85 000, or 170 000 µg/kg per day)*	Multiple systemic tumors in all exposed groups	Lynch et al., 1984
Mouse	Experimental (inhalation)	0, 50, 100 ppm	Multiple systemic tumors in all exposed groups	NTP, 1986
Rat	Experimental (oral)	0, 3000, or 12 000 µg/kg per day	Stomach, forestomach, and systemic tumors	Dunkelberg, 1982

* assuming a rat breathing rate of 12 L/hour.
** NR = not reported.

Conclusions

Ethylene oxide is a human carcinogen that is sometimes present as residual contamination in foods that are fumigated. However, the contribution to excess cancer risk from these residues has been estimated to be very small (i.e. in the 1×10^{-4} to 1×10^{-6} range using cancer potency estimates derived from animal studies). It also occurs as a byproduct of polysorbate emulsifiers and from degradation of polyethoxylated packaging materials and is produced from endogenous gut microflora reactions with ethylene. Estimates show that the total intake from all food sources is less than $1/200\,000$ the dose of some occupational groups that have been studied and found to have elevated cancer risks. These worst case exposure estimates from foods assume there is no loss of ETO through cooking, which is an overestimate of actual exposure, probably by several fold.

Following fumigation with ETO, data from the USA and New Zealand show that the breakdown products, ECH and EBH, remain at considerable concentrations in spices for a long time. Whether or not these breakdown products contribute to any potential cancer risk is unknown, as there have been no definitive assessments of their potential for carcinogenicity by the oral route. However, the information currently available suggests that any cancer risk posed by these breakdown products is negligible at current intake estimates. Nonetheless, the health effects and risks from the halohydrin breakdown products should be more fully explored.

References

ATSDR (Agency for Toxic Substances and Disease Registry) (1990) *Toxicological Profile for Ethylene Oxide*, Profile 137 (www.atsdr.cdc.gov/toxprofiles/tp137.html).

Benson, L.O. and Teta, M.J. (1993) Mortality due to pancreatic and lymphopoietic cancers in chlorohydrin production workers, *British Journal of Industrial Medicine*, **50**(8): 710–716.

Bisanti, L., Maggini, M., Raschetti, R., Spila, S., Ippolito, F.M., Caffari, B., Segnan, N., and Ponti, A. (1993) Cancer mortality in ethylene oxide workers, *British Journal of Industrial Medicine*, **50**: 317–324.

CARB (California Air Resources Board) (1987) *Staff Report: Initial Statement of Reasons for Rulemaking in the Identification of Ethylene Oxide as a Toxic Air Contaminant*. Sacramento, CA. 25 September.

Conan, L., Foucault, B., Siou, G., Chaigneau, M., and Le Moan, G. (1979) Contribution a la recherche d'une action mutagen des residus d'oxyde d'ethylene, d'ethylene glycol et de chloro-2-ethanol dansle materiel plastique sterilise par l'oxide d'ethylene, *Annals Fals. Exp. Chim.* **773**: 141–151 (cited in NTP, 1985).

Crump, K.S. (1984) An improved procedure for low-dose carcinogenic risk assessment from animal data, *Journal of Environmental Pathology and Toxicology*, **5**: 339–348.

Currier, M.F., Carlo, G.L., Poston, P.L., and Ledford, W.E. (1984) A cross sectional study of employees with potential occupational exposure to ethylene oxide, *British Journal of Industrial Medicine*, **41**: 492–498.

Dunkelberg, H. (1982) Carcinogenicity of ethylene oxide and 1,2-propylene oxide upon intragastric administration to rats, *British Journal of Cancer*, **46**: 924–933.

Ehrenberg, L. and Tornqvist, M. (1995) The research background for risk assessment of ethylene oxide: aspects of dose, *Mutation Research*, **330**: 41–54.

Epstein, S., Arnold, E., Andrea, J., Bass, W., and Bishop, Y. (1972) Detection of chemical mutagens by the dominant lethal assay in the mouse, *Toxicology and Applied Pharmacology*, **23**: 288–325.

European Commission (2002) Opinion of the Scientific Committee on Food on impurities of ethylene oxide in food additives, *Scientific Committee on Food*, SCF/CS/ADD/EMU/186 final, 6 May.

Food and Chemical News (1995) ASTA defends ethylene oxide use on spices, submits scientific review, **26**.

Fowles, J.R., Mitchell, J., and McGrath, H. (2001) Assessment of cancer risk from ethylene oxide residues in spices imported into New Zealand, *Food and Chemical Toxicology*, **39**: 1055–1062.

Granath, F., Rohlen, D., Goransson, C., Hansson, L., Magnusson, A.L., and Tornqvist, M. (1996) Relationship between dose in vivo of ethylene oxide and exposure to ethene in exposed workers, *Human and Experimental Toxicology*, **15**: 826–833.

Hogstedt, C. (1988) Epidemiological studies on ethylene oxide and cancer: an updating. IACR Scientific Publication No. 89. Symposium on detection of DNA damaging agents in man. Espoo, Finland. September 2–11, 1987.

Hogstedt, C., Malmqvist, N., and Wadman, B. (1979) Leukemia in workers exposed to ethylene oxide, *Journal of the American Medical Association*, **241**: 1132–1133.

Hogstedt, C., Aringer, L., and Gustavsson, A. (1986) Epidemiologic support for ethylene oxide as a cancer-causing agent, *Journal of the American Medical Association*, **255**: 1575–1578.

IARC (International Agency for Research on Cancer) (1994) *Monographs*, Vol. 60, p. 73. Updated 1997.

Isakova, G., Ekshtat, B., and Kerkis, Y. (1971) On studies of the mutagenic properties of chemical substances in the establishment of hygienic standards, *Hyg Sanit* (USSR) **36**: 178–84 (cited in NTP, 1985a).

Ivett, J.L., Brown, B.M., Rodgers, C., Anderson, B.E., Resnick, M.A., and Zeiger, E. (1989) Chromosomal aberrations and sister chromatid exchange tests in Chinese hamster ovary cells *in vitro*. IV. Results with 15 chemicals, *Environmental and Molecular Mutagenesis*, **14**(3): 165–187.

Johnson, M.K. (1967) Detoxication of ethylene chlorohydrin, *Food and Cosmetic Toxicology*, **5**: 449.

Lynch, D.W., Lewis, T.R., Moorman, W.J., Burg, J.R., Groth, D.H., Khan, A., Ackerman, L.J., and Cockrell, B.Y. (1984) Carcinogenic and toxicologic effects of inhaled ethylene oxide and propylene oxide in F344 rats, *Toxicology and Applied Pharmacology*, **76**: 69–84.

McGregor, D.B., Brown, A., Cattanach, P., Edwards, I., McBride, D., Riach, C., and Caspary, W.J. (1988) Responses of the L5178Y TK+/TK– mouse lymphoma cell forward mutation assay. 3.72 Coded chemicals, *Environmental and Molecular Mutagenesis*, **12**: 85–154.

Modderman, J. (1986) Telephone communication between John Modderman, U.S. Food and Drug Administration, and Ralph Propper, ARB, October 15, 1986 (cited in CARB, 1987).

Mstage (version 2.01) (1992) Cambridge Environmental, Inc., Cambridge, MA, 02141.

NTP (National Toxicology Program) (1985a) *Fourth Annual Report on Carcinogens*. Washington, DC: Department of Health and Human Services.

NTP (National Toxicology Program) (1985b) *NTP Technical Report on the Toxicology and Carcinogenesis Studies of 2-Chloroethanol (Ethylene Chlorohydrin) (CAS No. 107-07-3) in F344 Rats and Swiss CD-1 Mice (Dermal Studies)*, NIH Publication no. 86-2531. Washington, DC: Department of Health and Human Services.

NTP (National Toxicology Program) (1986) *NTP Technical Report on the Toxicology and Carcinogenesis Studies of Ethylene Oxide (CAS No. 75-21-8) in B6C3F1 Mice (Inhalation Studies)*, NIH Publication no. 86-2582. Washington DC: Department of Health and Human Services.

NTP (National Toxicology Program) (1998) *Eighth Report on Carcinogens*. Washington DC: Department of Health and Human Services.

Olsen, G.W., Lacey, S.E., Bodner, K.M., Chau, M., Arceneaux, T.G., Cartmill, J.B., Ramlow, J.M., and Boswell, J.M. (1997) Mortality from pancreatic and lymphopoietic cancer among workers in ethylene and propylene chlorohydrin production, *Occupational and Environmental Medicine*, **54**: 592–598.

Pfeiffer, E. and Dunkelberg, H. (1980) Mutagenicity of ethylene oxide and propylene oxide and of the glycols and halohydrins formed from them during the fumigation of foodstuffs, *Food and Cosmetic Toxicology*, **18**: 115–118.

Sheu, C., Cain, K., Gryder, R., and Generoso, W. (1983) Heritable translocations test with ethylene chlorohydrin in male mice, *Journal of the American College of Toxicology*, **2**: 221–223.

Shore, R.E., Gardner, M.J., and Pannett, B. (1993) Ethylene oxide: an assessment of the epidemiological evidence on carcinogenicity, *British Journal of Industrial Medicine*, **50**: 971–997.

Snellings, W.M., Weil, C.S., and Maronpot, R.R. (1981) *Ethylene Oxide: Two-year Inhalation Study on Rats*. Pittsburgh, PA: Bushy Run Research Center (Final Report no. 44-20).

Snellings, W.M., Weil, C.S., and Maronpot, R.R. (1984) A two-year inhalation study of the carcinogenic potential of ethylene oxide in Fischer 344 rats, *Toxicology and Applied Pharmacology*, **75**: 105–117.

Statistics New Zealand (1999) Official population figures for New Zealand as of November 1998.

Stayner, L., Steenland, K., Greife, A., Hornung, R., Hayes, R.B., Nowlin, S., Morawetz, J., Ringenburg, V., Elliot, L., and Halperin, W. (1993) Exposure–response analysis of cancer mortality in a cohort of workers exposed to ethylene oxide, *American Journal of Epidemiology*, **138**: 787–798.

Steenland, K., Stayner, H., Greife, A., Halperin, W., Mayes, R., Hornung, R., and Noalin, S. (1991) Mortality among workers exposed to ethylene oxide, *New England Journal of Medicine*, **324**: 1402–1407.

Stich, H., San, R., Lam, P., and Koropatnick, D. (1976) The detection of naturally occurring and man-made carcinogens and mutagens by the DNA repair assay, *Second Joint US/USSR Symposium on the Comprehensive Analysis of the Environment*, pp. 85–88 (cited in NTP, 1985).

Storer, R.D. and Conolly, R.B. (1985) An investigation of the role of microsomal oxidative metabolism in the *in vivo* genotoxicity of 1,2-dichloroethane, *Toxicology and Applied Pharmacology*, **77**: 36–46.

USEPA (United States Environmental Protection Agency) (1985) *Health Assessment Document for Ethylene Oxide*. Final Report. Washington, DC.

USEPA (United States Environmental Protection Agency) (1988) Memorandum from Leung Cheng, Health Effects Division, to Mark Boodee, Special Review Branch: Ethylene Oxide. *Dietary Exposure Assessment in Spices*. 16 November.

USEPA (United States Environmental Protection Agency) (1996) Memorandum from Leung Cheng, Health Effects Division, to Vivian Prunier, Special Review Branch: Ethylene Oxide. Case No. 2275. *Analytical Method, Residue Persistence in Herbs and Spices and Walnuts, and Cooking Study*. 28 March.

USEPA (United States Environmental Protection Agency) (1999a) *Integrated Risk Information System (IRIS)* (www.epa.gov/iris).

USEPA (United States Environmental Protection Agency) (1999b) Personal communication with Dr Lisa Niesensen, Director, Special Review & Reregistration Division, United States Environmental Protection Agency.

Van Duuren, B.L., Seidman, I., Melchionne, S., and Kline, S.A. (1985) Carcinogenicity bioassays of bromoacetaldehyde and bromoethanol – potential metabolites of dibromoethane, *Teratogenesis, Carcinogenesis and Mutagenesis* **5**: 393–403.

Weller, E., Long, N., Smith, A., Williams, P., Ravi, S., Gill, J., Henessey, R., Skornik, W., Brain, J., Kimmel, C., Kimmel, G., Holmes, L., and Ryan, L. (1999) Dose–rate effects of ethylene oxide exposure on developmental toxicity, *Journal of Toxicological Sciences*, **50**: 259–270.

WHO (World Health Organization) (1985) *Environmental Health Criteria 55: Ethylene oxide*. International Programme on Chemical Safety. Geneva: WHO.

18 Dietary patulin and its effects

Patrizia Restani

Introduction

Exposure to mycotoxins by food intake is considered an important risk for animal and human health. It had been suspected that moldy foods could cause illness in animals and humans before the existence of mycotoxins was experimentally demonstrated.

The occurrence of ergot intoxication (ergotism) is the oldest recognized mycotoxicosis in humans and animals. At present, more than 200 mycotoxins are know to exist and this number is continuously increasing so that the impact of these naturally occurring contaminants on human health cannot be assessed comprehensively. In some cases, toxic effects in human have been demonstrated after ingestion of mycotoxins with food or occasional inhalation. However, data on adverse effects are often lacking and association between a mycotoxin and an health disorder can only be hypothesized.

The tolerable daily intakes (TDIs) or provisional (maximum) tolerable daily intakes (PTDIs/PMTDIs) have been established by international toxicological committees only for the most well documented mycotoxins.

Another critical aspect in evaluating the possible risk due to dietetic intake of mycotoxins is the lack of data on actual exposure. Data on mycotoxin content in foods and on the consumption of these foods by general and geographically identified populations are necessary in order to perform reliable exposure analyses.

A considerable increase in patulin research has been seen in the past decade, and its presence in some foods has been well documented. On the basis of analytical data, food-borne exposure of human beings to patulin is likely to occur. This chapter evaluates data on occurrence, toxicological effects and estimated exposure.

Chemical aspects of patulin

Chemical structure of patulin

The chemical structure of patulin, 4-hydroxy-4H-furo[3,2-c] pyran-2(6H)-one, is shown in Figure 18.1; the mycotoxin is a secondary metabolite produced by

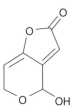

Figure 18.1 Chemical structure of patulin (4-hydroxy-4H-furo[3,2-c] pyran-2(6H)-one).

approximately 60 species of molds belonging to over 30 genera. Many fungi found in spoiled food such as *Penicillium* spp. and *Aspergillus* spp. (including *A. clavatus, A. terreus, P. patulum, P. aspergillus, P. urticae, P. expansum,* and *Byssochlamys nivea*) produce patulin frequently when they invade fruits (Davis and Diener, 1987; Lai *et al.*, 2000; Scott, 1994). In particular, *P. expansum*, a common post-harvest pathogen of apples and pears, is the most important producer of the mycotoxin detectable in fruits and juices (Paster *et al.*, 1995; Sommer *et al.*, 1974).

Patulin biosynthesis

The patulin biosynthesis is one of the best characterized pathways of fungal secondary metabolism. Patulin is biosynthetized by *Penicillium patulum* from the aromatic polyketide precursur 6-methylsalicylic acid (6-MSA), which is formed by condensation of one acetyl-CoA and three malonyl-CoA units with NADPH as a reducing factor (Murphy and Lynen, 1975). The portion of biosynthesis from gentisyl aldehyde to patulin is complex (Gaucher, 1979; Iijima *et al.*, 1983; Sekiguchi and Gaucher, 1979a, 1979b; Sekiguchi *et al.*, 1983) and the following patulin precursors have been identified:

- (+)-isoepoxydon (Sekiguchi and Gaucher, 1979a, 1979b)
- (−)-phyllostine (Sekiguchi and Gaucher, 1978, 1979b)
- neopatulin (Sekiguchi *et al.*, 1979)
- ascladiol (Sekiguchi *et al.*, 1983).

The hypothesized biosynthetic pathway of patulin from 6-MSA is illustrated in Figure 18.2. In 1989, Priest and Light observed that *m*-hydroxybenzaldehyde, gentisyl aldehyde, gentisyl quinone, and isoepoxydon could be branch products of 6-MSA degradation rather than obligatory intermediates in patulin biosynthesis.

Patulin occurrence

Although apples (Figure 18.3) and pears are the most usually contaminated, patulin can be detected in several fruits and cereals, while the growth of the

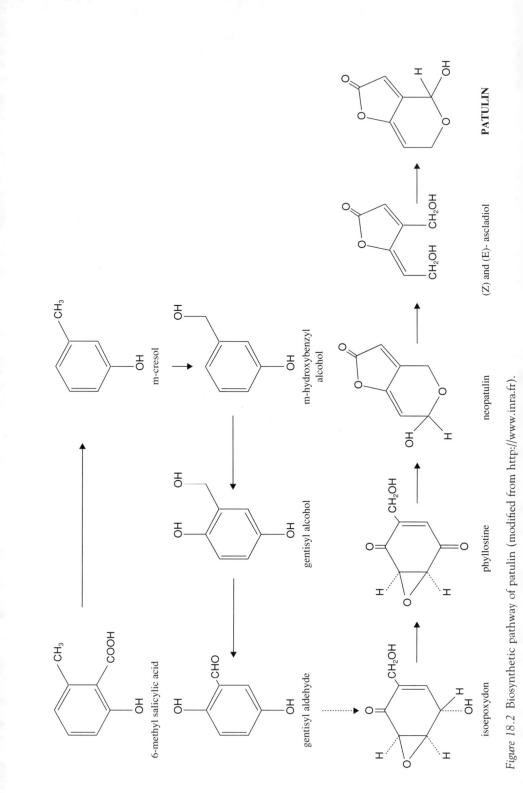

Figure 18.2 Biosynthetic pathway of patulin (modified from http://www.inra.fr).

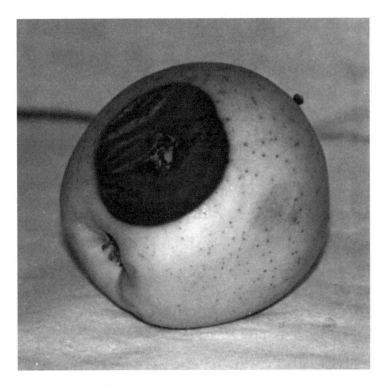

Figure 18.3 A golden apple with an area affected by patulin-producing fungi.

fungus has been detected in bananas, pineapples, grapes, peaches, and apricots. The foodstuffs where patulin or patulin-producing fungi have been identified are listed in Table 18.1.

Patulin in fruits and derivatives: role of storage conditions and technological processes

Penicillium expansum, the most important among fungi producing patulin, is often isolated from the surface of healthy fruit tissue; however, the growth of the blue mold (a distinctive characteristic of *P. expansum*), and subsequent production of patulin, normally occurs only in those cases where the surface tissue of fruit has been damaged (Buchanan *et al.*, 1974; Wilson and Nuovo, 1973). The surface damage may be precipitated by a number of vectors including insects, storm damage and handling procedures (Doores, 1983; Spotts and Cervantes, 1993).

It has been shown that the ability of different strains of *Penicillium expansum* to grow and produce patulin in pears and apples varies at different temperatures; some strains produce patulin between 0 and 25°C, the maximum production occurring at 25°C for pears and 17°C for apples (Paster *et al.*, 1995). The

Table 18.1 Foodstuffs where patulin or patulin-producing fungi have been detected

Group	Food	Reference
Fruit or fruit juices	Apples	Beretta *et al.*, 2000; Frank, 1977; Mortimer *et al.*, 1985; Mutti and Quintavalla, 1989; Thurm *et al.*, 1979
	Apricot	Frank *et al.*, 1977; Mutti and Quintavalla, 1989
	Banana	Frank *et al.*, 1977
	Blackcurrants	Larsen *et al.*, 1998
	Blueberries	Akerstrand *et al.*, 1976
	Cherries	Larsen *et al.*, 1998
	Grape	Abrunhosa *et al.*, 2001; Altmayer *et al.*, 1982, 1985; Benkhemmar *et al.*, 1993; Frank *et al.*, 1977; Rice, 1980
	Peaches	Frank *et al.*, 1977; Thurm *et al.*, 1979
	Pears	Buchanan *et al.*, 1974; Frank, 1977; Thurm *et al.*, 1979
	Pineapples	Frank *et al.*, 1977
	Plums	Thurm *et al.*, 1979
	Tropical fruits	Mutti and Quintavalla, 1989
Fruit derivatives	Cider	Frayssinet, 1988
Vegetables	Beetroot	Wisniewska and Piskorska-Pliszczynska, 1982
	Tomatoes	Thurm *et al.*, 1979
Cereals and derivatives	Barley	Lopez-Diaz and Flannigan, 1997
	Corn	Alp *et al.*, 1997; Lin *et al.*, 1993
	Sesame	Demirer *et al.*, 1989
	Wheat	Lopez-Diaz and Flannigan, 1997
	Bread and pastry	Bullerman and Hartung, 1973; Reiss, 1972
Milk and derivatives	Milk	Singh *et al.*, 1992
	Cheese	Bullerman 1976, 1980, 1984; Olivigni and Bullerman, 1978; Scott, 1989
Meat and derivatives	Meat products	Mintzlaff *et al.*, 1972a
	Sausages	Mintzlaff *et al.*, 1972b

production of patulin is also a function of water activity (a_w), which is the amount of water at microorganisms' disposal for their growth; patulin can be formed down to a_w 0.88 (Lotzsch and Trapper, 1978). For *Penicillium expansum*, *Penicillium patulum*, and *Aspergillus clavatus*, the lowest a_w values for patulin production were 0.99, 0.95, and 0.99, respectively (Northolt *et al.*, 1978). The lowest values for patulin production by *Byssochlamys nivea* were 0.978, 0.968, and 0.959 at 21, 30, and 37°C, respectively (Roland and Beuchat, 1984).

Patulin production can be totally inhibited when apples are stored under 3% CO_2/2% O_2 (25°C). On the other hand, under 3% CO_2/10% O_2 and 3% CO_2/ 20% O_2 some strains of fungi are still able to produce the mycotoxin in different amounts (Paster *et al.*, 1995). The production of patulin can be controlled by using sub-atmospheric pressure; incubation at 160 mm Hg significantly inhibits both patulin production and growth of *Penicillium patulum* and *Penicillium expansum* (Adams *et al.*, 1976). Buchanan *et al.* (1983) showed that caffeine inhibits the patulin production by *Penicillium orticae*.

Contamination of apples with patulin is normally associated with the areas of spoiled tissue, with penetration occurring up to approximately 1 cm into the surrounding healthy tissue (Taniwaki *et al.*, 1992). Beretta *et al.* (2000) showed that the amount of patulin was extraordinarily high in the rotten area of apple, but the mycotoxin could also be found in the part unaffected by mould. Removal of the decayed portions from raw fruit, prior to further processing, has been reported to reduce significantly patulin concentrations in the final juiced products (Lovett *et al.*, 1975; Sydenham *et al.*, 1995, 1997).

Although several chemical and physical procedures (Table 18.2) may be used to reduce further patulin concentration in pressed juice or fruit derivatives, the toxin remains relatively stable under acidic conditions (Damoglou and Campbell, 1986). In fact, patulin is quite stable in acidic media at temperature of 125°C with pH ranging between 3.5 and 5.5. Values for half-life are 64 h at pH 8 and 1310 h at pH 6 (Brackett and Marth, 1979c). Industrial processing for apple products, through concentration by vacuum distillation and high-temperature

Table 18.2 Biological, chemical and physical procedures to reduce patulin content in fruit derivatives

Class of treatment	Treatment	Reference
Adsorption processes	Activated carbon	Artik *et al.*, 1995; Leggott *et al.*, 2001
	Carbon composite material	Huebner *et al.*, 2000
	Charcoal	Sands *et al.*, 1976
Biological processes	Alcoholic fermentation	Stinson *et al.*, 1978
Chemical treatment	Ascorbic acid	Brackett and Marth, 1979b; Doyle *et al.*, 1982; Steiner *et al.*, 1999
	Benzoic acid	Girisham and Reddy, 1986
	Lemon oil	Hasan, 2000
	Oxidative degradation	McKenzie *et al.*, 1997
	Propionate	Lennox and McElroy, 1984
	SO_2	Adam, 1979; Adam and Koller, 1980; Doyle *et al.*, 1982; Roland *et al.*, 1984; Steiner *et al.*, 1999
	Sorbate	Lennox and McElroy, 1984; Sanchis *et al.*, 1991
Physical treatment	Irradiation	Bullerman and Hartung, 1975; Zegota *et al.*, 1988
	Microwaves	Niola *et al.*, 1990
	Ultraviolet radiation	Valletrisco *et al.*, 1990

short-time (HTST) pasteurization treatment at 90°C for 10s, decreased the patulin content to 18.4% and 18.8%, respectively. Yeast fermentation with two strains of *Saccharomyces cerevisiae* effectively removes patulin from English commercial cider (Burroughs, 1977; Burroughs and Whiteley, 1976).

Conventional clarification using gelatine, bentonite, and activated charcoal was found effective in removing patulin from apple juice; however, this technique causes a significant decrease in apple juice phenolic substances, adversely affecting the product authenticity (Gokmen *et al.*, 2001). Conventional clarification using a rotary vacuum pre-coat filter and ultrafiltration can be useful in removing patulin from apple juices; the average losses of patulin were 39% for conventional clarification with filtration and 25% for ultrafiltration. Washing and handling appear to be the most critical steps in removing patulin from apples, since up to 54% could be eliminated using high-pressure water spraying (Acar *et al.*, 1998).

There is little decrease in patulin content when apple juice is packed and stored (Lai *et al.*, 2000).

Methods for patulin quantification

Several methods have been developed to detect patulin in foodstuffs (Table 18.3); some reviews on mycotoxin determination have been published (Dorner, 1996; Ikins, 1991; Liu, 1990).

Toxicological aspects of patulin

Patulin is a toxic substance with suspected carcinogenic properties; patulin toxicity data have been reviewed in detail by IARC (1986), FAO/WHO (Wouters and Speijers, 1996) and the FDA (2001).

Absorption, distribution, and excretion

The toxicokinetic profile of patulin was studied in Sprague-Dawley rats after a single dose of 3 mg/kg bw of ^{14}C-patulin in citrate buffer.

The animals (17 males and 12 females) were placed in metabolic cages and feces, urine, and CO_2 were collected; one or two animals/sex were sacrificed after 4 h, 24 h, 48 h, 72 h, and seven days. The recovery of radioactivity within seven days from acute treatment is illustrated in Table 18.4. Most of the excretion of radioactivity occurred within the first 24 h; the major retention sites of patulin were erythrocytes and blood-rich organs (spleen, kidney, lung, and liver) (Dailey *et al.*, 1977a).

Effects on biochemical parameters

In vitro studies have been performed to identify modifications in biochemical parameters after treatment with patulin (Arafat *et al.*, 1985; Arafat and Musa, 1995;

Table 18.3 Analytical methods for patulin quantification in foodstuffs

Analytical method	Reference
Bioassays	Cardeilhac et al., 1972 Lenz et al., 1986 Lompe and von Milczewski, 1979 Reiss, 1975 Yates and Porter, 1982
Colorimetry	Subramanian, 1982
Capillary electrophoresis	Tsao and Zhou, 2000
Gas chromatography[a]	Beaver, 1986 Tarter and Scott, 1991
Gas chromatography/mass spectrometry[a]	Cole, 1986 Llovera et al., 1999 Roach et al., 2000 Rupp and Turnipseed, 2000 Sheu and Shyu, 1999
High performance liquid chromatography[b]	Brause et al., 1996 Gokmen and Acar, 1996 Machinski and Midio, 1998 Rovira et al., 1993
Immunoassays	McElroy and Weiss, 1993
Immunoelectrophoresis	Mehl et al., 1986
Isotope stable dilution (GC/MS)	Rychlik and Schieberle, 1999
Thin layer chromatography[a]	Abramson et al., 1989 Jonsyn, 1990 Miguel and de Andres, 1987 Nesheim and Trucksess, 1986 Prieta et al., 1992

[a] Only methods published after 1985 have been considered.
[b] Only methods published after 1990 have been considered.

Table 18.4 Recovery of the given radioactivity (^{14}C-patulin) within seven days from single dose treatment in rat (Dailey et al., 1977a)

Tissue or biologic fluid analyzed	Percentage of given radioactivity
Feces	49
Urine	36
Soft tissue and blood	2–3
Expired CO_2	1–2

Ashoor and Chu, 1973a, 1973b; Bourdiol et al., 1990; Braunberg et al., 1982; Burghardt et al., 1992; Fuks-Holmberg, 1980; Hayes, 1977; Miura et al., 1993; Moule and Hatey, 1977; Phillips and Hayes, 1978; Tashiro et al., 1979). In most cases, the observed adverse effects were associated with the capability of patulin in binding SH-groups of enzymes. In fact, several studies showed a multiple electrophilic reactivity of patulin towards simple thiol nucleophiles and the ability of the mycotoxin to covalently crosslink proteins (serum albumin, alfa and beta-tubulin) (Fliege and Metzler, 1999).

Table 18.5 summarizes the in vivo studies that have been performed to evaluate biochemical modifications.

Toxicological studies

Since the aim of this chapter is the evaluation of toxicological risk associated with the dietary intake of patulin, only the studies where the mycotoxin was administered by oral route will be discussed.

Acute toxicity studies

The data on experimental acute toxicity studies of patulin (LD_{50}) are summarized in Figure 18.4.

The adverse effects reported in the studies were agitation, in some cases convulsions, dyspnea, pulmonary congestion and edema, ulcerations, hyperemia and gastrointestinal distension. Histopathological alterations (ulceration and inflammation of gastrointestinal tract) were associated with the antibiotic activity of patulin on gastrointestinal flora. LD_{50} values ranged between 27.8 and 55 mg/kg bw for adult rat and between 17 and 48 mg/kg bw for adult mouse; in hamster the LD_{50} was 31.5 mg/kg bw (Hayes et al., 1978; McKinley and Carlton, 1980a, 1980b; McKinley et al., 1982). A higher value was found in weaning rats (108–118 mg/kg bw) (Hayes et al., 1978).

Several studies have been performed in breeding animals. Studies in sheep were performed by administering ethyl acetate extract of Byssochlamis nivea culture (containing patulin) either orally by syringe (11–20 mg/kg bw) or by esophageal tube (15–20 mg/kg bw). A dose of 20 mg/kg bw by syringe caused death in 5 h while the maximum dose by esophageal tube led only to slight temporary intoxication. Acute symptoms were nasal discharge, cessation of rumination, reduction of the pain threshold in the retro-sternal area, weight loss, and reduced food intake. Histological lesions of the kidneys and liver were described. Increased urea levels (50–200%) and reduced serum protein level were observed. No nervous signs developed during acute intoxication (Camguilhem et al., 1975, 1976).

Piglets aged 17–20 days were given patulin by oral route. A single dose of 2.5 mg/kg bw induced acute toxicosis, while doses of ≥5 mg/kg were lethal. Vomiting, salivation, anorexia, polypnea, weight loss, erythropenia, and leukocytosis

Table 18.5 *In vivo* studies on enzyme activity and other biochemical parameters

Biochemical parameter	Species/route	Dose (time)	Toxic effect	Reference
Acetylcholinesterase and Na-K-ATPase	Albino rat/intraperitoneal	1.6 mg/kg bw/day (one month)	Enzyme activity in cerebral hemisphere, cerebellum and medulla oblongata were inhibited	Devaraj *et al.*, 1982a
ATPase, Na-K-ATPase and alkaline phosphatase	Albino rat/intraperitoneal	1.6 mg/kg bw/day (one month)	Total activity reduced	Devaraj *et al.*, 1982b
Insulin, blood glucose	Rat/intraperitoneal	1 mg/kg bw on alternate days (3 months)	Elevated glucose curve; reduced insulin production (diabetogenic activity)	Devaraj *et al.*, 1986a
Lactate dehydrogenase and alanine amino transferase (GTP)	Pregnant Sprague-Dawley rat/os	3 mg/kg bw per day (days 1–19 gestation)	Increase of the liver lactate dehydrogenase and depression of placental GPT	Fuks-Holmberg, 1980
Plasma protein concentration, albumin fraction	Albino rat/intraperitoneal	0.1 mg on alternate days (15 doses)	Plasma total protein concentration and albumin fraction were decreased	Gopalakrishnan and Sakthisekaran, 1991
Liver mixed function oxidase and cytochrome P-450 activity	Male F344 rat/intraperitoneal	0 to 10 mg/kg bw (one dose)	Oxidative cleavage of phosphonothioate and aryl hydrocarbon hydrolase were elevated at 10 mg/kg	Kangsadalampai *et al.*, 1981
Glycogen phosphorylase, blood glucose	Male mouse/intraperitoneal	0.1 mg on alternate days (10 doses)	Enzyme activation in liver; 60% increasing of blood glucose level	Madiyalakan and Shanmugasundaram, 1978

Table 18.5 (cont'd)

Biochemical parameter	Species/route	Dose (time)	Toxic effect	Reference
Na-K-ATPase and Mg-ATPase	Male ICR mice/intraperitoneal	5.0–7.5 mg/kg bw (one dose)	Enzyme activity in liver, kidney, and brain preparations was inhibited after 48 h	Phillips and Hayes, 1977
Insulin-dependent enzymes	Albino rat/intraperitoneal	0.1 mg on alternate days (15 doses)	In liver, kidney and intestine, glycogen phosphorylase was markedly increased; the glycolytic enzymes hexokinase and aldolase were significantly lowered. Glucose 6-phosphatase and fructose 1,6 diphosphatase activities were increased	Sakthisekaran et al., 1989
Glycogen phosphorylase, hexokinase, glucose 6-phosphatase, fructose 1.6-diphosphatase and aldolase	Albino rat/intraperitoneal	0.1 mg on alternate days (15 doses)	Aldolase level in liver, kidney and intestine tissue was reduced	Sakthisekaran and Shanmugasundaram, 1990
Mixed function oxidase	Male ICR mouse/intraperitoneal	1–4.5 mg/kg bw (one dose) 1 mg/kg bw daily (5–14 doses)	Induction of mixed function oxidase	Siraj et al., 1980

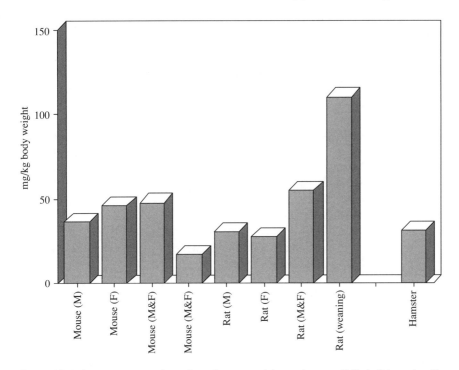

Figure 18.4 Acute toxicity of patulin administered by oral route (LD_{50}) (M, males; F, females). Data from Escoula *et al.*, 1977; Hayes *et al.*, 1978; McKinley and Carlton, 1980a, 1980b; McKinley *et al.* (1982).

were the principal clinical signs. Hemorrhagic enteritis, venous stasis and pulmonary edema were also observed (Obrazhei, 1987).

After overnight deprivation of food, varying doses of patulin were injected into the crops of White Leghorn cockerels; an LD_{50} dose of 170 mg/kg diet was found. Watery crop and fluid accumulation in the peritoneal cavity were found after 12 h in birds given a sublethal dose, and after 16–18 h digestive tract hemorrhages occurred (Lovett, 1972).

Short-term toxicity studies

MOUSE

When patulin was administered by gavage to Swiss ICR mice at doses of 0 to 36 mg/kg bw, daily or on alternate days for two weeks, body weight was depressed and mortality increased in a dose-dependent manner. Histopathological alterations found in the gastrointestinal tract were epithelial degeneration and desquamation, hemorrhage, ulceration, and exudation (McKinley and Carlton, 1980a).

RAT

When patulin was administered by gavage to Sprague-Dawley rats at doses of 28 or 41 mg/kg bw, daily or on alternate days for two weeks, no evidence of cumulative toxicity was found; gross and histopathological alterations were similar to those found in the LD_{50} studies. Histopathological lesions found in the stomach were ulceration of the mucosa, epithelial degeneration, hemorrhage, and neutrophil and mononuclear cell infiltration (McKinley *et al.*, 1982).

Female and male Wistar rats were given drinking-water containing patulin at 0, 25, 85, or 295 mg/L for four weeks. Compared with controls, a decrease in food and liquid intake was observed in groups receiving the mid and high doses. In the high-dose group the following adverse effects were observed:

1 body weight was decreased
2 creatinine clearance was lowered, without morphological glomerular damage
3 fundic ulcers in the stomach, and enlargement and activation of pancreatic–duodenal lymph nodes were noticed.

In both mid- and high-dose groups villous hyperemia was observed in the duodenum. Since no changes in the relative weight or histological appearance of the adrenal glands were observed, the authors suggested that the fundic ulcers in the stomach were due to a direct effect of patulin and not to an indirect stimulation by adrenal glands (stress). The no-observed-effect level (NOEL) in this study was 25 mg/L (Speijers *et al.*, 1988).

Weaning albino rats, weighing about 25 g each, received by gavage 0 or 100 μg patulin on alternate days for 30 days. At the end of the treatment period, the rats were sacrificed and intestinal tissue used to evaluate lipids and Na-K dependent ATPase. Total lipids, phospholipids and triglycerides decreased significantly whereas total cholesterol levels showed a 12.6% increase in the treated rats. Significant inhibition of membrane bound Na-K dependent ATPase was also observed in intestinal tissue (−32.4%) (Devaraj and Devaraj, 1987).

Administration of patulin (1 mg/kg bw) and *Penicillium patulum* (*P. griseofulvum*)-contaminated diet to weaning albino rats for three months produced a significant increase in blood glucose levels and a decrease in the activities of pancreatic lysosomal marker enzymes, namely cathepsin B and acid phosphatase. Authors suggested a relationship between the activities of lysosomal enzymes and production of insulin by islets of beta-cells (Devaraj *et al.*, 1986a).

Groups of Wistar rats were given drinking-water containing patulin at concentration of 0, 6, 30 or 150 mg/L for 13 weeks. No effect on the intestinal microflora was observed. In mid- and high-dose groups, the following adverse effects were observed:

1 a decrease in food and water intake
2 a slight impairment of the kidney function and villous hyperemia in the duodenum.

Only in the high-dose group, body weight gain was decreased and hematological parameters were slightly modified. The NOEL was 6 mg patulin/L drinking-water, corresponding to 0.8 mg/kg bw per day (Speijers *et al.*, 1986).

HAMSTER

When patulin was given by gavage to groups of Syrian hamsters at doses of 0, 16 or 24 mg/kg bw daily or on alternate days for 14 days, body weight decrease and higher mortality were observed in all treated groups. These effects showed no dose dependence. Gross lesions were found in the stomach and duodenum. Histopathological lesions were found in the gastrointestinal tract: epithelial degeneration, hemorrhage, and ulceration (McKinley and Carlton, 1980b).

CHICKEN

White leghorn chicks (51 days old) were given by gavage 0 or 100 µg patulin every 48 h. After 15 doses, the animals were sacrificed and organs were removed. The following enzymatic modifications were observed:

1 a reduction of total ATPase activity in kidney (−40%) and intestine (−52%)
2 a decrease of Na-K-dependent ATPase activity in kidney (−46%) and in intestine (−55%) (Devaraj *et al.*, 1986b).

For six weeks, groups of Mamoura chickens (30 months old) were given a commercial maize–soybean meal diet containing 0 or 100 mg/kg of patulin. Mycotoxin-contaminated diet influenced ash and calcium content of egg shells, blood urea, aspartate transaminase, alkaline phosphatase, relative organ weight, moisture, protein and fat content of red muscle, and texture and percentage of lean meat in red and white muscles (Abdelhamid and Dorra, 1990).

A group of 50 chickens (15 days old) received a control diet or a diet containing patulin at the concentrations found in feedstuffs during routine examinations. Bodyweight gain was significantly less for treated chickens. Liver and kidney lesions were observed (Bitany *et al.*, 1979).

MONKEY

Pigtail monkeys were given daily oral doses of patulin for four weeks. Four groups of monkeys received 0, 5, 50, or 500 µg/kg bw. After this period, the monkeys on 500 µg/kg bw were given 5 mg/kg bw per day for two additional weeks. No statistically significant changes were observed in hematological parameters, with the exception of alkaline phosphatase activities, which decreased as patulin dosage increased. The monkeys receiving 5 mg/kg bw per day of patulin rejected their food during the last three days of the experiment (Garza *et al.*, 1977).

Long-term toxicity and carcinogenicity studies

RAT

A series of twice weekly doses totalling 358 mg patulin/kg bw was administered by gavage to female rats from weaning over a period of 74 weeks. The dosages were 1 mg/kg bw for four weeks and 2.5 mg/kg bw for the following 70 weeks. Although there was a high spontaneous incidence of benign tumors, no carcinogenic action due to patulin was observed (Osswald *et al.*, 1978).

Groups of FDRL Wistar rats were given 0, 0.1, 0.5, or 1.5 mg patulin/kg bw per day by gavage three times per week for 24 months. The rats were derived from the F_1 generation of a one-generation reproductive toxicity study. Mortality increased in both sexes at the highest dose: all males had died by 19 months while 19% of females survived. The cause of death appeared to be increased pulmonary and laryngo-tracheal inflammation. Body weights of males were reduced at the mid and high doses, while female body weight was not affected. No consistent significant differences among groups were observed in the hematology, clinical chemistry or urine analysis parameters measured during or at the end of the study. No difference in tumor incidence was observed. The NOEL was 0.1 mg/kg bw administered three times weekly (Becci *et al.*, 1981).

Genotoxicity studies

Patulin was negative in mutagenicity tests with *Salmonella typhimurium* but was significantly positive in other *in vitro* assays. A summary of the results obtained in *in vitro* genotoxicity studies can be found in Wouters and Speijers (1996).

HAMSTER

Patulin induced chromosomal damage in bone marrow cells when Chinese hamsters were treated twice by gavage with 1, 10, and 20 mg patulin/kg bw (Korte, 1980). The rate of chromosomal aberration induced by the mycotoxin was significantly suppressed in animals given ethanol for nine weeks prior to exposure (Korte *et al.*, 1979).

The capability of patulin to induce chromosome damages *in vivo* was tested in the Chinese hamster by examination of bone marrow cells. Patulin caused chromosome aberrations when administered at the doses of 10 and 20 mg/kg bw (Matthiaschk and Korte, 1986; Roll *et al.*, 1990).

Reproductive toxicity studies

MOUSE

Pregnant mice received by gavage twice-daily doses of 2 mg/kg bw patulin on days 14–19 of pregnancy, giving a total dose of 24 mg/kg bw. Offspring of these mice showed no evidence of transplacental carcinogenicity at this dose, but during the neonatal period 11/52 females and 8/43 males born to the treated dams died. All showed similar signs of toxicity (Osswald *et al.*, 1978).

RAT

Patulin was administered to F_0 generation Sprague-Dawley rats at 0, 1, 1.5, 7.5, or 15 mg/kg bw by gavage five times/week before mating; the pregnant dams were treated daily at the same dosages during pregnancy. High mortality and insufficient progeny in groups receiving the two highest doses made continuing study impossible. Half of the dams were sacrificed on day 20 of gestation and used for a teratological evaluation. The remaining dams were allowed to produce an F_1 generation. Some control and treated (1.5 mg/kg bw) animals were maintained to produce an F_{2A} generation. The study continued for 20–23 weeks with F_{1A} generation animals given 0 or 1.5 mg/kg bw. The only lesion found at necroscopy that could be due to patulin administration was gaseous distension of the gastrointestinal tract, probably associated with the antibiotic activity of patulin on the intestinal flora. A decreased weight gain in males of F_0 generation was dose-related. An impairment in growth rates of F_{1A} and F_{2A} progeny of both sexes was statistically significant at the dose of 1.5 mg/kg bw. At the dose of 1.5 mg patulin/kg bw fetuses taken from treated dams on day 20 of pregnancy were noticeably smaller than controls and the difference was statistically significant for F_{2A} males (Dailey *et al.*, 1977b).

Rats were gavaged with 0, 0.1, 0.5, and 1.5 mg/kg of patulin three times/week. A dose-related decrease in growth and maturation was observed in the F_1 generation, but after six months of exposure little or no effect was observed (Gallo *et al.*, 1977).

Pregnant rats were treated daily by gavage from day 0 to day 19 of gestation with or without patulin. During the first seven days 3/7 treated animals died with gas-filled stomach; in the other four animals no significant resorption of fetuses was seen (Holmberg, 1979).

Groups of FDRL Wistar rats were given 0, 0.1, 0.5, or 1.5 mg patulin/kg bw per day by gavage three times/week for four weeks before mating; pregnant females were treated during gestation and lactation. The highest dose caused a significantly increased mortality rate as compared to control animals. There was no statistically significant difference among groups in the following reproductive parameters: mating success, litter size, fertility, gestation viability. No difference was observed in lactation indices and pup weight at birth, at four days and at weaning. Histopathological evaluation of grossly abnormal tissues of the F_0 generation did not show any effect associated with patulin treatment (Becci *et al.*, 1981).

In another study, effects of oral administration of patulin on reproductive performance of pregnant rats showed significant anti-implantational activity. Moreover, patulin administration showed a significant abortifacient activity (Choudhary *et al.*, 1992).

Teratogenicity and embryotoxicity studies

MOUSE

Twelve pregnant Swiss mice received 0 or 2 mg/kg bw per day of patulin by gavage for six days starting 14 days after mating. Mean survival time was significantly reduced in treated animals, while 2/12 control and 5/15 animals developed tumors. Of the offspring, 8/43 male and 11/52 female suckling mice died in the first six days of life, with hyperemia and bleeding localized in brain, lungs, and skin. When these early deaths were excluded from the calculations, patulin did not affect survival time in the animals exposed *in utero* (Osswald *et al.*, 1978).

Patulin was investigated in NMRI mice for embryotoxic and teratogenic activity. Animals received orally on day 12 and 13 of pregnancy 0 or 3.75 mg/kg bw of patulin. No effect was observed on the numbers of implantations, delivered fetuses, resorptions, dead fetuses, fetal weight or malformations of the skeleton and organs. Patulin was found to elevate the rate of cleft palates when administered intraperitoneally at a dose of 3.75 mg/kg bw (Matthiaschk and Korte, 1986; Roll *et al.*, 1990).

RAT

In a two-generation reproductive toxicity study, offspring of Sprague-Dawley female rats of the F_1 and F_2 generation exposed by gavage to 0 and 1.5 mg/kg bw/day of patulin were observed for teratogenic effects. Patulin caused an increase in resorption in the F_1 litters, but the same effect was not seen in the F_2 generation. The average weight of male fetuses of the F_2 litters was significantly lower than that of controls. No teratogenic effect was observed (Dailey *et al.*, 1977b).

Immunotoxicity studies

MOUSE

Swiss female mice receiving by gavage 10 mg/kg bw patulin for 1–4 days showed enhanced resistance to intraperitoneal challenge with viable *Candida albicans* at day 2. Immunoglobulins levels (IgA, IgM, and IgG) were markedly depressed (10–75%); the authors concluded that an increase in neutrophil count may be among the factors underlying the late increase in resistance to *C. albicans* after administration of patulin (Escoula *et al.*, 1988a).

Swiss female mice, receiving by gavage 10 mg patulin/kg bw from day 0 to day 4, were lymphopenic on days 5 and 10, but not on day 20. There was no effect on neutrophil count on day 5. A significant suppression of the chemiluminescence response of peritoneal leukocytes was observed. Spleen lymphocytes showed a decrease in absolute number, most pronounced for the B-cell population, whereas the T population showed a relative increase after patulin treatment. The mitogenic response to phytohemagglutinin, concanavaline A and, in particular, poke weed mitogen was also depressed by patulin. A parallel decrease in serum immunoglobulin levels was observed. The immunosupressive effect of patulin is reversible and probably due to interaction with cellular free SH groups, since the action of the mycotoxin can be partially prevented by the prior administration of cystein (Escoula *et al.*, 1988b).

Patulin was investigated on immunological responses of Balb/c mice. *In vivo* studies on immunity were performed in mice receiving *Bortedella pertussis* antigens and keyhole limpet hemocyanin (KLH). Patulin at dose levels of 2 and 4 mg/kg bw significantly reduced the delayed type hypersensitivity to *B. pertussis* antigen and did not reduce anti-KLH antibody production. Splenocytes were harvested in mice with or without antigen stimulation to assess mitogenic responses. Patulin generally increased splenocyte proliferation and strongly inhibited lymphocyte proliferation at higher concentration (ID_{50} from 0.02 to 0.24 µM depending on mitogens) (Paucoud *et al.*, 1990).

Patulin inhibited DNA synthesis in peripheral lymphocytes. These effects were reduced by cystein, which suggested a role of sulfydryl binding in patulin induced toxicity. In mice, an increased resistance to *Candida albicans* and decreased concentration of circulating immunoglobulins were observed (Sharma, 1993).

Female $B6C3F_1$ mice were exposed to patulin at dose levels of 0.08, 0.16, 0.32, 0.64, 1.28, and 2.56 mg/kg bw for 28 days by gavage. No effects were observed with the exposed animals on either body weight or body weight gain compared to the controls. No effect was observed on spleen, liver, lungs, thymus, or kidney weights. The only organ weight to show a change was absolute brain weight, which was increased 16% at the 0.64 mg/kg dose level. The erythrocyte count, hemoglobin, hematocrit, MCV, MCH, MCHC, platelets, and reticulocytes were unaffected. Leukocyte counts were decreased by 30% and 32% at the 1.28 mg/kg and 2.56 mg/kg dose levels, respectively. No effect was observed on the percentage of lymphocytes, neutrophils, or eosinophils in the leukocyte differential. However, when lymphocytes were evaluated as absolute numbers a 33% statistically significant reduction was seen in each of the two highest doses. Based on the leukocyte results, the NOEL for patulin was 0.64 mg/kg. However, based on the lack of effects on the functional assays, patulin was not immunosuppressive at dose levels of ≤2.56 mg/kg bw (Llewellyn *et al.*, 1998; NIH, 1997).

RABBIT

In rabbits, the administration of patulin reduced serum circulating immunoglobulins, blastogenesis of lymphocytes, and chemiluminescence of peritoneal leukocytes (Sharma, 1993).

Toxicological evaluation

In 1996, the Joint FAO/WHO Expert Committee on Food Additives (JECFA) established for patulin a provisional maximum tolerable daily intake (PMTDI) of 0.4 µg/kg bw (Wouters and Speijers, 1996). This value was based on a NOEL (no-observable-effect level) of 0.1 mg/kg bw per day from a study where patulin was administered three times per week (Becci *et al.*, 1981). The total weekly intake of 0.3 mg/kg bw was converted to a daily intake of 43 µg/kg bw per day by dividing it by 7. Using a safety factor of 100, a PMTDI of 0.43 µg/kg bw per day was established.

Assessment of exposure to patulin

Several papers containing data on patulin concentration in apple and fruit derivatives have been published (Table 18.6). Since apple juices are the major dietary source of patulin, these products seem the most important in estimating the actual exposure of consumers.

Surveys of apple juices for patulin

Up to now, patulin presence in apple derivatives has been subjected to statutory regulation only in some countries. However, the quality of fruit juices has been controlled in most industrialized countries by the setting of a guideline or a recommended maximum concentration, commonly set at 50 µg/L or 50 µg/kg.

In UK, surveys of patulin in apple juice have been carried out since 1992, when the problem of contamination above 50 mg/L was first identified (Food Standards Agency, 1999). The UK Committee on Toxicity of Chemicals in Food, Consumer Products and the Environment reviewed the available toxicity data on patulin in 1992 and recommended that the mycotoxin concentrations in food should be reduced to the lowest technologically achievable level. In 1993 a second survey of apple juice was performed to evaluate the effectiveness of industry actions to reduce patulin contamination of apple juices, and the control continued in the following years. As shown in Figure 18.5, the results of surveys indicate that there was a continued reduction in the number of juices containing patulin above the level of 50 µg/L.

Patulin concentration in apple juices has been evaluated in several countries. Figure 18.6 illustrates the results of apple juice analyses performed in the period 1998–2000; data are from China–Taiwan (Lai *et al.*, 2000), Italy (Beretta *et al.*, 2000), Sweden (Thuvander *et al.*, 2001), and the UK (Food Standards Agency, 1999).

In these countries, most apple juices presented a patulin concentration below the detection limit. Moreover, when detectable the toxin level in commercial products was normally below the suggested maximum limit of 50 µg/L.

Patulin content in various apple-based products

It has been shown that the presence of patulin in each apple product can be different, and a higher risk could be associated with some derivatives.

Table 18.6 Patulin content in apple and fruit products

Country	Product	Percentage of positive samples (number of samples)	Range of concentration (µg/L)	Percentage of sample with level >50 µg/L	Reference
Australia	Fruit juices and concentrates	57.4 (258)	5–1130	28.3	Burda, 1992
Brazil	Fruit juices	0 (125)	9–	0	De Sylos and Rodriguez-Amaya, 1999
China (Taiwan)	Apple baby-juices	0 (9)	–	0	Lai et al., 2000
	Juice drinks	0 (11)	–	0	
	Apple juices	16.9 (71)	15–49	0	
	Mixed juices	0 (14)	–	0	
Cuba	Preserved fruits	17.9 (230)	30–237	–	Sanchez Regueiro et al., 1991
Germany	Apple juices	–	0.02–0.3	0	Fritz et al., 1979
Finland	Apple juice concentrates	20.3 (64)	50–690	20.3	Lindroth and Niskanen, 1978
	Apple flavours	21.4 (14)	6–1770	–	
	Apple juices (home-made)	40.0 (20)	30–16 400	–	
Italy	Apple juices and fruit sauce	73.7 (19)	3.1–4.96	–	Plessi et al., 1998
Italy	Apple juices	53.8 (12)	0.14–28.2	0	Beretta et al., 2000
	Apple juice with pulp	77.8 (27)	1.2–1150	25.0	
	Baby foods	48.0 (165)	0.03–6.39	0	
Poland	Apple juices	56 (165)	traces–253	–	Kubacki, 1986
Poland	Apple juice concentrates	25.8 (31)	10–253	–	Lipowska et al., 1981
South Africa	Apple juice concentrates	33.3 (6)	5–45	0	Leggott and Shephard, 2001
	Apple whole fruit products	60.0 (10)	10	0	
	Infant fruit juices	45.5 (66)	5–20	0	
Sweden	Apple drinks	12.8 (34)	2.5–27	0	Josefsson and Andersson, 1976
Sweden	Apple juices	100 (215)	2–50	0	Thuvander et al., 2001
Turkey	Apple juice concentrates	100 (482)	7–376	43.5	Gokmen and Acar, 1998
Turkey	Apple juice concentrates	28.0 (300)	5–376	34.0	Gokmen and Acar, 2000
UK	Apple juices	25.0 (24)	15–171	2.5	Evans, 1999
UK	Apple juices	34.3 (862)	5–56	0.4	Mortimer et al., 1985
UK	Apple juices (cloudy)	31.3 (150)	10–490	3.5	Food Standards Agency, 1999
	Apple juices (clear)	57.5 (40)	10–118	1.3	
USA	Apple juices		traces–350	–	Brackett and Marth, 1979a

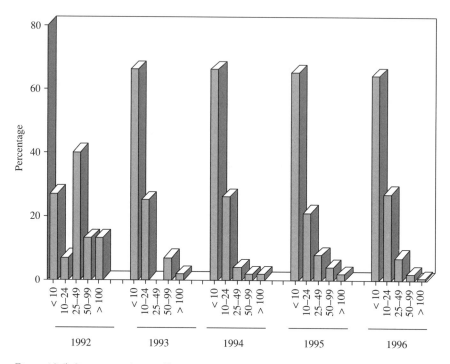

Figure 18.5 Summary of surveillance results for patulin content (μg/L) in apple juices analyzed in the UK, 1992–6 (Food Standards Agency, 1999).

Beretta *et al.* (2000) reported different ranges of patulin concentration in clear apple juices, apple juices with pulp, and baby foods (Figure 18.7).

The patulin level in clear apple juices ranged between values below the detection limit and 28.24 μg/L; in apple juices with pulp the patulin content was highly variable. Most samples (75%) had a patulin content ranging between undetectable values and 13.5 μg/L, but 25% of samples were above the Italian legal limit of 50 μg/L (Italian Ministry of Health, 1999) and two of them contained approximately 1 mg/L of the mycotoxin. The lower levels of patulin observed in clear juices could be explained by the clarification processes, which can remove high percentages of the mycotoxin (Acar *et al.*, 1998). In the case of baby foods, all samples were below the legal limit and the highest patulin content was 6.39 μg/L. The high controls performed on apples used in these products can explain the very low contamination level of baby foods.

Quality of apple-based products and relative contamination

Few data have been published on the role of apple quality control in reducing the patulin presence in apple-based products. Beretta *et al.* (2000) compared clear apple juices and baby foods from different agricultural strategies. No statistically significant difference was observed between the baby foods (strained) containing

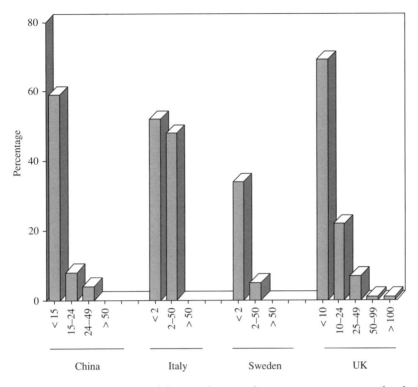

Figure 18.6 Patulin content (µg/L) in apple juices from various countries analyzed in 1998–2000. Data from Beretta *et al.*, 2000; Food Standards Agency, 1999; Lai *et al.*, 2000; Thuvander *et al.*, 2001.

apples from conventional Good Agricultural Practices (GAP) agriculture (2.25 µg/L ± 2.48, m ± SD) and from agriculture based on integrated pest management (1.70 µg/L ± 2.01, m ± SD). Clear apple juices from conventional agriculture presented patulin levels similar to those found in baby foods, while in organic products the amount of the mycotoxin was more variable. Although the patulin levels were always below the legal limit, a statistically significant difference was found between the juices containing apple from conventional and organic agriculture (1.01 µg/L ± 1.13 versus 7.69 µg/L ± 8.00, m ± SD).

Moreover, samples of juice with pulp having patulin level close to 1 mg/kg were from "discount" markets.

MAFF UK (Food Standards Agency, 1999) showed that patulin contamination above the advisory level is more likely to occur in directly produced juices made by small or farm producers. The cost and the time needed for analysis of patulin in apple juices effectively prevent small producers from testing each batch as should be recommended. Lindroth and Niskanen (1978) showed that the frequency of patulin in commercial and home-made juices was 20 and 40%, respectively.

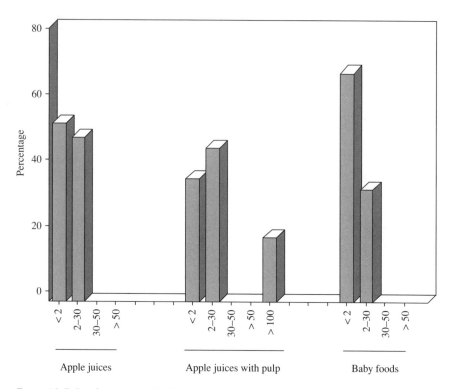

Figure 18.7 Patulin content (µg/L) in apple juices and baby foods analyzed in Italy in 1999 (Beretta *et al.*, 2000).

These data indicate the important role of quality control in reducing the patulin-associated risks for consumers: efforts must continually be made to encourage all manufacturers to keep patulin concentrations in their products to a minimum.

Assessment of exposure to patulin versus PMTDI

Considering that the tolerated patulin level is commonly set at 50 µg/L, the PMTDI would be reached by consuming about 500 ml of juice containing the highest tolerated quantity of patulin. This quantity is much higher than the usual consumption in some European countries; for example, fruit juice intake in Italy has been established at 7.5 g/day by the Ministry of Health, so that the risk for patulin intake seems limited to a very small percentage of the Italian population. A different situation was described in countries where the consumption of apple juice is high; Figure 18.8 shows the mean and 90th percentile apple juice intakes for the USA (FDA, 2001).

The juice intake data were taken from the 1994–1996 United States Department of Agriculture Nationwide Food Consumption Survey, which encompasses

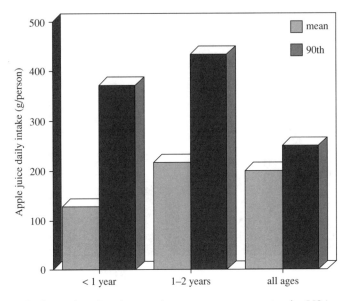

Figure 18.8 Daily intake of apple juice by various age groups in the USA: mean and 90th percentile (FDA, 2001).

the intake as pure juice as well as apple juice as an ingredient in other foods. Patulin occurrence data were taken from 2977 samples analyzed privately from US industries. To estimate exposure to dietary patulin, FDA used a probabilistic modeling method known as "Monte Carlo simulation" (Rubinstein, 1981). FDA estimated the exposure to patulin for apple juice drinkers of "all ages" and of two groups among small children: children less than one year old, and children 1–2 years old.

Figure 18.9 shows the estimated exposures to patulin (µg/kg bw per day) using the following body weights: 8 kg for children less than one year old, 12 kg for children 1–2 years old, and 64 kg for all age groups.

The estimated patulin exposure, calculated with data from all analyzed samples (Figure 18.9, left), likely exaggerates actual patulin intake since many commercial lots included in the study were rejected by the importers for excessive patulin content. For this reason a second estimation was made considering only those samples below the limit of 50 µg/L (Figure 18.9, right). The data illustrated in Figure 18.9 indicate that even though industries do not implement controls for patulin (all apple juices reaching the USA market), the estimated 90th percentile patulin exposure for apple juice consumers of all ages would be below the PMTDI of 0.43 µg/kg bw per day. However, the exposure for children under one year of age would be nearly three times the PMTDI and that for children 1–2 years old would be three times the PMTDI.

If the patulin level is controlled, all apple juices above the accepted limit would be rejected and the estimated 90th percentile patulin exposure for all the

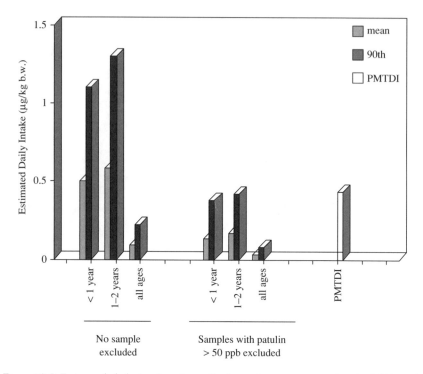

Figure 18.9 Estimated daily intake of patulin by various age groups in the USA with respect to the PMTDI: mean and 90th percentile (FDA, 2001).

age groups considered would not exceed the PMTDI of 0.43 µg/kg bw per day. The exposure for consumers of all ages would be five-fold less than the PMTDI, providing a 500-fold safety factor for lifetime consumption. The exposure would be only slightly below the PMTDI for children under one year of age, and essentially at the PMTDI for 1–2 years old children.

Conclusion

FDA concluded its document with the sentence: "The information presented in this paper supports a 50 µg/kg action level for patulin in apple juices, apple juice concentrates, and apple juice products based on the level found or calculated to be found in single strength apple juice or in the single strength apple juice component of the product" (FDA, 2001).

On the other hand, Codex Alimentarius (2001) reported that "Various recent exposure assessments indicate indeed that, although the average lifetime exposure is below the PMTDI, the exposure of children to patulin through the consumption of apple juices is in the range of, or even exceeds the PMTDI for a considerable period during childhood. Consequently, there is a need to further reduce patulin exposure and to achieve even lower contamination levels, in particular with regard to the protection of children."

The European Community is of the opinion that the exposure of children to patulin needs closer examination and has initiated a study in the framework of the scientific cooperation between Member States to evaluate the dietary intake of patulin of high-risk groups (mainly infants and children). In Italy, because of this uncertainty, the AIIPA (Italian Association of Food Industries) asked the Italian food industries to reduce the patulin contamination for baby foods below 25 μg/kg (AIIPA, 1996).

The author of this review is of the opinion that, pending an internationally accepted legal limit, two tolerated values could be considered for patulin: a level of 50 μg/L for apple juices, and a lower limit for baby foods

References

Abdelhamid, A.M. and Dorra, T.M. (1990) Study on effects of feeding laying hens on separate mycotoxins (aflatoxins, patulin or citrinin)-containing diets on the egg quality and tissue constituents, *Archives of Animal Nutrition*, **40**: 305–316.

Abramson, D., Thorsteinson, T., and Forest, D. (1989) Chromatography of mycotoxins on precoated reverse-phase thin-layer plates, *Archives of Environmental Contamination & Toxicology*, **18**: 327–330.

Abrunhosa, L., Paterson, R.R.M., Kozakiewicz, Z., Lima, N., and Venancio, A. (2001) Mycotoxin production from fungi isolated from grapes, *Letters in Applied Microbiology*, **32**: 240–242.

Acar, J., Gokmen, V., and Taydas, E.E. (1998) The effects of processing technology on the patulin content of juice during commercial apple juice concentrate production, *Zeitschrift fur Lebensmittel-Undersuchung und-Forschung A, Food Research and Technology*, **207**: 328–331.

Adam, R. (1979) Untersuchungen uber den Einfluss von Hydrogensulfitionen auf das Schimmelpilzgift Patulin. 2. Mitteilung: Versuche mit Apfelsaften [Influence of hydrogen sulphite on the mould toxin patulin. 2. Studies using apple juice], *Deutsche Lebensmittel-Rundschau*, **76**: 123–125.

Adam, R. and Koller, W.-D. (1980) Untersuchungen uber den Einfluss von Hydro-gensulfitionen auf das Schimmelpilzgift Patulin. 1. Versuche in wassrigen Losungen [Investigation on the effect of hydrogen sulphite ions on the mould toxin patulin. 1. Studies in acqueous solutions], *Deutsche Lebensmittel-Rundschau*, **75**: 254–256.

Adams, K.B., Wu, M.T., and Salunkhe, D.K. (1976) Effects of subatmospheric pressures on the growth and patulin production of *Penicillium expansum* and *Penicillium patulum*, *Lebensmittel-Wissenschaft & Technologie*, **9**: 153–155.

AIIPA (Italian Association of Food Industries) (1996) *Micotossine – Aggiornamento sui lavori della Commissione CE [Mycotoxins: about the EC recommendations]*, Circular no. 13233, 4 March.

Akerstrand, K., Molander, A., Andersson, A., and Nilsson, G. (1976) Mogel och patulin i djupfrysta blabar [Moulds and patulin in deep-frozen blueberries], *Var Foda*, **28**: 197–200.

Alp, M., Kocababli, N., Kahraman, R., and Yetim, M. (1997) Turkiye'de uretilen yemlik misir orneklerinin mantar ve mikotoksinler yonunden degerlendirilmesi [Evaluation of fungal and mycotoxin contamination in corn feed produced in Turkey], *Pendik Veteriner Mikrobiyoloji Dergisi*, **28**: 163–269.

Altmayer, B., Eichhorn, K.W., and Plapp, R. (1982) Untersuchungen über den Patulingehalt von Traubenmosten und Wein [Patulin content in grape juices and wine], *Zeitschrift fur Lebensmittel-Untersuchung und-Forschung*, **175**: 172–174.

Altmayer, B., Eichhorn, K.W., and Schwenk, S. (1985) Die Bedeutung mykotoxinbildener Pilzarten für den Weinbau [The importance of mycotoxin-producing fungus species for viticulture], *Nachrichtenblatt des Deutschen Pflanzenschutzdienstes*, **37**: 117–122.

Arafat, W. and Musa, M.N. (1995) Patulin-induced inhibition of protein synthesis in hepatoma tissue culture, *Research Communications in Molecular Pathology and Pharmacology*, **87**: 177–186.

Arafat, W., Kern, D., and Dirheimer, G. (1985) Inhibition of aminoacyl-tRNA synthetases by the mycotoxin patulin, *Chemical–Biological Interactions*, **56**: 333–349.

Artik, N., Cemeroglu, B., Aydar, G., and Saglam, N. (1995) Elma suyu konsantresinde aktif komur kullanimi uzerinde arastirmalar. II. Aktif komur kullanilarak elma suyu konsantresinde patulin miktarini azaltma olanaklari [Use of activated carbon for patulin control in apple juice concentrate], *Turkish Journal of Agriculture and Forestry*, **19**: 259–265.

Ashoor, S.H. and Chu, F.S. (1973a) Inhibition of alcohol and lactic dehydrogenase by patulin and penicillic acid *in vitro*, *Food and Cosmetic Toxicology*, **11**: 617–624.

Ashoor, S.H. and Chu, F.S. (1973b) Inhibition muscle aldolase by penicillic acid and patulin *in vitro*, *Food and Cosmetic Toxicology*, **11**: 995–1000.

Beaver, R.W. (1986) Gas chromatography in mycotoxin analysis. In: *Modern Methods in the Analysis and Structural Elucidation of Mycotoxins*, pp. 265–292. Orlando, FL: Academic Press.

Becci, P.J., Hess, F.G., Johnson, W.D., Gallo, M.A., Babish, J.G., Dailey, R.E., and Parent, R.A. (1981) Long-term carcinogenicity and toxicity studies of patulin in the rat, *Journal of Applied Toxicology*, **1**: 256–261.

Benkhemmar, O., Fremy, J.M., Lahlou, H., Bompeix, G., El-Mniai, H., and Boubekri, C. (1993) Production de la patuline par *Penicillium expansum* dans le jus de raisin de table [Production of patulin by *Penicillium expansum* in table grape juice], *Sciences des Aliments*, **13**: 149–154.

Beretta, B., Gaiaschi, A., Galli, C.L., and Restani, P. (2000) Patulin in apple-based foods: occurrence and safety evaluation, *Food Additives and Contaminants*, **17**: 399–406.

Bitany, Z., Glavits, R., and Sellvey, G. (1979) Takarmanyozasi kiserletek ochratoxin-A, patulin, T-2 toxin es butenolid hatasanak tanulmanyozasara broilercsirkeken [Feeding experiments with broiler chickens given ochratoxin A, patulin, T-2 toxin and butenolid], *Magyar Allatorvosok Lapja*, **34**: 417–422.

Bourdiol, D., Escoula, L., and Salvayre, R. (1990) Effect of patulin on microbicidal activity of mouse peritoneal macrophages, *Food and Chemical Toxicology*, **28**: 29–33.

Brackett, R.E. and Marth, E.H. (1979a) Patulin in apple juice from roadside stands in Wisconsin, USA, *Journal of Food Protection*, **42**: 862–863.

Brackett, R.E. and Marth, E.H. (1979b) Ascorbic acid and ascorbate cause disappearance of patulin from buffer solutions and apple juice, *Journal of Food Protection*, **42**: 864–866.

Brackett, R.E. and Marth, E.H. (1979c) Stability of patulin at pH 6.0–8.0 and 25 deg C, *Lebensmittel-Undersuchung und-Forschung*, **169**: 92–94.

Braunberg, R.C., Gantt, O.O., and Friedman, L. (1982) Toxicological evaluation of compounds found in food using rat renal explants, *Food and Chemical Toxicology*, **20**: 541–546.

Brause, A.R., Trucksess, M.W., Thomas, F.S., and Page, S.W. (1996) Determination of patulin in apple juice by liquid chromatography: a collaborative study, *Journal of AOAC International*, **79**: 451–455.

Buchanan, J.R., Sommer, N.F., Fortlage, R.J., Maxie, E.C., Mitchell, F.G., and Hsieh, D.P.H. (1974) Patulin from *Penicillium expansum* in stone fruits and pears, *Journal of the American Society for Horticultural Science*, **99**: 262–265.

Buchanan, R.L., Harry, M.A., and Gealt, M.A. (1983) Caffein inhibition of sterigmatocystin, citrinin, and patulin production, *Journal of Food Science*, **48**: 1226–1228.

Bullerman, L.B. (1976) Examination of Swiss cheese for incidence of mycotoxin producing molds, *Journal of Food Science*, **41**: 26–28.

Bullerman, L.B. (1980) Incidence of mycotoxin molds in domestic and imported cheeses, *Journal of Food Safety*, **2**: 47–58.

Bullerman, L.B. (1984) Effects of potassium sorbate on growth and patulin production by *Penicillium patulum* and *Penicillium roqueforti*, *Journal of Food Protection*, **47**: 312–315, 320.

Bullerman, L.B. and Hartung, T.E. (1973) Mycotoxin-producing potential of molds isolated from flour and bread, *Cereal Science Today*, **18**: 346–347.

Bullerman, L.B. and Hartung, T.E. (1975) Effect of low level gamma irradiation on growth and patulin production by *Penicillium patulum*, *Journal of Food Science*, **40**: 195–196.

Burda, K. (1992) Incidence of patulin in apple, pear, and mixed fruit products marketed in New South Wales, *Journal of Food Protection*, **55**: 796–798.

Burghardt, R.C., Barhoumi, R., Lewis, E.H., Bailey, R.H., Pyle, K.H., Clement, B.A., and Phillips, T.D. (1992) Patulin-induced cellular toxicity: a vital fluorescence study, *Toxicology and Applied Pharmacology*, **112**: 235–244.

Burroughs, L.F. (1977) Stability of patulin to sulphur dioxide and yeast fermentation, *Journal of the Association of Official Analytical Chemists*, **60**: 100–103.

Burroughs, L.F. and Whiteley, L.A. (1976) *Stability of Patulin to Sulphur Dioxide and Yeast Fermentation*, Long Aston Research Station, Report 1975, Bristol University, p. 161.

Camguilhem, R., Henry, M., and Escoula, L. (1975) An intoxication experiment on sheep by a semi-purified extract of *Byssochlamys nivea* (Patulin). I. Symptoms and lesions. *Twentieth World Veterinary Congress: Summaries*, Thessaloniki, Greece, Vol. 1: pp. 532–533.

Camguilhem, R., Escoula, L., and Henry, M. (1976) Toxines de *Byssochlamys nivea* Westling. I. Etude preliminaire de la toxicité chez le mouton [*Byssochlamys nivea* toxins. I. Preliminary study of the toxicity for sheep], *Annales de Recherches Veterinaires*, **7**: 177–183.

Cardeilhac, P.T., Nair, K.P.C., and Colwell, W.M. (1972) Tracheal organ cultures for the bioassays of nanogram quantities of mycotoxins, *Journal of the Association of the Official Analytical Chemists*, **55**: 1120–1121.

Codex Alimentarius (2001) Draft maximum level for patulin in apple juice and apple juice ingredients in other beverages. ALINORM 01/12 – Appendix X. European Community Comments of the Codex Alimentarius Commission, 24th Session, 2–7 July 2001, Geneva, Switzerland. http://europa.eu.int/comm/food/fs/ifsi/europositions/cac/cac_item10b_en.html

Choudhary, D.N., Sahay, G.R., and Singh, J.N. (1992) Effect of some mycotoxins on reproduction in pregnant albino rats, *Journal of Food Science and Technology – Mysore*, **29**: 264–265.

Cole, R.J. (1986) Gas chromatographic–mass spectrometric analysis of mycotoxins. In: *Modern Methods in the Analysis and Structural Elucidation of Mycotoxins*, pp. 335–351. Orlando, FL: Academic Press.

Dailey, R.E., Blaschka, A.M., and Brouwer, E.A. (1977a) Absorption, distribution and excretion of ^{14}C-patulin by rats, *Journal of Toxicology and Environmental Health*, **3**: 479–489.

Dailey, R.E., Brouwer, E., Blaschka, A.M., Reynaldo, E.F., Green, S., Monlux, W.S., and Ruggles, D.I. (1977b) Intermediate-duration toxicity study of patulin in rats, *Journal of Toxicology and Environmental Health*, **2**: 713–725.

Damoglou, A.P. and Campbell, D.S. (1986) The effect of pH on the production of patulin in apple juice, *Letters in Applied Microbiology*, **2**: 9–11.

Davis, N.D. and Diener, U.-L. (1987) Mycotoxins. In: *Food and Beverage Mycology* (ed. L.R. Beuchat), pp. 517–570. New York: Van Nostrand Reinhold.

Demirer, M.A., Dincer, B., Kaymaz, S., Alperden, I., Yalcin, S., and Ozer, E. (1989) Bazi gida maddelerinde mycoflora ve mycotoxin arastirmalari [Microflora and mycotoxins in some foodstuffs], *Veteriner Fakultesi Dersigi*, **36**: 85–107.

De Sylos, C.M. and Rodriguez-Amaya, D.B. (1999) Incidence of patulin in fruits and fruit juices marketed in Campinas, Brazil, *Food Additives and Contaminants*, **16**: 71–74.

Devaraj, H. and Devaraj, N. (1987) Rat intestinal lipid changes in patulin toxicity, *Indian Journal of Experimental Biology*, **25**: 637–638.

Devaraj, H., Shanmugasundaram, K.R., and Shanmugasundaram, E.R.B. (1982a) Neurotoxic effect of patulin, *Indian Journal of Experimental Biology*, **20**: 230–231.

Devaraj, H., Shanmugasundaram, K.R., and Shanmugasundaram, E.R.B. (1982b) Effect of patulin on intestinal amino acid uptake, *Current Science (Bangalore)*, **51**: 602–604.

Devaraj, H., Shanmugasundaram, K.R., and Shanmugasundaram, E.R.B. (1986a) Role of patulin as a diabetogenic lactone, *Indian Journal of Experimental Biology*, **24**: 458–459.

Devaraj, H., Suseela, R.E., and Devaraj, N. (1986b) Patulin toxicosis in chicks, *Current Science, India*, **55**: 998–999.

Doores, S. (1983) The microbiology of apples and apple products, *CRC Critical Reviews in Food Science and Nutrition*, **19**: 133–149.

Dorner, J.W. (1996) Mycotoxins in food: methods of analysis. In: *Handbook of Food Analysis. Volume 2: Residue and Other Food Component Analysis*, pp. 1089–1146. New York: Marcel Dekker.

Doyle, M.P., Applebaum, R.S., Brackett, R.E., and Marth, E.H. (1982) Physical, chemical and biological degradation of mycotoxins in foods and agricultural commodities, *Journal of Food Protection*, **45**: 964–971.

Escoula, L., Bourdiol, D., Linas, M.D., Recco, P., and Seguela, J.P. (1988a) Enhancing resistance and modulation of humoral immune response to experimental *Candida albicans* infection by patulin, *Mycopathologia*, **103**: 153–156.

Escoula, L., More, J., and Baradat, C. (1977) The toxins of *Byssochlamys nivea* Westling. I. Acute toxicity of patulin in adult rats and mice, *Annales de Recherches Veterinaires*, **8**: 41–49.

Escoula, L., Thomsen, M., Bourdiol, D., Pipy, B., Peuriere, S., and Roubinet, F. (1988b) Patulin immunotoxicology: effect on phagocyte activation and the cellular and humoral immune system of mice and rabbits, *International Journal of Immunopharmacology*, **10**: 983–989.

Evans, C. (1999) 1998 survey of apple juice for patulin, *Food Surveillance Information Sheet*, HMSO Publications Centre, London, no. 173, 1–50.

FDA (2001) Patulin in apple juice, apple juice concentrates and apple juice products. *Compliance Policy Guidance for FDA Staff: Apple Juice, Apple Juice Concentrates, and Apple Juice Products – Adulteration with Patulin*. US Food and Drug Administration, Center for Food Safety and Applied Nutrition, Office of Plant and Diary Foods and Beverages, September. http://www.cfsan.fda.gov

Food Standards Agency (1999) MAFF-UK – 1998 Survey of apple juice for patulin. No. 173, April. http://archive.food.gov.uk

Fliege, R. and Metzler, M. (1999) The mycotoxin patulin induces intra- and intermolecular protein crosslinks *in vitro* involving cysteine, lysine and histidine side chains, alfa-amino groups, *Chemico-Biological Interactions*, **123**: 85–103.

Frank, H.K. (1977) Occurrence of patulin in fruit and vegetables, *Annales de la Nutrition et de l'Alimentation*, **31**: 459–465.

Frank, H.K., Orth, R., and Figge, A. (1977) Patulin in Lebensmitteln pflanzlicher Herkunft. 2. Verschiedene Obstarten, Gemuse und daraus negergestellte Produkte [Patulin in foods of vegetable origin. 2. Several kinds of fruit and vegetable and fruit and vegetable products], *Zeitschrift fur Lebensmittel-Undersuchung und-Forschung*, **163**: 111–114.

Frayssinet, C. (1988) La patuline: un cancerogene dans les tonneaux normands [Patulin: a carcinogen in Normandy barrels], *Gazette Medicale de France*, **95**: 82–83.

Fritz, W., Buthig, C., and Engst, R. (1979) Zur analytik und lebensmittelhygienisch–toxikologischen Bedeutung von Patulin in Obst und Obstprodukten [On the determination and hygienic–toxicologic significance of patulin in fruits and fruit products], *Nahrung*, **23**: 159–167.

Fuks-Holmberg, D. (1980) The influence of patulin on rat fetus and rat and human placenta, *Toxicon*, **18**: 437–442.

Gallo, M.A., Bailey, D.E., Babish, J.G., Taylor, J.M., and Dailey, R.E. (1977) Toxicity and reproduction studies with patulin in the rat, *Toxicology and Applied Pharmacology*, **41**: 139.

Garza, H.C., Swanson, B.G., and Branen, A.L. (1977) Toxicological study of patulin in monkeys, *Journal of Food Science*, **42**: 1229–1231, 1235.

Gaucher, G.M. (1979) Mycotoxins – their biosynthesis in fungi: patulin and related carcinogenic lactones, *Journal of Food Protection*, **42**: 810–814.

Girisham, S. and Reddy, S.M. (1986) Efficacy of volatile compounds and food preservatives in the control of growth and patulin production by *Aspergillus terreus*. National Academy of Sciences, India, *Sciences Letters*, **9**: 373–374.

Gokmen, V. and Acar, J. (1996) Rapid reversed-phase liquid chromatographic determination of patulin in apple juice, *Journal of Chromatography A*, **730**: 53–58.

Gokmen, V. and Acar, J. (1998) Incidence of patulin in apple juice concentrates produced in Turkey, *Journal of Chromatography A*, **815**: 99–102.

Gokmen, V. and Acar, J. (2000) Long-term survey of patulin in apple juice concentrates produced in Turkey, *Food Additives and Contaminants*, **17**: 933–936.

Gokmen, V., Artik, N., Acar, J., Kahraman, N., and Poyrazoglu, E. (2001) Effects of various clarification treatments on patulin, phenolic compound and organic acid composition of apple juice, *European Food Research and Technology*, **213**: 194–199.

Gopalakrishnan, V.K. and Sakthisekaran, D. (1991) Effect of patulin on albumin fraction of plasma proteins studied in rats, *Biochemistry International*, **25**: 461–475.

Hasan, H.A.H. (2000) Patulin and aflatoxin in brown rot lesion of apple fruits and their regulation, *World Journal of Microbiology and Biotechnology*, **16**: 607–612.

Hayes, A.W. (1977) Effect of patulin on Krebs cycle intermediate-stimulated oxygen consumption, *Toxicology and Applied Pharmacology*, **41**: 165.

Hayes, A.W., Phillips, T.D., and Williams, W.L. (1978) Acute toxicity of patulin, *Toxicology and Applied Pharmacology*, **45**: 275–276.

Holmberg, D. (1979) The effect of patulin on placenta, fetus and yolk sac enzymes, *Toxicon*, **17**: 72.

Huebner, H.J., Mayura, K., Pallaroni, L., Ake, C.L., Lemke, S.L., Herrera, P., and Phillips, T.D. (2000) Development and characterization of a carbon-based composite material for reducing patulin levels in apple juice, *Journal of Food Protection*, **63**: 106–110.

IARC (International Agency for Research on Cancer) (1986) Some naturally occurring and synthetic food components, furocumarins and ultraviolet radiation, *Monographs on the Evaluation of Carcinogenic Risk of Chemicals to Man*, vol. 40, pp. 83–98.

Iijima, H., Noguchi, H., Ebizuka, Y., Sankawa, U., and Seto, H. (1983) The biosynthesis of patulin: the mechanism of oxidative aromatic ring cleavage and loss of side chain protons from aromatic intermediates, *Chemical and Pharmaceutical Bulletin*, **31**: 362–365.

Ikins, W.G. (1991) Modern methods of analysing mycotoxins in foods. In: *Instrumental Methods for Quality Assurance in Foods*, pp. 117–154. New York: Marcel Dekker.

Italian Ministry of Health (1999) *Direttiva in materia di controllo ufficiale sui prodotti alimentari: valori massimi ammissibili di micotossine nelle derrate alimentari di origine nazionale, comunitaria e Paesi terzi [Maximal acceptable mycotoxin concentrations in food of national and international origin]*. Circular dated 9 June.

Jonsyn, F. (1990) Using simple methods to derive qualitative and semiquantitative results of mycotoxins. A guide for scientists in developing countries, *Monatsschrift für Brauwissenschaft*, **43**: 250–253.

Josefsson, E. and Andersson, A. (1976) Patulin i appledrycker [Patulin in apple drinks], *Var Foda*, **28**: 189–196.

Kangsadalampai, K., Salunkhe, D.K., and Sharma, R.P. (1981) Patulin and rubratoxin B: interactions of toxic and hepatic effects and mutagenic potential, *Journal of Food Protection*, **44**: 39–42.

Korte, A. (1980) Chromosomal analysis in bone-marrow cells of Chinese hamsters after treatment with mycotoxins, *Mutation Research*, **78**: 41–49.

Korte, A., Slacik-Erben, R., and Obe, G. (1979) The influence of ethanol treatment on cytogenetic effects in bone marrow cells of Chinese hamsters by cyclophosphamide, aflatoxin B1 and patulin, *Toxicology*, **12**: 53–61.

Kubacki, S.J. (1986) The analysis and occurrence of patulin in apple juice. In: *Mycotoxins and Phycotoxins*. Sixth International IUPAC Symposium On Mycotoxins and Phycotoxins, Pretoria, Republic of South Africa, 22–25 July 1985, pp. 293–304. Amsterdam: Elsevier Science Publishers.

Lai, C-L., Fuh, Y-M., and Shih, D.Y-C. (2000) Detection of mycotoxin patulin in apple juice, *Journal of Food and Drug Analysis*, **8**: 85–96.

Larsen, T.O., Frisvad, J.C., Ravn, G., and Skaaning, T. (1998) Mycotoxin production by *Penicillium expansum* on blackcurrant and cherry juice, *Food Additives and Contaminants*, **15**: 671–675.

Leggott, N.L. and Shephard, G.S. (2001) Patulin in South African commercial apple products, *Food Control*, **12**: 73–76.

Leggott, N.L., Shepard, G.S., Stockenstrom, S., Staal, E., and van Schalkwyk, D.J. (2001) The reduction of patulin in apple juice by three different types of activated carbon, *Food Additives and Contaminants*, **18**: 825–829.

Lennox, J.E. and McElroy, L.J. (1984) Inhibition of growth and patulin synthesis in *Penicillium expansum* by potassium sorbate and sodium propionate in culture, *Applied and Environmental Microbiology*, **48**: 1031–1033.

Lenz, P., Sussmuth, R., and Seibel, E. (1986) Development of sensitive bacterial tests, exemplified by two mycotoxins, *Toxicology*, **40**: 199–205.

Lin, L.M., Zhang, J., Sui, K., and Sung, W.B. (1993) Simultaneous thin layer chromatographic determination of zearalenone and patulin in maize, *Journal of Planar Chromatography–Modern TLC*, **6**: 274–277.

Lindroth, S. and Niskanen, A. (1978) Comparison of potential patulin hazard in home made and commercial apple products, *Journal of Food Science*, **43**: 446–448.

Lipowska, T., Goszcz, H., and Kubacki, S.J. (1981) Wystepowanie patuliny w zageszczonych sokach jablkowych [Occurrence of patulin in concentrated apple juices], *Prace Instytutow i Laboratoriow Badawczych Przemyslu Spozywczego*, **34**: 111–117.

Liu, Y. (1990) Method for detecting special microbial toxins in food, *Journal of Toxicology, Toxin Reviews*, **9**: 121.

Llewellyn, G.C., McCay, J.A., Brown, R.D., Musgrove, D.L., Butterworth, L.F., Munson, A.E., and White, K.L. Jr (1998) Immunological evaluation of the mycotoxin patulin in female B6C3F1 mice, *Food and Chemical Toxicology*, **36**: 1107–1115.

Llovera, M., Viladrich, R., Torres, M., and Canela, R. (1999) Analysis of underivatized patulin by GC-MS technique, *Journal of Food Protection*, **62**: 202–205.

Lompe, A. and von Milczewski, K.-E. (1979) Ein Zellkulturfest fur den Nachweis von Mycotoxinen. I. Untersuchungen an Reinsubstanzen [A cell-culture assay for the detection of mycotoxins. I. Investigations with pure toxins], *Lebensmittel-Untersuchung und-Forschung*, **169**: 249–254.

Lopez-Diaz, T.M. and Flannigan, B. (1997) Production of patulin and cytochalasin E by 4 strains of *Aspergillus clavatus* during malting of barley and wheat, *International Journal of Food Microbiology*, **35**: 129–136.

Lotzsch, R. and Trapper, D. (1978) Bildung von Aflatoxinen und Patulin in Abhangigkeit von der Wasseraktivitat (aw-Wert) [Aflatoxin and patulin production as a function of water activity (aw value)], *Fleischwirtschaft*, **58**: 2001, 2007.

Lovett, J. (1972) Patulin toxicosis in poultry, *Poultry Science* **51**: 2097–2098.

Lovett, J., Thompson, R.G. Jr, and Boutin, B.K. (1975) Trimming as a means of removing patulin from fungus-rotted apples, *Journal of the Association of Official Analytical Chemists*, **58**: 909–911.

McElroy, L.J. and Weiss, C.M. (1993) The production of polyclonal antibodies against the mycotoxin derivative patulin hemiglutarate, *Canadian Journal of Microbiology*, **39**: 861–863.

Machinski, M. Jr and Midio, A.F. (1998) Validation of a simple and sensitive HPLC method for patulin in apple juice, *Alimentaria*, **298**: 23–25.

McKenzie, K.S., Sarr, A.B., Mayura, K., Bailey, R.H., Miller, D.R., Rogers, T.D., Norred, W.P., Voss, K.A., Plattner, R.D., Kubena, L.F., and Phillips, T.D. (1997) Oxidative degradation and detoxification of mycotoxins using a novel source of ozone, *Food and Chemical Toxicology*, **35**: 807–820.

McKinley, E.R. and Carlton, W.W. (1980a) Patulin mycotoxicosis in Swiss ICR mice, *Food and Cosmetic Toxicology*, **18**: 181–187.

McKinley, E.R. and Carlton, W.W. (1980b) Patulin mycotoxicosis in the Syrian hamster, *Food and Cosmetic Toxicology*, **18**: 173–179.

McKinley, E.R., Carlton, W.W., and Boon, G.D. (1982) Patulin mycotoxicosis in the rat: toxicology, pathology and clinical pathology, *Food and Chemical Toxicology*, **20**: 289–300.

Madiyalakan, R. and Shanmugasundaram, E.R. (1978) Effect of patulin on mouse liver glycogen phosphorylase, *Indian Journal of Experimental Biology*, **16**: 1084–1085.

Matthiaschk, G. and Korte, A. (1986) Studies on the embriotoxicity and mutagenicity of mycotoxins, *Mycotoxin Research*, **2**: 89–97.

Mehl, M., Starke, R., Jacobi, H.D., Schleinitz, K.D., and Wasicki, P. (1986) Immuno-logischer Nachweis des Mycotoxins Patulin [Immunological detection of the mycotoxin patulin], *Pharmazie*, **41**: 147–148.

Miguel, J.A. and de Andres, V. (1987) Metodo rapido de cromatografia en capa fina de alta eficacia para la determinacion de patulina y acido penicilico en granos [A rapid method for patulin and penicillic acid determination in grains by high performance thin layer chromatography], *Investigacion Agraria Produccion y Proteccion Vegetales*, **2**: 225–235.

Mintzlaff, H.-J., Ciegler, A., and Leistner, L. (1972a) Pathogene und toxinogene Hefen und Schimmelpilze in Fleisch und Fleischwaren [Pathogenic and toxigenic yeasts and mould fungi in meat and meat products], *Archiv fur Lebensmittelhygiene*, **23**: 287–291.

Mintzlaff, H.-J., Ciegler, A., and Leistner, L. (1972b) Potential mycotoxin problems in mould-fermented sausage, *Zeitschrift fur Lebensmittel-Untersuchung und-Forschung*, **150**: 133–137.

Miura, S., Hasumi, K., and Endo, A. (1993) Inhibition of protein phenylation by patulin, *FEBS Letters*, **318**: 88–90.

Mortimer, D.N., Parker, I., Shepherd, M.J., and Gilbert, J. (1985) A limited survey of retail apple and grape juices for the mycotoxin patulin, *Food Additives and Contaminants*, **2**: 165–170.

Moule, Y. and Hatey, F. (1977) Mechanism of the *in vitro* inhibition of transcription by patulin, a mycotoxin from *Byssochlamys nivea*, *FEBS Letters*, **74**: 121–125.

Murphy, G. and Lynen, F. (1975) Patulin biosynthesis: the metabolism of m-hydroxybenzyl alcohol and m-hydroxybenzaldehyde by particulate preparations from *Penicillium patulum*, *European Journal of Biochemistry*, **58**: 467–475.

Mutti, P. and Quintavalla, S. (1989) Presenza e stabilità della patulina in derivati della frutta [Occurrence and stability of patulin in fruit products], *Industria delle Conserve*, **64**: 251–254.

Nesheim, S. and Trucksess, M.K. (1986) Thin-layer chromatography/high performance thin-layer chromatography as a tool for mycotoxin determination. In: *Modern Methods in the Analysis and Structural Elucidation of Mycotoxins*, pp. 239–264. Orlando, FL: Academic Press.

NIH (1997) *Immunotoxicity of patulin (CAS No. 149-29-1) in female B6C3F$_1$ mice*. NTP Report IMM96010. http://ntp-server.niehs.nih.gov

Niola, I., Stefanelli, C., and Azzi, A. (1990) Impiego delle microonde nella destabilizzazione della patulina [Use of microwaves to destabilize patulin], *Industrie Alimentari*, **29**: 1104–1106.

Northolt, M.D., van Egmond, H.P., and Paulsch, W.E. (1978) Patulin production by some fungal species in relation to water activity and temperature, *Journal of Food Protection*, **41**: 885–890.

Obrazhei, A.F. (1987) Toxicity of patulin for swine, *Veterinariya (Moskow)*, **4**: 58–61.

Olivigni, F.J., and Bullerman, L.B. (1978) Production of penicillic acid and patulin by an atypical *Penicillium roqueforti* isolate, *Applied and Environmental Microbiology*, **35**: 435–438.

Osswald, H., Frank, H.K., Komitowski, D., and Winter, H. (1978) Long-term testing of patulin administered orally to Sprague-Dawley rats and Swiss mice, *Food and Cosmetic Toxicology*, **16**: 243–247.

Paster, N., Huppert, D., and Barkai-Golan, R. (1995) Production of patulin by different strains of *Penicillium expansum* in pear and apple cultivars stored at different temperatures and modified atmospheres, *Food Additives and Contaminants*, **12**: 51–58.

Paucoud, J.C., Krivobok, S., and Vidal, D. (1990) Immunotoxicity testing of mycotoxins T-2 and patulin on Balb/c mice, *Acta Microbiologica Hungarica*, **37**: 331–339.

Phillips, T.D. and Hayes, A.W. (1977) Effects of patulin on adenosine triphosphatase activities in the mouse, *Toxicology and Applied Pharmacology*, **42**: 175–187.

Phillips, T.D. and Hayes, A.W. (1978) Effects of patulin on the kinetics of substrate and cationic ligand activation of adenosine triphosphatase in mouse brain, *Journal of Pharmacology and Experimental Therapeutics*, **205**: 606–616.

Plessi, M., Bertelli, D., and Monzani, A. (1998) Valutazione del contenuto di patulina in prodotti per la prima infanzia a base di mela [Evaluation of the patulin content of apple-based baby-foods], *Rivista di Scienza dell'Alimentazione*, **27**: 237–243.

Priest, J.W. and Light, R.J. (1989) Patulin biosynthesis: epoxidation of toluquinol and gentisyl alcohol by particulate preparations from *Penicillium patulum*, *Biochemistry*, **28**: 9192–9200.

Prieta, J., Moreno, M.A., Blanco, J.L., Suarez, G., and Dominguez, L. (1992) Determination of patulin by diphasic dialysis extraction and thin-layer chromatography, *Journal of Food Protection*, **55**: 1001–1002.

Reiss, J. (1972) Nachweis von Patulin in spontan verschimmeltem Brot und Gebäck. Mycotoxine in Nahrungsmitteln. II [Detection of patulin in spontaneously moulded bread and pastry. Mycotoxins in food. II], *Naturwissenschaften*, **59**: 1–37.

Reiss, J. (1975) Mycotoxin bioassay, using *Bacillus stearothermophilus*, *Journal of the Association of Official Analytical Chemists*, **58**: 624–625.

Rice, S.L. (1980) Patulin production by *Byssochlamys* spp in canned grape juice, *Journal of Food Science*, **45**: 485–488, 495.

Roach, J.A.G., White, K.D., Trucksess, M.W., and Thomas, F.S. (2000) Capillary gas chromatography/mass spectrometry with chemical ionization and negative ion detection for confirmation of identity of patulin in apple juice, *Journal of AOAC International*, **83**: 104–112.

Roland, J.O. and Beuchat, L.R. (1984) Influence of temperature and water activity on growth and patulin production by *Byssochlamis nivea* in apple juice, *Applied and Environmental Microbiology*, **47**: 205–207.

Roland, J.O., Beuchat, L.R., Worthington, R.E., and Hitchcock, H.L. (1984) Effects of sorbate, benzoate, sulfur dioxide and temperature on growth and patulin production by *Byssochlamys nivea* in grape juice, *Journal of Food Protection*, **47**: 237–241.

Roll, R., Matthiaschk, G., and Korte, A. (1990) Embriotoxicity and mutagenicity of mycotoxins, *Journal of Environmental Pathology, Toxicology and Oncology*, **10**: 1–7.

Rovira, R., Ribera, F., Sanchis, V., and Canela, R. (1993) Improvements in the quantitation of patulin in apple juice by high-performance liquid chromatography, *Journal of Agricultural and Food Chemistry*, **41**: 214–216.

Rubinstein, R. (1981) *Simulation and the Monte Carlo Method*. New York: Wiley.

Rupp, H.S. and Turnipseed, S.B. (2000) Confirmation of patulin and 5-hydroxymethylfurfural in apple juice by gas chromatography/mass spectrometry, *Journal of AOAC International*, **83**: 612–620.

Rychlik, M. and Schieberle, P. (1999) Quantification of the mycotoxin patulin by a stable isotopic dilution assay, *Journal of Agricultural and Food Chemistry*, **47**: 3749–3755.

Sakthisekaran, D. and Shanmugasundaram, E.R. (1990) Effect of patulin on the kinetic properties of the enzyme aldolase studied in rat liver, *Biochemistry International*, **21**: 117–134.

Sakthisekaran, D., Shanmugasundaram, K.R.B., and Shanmugasundaram, E.R.B. (1989) Effect of patulin on some enzymes of carbohydrate metabolism studied in rats, *Biochemistry International*, **19**: 37–51.

Sanchez Regueiro, O., Alonso Jimenez, E., and Garcia Perez, A.W. (1991) Determinacion de patulina en frutas frescas y en conserva [Patulin determination in fresh and preserved fruits], *Revista Cubana de Alimentation y Nutricion*, **5**: 77–81.

Sanchis, V., Fons, E., Vinas, I., Torres, M., and Canela, R. (1991) Efectos del sorbato potasico en la produccion de patulina por cepas de *Penicillium griseofulvum* y *P. expansum*. [Effects of potassium sorbate on patulin production by strains of *Penicillium griseofulvum* and *P. expansum*], *Revista Iberoamericana de Micologia*, **8**: 66–69.

Sands, D.C., McIntyre, J.L., and Walton, G.S. (1976) Use of activated charcoal for the removal of patulin from cider, *Applied and Environmental Microbiology*, **32**: 388–391.

Scott, P.M. (1989) Mycotoxigenic fungal contaminants of cheese and other dairy products. In *Mycotoxins in Dairy Products*, pp. 193–259. London: Elsevier Applied Science.

Scott, P.M. (1994) Penicillium and Aspergillus toxins. In *Mycotoxins in Grain: Compounds other than Aflatoxin* (eds by J.D. Miller and H.L. Trenholm), pp. 261–285. St Paul, MN: Eagam Press.

Sekiguchi, J. and Gaucher, G.M. (1978) Identification of phyllostine as an intermediate of the patulin pathway in *Penicillium urticae*, *Biochemistry*, **17**: 1785–1791.

Sekiguchi, J. and Gaucher, G.M. (1979a) Isoepoxydon, a new metabolite of the patulin pathway in *Penicillium urticae*, *Biochemical Journal*, **182**: 445–453.

Sekiguchi, J. and Gaucher, G.M. (1979b) Patulin biosynthesis: the metabolism of phyllostine and isoepoxydon by cell-free preparations from *Penicillium urticae*, *Canadian Journal of Microbiology*, **25**: 881–887.

Sekiguchi, J., Gaucher, G.M., and Yamada, Y. (1979) Biosynthesis of patulin in *Penicillium orticae*: identification of isopatulin as a new intermediate, *Tetrahedron Letters*, **1**: 41–42.

Sekiguchi, J., Shimamoto, T., Yamada, Y., and Gaucher, G.M. (1983) Patulin biosynthesis: enzymatic and nonenzymatic transformations of the mycotoxin (E)-ascladiol, *Applied and Environmental Microbiology*, **45**: 1939–1942.

Sharma, R.P. (1993) Immunotoxicity of mycotoxins, *Journal of Dairy Science*, **76**: 892–897.

Sheu, F. and Shyu, Y.T. (1999) Analysis of patulin in apple juice by diphasic dialysis extraction with *in situ* acylation and mass spectrometric determination, *Journal of Agricultural and Food Chemistry*, **47**: 2711–2714.

Singh, R.S., Sharma, M.K., and Chander, H. (1992) Incidence of *Penicillium* toxins in milk and milk products, *Indian Journal of Animal Sciences*, **62**: 285–286.

Siraj, M.Y., Hayes, A.W., Takanaka, A., and Ho, I.K. (1980) Effect of patulin on hepatic mono-oxygenase in male mice, *Journal of Environmental Pathology and Toxicology*, **4**: 545–553.

Sommer, N.F., Buchanan, J.R., and Fortlage, R.J. (1974) Production of patulin by *Penicillium expansum*, *Applied Microbiology*, **28**: 589–593.

Speijers, G.J.A., Franken, M.A.M., van Leeuwen, F.X.R., van Egmond, H.P., Boot, R., and Loeber, J.G. (1986) *Subchronic oral toxicity study of patulin in the rat*, Report no. *618314 001*, Rijksinstituut voor Volksgezondheid en Milieuhygiene.

Speijers, G.J.A., Franken, M.A.M., and van Leeuwen, F.X.R. (1988) Subacute toxicity study on patulin in the rat: effects on kidney and gastro-intestinal tract, *Food and Chemical Toxicology*, **26**: 23–30.

Spotts, R.A. and Cervantes, L.A. (1993) Use of filtration for removal of conidia of *Penicillium expansum* from water in pome fruit packing houses, *Plant Diseases*, **77**: 828–830.

Steiner, I., Werner, D., and Washuttl, J. (1999) Patulin in Obstsaften – II. Patulinabbau [Patulin in fruit juices – II. Degradation of patulin], *Ernahrung*, **23**: 251–255.

Stinson, E.E., Osman, S.F., Huhtanen, C.N., and Bills, D.D. (1978) Disappearance of patulin during alcoholic fermentation of apple juice, *Applied Environmental Microbiology*, **36**: 620–622.

Subramanian, T. (1982) Colorimetric determination of patulin produced by *Penicillium patulum*, *Journal of the Association of Official Analytical Chemists*, **65**: 5–7.

Sydenham, E.W., Vismer, H.F., Marasas, W.F.O., Brown, N.L., Schlechter, M., and Rheeder, J.P. (1997) The influence of deck storage and initial processing on patulin levels in apple juice, *Food Additives and Contaminants*, **14**: 429–434.

Sydenham, E.W., Vismer, H.F., Marasas, W.F.O., Brown, N.L., Schlechter, M., van der Westhuizen, L., and Rheeder, J.P. (1995) Reduction of patulin in apple juice samples – influence of initial processing, *Food Control*, **6**: 195–200.

Taniwaki, M.H., Hoenderboom, C.J.M., De Almeida Vitali, A., and Uboldi Eiroa, M.E. (1992) Migration of patulin in apples, *Journal of Food Protection*, **55**: 902–904.

Tarter, E.J. and Scott, P.M. (1991) Determination of patulin by capillary gas chromatography of the heptafluorobutyrate derivative, *Journal of Chromatography A*, **538**: 441–446.

Tashiro, F., Hirai, K., and Ueno, Y. (1979) Inhibitory effects of carcinogenic mycotoxins on deoxyribonucleic acid-dependent ribonucleic acid polymerase and ribonuclease H, *Applied and Environmental Microbiology*, **38**: 191–196.

Thurm, V., Paul, P., and Koch, C.E. (1979) Zur hygienischen Bedeutung von Patulin in Lebensmittel. 2. Mitt. Zum Vorkommen von Patulin in Obst und Gemuse [On the hygienic significance of patulin in food. 2. On the occurrence of patulin in fruit and vegetable], *Nahrung*, **23**: 131–134.

Thuvander, A., Moller, T., Enghardt Barbieri, H., Jansson, A., Salomonsson, A.-C., and Olsen, M. (2001) Dietary intake of some important mycotoxins by the Swedish population, *Food Additives and Contaminants*, **18**: 696–706.

Tsao, R. and Zhou, T. (2000) Micellar electrokinetic capillary electrophoresis for rapid analysis of patulin in apple cider, *Journal of Agricultural and Food Chemistry*, **48**: 5231–5235.

Valletrisco, M., Casadio, S., and Stefanelli, C. (1990) Impiego di radiazioni UV per la degradazione delle micotossine [Use of ultraviolet radiation to break down mycotoxins], *Industrie Alimentari*, **29**: 1111–1112.

Wilson, D.M. and Nuovo, G.J. (1973) Patulin production in apples decayed by *Penicillium expansum*, *Applied Microbiology*, **26**: 124–125.

Wisniewska, H. and Piskorska-Pliszczynska, J. (1982) Natural occurrence of patulin in fodder beetroots, *Bulletin of the Veterinary Institute in Pulawy*, **25**: 38–42.

Wouters, M.F.A. and Speijers, G.J.A. (1996) Patulin. In: *Toxicological Evaluation of Certain Food Additives and Contaminants in Food*, WHO Food Additive Series, vol. 35, pp. 377–402.

Yates, I.E. and Porter, J.K. (1982) Bacterial bioluminescence as a bioassay for mycotoxins, *Applied and Environmental Microbiology*, **44**: 1072–1075.

Zegota, H., Zegota, A., and Bachman, S. (1988) Effect of irradiation on the patulin content and chemical composition of apple juice concentrates, *Zeitschrift fur Lebensmittel-Untersuchung und-Forschung*, **187**: 235–238.

19 Pesticide residues in food

Yumi Akiyama and Naoki Yoshioka

Summary

Monitoring data of pesticide residues in food are reviewed. We analyzed 1092 agricultural products collected in Hyogo prefecture, Japan during a period of seven years (April 1995–March 2002). Detection rates and concentration level of pesticide residues on each sample, and data from other countries' monitoring programs, are presented. In vegetables, cucumber, eggplant, sweet pepper, tomato, and celery showed relatively high detection rates. Pesticides frequently detected were iprodione, procymidone, acephate, methamidophos, and endosulfan. In fruits, most of the commodities except for watermelon, mandarin orange, and kiwi fruit showed high detection rates. Iprodione, captan and chlorpyrifos were frequently detected. Over 10% of fruit samples contained more than four different pesticides. Most of the residues were present at low concentrations, and the rates of violation (i.e. levels exceeding the maximum residue levels (MRLs) were within the low-level range (0.0 to 3.2%) for each sample group.

Introduction

A wide variety of pesticides are used: globally, more than 700 are applied to primary commodities. In Japan, about 360 kinds of pesticide are registered and permitted for use with agricultural products. To ensure food safety and consumer health, MRLs for pesticides in each commodity have been established in each country. For international standards, the Codex Alimentarius Commission established MRLs for about 200 pesticides. The Japanese Ministry of Health, Labour and Welfare, which accepts these Codex MRLs as far as possible, has been increasing the number of MRLs year by year, and at present the Food Sanitation Law regulates 229 pesticides (Notification No. 94 (13 March 2002)).

Monitoring programs have been conducted in many countries to investigate whether MRLs were observed satisfactorily. Results have been reported in papers (Dogheim *et al.*, 1999; Juhler *et al.*, 1999; Neidert and Saschenbrecker,

1996; Ripley *et al.*, 2000), in books (Japanese Consumers' Co-operative Union Laboratory, 1998; Standard Division of Food Safety Department, 2001) and online (US Department of Agriculture (USDA), 2002; US Food and Drug Administration (USFDA), 2000). We have reported the results of the monitoring program conducted in Hyogo Prefecture, Japan, from Fiscal Years (FYs) 1995 to 1999 (Akiyama *et al.*, 2002). In that paper, including our latest results during FYs 2000–2001, we described pesticide residues in agricultural products, meat, milk, and processed foods.

Pesticide classification

Pesticides can be classified by their constituent elements and structure and also by their application. We analyzed 228 pesticides simultaneously by GC/MS (Akiyama *et al.*, 2002) in the monitoring program of FY2001. They are classified and shown in Table 19.1. The toxicological properties of the main pesticides

Table 19.1 Classification of pesticides tested in our institute

Organophosphorus pesticides

Insecticides	EPN, acephate, azinphosmethyl, cadusafos, carbophenothion, chlorfenvinphos (-E, -Z), chlorpyrifos, chlorpyrifosmethyl, cyanofenphos, cyanophos, demeton-S-methyl, diazinon, dichlorvos, dimethoate, dimethylvinphos (-E, -Z), ethion, ethoprophos, etrimfos, fenitrothion, fensulfothion, fenthion, fonofos, fosthiazate, isofenphos, isoxathion, malathion, methacrifos, methamidophos, methidathion, monocrotophos, naled, omethoate, parathion, parathionmethyl, phenthoate, phorate, phosalone, phosmet, phosphamidon, phoxim, pirimiphosmethyl, profenofos, prothiofos, pyraclofos, quinalphos, tetrachlorvinphos, terbufos, thiometon, triazophos, trichlorfon, vamidothion
Fungicides	edifenphos, iprobenfos, tolclofosmethyl
Herbicide	butamifos

Organochlorine pesticides

Insecticides	BHC (α-, β-, γ-, δ-), DDT(*p,p′*-, *o,p′*-), aldrin, chlordane, chlorobenzilate, dicofol, dieldrin, endosulfan (α-, β-), endrin, heptachlor, heptachlor epoxide (endo, exo), hexachlorobenzene, methoxychlor, mirex, nonachlor
Fungicides	captafol, captan, chlorotalonil, phthalide, folpet, quintozene
Herbicide	indanofan

Pyrethroid pesticides

Insecticides	acrinathrin, allethrin, bifenthrin, bioresmethrin, cyfluthrin, cyhalothrin, cypermethrin, deltamethrin, ethofenprox, fenpropathrin, fenvalerate, flucythrinate, fluvalinate, halfenprox, permethrin, phenothrin, pyrethrins, silafluofen, tefluthrin, tetramethrin, tralomethrin

Table 19.1 (cont'd)

N-methylcarbamate pesticides

Insecticides   XMC, aldicarb, bendiocarb, carbaryl, carbofuran, ethiofencarb, fenobucarb, isoprocarb, methiocarb, methomyl, metolcarb, oxamyl, propoxur, xylylcarb

Herbicide   terbucarb

Organonitrogen pesticides

Insecticides   acetamiprid, buprofezin, chlorfenapyr, clofentezine, etoxazole, fipronil, pirimicarb, pymetrozine, pyridaben, pyrimidifen, pyriproxyfen, tebufenozide, tebufenpyrad

Fungicides   acibenzolar-S-methyl, azoxystrobin, bitertanol, carpropamid, cyproconazole, cyprodinil, dichlofluanid, diethofencarb, difenoconazole, dimethomorph, diphenylamine, fenarimol, fludioxonil, flusilazole, flutolanil, furametpyr, hexaconazole, imazalil, imibenconazole, iprodione, kresoximmethyl, mepanipyrim, mepronil, myclobutanil, penconazole, pencycuron, prochloraz, procymidone, propamocarb, propiconazole, pyrifenox (-E, -Z), pyrimethanil, tebuconazole, tetraconazole, thiabendazol, thifluzamide, tolylfluanid, triadimenol, triadimefon, trichlamide, tricyclazole, triflumizole, vinclozolin

Herbicides   EPTC, alachlor, atrazine, bifenox, bromacil, butachlor, butylate, cafenstrole, chlomethoxyfen, chlornitrofen, chlorprofam, clethodim, cyanazine, cyhalohopbutyl, desmedipham, diflufenican, dimethenamid, diphenamid, esprocarb, ethobenzanide, fenoxapropethyl, lenacil, mefenacet, methabenzthiazuron, metolachlor, metribuzin, nitrofen, pendimethalin, pentoxazone, pretilachlor, propanil, propyzamide, pyraflufenethyl, pyrazoxyfen, pyributicarb, pyriminobacmethyl (-E, -Z), quizalofopethyl, simazine, simethryne, swep, terbacil, thenylchlor, thiobencarb, trifluralin

Plant-growth   ethoxyquin, ethychlozate, paclobutrazol, uniconazol P
regulators

Other pesticides

Insecticides   bromopropylate, methoprene, piperonyl butoxide, propargite

Fungicides   diphenyl, isoprothiolane, *o*-phenylphenol

Herbicides   benfuresate, cinmethylin, dimethipin, phenothiol

---

are given in Table 19.2 (Agricultural Promotion Division, 2002; Food Hygienics Society of Japan, 2002; Shibuya *et al.*, 2002; Tomlin, 2000; Uesugi *et al.*, 1997).

Pesticide residues

During a seven-year monitoring survey (April 1995–March 2002) of pesticide residues in agricultural products, we analyzed 1092 samples collected in Hyogo prefecture, Japan. There were 701 domestic samples and 391 imported. Overall,

Table 19.2 Toxicological properties of main pesticides

Pesticide		Carcinogenicity IARC class[a]	Acute toxicity WHO class[b]	Acute toxicity Oral LD_{50}[c] (mg/kg)	Fish toxicity Class[d]	Fish toxicity TLm_{48}[e] (ppm)	ADI[f] (mg/kg per day)
Organophosphorus pesticides							
Insecticides	EPN	2B	Ia	♂36, ♀24	Bs	1–2	0.0023
	Acephate	3	III	♂1447, ♀1030	A		0.03
	Chlorpyrifos	3	II	♂163, ♀135	C	0.13	0.01
	Diazinon	3	II	1250	Bs	3.2	0.002
	Methamidophos		Ib	♂15.6, ♀13.0	–		0.004
Fungicides	Edifenphos		Ib	100–260	B	1.3–2	0.003
Herbicides	Butamifos		II	♂1070, ♀845	B	2.25	0.005
Organochlorine pesticides							
Insecticides	DDT	2B	II	♂113, ♀118	C	0.11	0.02
	Dicofol	3	III	♂595, ♀578	B	1.1	0.002
	Dieldrin	3	Ib	46	C	0.018	0.0001
	Endosulfan		II	70	D	7.2 ppb	0.006
Fungicides	Captan	3	III	9000	C	0.25	0.1
Herbicides	Indanofan			♂631, ♀460	B		0.0035
Pyrethroid pesticides							
Insecticides	Cypermethrin		II	250–4150	C	0.002	0.05
	Deltamethrin	3	II	135–>5000	–		0.01
	Ethofenprox		III (Table 5)	>42 880	B	5	0.03
	Fenvalerate	3	II	451	C	0.75 ppb	0.02
	Permethrin	3	II	430–4000	C		0.05
N-methylcarbamate pesticides							
Insecticides	Carbaryl	3	II	♂850, ♀500	B	>10	0.003
	Fenobucarb		II	♂623, ♀657	Bs	12.6	0.012
	Methomyl		Ib	♂34, ♀30	B	2.8	0.03
Herbicides	Terbucarb			>34 600	A	>40	–

Table 19.2 (cont'd)

Pesticide	Carcinogenicity IARC class[a]	Acute toxicity WHO class[b]	Acute toxicity Oral LD$_{50}$[c] (mg/kg)	Fish toxicity Class[d]	Fish toxicity TLm$_{48}$[e] (ppm)	ADI[f] (mg/kg per day)
Organonitrogen pesticides						
Insecticides						
Acetamiprid			♂217, ♀146	A	>100	0.066
Chlorfenapyr		II	♂441, ♀1152	C	0.11	0.026
Tebufenpyrad		III	♂595 ♀997	C	0.5	0.0021
Fungicides						
Bitertanol		III (Table 5)	>5000	B	2.5	0.01
Imazalil		II	227–343	–		0.03
Iprodione		III (Table 5)	>2000	A	16.6	0.06
Mepronil		III (Table 5)	>10 000	B	4.2	0.05
Procymidone		III (Table 5)	♂6800, ♀7700	A	11	0.1
Thiabendazol		III (Table 5)	3100	A	>40	0.1
Herbicides						
Chlorprofam		III (Table 5)	5000–7500	A	10–40	0.10
Pyrazoxyfen	3	III	♂1690, ♀1644	B	2.5	0.0015
Trifluralin		III (Table 5)	>5000	Bs	4.2	0.024
Plant-growth regulator						
Ethoxyquin	3	III	1920	–		0.005
Other pesticides						
Insecticides						
Bromopropylate		III	>5000	B	1.4	0.03
Fungicides						
o-Phenylphenol	3	III (Table 5)	2700	B	5.1	0.02
Herbicides						
Benfuresate		III (Table 5)	♂3536, ♀2031	A	50	0.0307

[a] International Agency for research on Cancer (IARC) carcinogenicity evidence classifications.
- Group 1: the agent is carcinogenic to humans.
- Group 2A: the agent is probably carcinogenic to humans.
- Group 2B: the agent is possibly carcinogenic to humans.
- Group 3: the agent is not classifiable as to its carcinogenicity to humans.
- Group 4: the agent is probably not carcinogenic to humans.

From *The Pesticide Manual*, 12th edn (2000).

b *WHO toxicity classification*

Class		LD$_{50}$ for the rat (mg/kg b.w.)			
		Oral		*Dermal*	
		Solids	*Liquids*	*Solids*	*Liquids*
Ia	Extremely hazardous	≤5	≤20	≤10	≤40
Ib	Highly hazardous	5–50	20–200	10–100	40–400
II	Moderately hazardous	50–500	200–2000	100–1000	400–4000
III	Slightly hazardous	≥501	≥2001	≥1001	≥4001
Table 5	Product unlikely to present acute hazard in normal use	≥2000	≥3000	–	–
Table 6	Not classified; believed obsolete				
Table 7	Fumigants not classified under WHO				

From *The Pesticide Manual*, 12th edn (2000).

c 50% lethal dose for the rat (♂male, ♀female). From *The Pesticide Manual*, 12th edn (2000) and *Pesticide Data Book*, 3rd edn (1997).

d *Fish toxicity classification set by the Japanese Agricultural Chemicals Regulation Law*

Class	TLm$_{48}$ (carp)	TLm$_3$ (daphnias)
A	>10 ppm	>0.5 ppm
B	0.5–10 ppm	≤0.5 ppm
Bs	Special attention is paid in Class B	
C	≤0.5 ppm	
D	Designated pesticides of water pollution	

From *Shibuya Index*, 9th edn (2002).

e Median tolerance limit during 48 h for the carp. From *Guideline for Control of Vermin and Weed of Agricultural Products in Hyogo Prefecture* (2002) and *Pesticide Data Book*, 3rd edn (1997).

f Acceptable daily intake set by FAO/WHO or Japanese Food Sanitation Committee. From *The Pesticide Manual*, 12th edn (2000) and *Journal of the Food Hygienics Society of Japan*, **43**: J-91 (2002).

Table 19.3 Distribution of pesticide residues detected above 0.01 µg/g by percentage of MRL

Sample group	Total residues (≥0.01 µg/g)	Percentage of MRLs				No MRLs
		<10%	<50%	<100%	≥100%	
Domestic						
Cereals	17	12	2	0	0	3
Beans	5	0	0	0	0	5
Vegetables	284	130	23	3	3	125
Teas	7	7	0	0	0	0
Fruits	191	117	20	1	0	53
Total	504	266	45	4	3	186
Rate(%)		52.8	8.9	0.8	0.6	36.9
Imported						
Cereals	0	0	0	0	0	0
Beans	1	0	1	0	0	0
Vegetables	38	13	1	1	0	23
Citrus fruits	359	121	177	15	0	46
Other fruits	133	61	28	4	1	39
Total	531	195	207	20	1	108
Rate(%)		36.7	39.0	3.8	0.2	20.3

The data are for FYs 1995–2001. Data for FYs 1995–1999 are reported in *Journal of AOAC International*, **85**: 692–703 (2002).

49% of domestic and 31% of imported samples contained no detectable residues. Multiple residues were detected in 218 (31%) of domestic and 207 (53%) of imported samples. The limit of quantitation (LOQ) was set at 0.01 µg/g and the limit of detection (LOD) was 0.001 µg/g.

Table 19.3 shows the distribution of pesticide residues detected above 0.01 µg/g by percentage of MRL. In domestic samples, the concentrations of 53% of the detectable residues were less than 10% of the MRL, and 9% were within the range of 10–50% of the MRL; there is no MRL for 37% of the total residues detected. In imported samples, 37% of the detectable residues were <10% of the MRL, and 39% were 10–50% of the MRL. Most of the residues distributed in the 10–50% section were antifungal agents used for citrus fruits.

We found violations of the MRL in four samples. They were diazinon in chrysanthemum (0.94 µg/g, MRL 0.1 µg/g), dieldrin in cucumber (0.03 µg/g, MRL 0.02 µg/g), EPN in eggplant (0.19 µg/g, MRL 0.1 µg/g), and bitertanol in banana (0.65 µg/g, MRL 0.5 µg/g). The rates of violation of the MRL are listed in Table 19.4, and compared with other countries' monitoring data. Though not only the kinds of pesticide tested but also the MRL allowed for a particular pesticide–commodity combination varied from country to country, all data showed low violation rates, ranging from 0.0 to 3.2%.

Table 19.4 Percentage of samples with residues exceeding MRL

Data origin (year tested)	Sample group		No. of samples tested	Samples exceeding MRL	
				No.	%
Hyogo, Japan (1995–2001)	Domestic	Vegetable	449	3	0.67
		Fruit	146	0	0.0
	Imported	Vegetable	79	0	0.0
		Fruit	275	1	0.36
USDA[a] (2000)		Vegetable	3488	11	0.32
		Fruit	4652	7	0.15
USFDA[b] (1999)	Domestic	Vegetable	1414	3	0.21
		Fruit	1063	4	0.38
	Imported	Vegetable	2768	16	0.58
		Fruit	2290	3	0.13
Ontario, Canada[c] (1991–1995)		Vegetable	1536	49	3.19
		Fruit	802	25	3.12
Egypt[d] (1995)		Vegetable	238	3	1.26
		Fruit	159	4	2.52
Denmark[e] (1995–1996)	Domestic	Vegetable and fruit	1078	6	0.56
	Imported	Vegetable and fruit	1437	14	0.97

[a] From http://www.ams.usda.gov/science/pdp/00summ.pdf.
[b] From http://www.cfsan.fda.gov/~dms/pes99rep.html.
[c] From *Journal of AOAC International*, **83**: 196–213 (2000).
[d] From *Journal of AOAC International*, **82**: 948–955 (1999).
[e] From *Journal of AOAC International*, **82**: 337–358 (1999).

Vegetables

Table 19.5 shows the detection rates of pesticide residues on each type of vegetable. Cucumber, eggplant, sweet pepper, tomato, and celery showed relatively high detection rates. The LOD of the analytical method for the pesticide residues as well as the number and kind of pesticides tested in a sample can easily affect the detection rates. The detection rates are likely to show high values as analytical technique improves.

The major residues detected on each commodity are listed in Table 19.6 with their concentration levels and detection rates. Iprodione, procymidone (fungicides), acephate, methamidophos and endosulfan (insecticide) were frequently detected. In our monitoring data (Hyogo, Japan), 70% of the detections in domestic vegetables were <0.05 µg/g, and 95% were <0.5 µg/g. Most of the residues were present at low concentrations.

Table 19.7 shows the distribution of multiple pesticide residues above LOQ for each commodity. Five or more kinds of pesticide were detected in 10% of tomato and 25% of baby pea samples. Overall, 3% of our samples and 11% of USDA samples contained more than four different pesticides. Details of pesticides

Table 19.5 Detection rates of pesticide residues on vegetables tested in various countries

Commodity	Hyogo, Japan (1995–2001)		USDA[a] (2000)	USFDA[b] (1999)		Ontario, Canada[c] (1991–1995)	Canada[d] (1992–1993)		Egypt[e] (1995)
	Domestic	Imported		Domestic	Imported		Domestic	Imported	
Cucumber	75.0		77.7	42.6	62.2	68.9	7.9	21.4	38.3
Eggplant	67.9			5.9	46.0			8.1	85.7
Okra		66.7		22.2	7.1				
Pumpkin	42.9	35.0		34.3	52.8			4.5	
Sweet pepper	83.3	100.0	70.1	23.7	40.8	56.7	21.4	39.9	37.5
Tomato	82.8			65.3	40.3	48.9	4.3	19.4	46.7
Asparagus	0.0	27.3		2.3	5.5	38.6			
Broccoli	0.0	43.3		12.0	28.6	50.0		4.8	
Cabbage	30.6			9.8	30.8	45.8	11.1	10.3	60.0
Cauliflower	28.6			6.7	0.0	35.2		2.4	0.0
Celery	87.5			88.9	57.1	95.2	34.3	31.5	
Chinese cabbage	53.3				57.1				
Chrysanthemum	70.0								
Komatsuna	77.8								
Lettuce	63.3		37.2	46.8	50.0	85.2	16.8	16.5	25.0
Spinach	60.0			56.8	57.5		25.0	31.8	
Burdock	44.4	0.0							
Carrot	52.4		80.4	45.7	16.7	60.3	10.8	20.8	9.5
Garden radish	24.1			33.3	26.3	43.4		4.3	
Onion	13.3	0.0		11.1	9.8	20.3	6.6	14.9	0.0
Welsh onion	28.6								
Potato	40.0		69.9	42.2	5.3	27.8	2.5	13.3	
Sweet potato	7.7			25.9	5.9			18.8	
Baby kidney bean	46.2		68.9	29.8	50.5	34.9	4.8	19.2	41.6
Baby pea	0.0	100.0		15.3	42.9			11.8	15.3
Mushroom	50.0	50.0		22.2	15.5	64.4	7.3	2.4	

[a] From http://www.ams.usda.gov/science/pdp/00summ.pdf.
[b] From http://www.cfsan.fda.gov/~dms/pes99rep.html.
[c] From Journal of AOAC International, **83**: 196–213 (2000).
[d] From Journal of AOAC International, ...

Table 19.6 Concentration level of pesticide residues detected on vegetables

Data origin (year tested)	Pesticide	Samples tested	Residue (μg/g)						Positive %
			<0.01	<0.05	<0.1	<0.5	<1	≥1	
Cucumber									
Hyogo, Japan Domestic (1995–2001)	Procymidone	16	1	2	3	3	0	0	56.3
	Endosulfan	20	1	1	1	1	0	0	20.0
	Ethofenprox	20	2	1	0	0	0	0	15.0
	Iprodione	24	1	1	1	0	0	0	12.5
USDA[a] (2000)	Endosulfan sulfate	737			(0.008~0.096)				55.4
	Endosulfan	737			(0.007~0.15)				43.7
	Dieldrin	737			(0.003~0.085)				16.3
	Metalaxyl	211			(0.017~0.072)				12.8
	Methamidophos	737			(0.002~0.69)				11.5
	Chlorotalonil	737			(0.007~0.47)				9.4
	Oxadixyl	211			(0.017~0.086)				7.6
Ontario, Canada[b] (1991–1995)	Endosulfan	103			(0.005~1.1)				56.3
	Dithiocarbamate	103			(0.1~1.5)				12.6
	Iprodione	103			(0.017~0.38)				9.7
	Captan	103			(0.006~0.032)				6.8
Canada[c] Domestic (1992–1993)	Endosulfan	356		3	4	6	1	0	3.9
	Dieldrin	356		6	2	0	0	0	2.2
Canada[c] Imported (1992–1993)	Endosulfan	721		26	36	36	1	0	13.7
	Methamidophos	721		23	4	11	0	0	5.3
Egypt[d] (1995)	Dithiocarbamate	16			(0.10~0.30)				56.3
	Dicofol	47			(0.04~0.10)				6.4

Table 19.6 (cont'd)

Data origin (year tested)	Pesticide	Samples tested	Residue (μg/g)						Positive %
			<0.01	<0.05	<0.1	<0.5	<1	≥1	
Eggplant									
Hyogo, Japan Domestic (1995–2001)	Iprodione	28	3	3	0	0	0	0	21.4
	Chlorfenapyr	19	2	2	0	0	0	0	21.1
	Procymidone	23	1	2	0	1	0	0	17.4
	EPN	28	1	1	1	1	0	0	14.3
	Bromopropylate	23	1	1	0	1	0	0	13.0
Canada Imported (1992–1993)	Methamidophos	86		4	0	0	0	0	4.7
	Endosulfan	86		0	1	1	0	0	2.3
Egypt (1995)	p,p'-DDE	7			(0.01~0.2)				42.9
	Dimethoate	7			(0.01~0.03)				42.9
Okra									
Hyogo, Japan Imported (2000–2001)	Methamidophos	3	0	0	0	2	0	0	66.7
	Cypermethrin	3	0	2	0	0	0	0	66.7
Pumpkin									
Hyogo, Japan Domestic (1995–2001)	Iprodione	7	0	0	0	2	0	0	28.6
	Procymidone	7	0	1	1	0	0	0	28.6
Hyogo, Japan Imported (1995–2001)	Methomyl	20	0	0	0	0	1	0	5.0
	Iprodione	20	0	0	0	1	0	0	5.0
	Acephate	20	0	0	0	1	0	0	5.0
Canada Imported (1992–1993)	Endosulfan	44		0	1	1	0	0	4.5

Sweet pepper

Hyogo, Japan Domestic (1995–2001)							
Procymidone	10	1		2	0	0	30.0
Iprodione	12	1		2	0	0	25.0
Permethrin	12	1		1	1	1	25.0
Hyogo, Japan Imported (2001)							
Tetraconazole	1	0		0	1	0	100.0
USDA (2000)							
Methamidophos	738		(0.003~0.47)				30.4
Acephate	738		(0.003~1.3)				20.5
Methomyl	738		(0.007~0.41)				16.9
Chlorpyrifos	738		(0.007~0.30)				14.5
Endosulfan	738		(0.008~1.1)				14.5
Endosulfan sulfate	738		(0.012~0.45)				13.9
Metalaxyl	738		(0.017~0.27)				12.6
Omethoate	738		(0.005~0.15)				8.5
Oxamyl	738		(0.008~0.21)				8.5
Dicofol	738		(0.017~1.21)				8.4
Ontario, Canada (1991–1995)							
Dithiocarbamate	104		(0.1~3.1)				29.8
Endosulfan	104		(0.006~0.92)				14.4
Captan	104		(0.005~0.14)				5.8
Carbaryl	104		(0.086~0.71)				5.8
Carbofuran	104		(0.01~0.18)				5.8
Canada Domestic (1992–1993)							
Acephate	42	0	1	2	0	0	7.1
Endosulfan	42	1	0	0	0	1	4.8
Methamidophos	42	1	0	1	0	0	4.8
Canada Imported (1992–1993)							
Methamidophos	933	53	19	39	4	1	12.4
Endosulfan	933	33	23	39	7	2	11.1
Acephate	933	8	16	21	10	6	6.5
Chlorpyrifos	933	8	21	13	0	0	4.5
Methomyl	933	9	9	11	2	0	3.3
Egypt (1995)							
Dicofol	8	(0.25~0.79)					25.0
Tetradifon	8	(0.09~0.17)					25.0

Table 19.6 (cont'd)

Data origin (year tested)	Pesticide	Samples tested	Residue (µg/g)						Positive %
			<0.01	<0.05	<0.1	<0.5	<1	≥1	
Tomato									
Hyogo, Japan Domestic (1995–2001)	Procymidone	20	3	2	1	2	0	0	40.0
	Diethofencarb	29	3	2	1	0	0	0	20.7
	Iprodione	29	2	2	0	2	0	0	20.7
	Ethofenprox	25	1	2	2	0	0	0	20.0
	Buprofezin	29	1	4	0	0	0	0	17.2
	Dichlofluanid	29	0	1	1	2	0	0	13.8
Ontario, Canada (1991–1995)	Dithiocarbamate	90			(0.1~1)				23.3
	Chlorothalonil	90			(0.005~3.7)				11.1
	Endosulfan	90			(0.007~0.5)				7.7
	Captan	90			(0.005~0.098)				6.7
	Iprodione	90			(0.058~0.22)				5.6
Canada Domestic (1992–1993)	Ethion	786		8	5	2	0	0	1.9
Canada Imported (1992–1993)	Methamidophos	1153		49	31	42	0	0	10.6
	Endosulfan	1153		12	15	28	2	0	4.9
Egypt (1995)	Dithiocarbamate	23			(0.1~0.7)				100.0
	Dicofol	62			(0.02~0.28)				14.5
	Profenofos	62			(0.04~2)				8.1

Asparagus

Origin (period)	Pesticide	n						%
Hyogo, Japan Imported (1995–2001)	Cypermethrin	11	1	1	0	0	0	18.2
	EPN	11	0	1	0	0	0	9.1
Ontario, Canada (1991–1995)	Dithiocarbamate	57			(0.1~1.5)			29.8
	Carbaryl	57			(0.42~6.8)			5.3

Broccoli

Origin (period)	Pesticide	n						%
Hyogo, Japan Imported (1995–2001)	Permethrin	30	1	4	0	0	0	16.7
	Fenvalerate	30	1	2	0	0	0	10.0
	DDT	30	3	0	0	0	0	10.0
Ontario, Canada (1991–1995)	Dithiocarbamate	52			(0.1~1.4)	0	0	32.7
	Endosulfan	52			(0.015~0.1)	0	0	13.5
	Carbaryl	52			(0.034~1.1)	0	0	5.8
	Methamidophos	52			(0.008~0.042)	0	0	5.8
Canada Imported (1992–1993)	Phorate	105	0	0	0	2	0	1.9

Cabbage

Origin (period)	Pesticide	n						%
Hyogo, Japan Domestic (1995–2001)	Iprodione	36	0	4	0	0	0	11.1
	Fluvalinate	36	4	0	0	0	0	11.1
	Permethrin	36	1	0	0	1	0	5.6
Ontario, Canada (1991–1995)	Dithiocarbamate	59			(0.1~3.7)			30.5
	Cypermethrin	59			(0.008~0.45)			15.3
	Endosulfan	59			(0.006~0.13)			6.8

Table 19.6 (cont'd)

Data origin (year tested)	Pesticide	Samples tested	Residue (μg/g)						Positive %
			<0.01	<0.05	<0.1	<0.5	<1	≥1	
Canada Domestic (1992–1993)	Methamidophos	9		1	0	0	0	0	11.1
Canada Imported (1992–1993)	Acephate	29		0	1	0	0	0	3.4
	Methamidophos	29		0	1	0	0	0	3.4
	γ-BHC	29		0	1	0	0	0	3.4
Egypt (1995)	Omethoate	5			(0.46)				20.0
	Dimethoate	5			(0.42)				20.0
	Pirimiphosethyl	5			(0.32)				20.0
	Dicofol	5			(0.03)				20.0
Cauliflower Hyogo, Japan Domestic (1995–2001)	Iprodione	7	0	1	0	0	0	0	14.3
Ontario, Canada (1991–1995)	Dithiocarbamate	54			(0.1~1.2)				25.9
	Diazinon	54			(0.008~0.069)				5.6
	Methamidophos	54			(0.005~0.009)				5.6
Celery Hyogo, Japan Domestic (1995–2001)	Chlorothalonil	6	0	0	0	2	1	0	50.0
	Procymidone	8	0	3	0	0	0	0	37.5
	Fenvalerate	8	1	0	0	1	0	0	25.0
	Malathion	8	0	1	0	1	0	0	25.0

Origin / Commodity (Year)	Pesticide	No. of samples							Detection (%)
Ontario, Canada (1991–1995)	Parathion	83			(0.003~0.38)				53
	Dithiocarbamate	83			(0.1~13)				49.4
	Diazinon	83			(0.003~0.21)				37.3
	Endosulfan	83			(0.017~1.7)				31.3
	Chlorothalonil	83			(0.019~9.7)				26.5
	Carbaryl	83			(0.02~2.7)				25.3
	Cypermethrin	83			(0.006~0.38)				24.1
	Malathion	83			(0.004~1)				22.9
	Captan	83			(0.005~2)				15.7
Canada Domestic (1992–1993)	Endosulfan	140		0	1	14	13	2	21.4
	Malathion	140		3	2	11	4	1	15.0
	Parathion	140		2	6	4	3	1	11.4
Canada Imported (1992–1993)	Chlorothalonil	305		17	5	8	4	0	11.1
	Dicloran	305		14	5	4	0	1	7.9
	Acephate	305		6	5	4	0	0	4.9
Chinese cabbage Hyogo, Japan Domestic (1995–2001)	Fenvalerate	30	1	3	0	2	0	0	20.0
	Permethrin	30	1	1	0	1	0	0	10.0
	Chlorothalonil	12	0	0	0	1	0	1	16.7
	Acetamiprid	22	0	0	0	2	0	0	9.1
	Captan	30				0	1	1	6.7
Chrysanthemum Hyogo, Japan Domestic (1995–2001)	Isoxathion	20	0	0	1	0	1	1	15.0
	Permethrin	20	2	0	0	0	1	0	15.0
	Efhofenprox	17	1	0	0	1	0	0	11.8
Komatsuna Hyogo, Japan Domestic (1995–2001)	Cypermethrin	9	0	1	0	0	2	0	33.3
	Chlorfenapyr	9	1	0	0	1	0	0	22.2
	Acetamiprid	9	0	0	0	0	1	0	11.1

Table 19.6 (cont'd)

Data origin (year tested)	Pesticide	Samples tested	Residue (μg/g)						Positive %
			<0.01	<0.05	<0.1	<0.5	<1	≥1	
Lettuce									
Hyogo, Japan Domestic (1995–2001)	Fenvalerate	30	0	2	3	2	0	0	23.3
	Acephate	30	0	3	1	0	1	0	16.7
	Methamidophos	30	2	2	0	0	0	0	13.3
	Fluvalinate	30	2	0	1	1	0	0	13.3
	Methomyl	30	0	4	0	0	0	0	13.3
	Procymidone	21	2	1	0	0	0	0	14.3
	Iprodione	30	0	2	0	1	0	0	10.0
USDA (2000)	Acephate	740			(0.003~0.16)				15.1
	Dimethoate	740			(0.003~0.12)				7.7
	Endosulfan sulfate	740			(0.012~0.48)				7.0
	Permethrin	392			(0.048~2.5)				5.6
	Methamidophos	740			(0.002~0.14)				5.3
Ontario, Canada (1991–1995)	Dithiocarbamate	325			(0.1~35)				62.5
	Parathion	325			(0.002~13)				32.3
	Diazinon	325			(0.001~1.8)				20.6
	Carbaryl	325			(0.003~11)				18.2
	Dimethoate	325			(0.002~5.2)				15.7
	Cypermethrin	325			(0.02~3.4)				12.3
Canada Domestic (1992–1993)	Dimethoate	380		2	8	14	4	0	7.4
	Methamidophos	380		6	5	2	1	0	3.7
	Endosulfan	380		0	1	6	5	0	3.2
	Parathion	380		0	1	5	4	0	2.6

		n							(%)
Canada Imported (1992–1993)	Permethrin	702		3	8	24	10	15	8.5
	Endsulfan	702		15	8	3	1	0	3.8
	Dimethoate	702		3	4	6	0	1	2.0
Egypt (1995)	Dimethoate	12			(0.17 0.25)				16.7
	Omethoate	12			(0.05)				8.3
Spinach									
Hyogo, Japan Domestic (1995–2001)	Methamidophos	20	0	4	1	0	0	0	25.0
	Acephate	20	0	3	1	0	1	0	25.0
	Cypermethrin	20	1	0	0	2	0	0	15.0
Canada Domestic (1992–1993)	Permethrin	4	1	0	0	1	0	0	25.0
Canada Imported (1992–1993)	Permethrin	264		6	21	3	6	25	23.1
	Endosulfan	264		5	2	7	1	0	5.7
	DDE	264		2	2	1	0	0	1.9
Burdock									
Hyogo, Japan Domestic (1995–2001)	Endosulfan	9	0	1	1	0	0	0	22.2
	Azoxystrobin	6	0	1	0	0	0	0	16.7
Carrot									
Hyogo, Japan Domestic (1995–2001)	Acephate	21	0	1	1	0	2	0	19.0
	Methamidophos	21	0	3	1	0	0	0	19.0
	Iprodione	21	1	2	0	0	0	0	14.3
USDA (2000)	Trifluralin	184			(0.002~0.16)				56.5
	Iprodione	184			(0.013~0.10)				31.5
	p,p'-DDE	184			(0.003~0.063)				22.3
	Linuron	184			(0.042~0.26)				10.9
	Diazinon	184			(0.007~0.039)				5.9

Table 19.6 (cont'd)

Data origin (year tested)	Pesticide	Samples tested	Residue (μg/g)						Positive %
			<0.01	<0.05	<0.1	<0.5	<1	≥1	
Ontario, Canada (1991–1995)	Parathion	58			(0.002~0.43)				29.3
	Dithiocarbamate	58			(0.1~1.2)				17.2
	Diazinon	58			(0.001~0.049)				15.5
	Phosmet	58			(0.006~0.11)				8.6
	Cypermethrin	58			(0.01~0.028)				8.6
	Iprodione	58			(0.031~0.14)				8.6
Canada Domestic (1992–1993)	Trifluralin	416		8	6	2	0	0	3.8
	Diazinon	416		3	2	2	0	0	1.7
Canada Imported (1992–1993)	Trifluralin	612		28	36	15	0	0	12.9
	DDE	612		14	7	15	0	0	5.9
	Captan	612		0	1	9	1	0	1.8
Egypt (1995)	Dicofol	21			(0.63)				4.8
	Triadimenol	21			(0.28)				4.8
	DDT	21			(0.07)				4.8
	Tetradifon	21			(0.05)				4.8
Garden radish									
Hyogo, Japan Domestic (1995–2001)	Acephate	29	1	1	0	0	0	0	6.9
	Methamidophos	29	1	1	0	0	0	0	6.9
Ontario, Canada (1991–1995)	Dithiocarbamate	23			(0.2~0.5)				17.4
	Diazinon	23			(0.089~0.31)				8.7
	Dimethoate	23			(0.008~0.053)				8.7

Canada Imported (1992–1993)	Carbaryl		47	0	0	1	0	0	2.1
	Chlortalonil		47	0	0	1	0	0	2.1
Onion									
Ontario, Canada (1991–1995)	Dithiocarbamate		74		(0.2~6.5)				12.2
	Cypermethrin		74		(0.014~0.45)				9.5
Canada Domestic (1992–1993)	Chlorpyrifos		137	0	2	2	0	0	2.9
	Diazinon		137	0	2	1	0	0	2.2
Canada Imported (1992–1993)	DDE		121	13	1	0	0	0	11.6
	Dieldrin		121	4	0	0	0	0	3.3
Welsh onion									
Hyogo, Japan Domestic (1995–2001)	Permethrin	1	21	0	0	0	0	1	9.5
	Triadimenol	0	21	0	1	1	0	0	9.5
	Iprodione	0	21	1	0	1	0	0	9.5
Potato									
Hyogo, Japan Domestic (1995–2001)	Acephate	1	20	1	1	1	0	0	20.0
	Methamidophos	1	20	2	0	0	0	0	15.0
USDA (2000)	Chlorprofam		369		(0.017~19)				64.8
Ontario, Canada (1991–1995)	Endosulfan		126		(0.006~0.17)				10.3
	Chlorpropham		126		(0.007~0.86)				10.3
	Dithiocarbamate		126		(0.1~1.1)				7.1

Table 19.6 (cont'd)

Data origin (year tested)	Pesticide	Samples tested	Residue (µg/g)							Positive %
			<0.01	<0.05	<0.1	<0.5	<1	≥1		
Canada Imported (1992–1993)	Chlopropham	225		5	2	8	5	8		12.4
Sweet potato										
Canada Imported (1992–1993)	Dicloran	85		0	0	9	2	1		14.1
	Chlorpyrifos	85		4	1	0	0	0		5.9
Baby kidney bean (green bean)										
Hyogo, Japan Domestic (1995–2001)	Chlorothalonil	4	0	0	1	0	0	0		25.0
	Procymidone	9	0	0	1	0	0	0		11.1
USDA (2000)	Methamidophos	720	(0.002~0.56)							27.2
	Acephate	720	(0.003~1.6)							26.7
	Endosulfan sulfate	720	(0.012~0.48)							26.5
	Endosulfan	720	(0.008~0.58)							19.3
	Iprodione	720	(0.020~0.47)							9.2
	Omethoate	720	(0.005~0.13)							8.9
	Dimethoate	720	(0.003~0.80)							8.5
	Chlorothalonil	209	(0.008~0.46)							8.1
	Esfenvalerate	466	(0.012~0.063)							6.2
	Quintozene	720	(0.005~0.017)							5.1
	Vinclozolin	720	(0.012~0.30)							5.0

Origin (year)	Pesticide	No. of samples						%
Ontario, Canada (1991–1995)	Dithiocarbamate	43		(0.2~2.2)		0	0	16.3
	Captan	43		(0.005~0.014)		0	0	7
Canada Domestic (1992–1993)	Dimethoate	165	2	1	0	0	0	1.8
	Captan	165	0	0	2	0	0	1.2
Canada Imported (1992–1993)	Endosulfan	630	8	12	25	0	1	7.3
	Methamidophos	630	9	8	11	0	0	4.4
	Acephate	630	7	3	11	4	2	4.3
	Dimethoate	630	1	1	10	1	0	2.1
Egypt (1995)	Dicofol	24		(0.05~1.4)				20.8
	Dimethoate	24		(0.05~0.14)				12.5
Baby pea Hyogo, Japan Imported (2000–2001)	Fenvalerate	4	3	0	0	0	0	100.0
	Triadimenol	4	0	1	2	0	0	75.0
	Methamidophos	4	0	0	1	0	0	75.0
	Omethoate	4	1	2	0	0	0	75.0
Canada Imported (1992–1993)	Dimethoate	195	2	3	3	1	2	5.6
	Carbaryl	195	1	0	2	1	2	3.1
Egypt (1995)	Dithiocarbamate	8		(0.14)				12.5
	Dimethoate	13		(0.28)				7.7
	Omethoate	13		(0.09)				7.7
	Dicofol	13		(0.08)				7.7
	Omethoate	4	1	2			0	75.0

Table 19.6 (cont'd)

Data origin (year tested)	Pesticide	Samples tested	Residue (μg/g)						Positive %
			<0.01	<0.05	<0.1	<0.5	<1	≥1	
Mushroom									
Hyogo, Japan Domestic (1995–2001)	Fluvalinate	8	1	1	0	0	0	0	25.0
Hyogo, Japan Imported (1995–2001)	Thiodicarb	4	0	0	0	1	0	0	25.0
	Bitertanol	4	0	1	0	0	0	0	25.0
Ontario, Canada (1991–1995)	Diazinon	45			(0.003~0.45)				51.1
	Dithiocarbamate	45			(0.1~1.4)				17.8
	Endosulfan	45			(0.028~0.6)				8.9
Canada Domestic (1992–1993)	Diazinon	96		5	2	0	0	0	7.3

[a] From http://www.ams.usda.gov/science/pdp/00summ.pdf.
[b] From Journal of AOAC International, **83**: 196–213 (2000).
[c] From Journal of AOAC International, **79**: 549–566 (1996).
[d] From Journal of AOAC International, **82**: 948–955 (1999).

Data origin (year tested)	Commodity	Samples tested	Percentage of samples detected with each no. of residues (≥LOQ)						
			1	2	3	4	5	6	≥7
Hyogo, Japan Domestic (1995–2001)	Celery	8	12.5	25.0	12.5	25.0	0.0	0.0	0.0
	Sweet pepper	12	33.3	8.3	8.3	0.0	8.3	0.0	0.0
	Tomato	29	34.5	13.8	3.4	6.9	3.4	6.9	0.0
	Komatsuna	9	44.4	22.2	0.0	0.0	0.0	0.0	0.0
	Cucumber	24	37.5	20.8	8.3	4.2	0.0	0.0	0.0
	Chrysanthemum	20	25.0	10.0	0.0	0.0	5.0	0.0	0.0
	Eggplant	28	35.7	10.7	3.6	0.0	0.0	3.6	0.0
	Lettuce	30	20.0	20.0	13.3	0.0	0.0	0.0	0.0
	Spinach	20	25.0	20.0	5.0	0.0	0.0	0.0	0.0
	Chinese cabbage	30	26.7	13.3	6.7	0.0	0.0	0.0	0.0
	Carrot	21	14.3	19.0	0.0	0.0	0.0	0.0	0.0
	Japanese mashroom	8	12.5	0.0	0.0	0.0	0.0	0.0	0.0
	Baby kidney bean	13	15.4	7.7	0.0	0.0	0.0	0.0	0.0
	Burdock	9	33.3	0.0	0.0	0.0	0.0	0.0	0.0
	Pumpkin	7	14.3	14.3	0.0	14.3	0.0	0.0	0.0
	Potato	20	5.0	10.0	0.0	0.0	0.0	0.0	0.0
	Cabbage	36	13.9	8.3	0.0	0.0	0.0	0.0	0.0
	Welsh onion	21	4.8	14.3	4.8	0.0	0.0	0.0	0.0
	Cauliflower	7	14.3	0.0	0.0	0.0	0.0	0.0	0.0
	Garden radish	29	6.9	6.9	0.0	0.0	0.0	0.0	0.0
	Onion	30	0.0	0.0	0.0	0.0	0.0	0.0	0.0
	Sweet potato	13	0.0	0.0	0.0	0.0	0.0	0.0	0.0
Hyogo, Japan Imported (1995–2001)	Baby pea	4	25.0	25.0	0.0	25.0	0.0	25.0	0.0
	Okra	3	0.0	33.3	0.0	33.3	0.0	0.0	0.0
	Japanese mushroom	4	50.0	0.0	0.0	0.0	0.0	0.0	0.0
	Pumpkin	20	20.0	5.0	0.0	0.0	0.0	0.0	0.0
	Broccoli	30	16.7	0.0	3.3	0.0	0.0	0.0	0.0
	Asparagus	11	18.2	0.0	0.0	0.0	0.0	0.0	0.0
	Burdock	4	0.0	0.0	0.0	0.0	0.0	0.0	0.0
USDA[a] (2000)	Carrot	184	31.0	27.7	13.6	5.4	1.6	1.1	0.0
	Cucumber	737	21.4	14.1	25.0	10.6	5.3	1.2	0.1
	Sweet pepper	738	17.6	20.3	10.8	5.6	4.7	5.0	6.0
	Potato	369	58.3	9.5	1.9	0.3	0.0	0.0	0.0
	Green bean	720	19.6	18.3	16.7	6.3	4.9	2.4	0.8
	Lettuce	740	20.8	9.7	4.3	1.6	0.5	0.1	0.0

[a] From http://www.ams.usda.gov/science/pdp/00summ.pdf.

Table 19.8 Multiple pesticide residues detected on vegetables

Commodity (month tested)	Multiple pesticide residues from one sample ($\mu g/g$)	
	Insecticide	Fungicide
[Domestic]		
Celery (2000.5)	Acephate 0.31, Methamidophos 0.04, Malathion 0.01, Fenvalerate Tr.	Procymidone 0.01, Diphenyl Tr.
Chrysanthemum (1997.12)	Diazinon 0.94, Isoxathion 4.64, Dimethoate 1.28, Omethoate 0.25, Permethrin 0.52, Phenthoate Tr.	Diphenyl Tr.
Cucumber (1996.9)	Acephate 0.08, Methamidophos 0.02, Dieldrin 0.03	Captan 0.11, Iprodione Tr., Triflumizole Tr.
Egg plant (1998.11)	Prothiofos 0.12, Methomyl 0.04, Fenobucarb 0.02, Endosulfan 0.09, Chlorfenapyr 0.03	Fludioxonil 0.04
Pumpkin (1999.2)	Chlorphenapyr 0.02, Fluvalinate 0.01, Ethofenprox Tr.	Procymidone 0.07, Triflumozole 0.01, Triadimenol Tr.
Sweet pepper (1998.6)	Acrinathrin 0.08, Cypermethrin 0.03, Endosulfan 0.06, Chlorfenapyr 0.22	Procymidone 0.03
Tomato (1999.2)	Acephate 0.08, Methamidophos 0.07, Methidathion 0.02, Buprofezin 0.01	Dichlofluanid 0.40, Diethofencarb 0.01
[Imported]		
Baby pea (2000.12)	Chlorpyrifos Tr., Dimethoate Tr., Omethoate 0.06, Methamidophos 0.12, Dicofol Tr., Cypermethrin 0.03, Fenpropathrin Tr., Fenvalerate 0.01, Chlorfenapyr 0.01	Triadimenol 0.18
Okra (2001.12)	Acephate 0.03, Methamidophos 0.16, Cypermethrin 0.01, Fenvalerate 0.03	Iprodione Tr.

Tr. indicates that trace level residue (0.001–0.01 µg/g) was detected. Partial data were reported in *Journal of AOAC International,* **85**: 692–703 (2002).

detected and their levels for typical samples containing multiple residues are shown in Table 19.8.

Fruits

Table 19.9 shows the detection rates of pesticide residues on each type of fruit. Most of the commodities except for watermelon, mandarin orange, and kiwi fruit showed high detection rates. Whether or not the specimens supplied for the tests contain peel markedly affects largely the detection rates.

The major residues detected on each commodity are listed in Table 19.10 with their concentration level and detection rates. Iprodione, captan (fungicides), and chlorpyrifos (insecticide) were frequently detected. In our monitoring data (Hyogo, Japan), 74% of the detections in domestic fruits were <0.05 µg/g, and 97% were <0.5 µg/g. From the imported citrus fruits, imazalil, thiabendazol, and o-phenylphenol (antifungal agents used as post-harvest pesticides) were often

Table 19.9 Detection rates of pesticide residues on fruits tested in various countries

Commodity	Percentage of samples with residues detected								
	Hyogo, Japan (1995–2001)		USDA[a] (2000)	USFDA[b] (1999)		Ontario, Canada[c] (1991–1995)	Canada[d] (1992–1993)		Egypt[e] (1995)
	Domestic	Imported		Domestic	Imported		Domestic	Imported	
Apple	87.0		78.8	62.4	65.2	87.2	20.3	22.5	46.2
Pear	88.9			71.4	69.7	85.5	21.4	23.4	
Peach	100.0		93.3	78.8	59.3	98.6	27.5	18.2	27.3
Plum	100.0			57.1	61.9	91.1	11.5	14.6	
Cherry		85.7	94.2	84.6	60.0	98.3	71.1	5.0	
Grape	76.2	100.0	69.0	50.0	65.2	97.4		21.3	80.0
Strawberry	66.7	100.0	90.9	77.6	69.5	90.2	14.2	49.8	86.4
Melon	90.0	80.0	57.3	29.2	70.5			9.4	38.5
Watermelon	36.4			9.7	36.4				
Japanese persimmon	77.8								
Mandarin orange	27.8								
Orange		98.0	79.7	66.2	57.1			20.3	46.2
Grapefruit		91.1		83.3	0.0			17.9	
Lemon		85.4		77.8	62.5			16.3	
Banana		97.9		40.0	56.2			1.4	
Pineapple		80.0	5.5		22.2			1.4	
Kiwi fruit		16.0			27.1			17.9	

[a] From http://www.ams.usda.gov/science/pdp/00summ.pdf.
[b] From http://www.cfsan.fda.gov/~dms/pes99rep.html.
[c] From Journal of AOAC International, **83**: 196–213 (2000).
[d] From Journal of AOAC International, **79**: 549–566 (1996).
[e] From Journal of AOAC International, **82**: 948–955 (1999).

Table 19.10 Concentration levels of pesticide residues detected on fruits

Data origin (year tested)	Pesticide	Samples tested	Residue (µg/g)						Positive %
			<0.01	<0.05	<0.1	<0.5	<1	≥1	
Apple									
Hyogo, Japan Domestic (1995–2001)	Chlorpyrifos	23	7	6	0	0	0	0	56.5
	Tebfenpyrad	20	6	3	2	0	0	0	55.0
	Bifenthrin	14	5	2	0	0	0	0	50.0
	Captan	23	1	2	1	3	1	1	39.1
	Propargite	20	0	0	1	6	0	0	35.0
	Carbaryl	23	1	1	1	2	0	0	21.7
	Iprodione	23	2	1	0	0	1	0	17.4
USDA[a] (2000)	Azinphosmethyl	184			(0.018–0.23)				42.4
	Diphenylamine	184			(0.042–2.1)				33.2
	Thiabendazol	184			(0.036–2.4)				32.6
	Captan	184			(0.020–1.1)				13.6
	Chlorpyrifos	184			(0.007–0.089)				11.9
	Phosmet	184			(0.018–0.55)				11.9
Ontario, Canada[b] (1991–1995)	Captan	125			(0.004–0.84)				56.8
	Dithiocarbamate	125			(0.1–1.9)				37.6
	Phosmet	125			(0.004–2)				35.2
	Phosalone	125			(0.006–3.7)				23.2
	Azinphosmethyl	125			(0.009–0.58)				21.6
	Dicofol	125			(0.007–1)				10.4
	Diphenylamine	125			(0.005–1.8)				10.4
Canada[c] Domestic (1992–1993)	Phosalone	795		2	10	25	13	5	6.9
	Dimethoate	795		5	4	8	2	0	2.4
	Azinphosmethyl	795		0	3	12	3	1	2.4
	Captan	795		0	5	12	1	0	2.3
	Diphenylamine	795		2	2	6	3	3	2.0

Canada[c] Imported (1992–1993)	Diphenylamine	841	2	6		33	18	28	10.3
	Carbaryl	841	5	9		19	4	1	4.5
	Chlorpyrifos	841	9	8		9	0	0	3.1
	Captan	841	0	4		12	1	0	2.0
Egypt[d] (1995)	Dicofol	13			(0.5~0.77)				38.5
	Tetradifon	13			(0.06~0.18)				23.1
	Dimethoate	13			(0.03~0.05)				15.4
Pear									
Hyogo, Japan Domestic (1995–2001)	Iprodione	18	4	5		0	0	0	50.0
	Bromopropylate	12	3	4		1	0	0	66.7
	Cyanophos	15	1	2		0	0	0	20.0
	Captan	18	0	1		0	1	0	11.1
	Dicofol	18	0	1		1	0	0	11.1
Ontario, Canada (1991–1995)	Captan	69			(0.005~2.5)				72.4
	Dithiocarbamate	69			(0.1~2.7)				42
	Azinphosmethyl	69			(0.006~3.7)				37.7
	Phosmet	69			(0.006~2.8)				34.8
	Endosulfan	69			(0.015~0.74)				23.2
	Cypermethrin	69			(0.015~0.27)				18.8
	Dicofol	69			(0.03~3.6)				11.6
	Iprodione	69			(0.006~0.24)				11.6
Canada Domestic (1992–1993)	Dicofol	238	4	7		11	2	1	10.5
	Endosulfan	238	4	6		4	1	0	6.3
	Phosalone	238	3	0		1	2	1	2.9
	Phosmet	238	3	1		2	0	0	2.5
	Captan	238	0	0		4	1	0	2.1
Canada Imported (1992–1993)	Phosmet	775	30	11		19	1	0	7.9
	Endosulfan	775	5	7		11	1	0	3.1
	Diphenylamine	775	12	3		6	2	0	3.0
	Dicofol	775	5	2		13	1	0	2.7

Table 19.10 (cont'd)

Data origin (year tested)	Pesticide	Samples tested	Residue (µg/g)						Positive %
			<0.01	<0.05	<0.1	<0.5	<1	≥1	
Peach									
Hyogo, Japan Domestic (1995–2001)	Acephate	9	1	1	0	1	0	0	33.3
	Methamidophos	9	0	1	1	0	0	0	22.2
	Carbaryl	9	1	1	0	0	0	0	22.2
USDA (2000)	Iprodione	534	(0.025~19)						63.5
	Azinphosmethyl	534	(0.010~0.65)						40.8
	Phosmet	534	(0.010~2.4)						35.2
	Chlorpyrifos	534	(0.002~0.10)						28.5
	Dicloran	534	(0.003~1.9)						15.4
	Carbaryl	534	(0.010~2.7)						14.8
	Fenvalerate	534	(0.003~0.085)						10.7
Ontario, Canada (1991–1995)	Captan	168	(0.004~17)						97.6
	Phosmet	168	(0.012~9)						57.1
	Azinphosmethyl	168	(0.003~1)						50.6
	Cypermethrin	168	(0.016~0.49)						39.3
	Iprodione	168	(0.019~8)						32.7
	Dithiocarbamate	168	(0.1~3.8)						19.6
	Dicloran	168	(0.007~6.9)						17.9
	Folpet	168	(0.005~0.29)						11.9
	Pirimicarb	168	(0.005~0.07)						11.3
Canada Domestic (1992–1993)	Phosmet	40		0	0	0	0	4	10.0
	Captan	40		0	0	2	0	1	7.5
	Dicloran	40		1	0	1	1	0	7.5
Canada Imported (1992–1993)	Phosmet	143		2	3	5	1	0	7.7
	Disulfoton	143		1	1	1	0	0	2.1

Origin (Year)	Pesticide	N						%
Egypt (1995)	Dimethoate	11			(0.62)			9.1
	Omethoate	11			(0.14)			9.1
	Permethrin	11			(0.11)			9.1
Plum								
Hyogo, Japan Domestic (1995–2001)	Bitertanol	3	1	2	0	0	0	100.0
	Iprodione	3	0	1	0	1	0	66.7
Ontario, Canada (1991–1995)	Captan	79			(0.002~2.5)			81
	Phosmet	79			(0.008~0.92)			43
	Azinphosmethyl	79			(0.004~1.3)			40.5
	Dithiocarbamate	79			(0.1~1.8)			12.7
Canada Domestic (1992–1993)	Endosulfan	26	0	0	1	1	0	7.7
	Dicloran	26	0	0	0	1	0	3.8
Canada Imported (1992–1993)	Dicloran	267	2	2	13	6	6	10.9
Cherry								
Hyogo, Japan Imported (1995–2001)	Myclobutanil	7	2	1	1	0	0	71.4
	Iprodione	7	1	2	1	0	0	57.1
	Carbaryl	7	0	0	2	0	0	28.6
USDA (2000)	Azinphosmethyl	275			(0.010~0.44)			59.3
	Myclobutanil	275			(0.008~0.32)			50.5
	Carbaryl	275			(0.010~3.0)			42.5
	Propiconazole	245			(0.025~0.26)			29.8
	Iprodione	275			(0.025~2.2)			29.5
	Tebuconazole	275			(0.025~1.2)			21.5
	Malathion	275			(0.003~0.063)			16

Table 19.10 (cont'd)

Data origin (year tested)	Pesticide	Samples tested	Residue (μg/g)						Positive %
			<0.01	<0.05	<0.1	<0.5	<1	≥1	
Ontario, Canada (1991–1995)	Captan	120			(0.005~4.8)				84.2
	Iprodione	120			(0.025~4.7)				45.8
	Phosalone	120			(0.011~5.9)				45.8
	Carbaryl	120			(0.003~5.3)				30.8
	Dithiocarbamate	120			(0.063~1.3)				30.8
	Azinphosmethyl	120			(0.004~1.6)				29.2
	Phosmet	120			(0.005~1.2)				20
Canada Domestic (1992–1993)	Dimethoate	38		2	3	17	2	0	63.2
	Phosalone	38		2	1	2	0	0	13.2
	Captan	38		0	0	2	1	0	7.9
Canada Imported (1992–1993)	Iprodione	19		0	0	1	0	0	5.3
Grape									
Hyogo, Japan Domestic (1995–2001)	Iprodione	21	1	0	1	8	2	0	57.1
	Permethrin	21	1	4	1	0	0	0	28.6
	Cyfluthrin	21	0	4	1	0	0	0	23.8
	Triflumizole	19	0	3	1	0	0	0	21.1
	Acephate	21	0	2	0	0	1	0	14.3
Hyogo, Japan Imported (1995–2001)	Iprodione	5	2	0	1	1	0	0	80.0
	Captan	5	0	0	1	1	0	0	40.0
	Methomyl	5	1	0	0	1	0	0	40.0

	Pesticide	n						Range	(%)
USDA (2000)	Captan	741						(0.013~0.75)	28.1
	Iprodione	741						(0.023~1.8)	27.9
	Myclobutanil	741						(0.030~0.54)	20.5
	Omethoate	741						(0.007~0.27)	13.9
	Dimethoate	741						(0.003~0.96)	11.9
Ontario, Canada (1991–1995)	Dithiocarbamate	114						(0.1~7)	74.6
	Captan	114						(0.005~3.2)	52.6
	Folpet	114						(0.003~5.3)	50.9
	Azinphosmethyl	114						(0.011~7.7)	38.6
	Iprodione	114						(0.007~2.2)	27.2
	Parathion	114						(0.002~0.25)	24.6
	Myclobutanil	114						(0.005~0.34)	19.3
	Endosulfan	114						(0.05~0.37)	14.9
	Carbaryl	114						(0.006~3.3)	14
Canada Imported (1992–1993)	Captan	971	7	8	50	18	14		10.0
	Vinclozolin	971	4	14	8	1	0		2.8
	Methomyl	971	4	5	11	0	0		2.1
Egypt (1995)	Dithiocarbamate	32						(0.13~6.8)	100.0
	Dicofol	65						(0.05~3.3)	20.0
	Malathion	65						(0.02~0.2)	16.9
	Dimethoate	65						(0.06~1.53)	12.3
Strawberry Hyogo, Japan Domestic (1995–2001)	Procymidone	6	1	1	0	0	0		50.0
	Triflumizole	5	1	0	1	0	0		40.0
	Ethiofencarb	6	0	0	0	0	1		16.7
Hyogo, Japan Imported (1995–2001)	Carbaryl	4	0	1	1	0	2		100.0
	Iprodione	4	1	0	0	0	0		75.0

Table 19.10 (cont'd)

Data origin (year tested)	Pesticide	Samples tested	Residue (µg/g)						Positive %
			<0.01	<0.05	<0.1	<0.5	<1	≥1	
USDA (2000)	Captan	518			(0.020~7.6)				61.0
	Iprodione	518			(0.035~3.0)				40.9
	Benomyl	476			(0.083~2.4)				18.3
	Malathion	518			(0.007~0.23)				17.8
	Carbaryl	518			(0.013~4.4)				17.2
	Myclobutanil	518			(0.033~0.56)				13.7
	Methomyl	518			(0.020~3.0)				12.7
Ontario, Canada (1991–1995)	Captan	51			(0.009~4.7)				68.6
	Endosulfan	51			(0.007~0.43)				47.1
	Iprodione	51			(0.014~0.75)				19.6
	Dithiocarbamate	51			(0.1~1.7)				19.6
	Azinphosmethyl	51			(0.005~0.061)				15.7
	Folpet	51			(0.028~0.4)				11.8
Canada Domestic (1992–1993)	Captan	246		1	1	5	6	10	9.3
	Endosulfan	246		2	2	3	0	0	2.8
Canada Imported (1992–1993)	Captan	275		11	1	9	6	78	38.2
	Vinclozolin	275		3	1	6	0	3	4.7
	Endosulfan	275		3	2	5	1	0	4.0
	Methomyl	275		4	3	3	1	0	4.0
	Carbaryl	275		2	2	1	1	0	2.2
Egypt (1995)	Dicofol	22			(0.02~1.4)				59.1
	Tetradifon	22			(0.1~0.69)				27.3
	Dithiocarbamate	22			(0.1~0.12)				13.6

Melon

Hyogo, Japan — Domestic (1995–2001)

Pesticide			n				(%)
Procymidone	1	3	8		0	0	50.0
Ethofenprox	0	2	9		0	0	22.2
Fenobucarb	0	2	10		0	0	20.0

Hyogo, Japan — Imported (1995–2001)

Pesticide			n				(%)
Endosulfan	0	4	8	0	0	0	50.0
Methamidophos	0	1	10	1	0	0	20.0

USDA (2000)

Pesticide			n				(%)
Endosulfan sulfate			406	(0.008~0.068)			41.6
Thiabendazol			408	(0.042~0.39)			11.8
Methamidophos			406	(0.002~0.32)			11.1

Canada — Imported (1992–1993)

Pesticide			n				(%)
Methamidophos	4	4	192	1	0	0	4.7
Endosulfan	0	6	192	1	0	0	3.6

Egypt (1995)

Pesticide			n				(%)
Dicofol			13	(0.05~0.15)			23.1
Tetradifon			13	(0.02~0.05)			23.1

Watermelon

Hyogo, Japan — Domestic (1995–2001)

Pesticide			n				(%)
Methomyl	0	3	22	1	0	0	18.2
Procymidone	2	1	16	0	0	0	18.8
Iprodione	0	2	22	0	0	0	9.1

Japanese persimmon

Hyogo, Japan — Domestic (1995–2001)

Pesticide			n				(%)
Fenvalerate	1	1	9	0	1	0	33.3
Silafluofen	0	1	4	1	0	0	50.0
Cypermethrin	0	2	9	0	0	0	22.2

Mandarin orange

Hyogo, Japan — Domestic (1995–2001)

Pesticide			n				(%)
Acephate	0	0	18	3	0	0	16.7
Methamidophos	2	1	18	0	0	0	16.7
Dicofol	0	1	18	1	0	0	11.1

Table 19.10 (cont'd)

Data origin (year tested)	Pesticide	Samples tested	Residue (μg/g) <0.01	<0.05	<0.1	<0.5	<1	≥1	Positive %
Orange									
Hyogo, Japan	Imazalil	49	0	1	1	4	17	22	91.8
Imported	Thiabendazol	49	0	2	1	5	7	20	71.4
(1995–2001)	Chlorpyrifos	49	2	8	7	7	0	0	49.0
	o-Phenylphenol	49	2	1	1	6	3	0	26.5
	Pyriproxyfen	35	2	5	0	0	0	0	20.0
	Dicofol	49	1	2	2	1	0	0	12.2
USDA	Imazalil	744			(0.010~0.50)				64.4
(2000)	Thiabendazol	744			(0.010~0.68)				29.7
Canada	Methidathion	1858		11	17	67	18	4	6.3
Imported	Chlorpyrifos	1858		28	41	42	2	0	6.1
(1992–1993)	Ethion	1858		10	17	38	4	0	3.7
	Carbaryl	1858		0	1	10	8	8	1.9
Egypt	Dicofol	13			(0.03~0.14)				23.1
(1995)	Dimethoate	13			(0.02~0.07)				15.4
Grapefruit									
Hyogo, Japan	Thiabendazol	56	0	2	1	4	7	29	76.8
Imported	Imazalil	56	0	2	1	10	10	14	66.1
(1995–2001)	o-Phenylphenol	56	1	1	2	6	1	1	21.4
	Chlorpyrifos	56	3	5	2	2	0	0	21.4
	Ethion	47	0	2	5	4	0	0	23.4
	Carbaryl	56	0	1	3	0	2	0	10.7
Canada	Ethion	290		8	9	12	2	3	11.7
Imported (1992–1993)	Carbaryl	290		0	0	10	0	1	3.8

Sample / Period	Pesticide								%
Lemon									
Hyogo, Japan Imported (1995–2001)	Thiabendazol	48	2	2	0	4	4	20	66.7
	Imazalil	48	0	2	0	4	7	15	58.3
	o-Phenylphenol	48	0	1	3	9	4	0	35.4
	Chlorpyrifos	48	2	3	4	4	0	0	27.1
	Dicofol	48	1	1	2	0	0	0	8.3
Canada Imported (1992–1993)	Chlorpyrifos	96		6	2	0	0	0	8.3
	Methidathion	96		0	0	3	0	0	3.1
	Bromopropyrate	96		0	0	1	1	0	2.1
Banana									
Hyogo, Japan Imported (1995–2001)	Chlorpyrifos	47	12	24	6	0	0	0	89.4
	Bitertanol	47	4	10	7	8	1	0	63.8
	Deltamethrin	47	5	3	0	0	0	0	17.0
	Iprodione	47	0	0	0	2	1	3	12.8
Canada Imported (1992–1993)	BHC	439	5	5	0	0	0	0	1.1
Pineapple									
Hyogo, Japan Imported (1995–2001)	Triadimenol	20	2	4	3	5	0	0	70.0
	Triadimefon	20	2	7	1	4	0	0	70.0
	Triflumizole	16	0	1	1	1	0	0	18.8
Kiwi fruit									
Hyogo, Japan Imported	Iprodione	25	2	2	0	0	0	0	16.0
Canada Imported (1992–1993)	Pirimiphosmethyl	106		1	3	2	1	0	6.6
	Vinclozolin	106		1	1	3	0	0	4.7
	Diazinon	106		4	0	0	0	0	3.8
	Chlorpyrifos	106		0	2	1	0	0	2.8

a From http://www.ams.usda.gov/science/pdp/00summ.pdf.
b From Journal of AOAC International, **83**: 196–213 (2000).
c From Journal of AOAC International, **79**: 549–566 (1996).
d From Journal of AOAC International, **82**: 948–955 (1999).

detected. Although residue levels of antifungal agents were not violative, 93% of detected residues were ≥0.1 µg/g. For the other imported fruits, the concentrations of 65% of the detections were <0.05 µg/g, and 96% were <0.5 µg/g. Bitertanol was detected in bananas, and triadimenol and triadimefon were detected in pineapples.

Table 19.11 shows the distribution of multiple pesticide residues above LOQ for each commodity. Five or more kinds of pesticide were detected in over 20% of apple, strawberry, and Japanese plum samples. Overall, 11% of our samples and 15% of USDA samples contained more than four different pesticides. Details of pesticides detected and their levels for typical samples containing multiple residues are shown in Table 19.12.

Cereals

Table 19.13 shows the detection rates of pesticide residues for each type of cereal. The number of pesticide residues detected above LOQ was only one or two for most of the positive samples. The major residues detected on each commodity are listed in Table 19.14 with their concentration levels and detection rates. In Japanese rice, the detection rates of mepronil, flutolanil (fungicides) and fenobucarb (insecticide) were relatively high, but residue levels were low.

Meat and milk

For meat and milk, the highly persistent organochlorine pesticides were objects of the monitoring. The detection rates and residue levels are shown in Table 19.15. The LODs of our data (Hyogo, Japan) were 0.01 µg/g for meat and 0.001 µg/g for milk. The Danish data showed that residues <0.01 µg/g remained in more than half of fat samples from cattle and pigs, but no results exceeding MRL were detected (Juhler et al., 1999).

Processed foods

We analyzed several processed foods by our multi-residue screening method. The results are shown in Table 19.16. Organophosphorus insecticides detected in pasta were considered to be used for wheat flour as post-harvest application. All the imported frozen potatoes contained chloropropham, but residue levels were under the MRL (50 µg/g) set for potatoes in Japan.

Conclusions

Monitoring programs of pesticide residues in food have been conducted in many countries. The detection rates of residues have increased with the improvement of analytical technique. We have presented the kinds and residue levels of major pesticides detected in each sample of a commodity. Concentration of most of the residues was low, and the rates of violation of the MRL ranged from 0.0 to 3.2% for each sample group.

Table 19.11 Distribution of multiple pesticide residues on fruits

Data origin (year tested)	Commodity	Samples tested	Percentage of samples detected with each no. of residues (≥LOQ)						
			1	2	3	4	5	6	≥7
Hyogo, Japan Domestic (1995–2001)	Peach	9	22.2	11.1	11.1	0.0	0.0	0.0	0.0
	Melon	10	40.0	30.0	20.0	0.0	0.0	0.0	0.0
	Japanese pear	18	38.9	16.7	11.1	0.0	5.6	0.0	0.0
	Apple	23	17.4	21.7	8.7	4.3	21.7	0.0	0.0
	Japanese persimmon	9	44.4	33.3	0.0	0.0	0.0	0.0	0.0
	Grape	21	28.6	23.8	9.5	9.5	4.8	0.0	0.0
	Strawberry	6	16.7	0.0	0.0	0.0	33.3	16.7	0.0
	Watermelon	22	27.3	0.0	4.5	0.0	0.0	0.0	0.0
	Mandarin orange	18	5.6	16.7	0.0	0.0	0.0	0.0	0.0
	Japanese plum	3	33.3	0.0	0.0	33.3	33.3	0.0	0.0
Hyogo, Japan Imported (1995–2001)	Strawberry	4	25.0	25.0	0.0	25.0	25.0	0.0	0.0
	Grape	5	40.0	40.0	0.0	0.0	0.0	0.0	0.0
	Orange	49	8.2	24.5	36.7	24.5	4.1	0.0	0.0
	Banana	47	46.8	29.8	8.5	2.1	0.0	0.0	0.0
	Grapefruit	56	7.1	46.4	19.6	8.9	3.6	1.8	0.0
	Cherry	7	42.9	14.3	28.6	0.0	0.0	0.0	0.0
	Lemon	48	22.9	31.3	18.8	8.3	4.2	0.0	0.0
	Pineapple	20	20.0	55.0	5.0	0.0	0.0	0.0	0.0
	Melon	10	20.0	20.0	0.0	0.0	0.0	0.0	0.0
	Kiwi fruit	25	12.0	0.0	0.0	0.0	0.0	0.0	0.0
USDA[a] (2000)	Nectarine	346	12.1	28.6	24.9	15.6	9.0	4.6	3.2
	Cherry	275	14.2	15.6	26.5	19.6	11.6	4.4	2.2
	Peach	534	11.8	18.9	21.5	17.2	11.8	6.0	6.0
	Strawberry	518	25.1	33.0	22.6	7.5	1.9	0.6	0.2
	Orange	744	56.5	21.5	1.7	0.0	0.0	0.0	0.0
	Apple	184	29.3	28.3	9.8	8.2	2.2	1.1	0.0
	Grape	741	32.5	17.5	9.3	6.7	2.3	2.3	0.5
	Melon	410	37.1	14.1	4.6	1.5	0.0	0.0	0.0
	Pineapple	364	4.7	0.8	0.0	0.0	0.0	0.0	0.0

[a] From http://www.ams.usda.gov/science/pdp/00summ.pdf.

Table 19.12 Multiple pesticide residues detected on fruits

Commodity (month tested)	Multiple pesticide residues from one sample ($\mu g/g$)	
	Insecticides	Fungicides
[Domestic]		
Apple (2002.1)	Chlorpyrifos 0.02, Fenpropathrin Tr., Bifentrin Tr., Carbaryl 0.22, Chlorfenapyr 0.02, Propargite 0.20	Captan 1.13
Grape (2001.8)	Acephate 0.02, Methamidophos C.01, Cyfluthrin 0.02	Iprodione 0.36, Kresoximmethyl 0.13
Japanese pear (2000.9)	Dicofol 0.33, Silafluofen 0.03, Methomyl 0.05	Captan 0.69, Iprodione 0.01, Difenoconazole Tr.
Japanese plum (1999.7)	Fenitrothion 0.01, Fenvalerate 0.08, Cypermethrin 0.01	Iprodione 0.43, Bitertanol 0.02
Strawberry (1998.5)	Pyridaben 0.08, Tebufenpyrad 0.05, Acetamiprid 0.02	Iprodione 0.26, Triflumizole 0.02, Procymidone 0.02
[Imported]		
Banana (2000.7)	Chlorpyrifos 0.01, Methamidophos 0.06, Bifentrin Tr.	Bitertanol 0.01, Iprodione 0.54
Grapefruit (2002.1)	Chlorpyrifos 0.06, Methidathion 0.36	Azoxystrobin 0.04, Imazalil 0.82, Thiabendazol 1.00, o-Phenylphenol 0.08
Lemon (1999.2)	Malathion 0.02, Carbaryl 0.05	Imazalil 0.32, Thiabendazol 2.49, o-Phenylphenol 0.66
Orange (1995.11)	Chlorpyrifos 0.03, Dicofol 0.35	Imazalil 0.64, Thiabendazol 1.74, o-Phenylphenol 0.27
Strawberry (1997.8)	Malathion 0.01, Carbaryl 0.41, Dicofol 0.02	Myclobutanil 0.04, Iprodione 0.01

Tr. indicates that trace level residue (0.001–0.01 $\mu g/g$) was detected. Partial data were reported in *Journal of AOAC International*, **85**: 692–703 (2002).

Table 19.13 Detection rates and distribution of multiple pesticide residues on cereals

Data origin (year tested)	Commodity	Samples tested	Total positive samples		No. of detected residues (≥LOQ)					
			No.	%	1	2	3	4	5	≥6
Hyogo, Japan Domestic (1995–2001)	Rice	47	23	48.9	9	2	1	0	0	0
	Buckwheat	10	4	40.0	1	0	0	0	0	0
	Corn	4	1	25.0	0	0	0	0	0	0
	Wheat	3	0	0.0	0	0	0	0	0	0
Hyogo, Japan Imported (1995–2001)	Rice	12	4	33.3	0	0	0	0	0	0
	Corn	2	0	0.0	0	0	0	0	0	0
USDA[a] (2000)	Rice	178	58	32.6	48	10	0	0	0	0
USFDA[b] Domestic (1999)	Rice	55	17	30.9						
	Corn	41	12	29.3						
	Wheat	234	123	52.6						
USFDA[b] Imported (1999)	Rice	99	7	7.1						
	Corn	6	2	33.3						
	Wheat	42	21	50.0						

[a] From http://www.ams.usda.gov/science/pdp/00summ.pdf.
[b] From http://www.cfsan.fda.gov/~dms/pes99rep.html.

Table 19.14 Concentration level of pesticide residues detected on cereals

Data origin (year tested)	Pesticide	Samples tested	Residue (µg/g)						Positive %
			<0.01	<0.05	<0.1	<0.5	<1	≥1	
Rice									
Hyogo, Japan Domestic (1995–2001)	Mepronil	47	0	9	0	0	0	0	19.1
	Fenobucarb	47	5	1	0	0	0	0	12.8
	Flutolanil	47	4	1	1	0	0	0	10.6
	Isoprothiolane	47	1	1	1	1	0	0	6.4
	Dichlorvos	47	1	1	0	0	0	0	4.3
	Ediphenphos	47	1	1	0	0	0	0	4.3
	Silafluofen	47	2	0	0	0	0	0	4.3
	Fenitrothion	47	0	1	1	0	0	0	2.1
Food Agency[a] (Japan) Domestic (2001)	Fenobucarb	995			(0.011~0.34)				5.2
	Mepronil	995			(0.014~0.23)				1.5
	Fenitrothion	995			(0.015~0.16)				1.2
	Flutolanil	995			(0.028~0.16)				0.9
	Ediphenphos	995			(0.021~0.16)				0.8
	Tricyclazole	995			(0.028~0.11)				0.6
USDA[b] (2000)	Malathion	178			(0.008~0.13)				17.4
	Piperonil butoxide	178			(0.033~0.20)				13.5
	Methoxychlor	178			(0.017)				3.4
	Carbaryl	178			(0.010~0.040)				1.7
Wheat									
Food Agency (Japan) Imported (2001)	Malathion	272			(0.01~0.22)				75.7
	Chlorpyrifosmethyl	272			(0.01~1.17)				51.8
	Glyphosate	272			(0.01~3)				47.4
	Bromide ion	272			(1~15)				98.2

[a] From http://www.syokuryo.maff.go.jp/archives/data/pure9.htm.
[b] From http://www.ams.usda.gov/science/pdp/00summ.pdf.

Table 19.15 Detection rates and levels of pesticide residues on meat and milk

Data origin (year tested)	Pesticide	Samples tested	Percentage of samples detected with each level of residues		Residue (µg/g)		MRL (µg/g)
			<0.01 µg/g	≥0.01 µg/g	min.	max.	
Fat from cattle (domestic)							
Hyogo, Japan (1998–2002)	DDT[b]	24		33.3	0.010	0.090	5
	Dieldrin	24		0.0			0.2
	Heptachlor	24		0.0			0.2
	β-BHC	8		12.5	0.099		
	γ-BHC	8		0.0			
	Endrin	8		0.0			
	Chlorpyrifosmethyl	8		0.0			
Denmark[a] (1995–1996)	DDT	235	55.9	3.8	0.004	0.036	1.0
	Dieldrin	235	1.7	0.0	0.006	0.007	0.2
	α-BHC	235	1.7	0.0	0.003		0.2
	γ-BHC	235	2.5	0.4	0.004	0.012	1.0
	HCB[c]	235	52.5	1.3	0.003	0.031	0.2
Fat from pigs (domestic)							
Hyogo, Japan (1998–2002)	DDT	18		0.0			5
	Dieldrin	18		0.0			0.2
	Heptachlor	18		0.0			0.2
Denmark (1995–1996)	DDT	240	51.7	5.8	0.004	0.032	1.0
	Dieldrin	240	2.5	0.0	0.006	0.008	0.2
	α-BHC	240	0.8	0.0	0.004		0.2
	HCB	240	2.5	0.0	0.003	0.005	0.2

Table 19.15 (cont'd)

Data origin (year tested)	Pesticide	Samples tested	Percentage of samples detected with each level of residues		Residue (μg/g)		MRL (μg/g)
			<0.01 μg/g	≥0.01 μg/g	min.	max.	
Fat from poultry (domestic)							
Hyogo, Japan (1998–2002)	DDT	18		11.1	0.017	0.048	5
	Dieldrin	18		5.6		0.036	0.2
	Heptachlor	18		0.0			0.2
Denmark (1995–1996)	DDT	48	0.0	2.1		0.012	1.0
	γ-BHC	48	0.2	6.3	0.004	0.063	1.0
Milk (domestic)							
Hyogo, Japan (2001–2002)	DDT	20	0.0	0.0			0.05
	Dieldrin	20	0.0	0.0			0.005
	Heptachlor	20	0.0	0.0			
	β-BHC	20	0.0	0.0			0.2
	γ-BHC	20	0.0	0.0			
	Chlorpyrifosmethyl	20	0.0	0.0			

[a] From *Journal of AOAC International*, **82**: 337–358 (1999).
[b] Sum of p,p'-DDD, p,p'-DDE, and p,p'-DDT.
[c] Hexachlorobenzene.

Table 19.16 Pesticide residues detected on processed foods

Commodity (year tested)	No. of samples Tested	Positive	Pesticide	Residue (μg/g) <0.01	<0.05	<0.1	<0.5	<1	≥1
Tomato porducts (whole tomato, sauce, juice, and ketchup) (2000)	(domestic) 7	0							
	(imported) 6	5	Ethoxyquin	0	1	0	0	0	0
			o-Phenylphenol	3	1	0	0	0	0
			Procymidone	1	0	0	0	0	0
			Azoxystrobin	1	0	0	0	0	0
Pasta (spaghetti and penne) (2000)	(domestic) 3	3	Malathion	3	0	0	0	0	0
	(imported) 15	15	Pirimiphosmethyl	6	5	1	0	0	0
			Chlorpyrifosmethyl	4	0	0	0	0	0
			Chlorpyrifos	2	0	0	0	0	0
Frozen potato (2001)	(domestic) 3	0							
	(imported) 12	12	Chloropropham	0	1	0	7	0	4
Beer (2001)	(domestic) 12	0							
	(imported) 3	3	o-Phenylphenol	0	3	0	0	0	0
Yogurt (2001)	(domestic) 10	0							

References

Agricultural Promotion Division (2002) *Guideline for Control of Vermin and Weed of Agricultural Products in Hyogo Prefecture*. Agriculture, Forestry and Fisheries Department of Hyogo Prefecture, Japan.

Akiyama, Y., Yoshioka, N., and Tsuji, M. (2002) Pesticide residues in agricultural products monitored in Hyogo prefecture, Japan, FYs 1995–1999, *Journal of AOAC International*, **85**: 692–703.

Dogheim, S.M., Gad Alla, S.A., El-Marsafy, A.M., and Fahmy, S.M. (1999) Monitoring pesticide residues in Egyptian fruits and vegetables in 1995, *Journal of AOAC International*, **82**: 948–955.

Food Agency, Japan (2002) Investigation results of pesticide residues in rice and wheat. http://www.syokuryo.maff.go.jp/archives/data/pure9.htm (accessed 15 July 2002).

Food Hygienics Society of Japan (2002) Acceptable daily intake (ADI) of pesticides, *Journal of the Food Hygienics Society of Japan*, **43**: J-91.

Japanese Consumers' Co-operative Union Laboratory (1998) *Data Book for Pesticide Residues*. Tokyo: Coop Press.

Juhler, R.K., Lauridsen, M.G., Christensen, M.R., and Hilbert, G. (1999) Pesticide residues in selected food commodities: results from the Danish National Pesticide Monitoring Program 1995–1996, *Journal of AOAC International*, **82**: 337–358.

Neidert, E. and Saschenbrecker, P.W. (1996) Occurrence of pesticide residues in selected agricultural food commodities available in Canada, *Journal of AOAC International*, **79**: 549–566.

Notification No. 94 (13 March 2002), Ministry of Health, Labour and Welfare, Japan.

Ripley, B.D., Lissemore, L.I., Leishman, P.D., Denomme, M.A., and Ritter, L. (2000) Pesticide residues on fruits and vegetables from Ontario, Canada, 1991–1995, *Journal of AOAC International*, **83**: 196–213.

Shibuya, S., Kawahata, Y., Kawahata, M., and Shimazaki, I. (eds) (2002) *Shibuya Index*, 9th edn. Tokyo: Shibuya Index Research Group.

Standard Division of Food Safety Department (2001) *Pesticide Residues in Food*. Pharmaceutical and Food Safety Bureau, Ministry of Health, Labour and Welfare, Japan.

Tomlin, C.D.S. (ed.) (2000) *The Pesticide Manual*, 12th edn. Farnham: British Crop Protection Council.

Uesugi, Y., Ueji, M., and Koshioka, M. (eds) (1997) *Pesticide Data Book*, 3rd edn. Tokyo: Soft Science Publications.

US Department of Agriculture (2002) Pesticide Data Program – Annual Summary Calendar Year 2000. http://www.ams.usda.gov/science/pdp/00summ.pdf (accessed 15 July 2002).

US Food and Drug Administration (2000) Pesticide Program: Residue Monitoring 1999. http://www.cfsan.fda.gov/~dms/pes99rep.html (accessed 15 July 2002).

Index